Atopic Dermatitis: Disease and Management

Atopic Dermatitis: Disease and Management

Edited by **Heidi Mueller**

FOSTER ACADEMICS

New Jersey

Published by Foster Academics,
61 Van Reypen Street,
Jersey City, NJ 07306, USA
www.fosteracademics.com

Atopic Dermatitis: Disease and Management
Edited by Heidi Mueller

International Standard Book Number: 978-1-63242-058-9 (Hardback)

Printed in China.

Contents

Preface

This book discusses various aspects of atopic dermatitis and different strategies for its management. Atopic dermatitis is a disease characterized by reddened, itching and dry skin. This allergic disorder has a complicated etiology and shows an extremely high clinical heterogeneity which complicates its treatment procedure. This book discusses some of the physiological mechanisms of this disorder and the important role of host-microorganism interactions. An analysis of the clinical diagnostic procedure and the disease management protocols normally used are included within the book. It also elaborates on the therapeutic approaches which show clinical benefits.

This book is a result of research of several months to collate the most relevant data in the field.

When I was approached with the idea of this book and the proposal to edit it, I was overwhelmed. It gave me an opportunity to reach out to all those who share a common interest with me in this field. I had 3 main parameters for editing this text:

1. Accuracy – The data and information provided in this book should be up-to-date and valuable to the readers.
2. Structure – The data must be presented in a structured format for easy understanding and better grasping of the readers.
3. Universal Approach – This book not only targets students but also experts and innovators in the field, thus my aim was to present topics which are of use to all.

Thus, it took me a couple of months to finish the editing of this book.

I would like to make a special mention of my publisher who considered me worthy of this opportunity and also supported me throughout the editing process. I would also like to thank the editing team at the back-end who extended their help whenever required.

Editor

Part 1

Disease Etiology

1

Mouse Models for Atopic Dermatitis Developed in Japan

Hiromichi Yonekawa[1], Toyoyuki Takada[2], Hiroshi Shitara[1], Choji Taya[1], Yoshibumi Matsushima[3], Kunie Matsuoka[4] and Yoshiaki Kikkawa[4]
[1]*Center for Basic Technology Research*
Tokyo Metropolitan Institute of Medical Science, Tokyo
[2]*Mammalian Genetics Laboratory, National Institute of Genetics, Mishima*
[3]*Research Institute for Clinical Oncology, Saitama Cancer Center, Saitama*
[4]*Mammalian Genetics Project, Tokyo Metropolitan Institute of Medical Science, Tokyo*
Japan

1. Introduction

The term atopic dermatitis (AD) was first proposed by Wise & Sulzberger (Wise, 1993), who defined the condition as "confusing types of localized and generalized lichenification, generalized neurodermatitis or a manifestation of atopy." AD (or atopic eczema) is recognized as a very common disease that affects at least 15% of children and is strongly associated with cutaneous hyper-reactivity to environmental triggers (Geha, 2003, Leung and Bieber, 2003, Novak et al., 2003). AD is characterized by complex symptoms, including chronic relapsing, extreme pruritus and eczematous skin disease, all of which are frequently associated with IgE hyperresponsiveness to environmental allergens (Hanifin, 1980, Larsen et al., 1986, Schultz Larsen, 1993). The rapid increase in the prevalence of AD over the past three decades has resulted in an intense effort to elucidate the underlying pathogenesis and in the use of radical treatments for this disorder (Taylor et al., 1984, Larsen et al., 1986, Geha, 2003). The causative factors for AD generally fall into two categories: environmental and genetic factors. House dust mites and air pollution are included in the environmental category, and their involvement in the disease has been strongly suggested by epidemiological studies (Hanifin, 1982). Alternatively, genetic factors, including several different candidate regions, have been suggested from linkage studies on atopic and non-atopic phenotypes see Morar et al., (2006) and references therein). The fact that multiple linkage regions have been associated with the disease might be due to: 1) the disease is polygenic and many different genetic factors may be affected with the diseases, 2) the disease is clinically heterogeneous and different subphenotypes are influenced by different risk loci, which is not always followed by one-to-one correspondence, 3) different populations have a different genetic pool and may have different genetic factors for the disease, and consequently genetic studies are still not good enough to correspond to these situations. Additionally, there is a lack of appropriate animal models for human AD except for the flaky tail (*Flg^{ft}*) mouse. The *Flg^{ft}* mouse carries a loss-of-function (LOF) mutation in the gene encoding filaggrin (FLG), and this LOF mutation causes the barrier abnormality.

The barrier abnormality is recently discovered to be linked to the incidence of AD (Oyoshi et al., 2009, Vercelli, 2009, Moniaga et al., 2010, O'Regan and Irvine, 2010).

2. Mouse models for human AD

To date, at least four mouse models for human AD have been developed in Japan. Two of four models, NC (NC/Nga) and NOA, are controlled by multiple genes, whereas the other two, DS-*Hm* and KOR-*adjm*, are controlled by a single gene. No responsible genes have been isolated yet from the polygenic AD models, even though the genetic loci were identified a decade ago. In contrast, the responsible genes for the monogenic AD models have been identified. Interestingly, the functions of the respective genes are completely different; one is a thermosensor in keratinocytes, whereas the other is an adapter protein in the NF-κB signaling pathway.

2.1 Polygenic mouse models for human AD: NC and NOA

Two promising mouse models for human AD are the inbred strains named Nishiki Nezumi Cinnamon (NC) (Matsuda et al., 1997) and Naruto Research Institute Otsuka Atrichia (NOA) (Natori et al., 1999). The NC strain was originally established in 1957 by Prof. K. Kondo of Nagoya University from a stock derived from Japanese fancy mice, called Nishiki Nezumi (Kondo et al., 1969, Kondo, 1983, Festing, 1996). The NC mice spontaneously develop severe dermatitis in the presence of nonspecific allergens. Morbid NC mice exhibit AD symptoms, including itching, erythema, hemorrhage, edema, crust, drying, and excoriation/erosion hyperplasia of the epidermis region of the face, neck, and/or back, and the symptoms are exacerbated by aging (Matsuda et al., 1997). Furthermore, NC mice display some of the characteristic histopathological features of AD, such as macrophage and eosinophil invasion into the dermis, increased numbers and activation of mast cells and lymphocytes, a reduction in ceramide (Aioi et al., 2001), the appearance of activated mast cells, and $CD4^+$ T cells in the lesion. These lines of evidence suggest that the symptoms shown by NC mice are quite similar to those of human AD from the clinical, pathological, and immunological perspective.

As an alternative to the NC model, the NOA strain was derived from a male spontaneous mutant with sparse coat hair, which was obtained in 1982 by cross breeding between a female C3H/He mouse and a male ddY mouse at the animal facility of Naruto Research Institute, Otsuka Pharmaceutical Factory, Inc. and was then established as an inbred strain. The visible characteristic phenotype of the NOA mouse is that the mouse becomes completely hairless and smooth-skinned in adulthood until the development of skin lesions. In particular, ulcerative skin lesions are observed with a prevalence of 30% by the 10th week of age and 90% by the 20th week of age. In severe cases, the lesions extend to cover almost 20% of surface area of the body. In addition, serological examination showed increased IgE levels, with significantly higher levels in the mice with ulcerative skin lesions, suggesting that IgE is also involved in the development of the lesions (Kondo et al., 1997). The susceptibility of NOA mice to AD is increased by *S. aureus* colonization of the skin, suggesting that the NOA model is a potentially useful animal model for evaluating the effects of antiseptic treatments on the disease (Kondo et al., 2006). NOA mice have also been subjected to therapy by Chinese herbal medicine (Lee et al., 2006) to survey factors associated with AD (Watanabe et al., 1999).

2.2 Details of the NC model

Of the two models, the NC model has been more widely used to compare the phenotype between human AD patients and the mice, to explore causative genes (Ito et al., 2004, Ogawa et al., 2005, Fallon et al., 2009, Jung et al., 2011) and genetic loci (Kohara et al., 2001), and for drug development (Yamamoto et al., 2007, Shah et al., 2010, Tanaka and Matsuda, 2011) and the therapy of human AD (Takeda and Gelfand, 2009). Therefore, the immunological, pathological and genetic characteristics have been extensively examined in detail.

To perform preclinical trials or to survey potential drug targets for AD using mice, a high incidence of AD onset is required. Thus, there is a drawback to using NC mice, namely, that the NC mice exhibit a very low rate of the spontaneous onset of AD under specific pathogen-free (SPF) conditions. Even under conventional (non-SPF) conditions, the incidence rates of AD are variable and depend on the circumstances of the animal facility in which the NC mice have been bred (Kikkawa et al., unpublished results). Therefore, experimental conditions for the onset of AD are necessary for a high and stable incidence of AD. Although hypersensitivity to some environmental factors is suggested to cause dermatitis, the precise factor remains unclear. The breakthrough identification of conditions to induce AD in NC mice was made by Morita and colleagues, who discovered that fur mites induced dermatitis associated with IgE hyperproduction in a substrain of mice, NC/Kuj (Morita et al., 1999), and the mite antigen-induced dermatitis was subsequently confirmed (Sasakawa et al., 2001). These lines of evidence suggested a new model system for antigen-induced dermatitis. Alternatively, dermatitis can also be induced in NC mice by a hapten, such as 2,4-dinitrofluorobenzene (DNFB) (Tomimori et al., 2002, Tomimori et al., 2005), trinitrochlorobenzene (TNCB) (Taniguchi et al., 2003), or FITC (Hvid et al., 2009). Using these induced dermatitis models in NC mice, extensive surveys for therapeutic agents, both chemicals and herbal medicine, have been performed(Kobayashi et al., 2003, Lee et al., 2007, Jiang et al., 2009, Joo et al., 2009, Lee et al., 2010, Choi et al., 2011, Kim et al., 2011, Park et al., 2011, Sung et al., 2011a, Sung et al., 2011b, Wu et al., 2011).

2.3 Establishment of hairless NC mice for the development of drugs and comprehensive therapy for human AD

Although the NC model is a promising mouse model for AD, it has another serious drawback, namely the existence of dense hair on the body. The dense hair disturbs the pathological observation of the symptoms in the earlier stages of AD onset and without hair shaving also interferes with the painting of an ointment to test its efficacy. Hair shaving itself leads to another severe problem, laboratory animal allergy (LAA). LAA is a form of occupational allergic disease. The development of LAA is due to the presence of IgE antibodies directed against animal proteins, and incidence rates are rapidly increasing. Hair shaving increases the chance of direct exposure of the researcher to the animal proteins, and the worst possible outcome of LAA is death by anaphylactic shock (Pacheco et al., 2003, Schweitzer et al., 2003, Matsui et al., 2004, Curtin-Brosnan et al., 2010). Therefore, a hairless model on an AD-prone genetic background would be an ideal and powerful tool for basic research, such as the discovery of the genes responsible for AD, and for drug development, such as the development of new ointment for the treatment of AD.

We have generated a hairless mouse model for AD on the NC genetic background to study the pathophysiology of the disease and to screen ointment compounds as novel therapies for skin lesions. To generate the hairless mice, we applied a novel method that we recently developed for the ablation of specific cell lineages using diphtheria toxin (DT), also known as the TRECK (Toxin receptor mediated cell knockout) method (Saito et al, 2001). To achieve the specific ablation of hair shafts, we used the promoter of the keratin 71 (*Krt71*/formerly *krt2-6g* or *mK6irs1*) gene, which encodes a type 2 keratin filament protein. The *Krt71* gene is involved in hair development, and mutation of the gene affects the morphology of the coat hair because the gene product is expressed in the cells of the inner root sheath (IRS). Several allelic mutations found in the Caracul (*Ca*) phenotype are morphologically very similar to the classic wavy coat mutation in laboratory mice (Kikkawa et al., 2003). Therefore, we constructed a minigene in which the expression of the human DT receptor, the intrinsic mechanism of which is to bind the heparin-binding EGF (Naglich et al., 1992a, Naglich et al., 1992b), is driven by the promoter of the *Krt71* gene (Fig. 1A). The minigene was introduced directly into pronucleus-stage eggs of the NC strain to generate 'NC/Nga-*Krt71*-TRECK'-transgenic (Tg) mice. Unexpectedly, NCN24, one of the two NC Tg founder lines, exhibited a dominant hairless phenotype without the administration of DT (Fig. 1B). Furthermore, a predisposition to atopic dermatitis-like symptoms and the elevation of IgE levels were observed in both the NCN24 and the wild type NC strain (Fig. 2). Our newly developed NCN24 mice will be useful to assess drugs for AD therapy because they allow the monitoring of skin inflammation without shaving (Takada et al., 2008b). DT is highly

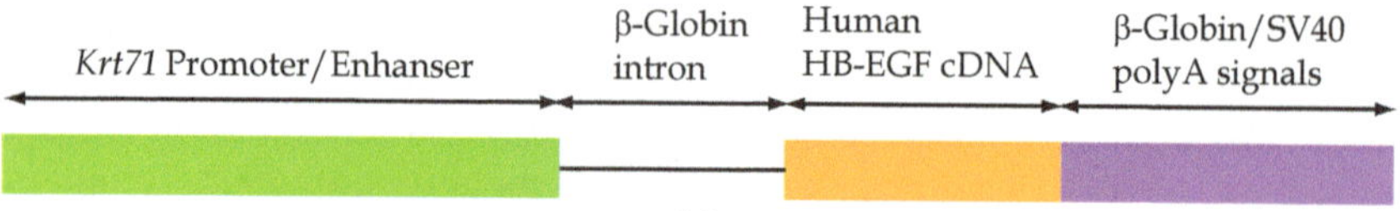

(a)

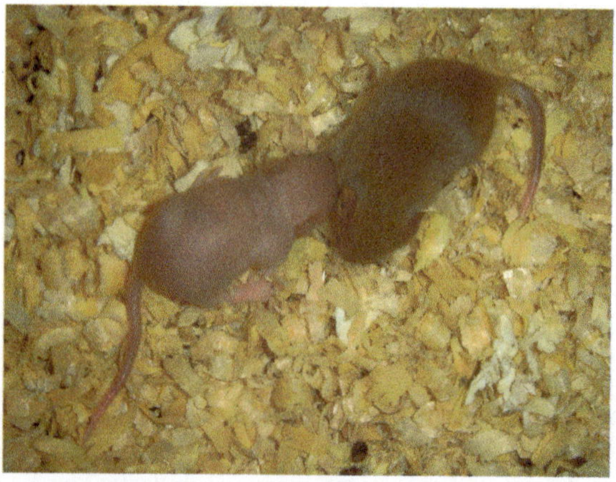

(b)

(a) Approximately 9 kb of the *Krt71* promoter region was amplified by PCR using genomic C57BL/6J mouse DNA. The *Krt71* promoter was cloned into the *Bam*HI and *Not*I sites of the TRECK vector (Saito et al. 2001). The 11-kb *Not*I/*Xho*I fragment containing the *Krt71* promoter, the β-globin intron, and human HB-EGF cDNA was excised, purified and used for microinjection.

(b) NC/Nga-Tg(Krt71-HBEGF)24Rin (NCN24) mice at postnatal day 14 (P14) exhibit a hairless phenotype over the whole body without DT treatment compared with the wild type littermates.

Fig. 1. Generation of *Krt71* promoter/human HB-EGF transgenic NC mice

toxic to humans, and therefore, it is not an appropriate agent to use in experimental models intended to investigate the pathogenic aspects relevant to human disease. DT treatment and the attention required for DT administration in mice would no longer be needed if the novel hairless Tg mice were used.

The NCN24 strain is co-isogenic to the wild type NC strain because the minigene was directly introduced into the NC genome by microinjection as described earlier. This means that, with the exception of coat hair, no phenotypic differences are expected between NCN24 mice and the original NC mice. We confirmed this by comparing the coat hair, the time to AD onset, the progression of AD, the serum IgE level and its change over time, and the composition of the immune cell populations in the bone marrow, spleen and thymus (Table 1) between NCN24 mice and the original NC mice (Takada et al., 2008b). As expected, there were no differences between the two strains except for coat hair. Therefore, we conclude that NCN24 mice will be useful for assessing the efficacy of drugs and for developing AD therapy because the model enables researchers to monitor skin inflammation without shaving.

A remaining issue is why the hairless phenotype occurred in the NCN24 line without the administration of DT because the TRECK method upon which the model was designed is based on the aberration of a cell lineage by DT through the human DT receptor (DTR) driven by a tissue-specific promoter introduced into the transgenic minigene (Saito et al, 2001). The key evidence for this phenomenon, namely, hairless phenotype without DT administration is that the original cellular function of DTR is heparin-binding EGF, an important role of which is the molecular regulation of the hair cell cycle (Mak and Chan, 2003). From the P1 to P12 stages in the NCN24 mice, we only observed immature or irregular hair follicles distributed in the skin sections, indicating that the proper processes

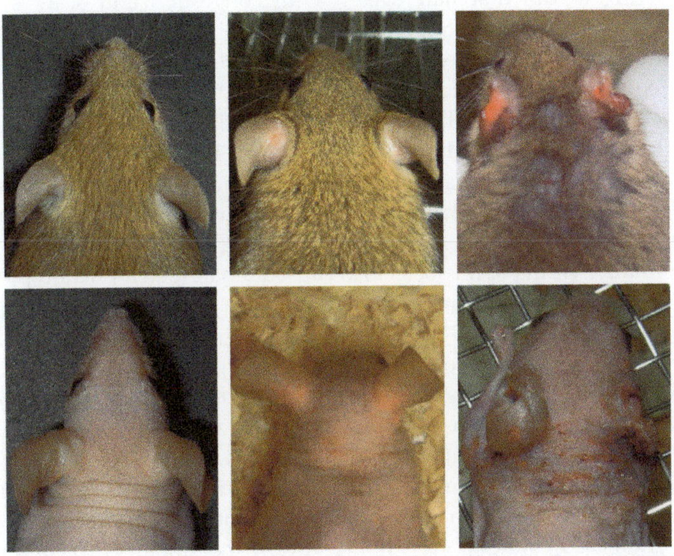

Fig. 2. The severity and histological features of the atopic dermatitis-like skin lesions in wild type (upper row) and NCN24 (lower row) mice during the progression of AD. The atopic dermatitis-like skin lesions were observed in the pinnae and scapula of the dorsal area along with congestion and scaly symptoms, and advanced dermatitis was seen in the middle- and right-side photographs in both wild type NC/Nga (upper low) and NCN24 mice (lower low).

Imune cells	Bone Marrow (× 10⁶) WT	Bone Marrow (× 10⁶) NCN24	Spleen (× 10⁶) WT	Spleen (× 10⁶) NCN24	Thymus (× 10⁶) WT	Thymus (× 10⁶) NCN24
Total cell number	33.00	34.80	56.40	63.10	84.60	98.55
B lineage cells	8.28	9.12	27.25	21.09	-	-
Dendritic cells	-	-	0.60	0.48	-	-
Myeloid cells	10.24	11.38	2.98	2.10	-	-
NK cells	0.14	0.09	1.40	1.16	-	-
NKT cells	0.07	0.05	0.27	0.22	-	-
T lineage cells	0.28	0.12	9.25	6.19	10.58	10.67
$CD4^+$ cells	-	-	7.20	4.56	6.23	5.72
$CD8^+$ cells	-	-	2.36	1.57	1.93	2.22
$CD4^+CD8^+$ cells	-	-	-	-	75.35	89.58
$CD4^+CD25^+$ cells	-	-	0.27	0.27	0.46	0.37

B lineage cells ($CD19^+$), Dendritic cells ($CD11c^+$), Myeloid cells ($Gr\text{-}1^+$), NK cells ($NK1.1^+DX5^+$), NKT cells ($NK1.1^+CD3^+$), T lineage cells ($CD3^+$). Data shown are the mean from two littermates.

Table 1. The number of immune cells in wild-type (wt) and NCN24 mice.

were not occurring in the first hair cycles, with congestion and scaly symptoms, and advanced dermatitis was seen in both wild type and NCN24. starting from the early anagen phase. The mechanisms that potentially cause the hairless phenotype could be simple; specifically, it could be the ectopic expression of the DTR (HB-EGF) driven by the *Krt71* promoter in the inner root sheath (IRS). As described earlier, HB-EGF is the major molecular regulator for the hair cell cycle (Mak and Chan, 2003). Transgenic mice in which HB-EGF was overexpressed by a ubiquitous expression vector showed hair abnormalities, including a bare-patch phenotype. This phenotype was attributed to the ectopic and irregular overexpression of HB-EGF in the IRS of the Tg mice (Takada et al., 2008b). Similarly, a spontaneous mutation at the *Krt71* locus also caused a bare-patch phenotype (Poirier et al., 2002). Therefore, the most likely mechanism causing the hairless phenotype in our Tg mice is the ectopic overexpression of HB-EGF, which disturbs the initiation of the normal hair cell cycle. Specifically, the *Krt71* promoter in the transgene guaranteed the IRS-specific expression of HB-EGF, which augmented the ectopic expression of HB-EGF in the IRS. Several mechanisms have previously been reported in which molecular signaling via the ErbB family, the members of which are involved downstream of HB-EGF signaling, is critical for skin and hair development during the neonatal period. HB-EGF is an essential molecule for the initiation of hair growth and for entry into the appropriate phase of the hair cycle (Mak & Chan 2003), although it is not clear how the human HB-EGF transcript might affect the development of the hair follicles in the neonatal period of NCN24 mice.

Evidence of an alternative explanation is that the phenotype we described partially resembles several phenotypic features that were reported in studies of the hairless mouse harboring a *hr/hr* mutation (Brooke, 1926). The hairless (*hr*) mutant mice have been well characterized and exhibit a hairless phenotype due to a failure of the follicular papilla to

ascend to the permanent portion of the hair follicle during the first catagen phase (Panteleyev et al., 1999). Therefore, we considered that a functional defect in the follicular papilla early in the anagen phase of NCN24 mice could cause an irregular sorting of the melanin granules and the weak and degraded features of the hair shaft. Unlike in the *hr* phenotype mice, hair degradation was observed in the newborn animals of the NCN24 line, demonstrating that in these hairless mice, the development of the hair follicles progressed normally, while the first cycle of the anagen phase was impaired (Takada et al., 2008b).
A third possibility is that the insertion disrupted a gene (s) that is indispensable for hair development. However, this is very unlikely because fluorescence in situ hybridization (FISH) analysis revealed that the transgene was detected in the telomeric region of chromosome 14, where no indispensable genes have been reported thus far (Takada et al., 2008b).

2.4 Attempts to identify the genes responsible for AD using polygenic AD models

Linkage analyses and a quantitative traits loci (QTL) analysis have been performed for the two models for human AD, NC and NOA, to identify the genetic loci responsible for AD. Using intercrossing or backcrossing between an AD model and a non-AD counterpart, the segregation ratio of F_2 or N_2 progeny was examined, and it was discovered that the segregation ratios did not follow Mendelian inheritance, suggesting that the AD phenotype is controlled by multiple genes. In fact, several loci were identified in both NC and NOA, as discussed below (Natori et al., 1999, Kohara et al., 2001, Watanabe et al., 2001). Despite extensive attempts spanning a decade, no responsible genes have yet been identified by positional cloning.

2.4.1 Linkage analyses for AD in NOA

Detailed linkage analyses revealed a significant co-segregation between ulcerative skin lesions and markers on murine chromosome 14. A statistical analysis indicated that the critical region was in the vicinity of *D14Mit236* and *D14Mit160* (Natori et al., 1999). These analyses also identified two additional modifier genes: one in the middle of chromosome 7 and the other in the telomeric region of chromosome 13 (Watanabe et al., 2001).

2.4.2 Linkage analyses for AD in NC

We performed a linkage disequilibrium analysis between AD or hyper-IgE-emia and chromosome-specific microsatellite loci in the backcrossed progeny of NC and MSM/Ms (MSM) mice. The MSM line originated from Japanese wild mice, *Mus musculus molossinus* (Moriwaki et al., 2009), and maintains a very large amount of genetic diversity in the genome (Kikkawa et al., 2001, Sakai et al., 2005, Takada et al., 2008a) compared with other classical inbred strains, such as BALB/c and C57BL/6, and we often use the MSM strain to perform finer genetic mapping. This analysis led to two important observations: 1) the occurrence of dermatitis is not associated with an elevated serum IgE level (Kohara et al. unpublished); and 2) the major locus responsible for dermatitis (the *derm1* locus) is located on the middle of chromosome 9 (Fig. 3). We also discovered additive (potentially modifier) loci with suggestive level on a few chromosomes (Kikkawa et al., unpublished). This genetic status resembles that of human AD because human AD is also polygenic, and mono- or oligogenic AD has not yet been reported. Furthermore, the association between hyper-IgE-emia and dermatitis/eczema is not always observed in humans. Unfortunately, we have not found any significant or suggestive loci for hyper-IgE-emia.

2.5 Monogenic mouse models for human AD: DS-*Nh* and KOR-*adjm*

In contrast to the polygenic AD models, there are two models in Japan that are the result of a single mutation. One is DS-*Nh*, and the other is KOR-*adjm*. Unlike the mouse models with polygenic factors, the genes responsible for dermatitis, DS-*Nh* and KOR-*adjm*, have been identified from the monogenic AD models.

2.5.1 The DS-*Nh* gene is the transient receptor potential cation channel, subfamily V member 3 (TRPV3)

A spontaneous mutant strain with a hairless phenotype (DS-*Nh*) was isolated from an inbred strain, DS, which was developed in 1954 from an outbred dd stock of the Central Institute for Experimental Animals, Tokyo, Japan. The DS-Nh mice exhibit ulcerative skin lesions on the cheek, neck and shoulder as initial symptoms when the mice are transferred from SPF to conventional conditions. The skin lesions have been associated with hyper-IgE-emia triggered by *Staphylococcus aureus* infection (Watanabe et al., 2003a, Watanabe et al., 2003b). The DS-*Nh* mice also exhibit heavy scratching behavior to itching, which is associated with elevated levels of histamine and nerve growth factor in the serum and/or skin tissues (Yoshioka et al., 2006). Furthermore, the DS-*Nh* mice exhibit other features that resemble human AD, such as significantly increased serum levels of IL-4 and IL-13 (Hikita et al., 2002) and increased numbers of whole mast cells and CD4$^+$ T cells (Yoshioka et al., 2006). Therefore, the DS-Nh mouse is a model of the pruritus associated with human AD.

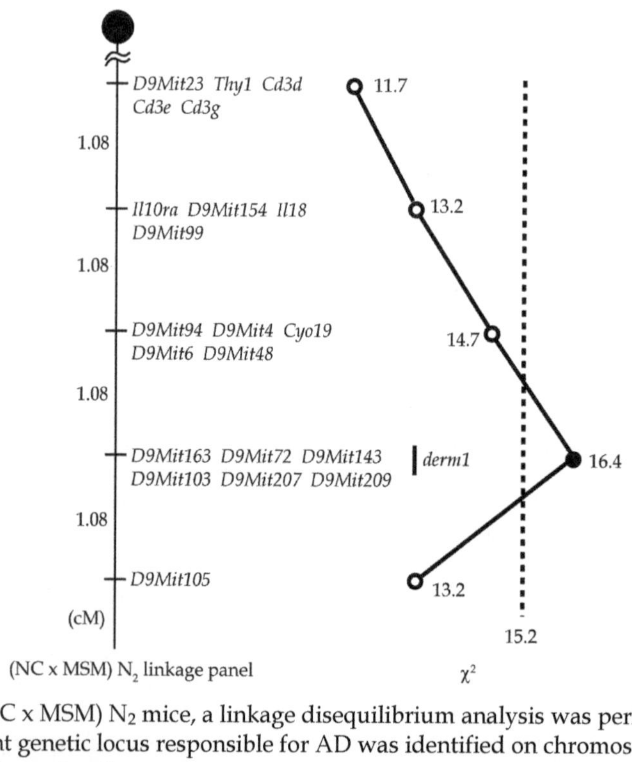

Fig. 3. Using (NC x MSM) N_2 mice, a linkage disequilibrium analysis was performed, and a single significant genetic locus responsible for AD was identified on chromosome 9. We designated the locus *derm1*.

The *Nh* mutation is controlled by a single dominant mutation that occurred in the transient receptor potential (TRP) cation channel, subfamily V member 3 (*Trpv3*). The TRP channels are expressed ubiquitously in the body and are thought to have important roles in maintaining proper vital status (Okuhara et al., 2007) because they are critical mediators in sensory systems and respond to temperature, touch, pain and other important stimuli. TRP channels are divided into six main subfamilies, including TRPV (Clapham, 2003). The TRPV subfamily is expressed in the skin, keratinocytes and hair follicles and is activated by temperatures higher than 32-39°C (Peier et al., 2002). The Gly573Ser substitution of *Trpv3* leads to increased ion-channel activity in keratinocytes, which influences the hair growth cycle in mice (Imura et al., 2007). By studying dermatitis in DS-*Nh* mice, two major pathways have been identified; one is the interaction between the gain-of-function *Trpv3* mutation and NKT cells with the T-cell receptor Vβ, and the other is the synergistic production of interleukin-13 (IL-13) through the activation of Toll-like receptor 2 by staphylococcal enterotoxin C-producing *S. aurous* (Yoshioka et al., 2007, Imura et al., 2008, Imura et al., 2009, Yoshioka et al., 2009).

2.5.2 The KOR-*adjm* gene is TNFR-associated factor 3-interacting protein 2 (TRAF3IP2)

Recently, we identified a new mouse model for human atopic dermatitis, the phenotype of which is controlled by a single recessive mutation. The spontaneous mutant mice, which exhibited high levels of serum IgE and an atopic dermatitis (AD)-like skin disease, were identified from a colony of the KOR inbred strain, which was derived from Japanese wild mice (Figs. 4, 5). No segregation was observed between hyper-IgE–emia and dermatitis in BALB/c x KOR mutant N_2 mice. Furthermore, linkage analysis showed that both phenotypes are controlled by a same single recessive locus, and thus we designated the

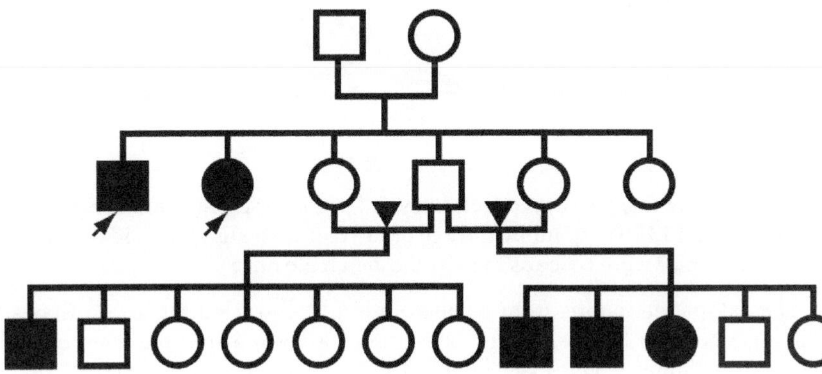

(a)

(a) Phenotype segregation in the KOR colony. A pedigree of the KOR strain in which *adjm* mutant mice were first discovered (shown by arrows). The squares and circles represent males and females, respectively. The closed and open symbols represent affected and non-affected individuals, respectively.

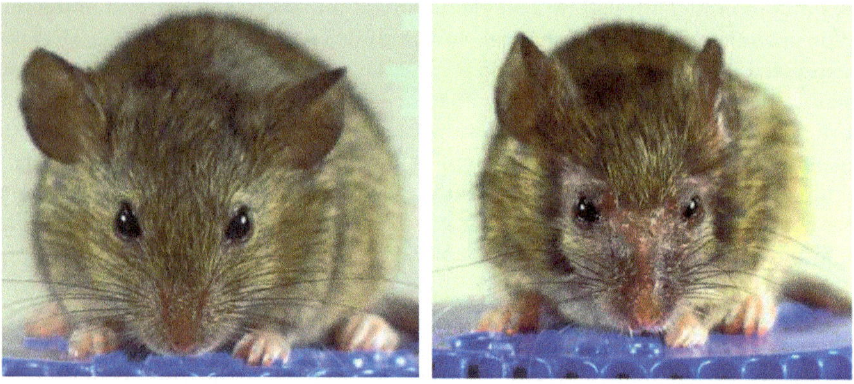

(b)

(b) The appearance of a healthy (left) KOR-*adjm*/*adjm* mouse after KOR-*adjm*/+ mouse disease onset is shown (right).

Fig. 4. *adjm* mutation identified from the KOR mouse colony.

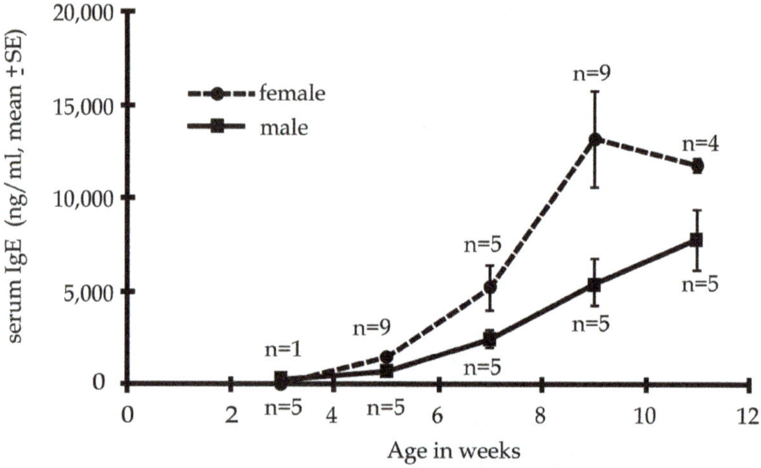

Fig. 5. Age-dependent increase in serum IgE level. The increase began at 5 weeks of age, and the IgE level reached 13,104 ng/ml by the age of 11 weeks. The IgE levels in female mutant (KOR-*adjm*/*adjm*) mice were twice as high as those in male mice

locus as *adjm* (atopic dermatitis from Japanese mice). We isolated the gene responsible for the AD-like phenotypes by positional cloning and discovered that the gene is the mouse homologue of the human TNFR-associated factor 3-interacting protein 2 (TRAF3IP2), which has formerly been called ACT1 (Li et al., 2000) or CIKS (Leonardi et al., 2000) protein. Furthermore, the gene included a single point mutation leading to the substitution of a stop codon for glutamine at amino acid position 214 (Fig. 6) (Matsushima et al., 2010). TRAF3IP2 was first reported as an adopter protein that is associated with and activates IB kinase and stimulates both the NF-B and the JNK signaling pathways (Li, 2008). It has been shown to function as an adaptor protein in signaling pathways mediated by the TNFR superfamily members CD40 and B cell-activating factor in epithelial cells and B cells as well as in the IL-17 -mediated signaling pathway (Li et al., 2000). Our results suggest that dysfunction of the TRAF3IP2 protein causes hyper-IgE-emia through the CD40- and B cell-activating factor-mediated pathway in B cells and causes skin inflammation through the IL-17-mediated pathway. This study demonstrates that the TRAF3IP2 protein has an important role in AD and suggests that the protein could be a therapeutic target for the treatment of AD (see Matsushima et al. (2010) and references therein).

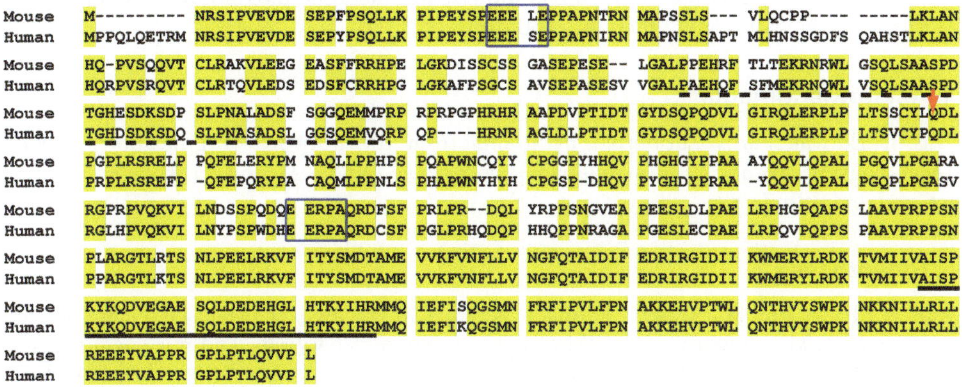

(a)

(a) Comparison of the mouse and human TRAF3IP2 protein sequences. The amino acid sequences in open boxes or underlined with broken or solid lines are the TRAF binding sites, the helix-loop-helix domain, and the coiled-coil domain, respectively.

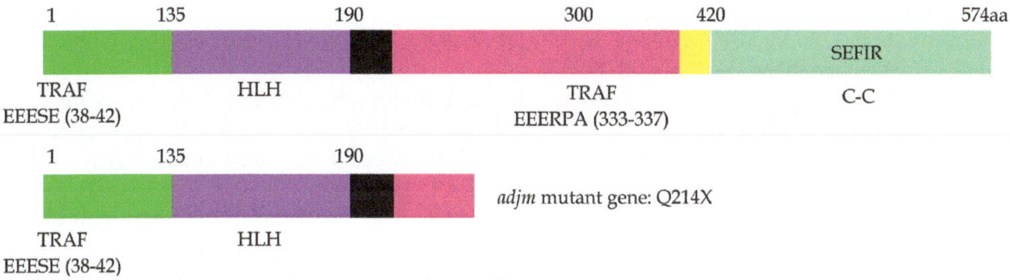

(b)

(b) The domain structure of the TRAF3IP2 protein. The *adjm* mutation causes the truncation of the TRAF3IP2 protein at amino acid 214. The truncated form lacks a C-terminal TRAF-binding site and a C-terminal coiled-coil domain.

Fig. 6. Alignment of amino acid sequence between mouse and human of TRAF3IP2 protein and the predicted structure of TRAF3IP2 protein in wild-type and *adjm* mutant

3. Conclusion

Four promising mouse models for human AD have been established thus far in Japan. Two models are polygenic, and the pathology and the onset of the disease are very similar to human AD, although no responsible genes have been isolated. In contrast, the other two models are monogenic, and the responsible genes have been identified. One, DS-*Nh*, is a gain-of-function mutation in the *Trpv3* locus, whereas the other, KOR-*adjm*, is a loss-of-function mutation in the *Traf3ip2* locus. The former mutation demonstrated the strong involvement of IL-13 in association with the *Trpv3* locus and the TCRVβ^b (NKT cell) haplotype. The latter mutation demonstrated the involvement of CD40L/BAFF signaling for B cell activation and of the IL-17 signaling pathway for the autoimmune and inflammatory responses through the activation of NF-κB. The involvement of the NF-κB pathway to AD is commonly suggested in both human and mouse, and therefore the finding shown here will facilitate the development of therapies and drugs.

4. Acknowledgments

This work was partly supported by grants from the Ministry of Education, Science, Technology, Sports and Culture of Japan Science (to H.Y and Y.M) and a Takeda Foundation research grant (to H.Y.).

5. References

Aioi, A., Tonogaito, H., Suto, H., Hamada, K., Ra, C.R., Ogawa, H., Maibach, H. & Matsuda H. (2001). Impairment of skin barrier function in NC/Nga Tnd mice as a possible model for atopic dermatitis. *The British Journal of Dermatology*, Vol.144, No.1, (January 2001), pp. 12-18, ISSN 0007-0963

Brooke, H.C. (1926). Hairless mice. *Journal of Heredity*, Vol.17, p. 173, ISSN 0022-1503

Choi, S.E., Park, K.H., Jeong, M.S., Kim, H.H., Lee do, I., Joo, S.S., Lee, C.S., Bang, H., Choi, Y.W., Lee, M.K., Seo, S.J. & Lee, M.W. (2011) Effect of Alnus japonica extract on a model of atopic dermatitis in NC/Nga mice. *Journal of Ethnopharmacology*, Vol. 136, No. 3 (July 2011), pp.406-413, ISSN 0378-8741

Clapham, D.E. (2003). TRP channels as cellular sensors. *Nature*, Vol.426, No.6966, (December 2003), pp. 517-524, ISSN 0028-0836

Curtin-Brosnan, J., Paigen, B., Hagberg, K.A., Langley, S., O'Neil, E.A., Krevans, M., Eggleston, P.A. & Matsui, E.C. (2010). Occupational mouse allergen exposure among non-mouse handlers. *Journal of Occupational & Environmental Hygiene*, Vol.7, No.12, (December 2010), pp. 726-734, ISSN 1545-9624

Fallon, P.G., Sasaki, T., Sandilands, A., Campbell, L.E., Saunders, S.P., Mangan, N.E., Callanan, J.J., Kawasaki, H., Shiohama, A., Kubo, A., Sundberg, J.P., Presland, R.B., Fleckman, P., Shimizu, N., Kudoh, J., Irvine, A.D., Amagai, M. & McLean, W.H. (2009). A homozygous frameshift mutation in the mouse Flg gene facilitates enhanced percutaneous allergen priming. *Nature Genetics* Vol.41, No.5, (April 2009) pp. 602-608, ISSN 1061-4036

Festing, M.F.W. (1996). Origins and characteristics of inbred strains of mice, In: *Genetic Variants and Strains of the Laboratory Mouse*, M.F. Lyon, S. Rastan & S.D.M. Brown, (Ed(s).), pp. 1537-1576, Oxford University Press, ISBN 9780198548690, Oxford

Geha, R.S. (2003). Allergy and hypersensitivity. Nature versus nurture in allergy and hypersensitivity. *Current Opinion in Immunology*, Vol.15, No.6, (December 2003), pp. 603-608, ISSN 0952-7915

Hanifin, J.M. (1982). Atopic dermatitis. *Journal of the American Academy of Dermatology*, Vol.6, No.1, (January 1982), pp. 1-13, ISSN 0190-9622

Hanifin, J.M. & Rajka, G. (1980). Diagnostic features of atopic dermatitis. *Acta Dermato-Venereologica - Supplementum*, Vol.92, pp. 44-47, ISSN 0365-8341

Haraguchi, M., Hino, M., Tanaka, H. & Maru M. (1997). Naturally occurring dermatitis associated with *Staphylococcus aureus* in DS-Nh mice. *Experimental Animals*, Vol.46, No.3, (July 1997), pp. 225-229, ISSN 1341-1357

Hikita, I., Yoshioka, T., Mizoguchi, T., Tsukahara, K., Tsuru, K., Nagai, H., Hirasawa, T., Tsuruta, Y., Suzuki, R., Ichihashi, M. & Horikawa T. (2002). Characterization of dermatitis arising spontaneously in DS-Nh mice maintained under conventional conditions: another possible model for atopic dermatitis. *Journal of Dermatological Science*, Vol.30, No.2, (November 2002), pp142-153, ISSN 0923-1811

Hvid, M., Jensen, H.K., Deleuran, B., Kemp, K., Andersson, C., Deleuran, M. & Vestergaard, C. (2009). Evaluation of FITC-induced atopic dermatitis-like disease in NC/Nga mice and BALB/c mice using computer-assisted stereological toolbox, a computer-aided morphometric system. *International Archives of Allergy & Immunology*, Vol.149, No.3, (February 2009), ISSN 1018-2438

Imura, K., Yoshioka, T., Hikita, I., Hirasawa, T., Sakata, T., Matsutani, T., Horikawa, T. & Arimura, A. (2008). Association of T-cell receptor Vbeta haplotypes with dry skin in DS-Nh mice. *Clinical & Experimental Dermatology*, Vol.34, No.1, (November 2008), pp. 1365-2230, ISSN 0307-6938

Imura, K., Yoshioka, T., Hikita, I., Tsukahara, K., Hirasawa, T., Higashino, K., Gahara, Y., Arimura, A. & Sakata, T. (2007). Influence of TRPV3 mutation on hair growth cycle in mice. *Biochemical & Biophysical Research Communications*, Vol.363, No.3, (September 2007), pp. 479-483, ISSN 0006-291X

Imura, K., Yoshioka, T., Hirasawa, T. & Sakata, T. (2009). Role of TRPV3 in immune response to development of dermatitis. *Journal of Inflammation*, Vol.6, (May 2009) p. 17, ISSN 1476-9255

Ito, M., Ogawa, K., Takeuchi, K., Nakada, A., Heishi, M., Suto, H., Mitsuishi, K., Sugita, Y., Ogawa, H. & Ra, C. (2004). Gene expression of enzymes for tryptophan degradation pathway is upregulated in the skin lesions of patients with atopic dermatitis or psoriasis. *Journal of Dermatological Science*, Vol.36, No.3, (December 2004), pp. 157-164, ISSN 0923-1811

Jiang, J., Yamaguchi, T., Funakushi, N., Kuhara, T., Fan, P. S., Ueki, R., Suto, H., Kase, Y., Ikeda, S. & Ogawa, H. (2009) Oral administration of Yokukansan inhibits the development of atopic dermatitis-like lesions in isolated NC/Nga mice. *Journal of Dermatological Science*, Vol. 56, No. 1 (October 2009), pp.37-42, ISSN 0923-1811

Joo, S.S., Won, T.J., Nam, S.Y., Kim, Y.B., Lee, Y.C., Park, S.Y., Park, H.Y., Hwang, K.W. & Lee do, I. (2009) Therapeutic advantages of medicinal herbs fermented with *Lactobacillus plantarum*, in topical application and its activities on atopic dermatitis. *Phytotherapy Research*, Vol. 23, No. 7, (July 2009), pp.913-919, ISSN 0951-418X

Jung, K., Tanaka, A., Fujita, H., Matsuda, A., Oida, K., Karasawa, K., Okamoto, N., Ohmori, K., Jee, Y., Shin, T. & Matsuda, H. (2011). Peroxisome proliferator-activated receptor gamma-mediated suppression of dendritic cell function prevents the onset of atopic dermatitis in NC/Tnd mice. *The Journal of Allergy & Clinical Immunology*, Vol.127, No.2, (January 2011), pp. 420-429, ISSN 0091-6749

Kikkawa, Y., Miura, I., Takahama, S., Wakana, S., Yamazaki, Y., Moriwaki, K., Shiroishi, T. & Yonekawa, H. (2001). Microsatellite database for MSM/Ms and JF1/Ms, molossinus-derived inbred strains. *Mammalian Genome*, Vol.12, No.9, (September 2001), pp. 750-752, 0938-8990 (Print)

Kikkawa, Y., Oyama, A., Ishii, R., Miura, I., Amano, T., Ishii, Y., Yoshikawa, Y., Masuya, H., Wakana, S., Shiroishi, T., Taya, C. & Yonekawa, H. (2003). A small deletion hotspot in the type II keratin gene *mK6irs1/Krt2-6g* on mouse chromosome 15, a candidate for causing the wavy hair of the caracul (*Ca*) mutation. *Genetics*, Vol.165, No.2, (October 2003), pp. 721-733, ISSN 0016-6731

Kim, M.S., Hur, Y.G., Kim, W.G., Park, B.W., Ahn, K.S., Kim, J.J. & Bae, H. (2011) Inhibitory effect of *Platycodon grandiflorum* on T(H)1 and T(H)2 immune responses in a murine model of 2,4-dinitrofluorobenzene-induced atopic dermatitis-like skin lesions. *Annals of Allergy, Asthma & Immunology*, vol. 106, No. 1 (January 2011), pp.54-61, ISSN 1081-1206

Kobayashi, H., Mizuno, N., Kutsuna, H., Teramae, H., Ueoku, S., Onoyama, J., Yamanaka, K., Fujita, N. & Ishii, M. (2003) Hochu-ekki-to suppresses development of dermatitis and elevation of serum IgE level in NC/Nga mice. *Drugs under Experimental and Clinical Research*, vol. 29, No. 2, (September 2003), pp.81-84, ISSN 0378-6501

Kohara, Y., Tanabe, K., Matsuoka, K., Kanda, N., Matsuda, H., Karasuyama, H. & Yonekawa, H. (2001). A major determinant quantitative-trait locus responsible for atopic dermatitis-like skin lesions in NC/Nga mice is located on Chromosome 9. *Immunogenetics*, Vol. 53, No.9, (February 2001), pp. 15-21, ISSN 0093-7711

Kondo, K., Tomita, T., Esaki, K., & Hayakawa, J. (March 1983). *Genetic Control of Laboratory Animals* (In Japanese), K., Kondo, T., Tomita, K., Esaki, & J., Hayakawa (Ed(s).). Soft Science, Inc., Tokyo.

Kondo, K., Nagami, T. & Teramoto, S. (1969). Differences in hematopoietic death among inbred strains of mice. In: *Comparative Cellular & Species Radiosensitivity* (V.P., Bond & T, Sugahara), (Ed(s).), pp. 20-29, Igakushoin, Tokyo

Kondo, T., Ohno, H., Taguchi, K., Satode, R. & Shiomoto, Y. (2006). Increased susceptibility to *Staphylococcus aureus* colonization of the skin of the NOA mouse: a potentially useful animal model for evaluating antiseptic effects. *Experimental Animals*, Vol.55, No.1, (January 2006), pp. 49-56, ISSN 1341-1357

Kondo, T., Shiomoto, Y., Kondo, T. & Kubo, S. (1997). The "NOA" mouse; a new hair-deficient mutant (a possible animal model of allergic dermatitis). *Mouse Genome*, Vol.95, No.3, (1997), pp. 698-700, ISSN 0959-0587.

Larsen, F.S., Holm, N.V. & Henningsen, K. (1986). Atopic dermatitis. A genetic-epidemiologic study in a population-based twin sample. *Journal of the American Academy of Dermatology*, Vol.15, No.3, (September 1986), pp. 487-494, ISSN 0190-9622

Lee, H.S., Kim, S.K., Han, J.B., Choi, H.M., Park, J.H., Kim, E.C., Choi, M.S., An, H.J., Um, J.Y., Kim, H.M. & Min, B.I. (2006). Inhibitory effects of *Rumex japonicus* Houtt. on the development of atopic dermatitis-like skin lesions in NC/Nga mice. *The British Journal of Dermatology*, Vol.155, No.1, (July 2006), pp. 33-38, ISSN 0007-0963

Lee, J.K., Ha, H., Lee, H.Y., Park, S.J., Jeong, S.L., Choi, Y.J. & Shin, H.K. (2010) Inhibitory effects of heartwood extracts of *Broussonetia kazinoki* Sieb on the development of atopic dermatitis in NC/Nga mice. *Bioscience, Biotechnology, and Biochemistry*, Vol. 74, No. 9, (September 2010), pp.1802-1806, ISSN 0916-8451

Lee, S.J., Oh, S.G., Seo, S.W., Ahn, H.J., Geum, D., Cho, J.J. & Park, C.S. (2007) Oral administration of *Astragalus membranaceus* inhibits the development of DNFB-induced dermatitis in NC/Nga mice. *Biological & Pharmaceutical Bulletin*, Vol. 30, No. 8 (August 2007), pp.1468-1471, ISSN 0918-6158

Leonardi, A., Chariot, A., Claudio, E., Cunningham, K. & Siebenlist, U. (2000). CIKS, a connection to Ikappa B kinase and stress-activated protein kinase. *Proceedings of the*

National Academy of Sciences of the United States of America, Vol.97, No.19, (September 2000), pp. 10494-10499, ISSN 0027-8424

Leung, D.Y. & Bieber, T. (2003). Atopic dermatitis. *Lancet*, Vol.361, No.9352 (January 2003), pp. 151-160, ISSN 0140-6736

Li, X. (2008). Act1 modulates autoimmunity through its dual functions in CD40L/BAFF and IL-17 signaling. *Cytokine*, Vol.41, No.2, (February 2008) pp. 105-113, ISSN 1043-4666.

Li X., Commane, M., Nie, H., Hua, X., Chatterjee-Kishore, M., Wald, D., Haag, M. & Stark, G.R. (2000). Act1, an NF-kappa B-activating protein. *Proceedings of the National Academy of Sciences of the United States of America*, Vol. 97, No.19, (September 2000), pp. 10489-10493, ISSN 0027-8424

Mak, K.K. & Chan, S.Y. (2003). Epidermal growth factor as a biologic switch in hair growth cycle. *The Journal of Biological Chemistry*, Vol.278, No.28, (July 2003), pp.26120-26126, ISSN 0021-9258

Matsuda, H., Watanabe, N., Geba, G.P., Sperl, J., Tsudzuki, M., Hiroi, J., Matsumoto, M., Ushio, H., Saito, S., Askenase, P.W. & Ra, C. (1997). Development of atopic dermatitis-like skin lesion with IgE hyperproduction in NC/Nga mice. *International Immunology*, vol.9, No.3, (March 1997), pp. 461-466, ISSN 0953-8178

Matsui, E.C., Krop, E.J., Diette, G.B., Aalberse, R.C., Smith, A.L. & Eggleston, P.A. (2004). Mouse allergen exposure and immunologic responses: IgE-mediated mouse sensitization and mouse specific IgG and IgG4 levels. *Annals of Allergy, Asthma, & Immunology*, Vol.93, No.2, (August 2004), pp.171-178, ISSN 1081-1206

Matsushima, Y., Kikkawa, Y., Takada, T., Matsuoka, K., Seki, Y., Yoshida, H., Minegishi, Y., Karasuyama, H. & Yonekawa, H. (2010). An atopic dermatitis-like skin disease with hyper-IgE-emia develops in mice carrying a spontaneous recessive point mutation in the *Traf3ip2* (Act1/CIKS) gene. *Journal of Immunology*, Vol.185, No.4, (August 2010), pp.2340-2349, ISSN 0022-1767

Moniaga, C.S., Egawa, G., Kawasaki, H., Hara-Chikuma, M., Honda, T., Tanizaki, H., Nakajima, S., Otsuka, A., Matsuoka, H., Kubo, A., Sakabe, J., Tokura, Y., Miyachi, Y., Amagai, M. & Kabashima, K. (2010) Flaky tail mouse denotes human atopic dermatitis in the steady state and by topical application with *Dermatophagoides pteronyssinus* extract. *The American Journal of Pathology*, Vol. 176, No. 5 (May 2010), pp.2385-2393, ISSN 0002-9440.

Morar, N., Willis-Owen, S.A., Moffatt, M.F. & Cookson, W.O. (2006). The genetics of atopic dermatitis. *The Journal of Allergy & Clinical Immunology*, Vol.118, No.1, (July 2006), pp. 24-34, ISSN 0091-6749

Morita, E., Kaneko, S., Hiragun, T., Shindo, H., Tanaka, T., Furukawa, T., Nobukiyo, A. & Yamamoto, S. (1999). Fur mites induce dermatitis associated with IgE hyperproduction in an inbred strain of mice, NC/Kuj. *Journal of Dermatological Science* Vol.19, No.1, (January 1999), pp. 37-43, ISSN 0923-1811

Moriwaki, K., Miyashita, N., Mita, A., Gotoh, H., Tsuchiya, K., Kato, H., Mekada, K., Noro, C., Oota, S., Yoshiki, A., Obata, Y., Yonekawa, H. & Shiroishi, T. (2009). Unique inbred strain MSM/Ms established from the Japanese wild mouse. *Experimental Animals*, Vol. 58, No.2, (April 2009), pp. 123-134, ISSN 1341-1357

Naglich, J.G., Metherall, J.E., Russell, D.W. & Eidels, L. (1992a). Expression cloning of a diphtheria toxin receptor: identity with a heparin-binding EGF-like growth factor precursor. *Cell*, Vol.69, No.6, (June 1992), pp. 1051-1061, ISSN 0092-8674

Naglich, J.G., Rolf, J.M & Eidels, L. (1992b). Expression of functional diphtheria toxin receptors on highly toxin-sensitive mouse cells that specifically bind radioiodinated toxin. *Proceedings of the National Academy of Sciences of the United States of America*, Vol.89, No.6, (March 1992), pp. 2170-2174, ISSN 0027-8424

Natori, K., Tamari, M., Watanabe, O., Onouchi, Y., Shiomoto, Y., Kubo, S. & Nakamura, Y. (1999). Mapping of a gene responsible for dermatitis in NOA (Naruto Research Institute Otsuka Atrichia) mice, an animal model of allergic dermatitis. *Journal of Human Genetics*, Vol.44, No.6, (August 1999), pp. 372-376, ISSN 1434-5161

Novak, N., Bieber, T. & Leung, D.Y. (2003). Immune mechanisms leading to atopic dermatitis. *The Journal of Allergy and Clinical Immunology*, Vol.112, No.6 Suppl, (December 2003), pp. S128-139, ISSN 0091-6749

Ogawa, K., Ito, M., Takeuchi, K., Nakada, A., Heishi, M., Suto, H., Mitsuishi, K., Sugita, Y., Ogawa, H. & Ra, C. (2005). Tenascin-C is upregulated in the skin lesions of patients with atopic dermatitis. *Journal of Dermatological Science*, Vol.40, No.1, (October 2005), pp. 35-41, ISSN 0923-1811

Okuhara, D.Y., Hsia, A.Y. & Xie, M. (2007). Transient receptor potential channels as drug targets. *Expert Opinion on Therapeutic Targets*, Vol.11, No.3, (March 2007), pp. 391-401, ISSN 1472-8222

O'Regan, G.M. & Irvine, A.D. (2010) The role of filaggrin in the atopic diathesis. *Clinical and Experimental Allergy : Journal of the British Society for Allergy and Clinical Immunology*, Vol. 40, No. 7 (July 2010) pp.965-972, ISSN 0954-7894.

Oyoshi, M.K., Murphy, G.F. & Geha, R.S. (2009) Filaggrin-deficient mice exhibit TH17-dominated skin inflammation and permissiveness to epicutaneous sensitization with protein antigen. *The Journal of Allergy and Clinical Immunology* Vol.124, No. 3, (September 2009) p.p. 485-493, 493 e481, ISSN 0091-6749.

Pacheco, K.A., McCammon, C., Liu, A.H., Thorne, P.S., O'Neill, M.E., Martyny, J., Newman, L.S., Hamman, R.F. & Rose, C.S. (2003). Airborne endotoxin predicts symptoms in non-mouse-sensitized technicians and research scientists exposed to laboratory mice. *American Journal of Respiratory & Critical Care Medicine*, Vol.167, No.7, (April 2003), pp. 983-990, ISSN 1073-449X

Panteleyev, A.A., Botchkareva, N.V., Sundberg, J.P., Christiano, A.M. & Paus, R. (1999). The role of the hairless (*hr*) gene in the regulation of hair follicle catagen transformation. *The American Journal of Pathology*, Vol.155, No.1, (July 1999), pp. 159-171, ISSN 0002-9440

Park, K.H., Choi, S.E., Choi, Y.W., Lee D.I., Joo, S.S., Jeong, M.S., Bang, H., Lee, C.S., Seo, S.J. & Lee, M.W. (2011) Topical application of two condensed tannins from the root of *Rosa multiflora* Thunberg for the treatment of atopic dermatitis (AD) in NC/Nga Mice. *Phytotherapy Research*, (June 2011), ISSN 0951-418X

Peier, A.M., Reeve, A.J., Andersson, D.A., Moqrich, A., Earley, T.J., Hergarden, A.C., Story, G.M., Colley, S., Hogenesch, J.B., McIntyre, P., Bevan, S. & Patapoutian, A. (2002). A heat-sensitive TRP channel expressed in keratinocytes. *Science* Vol.296, No.5575, (June 2002), pp. 2046-2049, ISSN 0193-4511

Poirier, C., Yoshiki, A., Fujiwara, K., Guenet, J.L. & Kusakabe M. (2002). Hague (*Hag*). A new mouse hair mutation with an unstable semidominant allele. *Genetics*, Vol.162, No.2, (October 2002), pp. 831-840, ISSN 0016-6731

Saito, M., Iwawaki, T., Taya, C., Yonekawa, H., Noda, M., Inui, Y., Mekada, E., Kimata, Y., Tsuru, A. & Kohno K. (2001). Diphtheria toxin receptor-mediated conditional and targeted cell ablation in transgenic mice. *Nature Biotechnology*, Vol.19, No.8, (August 2001), pp. 746-750, ISSN 1087-0156

Sakai, T., Kikkawa, Y., Miura, I., Inoue, T., Moriwaki, K., Shiroishi, T., Satta, Y., Takahata, N. & Yonekawa, H. (2005). Origins of mouse inbred strains deduced from whole-genome scanning by polymorphic microsatellite loci. *Mammalian Genome*, Vol.16, No.1, (January 2005), pp. 11-19, ISSN 0938-8990

Sasakawa, T., Higashi, Y., Sakuma, S., Hirayama, Y., Sasakawa, Y., Ohkubo, Y., Goto, T., Matsumoto, M. & Matsuda H. (2001). Atopic dermatitis-like skin lesions induced by topical application of mite antigens in NC/Nga mice. *International Archives of Allergy & Immunology*, Vol.126, No.3, (November 2001), pp. 239-247, ISSN 1018-2438

Schultz Larsen, F. (1993). Atopic dermatitis: a genetic-epidemiologic study in a population-based twin sample. *Journal of the American Academy of Dermatology*, Vol.28, No. 5 Pt 1, (May, 1993), pp. 719-723, ISSN 0190-9622

Schweitzer, I.B., Smith, E., Harrison, D.J., Myers, D.D., Eggleston, P.A., Stockwell, J.D., Paigen, B. & Smith, A.L. (2003). Reducing exposure to laboratory animal allergens. *Comparative Medicine*, Vol.53, No.5, (October 2003), pp. 487-492, ISSN 1532-0820

Shah, M.M., Miyamoto, Y., Yamada, Y., Yamashita, H., Tanaka, H., Ezaki, T., Nagai, H. & Inagaki, N. (2010). Orally supplemented *Lactobacillus acidophilus* strain L-92 inhibits passive and active cutaneous anaphylaxis as well as 2,4-dinitroflurobenzene and mite fecal antigen induced atopic dermatitis-like skin lesions in mice. *Microbiology and Immunology*, Vol.54, No.9, (September 2010), pp. 523-533, ISSN 0385-5600

Sung, Y.Y., Yoon, T., Jang, J.Y., Park, S.J., Jeong, G.H. & Kim, H.K. (2011a) Inhibitory effects of *Cinnamomum cassia* extract on atopic dermatitis-like skin lesions induced by mite antigen in NC/Nga mice. *Journal of Ethnopharmacology*, Vol.133, No. 2 (January 2010), pp. 621-628, ISSN 0378-8741

Sung, Y.Y., Yoon, T., Jang, J.Y., Park, S.J. & Kim, H.K. (2011b) Topical application of *Rehmannia glutinosa* extract inhibits mite allergen-induced atopic dermatitis in NC/Nga mice. *Journal of Ethnopharmacology*, Vol. 134, No. 1 (March 2010), pp.37-44, ISSN 0378-8741

Takada, T., Mita, A., Maeno, A., Sakai, T., Shitara, H., Kikkawa, Y., Moriwaki, K., Yonekawa, H. & Shiroishi, T. (2008a). Mouse inter-subspecific consomic strains for genetic dissection of quantitative complex traits. *Genome Research*, Vol.18, No.3, (March 2008), pp. 500-508, ISSN 1088-9051

Takada, T., Shitara, H., Matsuoka, K., Kojima, E., Ishii, R., Kikkawa, Y., Taya, C., Karasuyama, H., Kohno, K. & Yonekawa, H. (2008b). A novel hairless mouse model on an atopic dermatitis-prone genetic background generated by receptor-mediated transgenesis. *Transgenic Research*, Vol.17, No.6, (December 2008), pp. 1155-1162, ISSN 0962-8819

Takeda, K. & Gelfand, E.W. (2009). Mouse models of allergic diseases. *Current Opinion in Immunology*, Vol.21, No.6, (December 2009), pp. 660-665, ISSN 0952-7915

Tanaka, A. & Matsuda, H. (2011). Evaluation of itch by using NC/NgaTnd mice: a model of human atopic dermatitis. *Journal of Biomedicine & Biotechnology*, Vol.2011, (December 2010), 790436, ISSN 1110-7243

Taniguchi, Y., Kohno, K., Inoue, S., Koya-Miyata, S., Okamoto, I., Arai, N., Iwaki, K., Ikeda, M. & Kurimoto, M. (2003). Oral administration of royal jelly inhibits the development of atopic dermatitis-like skin lesions in NC/Nga mice. *International Immunopharmacology*, Vol.3, No.9, (September 2003), pp. 1313-1324, ISSN 1567-5769

Taylor, B., Wadsworth, J., Wadsworth, M. & Peckham, C. (1984) Changes in the reported prevalence of childhood eczema since the 1939-45 war. *Lancet*, Vol.2, No.8414, (December 1984), pp. 1255-1257, ISSN 0140-6736

Tomimori, Y., Muto, T., Fukami, H., Saito, K., Horikawa, C., Tsuruoka, N., Saito, M., Sugiura, N., Yamashiro, K., Sumida, M., Kakutani, S. & Fukuda, Y. (2002). Chymase participates in chronic dermatitis by inducing eosinophil infiltration. *Laboratory*

Investigation; a Journal of Technical Methods and Pathology, Vol. 82, No.6, (June 2002), pp. 789-794, ISSN 0023-6837

Tomimori, Y., Tanaka, Y., Goto, M. & Fukuda, Y. (2005). Repeated topical challenge with chemical antigen elicits sustained dermatitis in NC/Nga mice in specific-pathogen-free condition. *The Journal of Investigative Dermatology*, Vol.124, No.1, (January 2005), pp. 119-124, ISSN 0022-202X

Vercelli, D. (2009) Of flaky tails and itchy skin. *Nature Genetics*, Vol.41, No. 5, (May 2009), pp.512-513, ISSN 1061-4036.

Watanabe, A., Takeuchi, M., Nagata, M., Nakamura, K., Hirasawa, T., Nakao, H., Makino, S. & Harada, M. (2003a). Spontaneous development of dermatitis in DS-Nh mice under specific pathogen-free conditions. *Experimental Animals*, Vol.52, No.1, (January 2003), pp. 77-80, ISSN 1341-1357

Watanabe, A., Takeuchi, M., Nagata, M., Nakamura, K., Nakao, H., Yamashita, H., Makino, S., Harada, M. & Hirasawa, T. (2003b). Role of the Nh (Non-hair) mutation in the development of dermatitis and hyperproduction of IgE in DS-Nh mice. *Experimental Animals*, Vol. 52, No.5, (October 2003), pp. 419-423, ISSN 1341-1357

Watanabe, O., Natori, K., Tamari, M., Shiomoto, Y., Kubo, S. & Nakamura Y. (1999) Significantly elevated expression of PF4 (platelet factor 4) and eotaxin in the NOA mouse, a model for atopic dermatitis. *Journal of Human Genetics*, Vol.44, No.3, (January 1999), 173-176, ISSN 1434-5161

Watanabe, O., Tamari, M., Natori, K., Onouchi, Y., Shiomoto, Y., Hiraoka, I. & Nakamura, Y. (2001). Loci on murine chromosomes 7 and 13 that modify the phenotype of the NOA mouse, an animal model of atopic dermatitis. *Journal of Human Genetics*, Vol.46, No.4, (January 2001), pp. 221-224, ISSN 1434-5161

Wise, F. & Sulzberger, M.B. (1993). Footnote on problems of eczema, neurodermatitis and lichenification. In: *Year Book of Dermatology & Syphilology*, F., Wise & M.B., Sulzberger, (Ed(s).), pp. 38-39, Year Book Publishers, ISBN 0093-3627, Chicago

Wu, G., Li, L., Sung, G.H., Kim, T.W., Byeon, S.E., Cho, J.Y., Park, C.W. & Park, H.J. (2011) Inhibition of 2,4-dinitrofluorobenzene-induced atopic dermatitis by topical application of the butanol extract of *Cordyceps bassiana* in NC/Nga mice. *Journal of Ethnopharmacology*, Vol. 134, No. 2, (March 2010), pp.504-509, ISSN 0378-8741

Yamamoto, M., Haruna, T., Yasui, K., Takahashi, H., Iduhara, M., Takaki, S., Deguchi, M. & Arimura, A. (2007). A novel atopic dermatitis model induced by topical application with *Dermatophagoides farinae* extract in NC/Nga mice. *Allergology International*, Vol.56, No.2, (June 2007), pp. 139-148, ISSN 1323-8930

Yoshioka, T., Hikita, I., Asakawa, M., Hirasawa, T., Deguchi, M., Matsutani, T., Oku, H., Horikawa, T. & Arimura, A. (2006). Spontaneous scratching behaviour in DS-Nh mice as a possible model for pruritus in atopic dermatitis. *Immunology*, Vol. 118, No.3, (July 2006), pp. 293-301, ISSN 0019-2805

Yoshioka, T., Imura, K., Asakawa, M., Suzuki, M., Oshima, I., Hirasawa, T., Sakata, T., Horikawa, T. & Arimura, A. (2009). Impact of the Gly573Ser substitution in TRPV3 on the development of allergic and pruritic dermatitis in mice. *The Journal of Investigative Dermatology*, Vol.129, No.3, (March, 2009), pp. 714-722, ISSN 0022-202X

Yoshioka, T., Imura, K., Hikita, I., Hirasawa, T., Sakata, T., Matsutani, T., Horikawa, T. & Arimura, A. (2007). Impact of T-cell receptor Vbeta haplotypes on the development of dermatitis in DS-Nh mice: synergistic production of interleukin-13 caused by staphylococcal enterotoxin C and peptide glycans from *Staphylococcus aureus*. *Immunology*, vol. 121, No.1, (May 2007), pp 51-61, ISSN 0019-2805

2

Flaky Tail Mouse as a Novel Animal Model of Atopic Dermatitis: Possible Roles of Filaggrin in the Development of Atopic Dermatitis

Catharina Sagita Moniaga and Kenji Kabashima
Department of Dermatology, Kyoto University Graduate School of Medicine
Japan

1. Introduction

Understanding of human diseases has been enormously expanded by the use of animal models, because they allow for in-depth investigation of pathogenesis and provide invaluable tools for diagnostic and pharmaceutical purposes. Atopic dermatitis (AD) is a chronic, relapsing form of skin inflammation, a disturbance of epidermal-barrier function that culminates in dry skin, pruritus, and IgE-mediated sensitization to food and environmental allergens (Bieber, 2008, Mori, et al., 2010, Tokura, 2010). AD is a common disease with no satisfactory form of therapy; therefore, understanding the mechanism of AD through animal models is an urgent issue to be solved (Jin, et al., 2009, Matsuda, et al., 1997, Shiohara, et al., 2004). The complexity and variability of AD and multiple genetic and environmental factors underlying AD make creating a reproducible, accessible, and relevant animal model of AD particularly challenging (Scharschmidt &Segre, 2008).

Thus far, a number of mouse models have been developed. These models can be categorized into three groups: (1) models induced by epicutaneous application of sensitizers; (2) transgenic mice that either overexpress or lack selective molecules; and (3) mice that spontaneously develop AD-like skin lesions. These models display many features of human AD, and their studies have resulted in a better understanding of the pathogenesis of AD. They allow for an in-depth dissection of the mediators and cells that are critical for the development of allergic responses (Jin, et al., 2009).

Located at the interface between the body and the environment, the epidermis is an elaborate structure that shares few properties with other biological barriers. Key functions include providing physical and biochemical protection (O'Regan &Irvine, 2010), and playing important roles in host defense, inflammation, and regulation of immune responses (Schleimer, et al., 2007). Patients with AD exhibit impaired skin barrier functions and abnormal structure and chemistry of the stratum corneum (SC) (Leung &Bieber, 2003). Alteration of the skin barrier in AD is evidenced by reduction in the water content of the SC and by increased transepidermal water loss (TEWL) (Aioi, et al., 2001). Skin barrier dysfunction has emerged as a critical driving force in the initiation and exacerbation of AD and as "driver" of disease activity (Cork, et al., 2009, Elias, et al., 2008), although it has once been noted as a disease of immunological etiology (Leung &Bieber, 2003).

Elias et al. proposed the outside-to-inside pathogenic mechanisms in AD for the following reasons: (1) the extent of the permeability barrier abnormality parallels the severity of the disease phenotype in AD; (2) both the clinically uninvolved skin sites and the skin cleared of inflammation continue to display significant barrier abnormalities; (3) emollient therapy comprises effective ancillary therapy; and (4) specific replacement therapy which targets the prominent lipid abnormalities that account for barrier abnormality in AD, not only corrects the permeability-barrier abnormality but also comprises an effective anti-inflammatory therapy for AD (Elias, et al., 2008).

The evidence for a primary structural abnormality of the SC in AD is derived from a recently discovered link between the incidence of AD and loss-of-function mutations in the gene encoding filaggrin (*FLG*). Genetic studies have shown a strong association between AD and this mutation (Jin, et al., 2009). Moreover, there is a dose-response relationship between *FLG* deficiency and disease severity, such that patients with double-allele or compound heterozygote mutation in *FLG* display more severe and earlier-onset AD and an increased propensity for AD to persist into adulthood (Brown, et al., 2008, Irvine &McLean, 2006). This rapidly growing body of work has led to a paradigm shift in conception of AD pathogenesis, with increasing weight being placed on the role of a primary barrier abnormality that then precipitates downstream causing immunologic abnormalities as proposed (Elias, et al., 2008).

Based on these findings, it is assumed that mice that have a genetic defect in barrier function will provide a model of AD closer to the human disease than models provided by epidermal sensitization with allergens or haptens or by transgenic overexpression of cytokines in the skin or disruption of immune genes, and that these mice will have an advantage over NC/Nga mice in which the genetic defect is not known. Application of the knowledge gained from existing mouse models of AD to mice with genetic defects in skin barrier function should provide us with AD models that closely mimic human disease (Jin, et al., 2009).

2. Filaggrin and atopic dermatitis

2.1 Filaggrin mutation and atopic dermatitis

Filaggrin protein is localized in the granular layers of the epidermis. Profilaggrin, a 400-kDa polyprotein, is the main component of keratohyalin granules (Candi, et al., 2005, Listwan & Rothnagel, 2004). In the differentiation of keratinocytes, profilaggrin is dephosphorylated and cleaved into 10-12 essentially identical 27-kDa filaggrin molecules, which aggregates in the keratin cytoskeleton system to form a dense protein-lipid matrix in humans (Candi, et al., 2005). This structure is thought to prevent epidermal water loss and impede the entry of external stimuli, such as allergens, toxic chemicals, and infectious organisms. Therefore, filaggrin is a key protein in the terminal differentiation of the epidermis and in skin-barrier function (Gan, et al., 1990).

The genetic contribution of *FLG* loss-of-function mutations to AD is now well established. *FLG* mutation was first identified in ichthyosis vulgaris (IV), a common keratinizing disorder (Irvine &McLean, 2006). In 2006, Palmer et al. first identified two such mutations within the *FLG* gene, which strongly predispose to AD as well as IV (Palmer, et al., 2006). Since then, several additional studies have confirmed this association and discovered other mutations within this gene that predispose to AD. To date, approximately 40 loss-of-function *FLG* mutations have been identified in IV and/or AD in European and Asian populations. (Brown, et al., 2008, Marenholz, et al., 2006, Nomura, et al., 2007, Rodriguez, et al., 2009, Sandilands, et al., 2006, Sandilands, et al., 2007). Major differences exist in the spectra of *FLG* mutations observed between different ancestral groups, and each population is likely to have a unique set of *FLG* mutations (Osawa, et al., 2011).

Typically atopic manifestations follow a certain sequence, called the atopic march, beginning with AD in early infancy, followed by food allergy, asthma and the development of allergic rhinitis (Illi, et al., 2004). The association of *FLG* mutation with atopic march has been reported in cases involving pediatric asthma (Muller, et al., 2009), peanut allergy (Brown, et al., 2011), atopic asthma (Poninska, et al., 2011), allergic rhinitis (Poninska, et al., 2011) and nickel allergy (Novak, et al., 2008).

In addition, epidemiological studies have identified extremely significant statistical association between *FLG* mutation and AD. Intriguingly, these mutations are highly associated with several characteristics in AD patients, such as reduced level of natural moisturizing factor (NMF) in the SC (Kezic, et al., 2008), increased incidence of dry and sensitive skin (Sergeant, et al., 2009), clinical severity and barrier impairment (Nemoto-Hasebe, et al., 2009), allergen sensitization and subsequent development of asthma associated with eczema (Weidinger, et al., 2008), and serum levels of IgE (Wang, et al., 2011). On the other hand, several studies failed to identify an effect of *FLG* mutations on AD, such as skin conditions assessed by clinical scoring of AD and measurement of TEWL in a French population (Hubiche, et al., 2007). A similar lack of association was reported in contact allergy (Carlsen, et al., 2011) and pediatric eczema (O'Regan, et al., 2010).

As the conceptual framework underlying AD moves from solely immunological to epidermal barrier defects, the role of filaggrin and its putative mechanisms in priming AD have come under closer scrutiny. *FLG* mutations are postulated to have wide-ranging downstream biological effects, which include altered pH of SC, cutaneous microflora and aberrant innate and adaptive immune responses (O'Regan &Irvine, 2010).

2.2 Filaggrin and altered skin barrier function

AD is characterized by eczematous skin lesion, dry skin, pruritus, increased TEWL, and enhanced percutaneous penetration of both lipophilic and hydrophilic compounds (Jakasa, et al., 2011, Wollenberg &Bieber, 2000). The skin barrier defect is one of the primary events that initiate disease pathogenesis, allowing the entrance of numerous antigens into the epidermis in patients with AD (Onoue, et al., 2009, Osawa, et al., 2011). The *FLG* mutation carriers have demonstrated elevated TEWL (Jungersted, et al., 2010, Kezic, et al., 2008), basal erythema, skin hydration, increased skin pH (Jungersted, et al., 2010, Nemoto-Hasebe, et al., 2009), SC thickness (Nemoto-Hasebe, et al., 2009), impaired SC integrity upon repeated tape stripping (Angelova-Fischer, et al., 2011), and increased diffusivity of PEG 370 (Jakasa, et al., 2011) compared to healthy donors. Nevertheless, these alterations found in *FLG* mutation carriers are not consistently correlated with AD since AD patients without *FLG* mutation might also share some similar features. (Hubiche, et al., 2007, Jakasa, et al., 2011, Jungersted, et al., 2010, Kezic, et al., 2008). It is, therefore, suggested that other factors besides *FLG* loss-of-function mutations modulate skin barrier integrity, especially in AD.

Since the skin barrier is related to intercellular lipid bilayers of the SC, it might be interesting to examine the composition and the organization of intercellular lipids of the SC in AD patients in relation to *FLG* genotype and disease severity (Jakasa, et al., 2011). Carriers of *FLG* mutations showed significantly reduced levels of NMF in the SC (Kezic, et al., 2008). Similar lipid composition of *FLG* mutation carriers and individuals with normal filaggrin was observed (Angelova-Fischer, et al., 2011, Jungersted, et al., 2010), but a lower cermide/cholesterol ratio was detected in the former group (Angelova-Fischer, et al., 2011). Filaggrins proteolytically degraded into a pool of free amino acids including histidine and glutamine which are further converted to, respectively, urocanic acid (UCA) and 2-

pyrrolidone-5-carboxylic acid (PCA). The concentrations of UCA and PCA in SC in the carriers of *FLG* mutations were significantly lower than those in healthy donors (Kezic, et al., 2009). Therefore, filaggrin deficiency is sufficient to impair epidermal barrier formation.

An *in vitro* experiment using filaggrin knocked down human organotypic skin cultures showed enhanced penetration of hydrophilic dye Lucifer yellow, smaller lamellar bodies, and deficiency of their typical lamellae without altered lipid composition (Mildner, et al., 2010). In addition, UCA, one of the filaggrin-derived free amino acids and as an important UV absorbent within SC, was decreased following filaggrin knocked down, leading to increased sensitivity to UVB-induced keratinocyte (KC) damage (Mildner, et al., 2010).

2.3 Filaggrin and altered immunobiology

The SC serves as a biosensor of the external environment and a link between innate and adaptive immune systems (Vroling, et al., 2008). The critical association between the abnormal barrier in AD and Th2 polarization may in part be explained by the production of the cytokine, thymic stromal lymphopoietin (TSLP) (Ebner, et al., 2007). TSLP is expressed by epithelial cells, with the highest levels seen in lung-derived and skin-derived epithelial cells (Soumelis, et al., 2002, Ziegler, 2010), and is highly detected in the lesional skin of AD (Soumelis, et al., 2002) Inducible TSLP transgene specifically in the skin leads to the development of a spontaneous Th2-type skin inflammatory disease with the hallmark features of AD (Yoo, et al., 2005).

TSLP has been shown to activate dendritic cells to drive Th2 polarization, through upregulation of the co-stimulatory molecules CD40, CD80, and OX40L, triggering the differentiation of allergen-specific naïve $CD4^+$ T cells to Th2 cells that produce IL-4, IL-5, and IL-13 (Ebner, et al., 2007, Soumelis, et al., 2002).

Patients with Netherton syndrome (NS), a severe ichthyosis in which affected individuals experience a significant predisposition for AD, have elevated levels of TSLP in their skin. Upregulated kallikrein (KLK) 5 in the skin of NS patients directly activates proteinase-activated receptor 2 (PAR-2) and induces nuclear factor kappaB-mediated overexpression of TSLP, intercellular adhesion molecule 1, TNF-α, and IL-8. This phenomenon occurs independently of the environment, adaptive immune system and underlying epithelial barrier defect (Briot, et al., 2009, Briot, et al., 2010). *In vitro* study using human keratinocyte cell line HaCaT cells and reconstituted human epidermal layers transfected with filaggrin siRNA showed increased production of TSLP via toll-like receptor (TLR) 3 stimulation (Lee, et al., 2011). These findings suggest that reduced filaggrin levels may influence innate immune response via TLR stimuli and elevate TSLP, leading to AD-like skin lesions.

AD is one of the emerging diseases in which epidermal dysfunction increases allergen and microbial penetration in the skin, with the consequent development of adaptive Th2 immune responses (Kondo, et al., 1998) within regional lymphoid tissue. The resultant Th2 cells may then home back to the skin or lungs, where they recognize allergen in the skin (McPherson, et al., 2010), which leads to local Th2 inflammation, reduced antimicrobial peptide expression (Nomura, et al., 2003), and filaggrin downregulation (Howell, et al., 2007). Indeed, the induction of circulating allergen-specific $CD4^+$ T cells may be an important prerequisite underlying the pathogenesis of the atopic march (O'Regan, et al., 2009). Among moderate-to-severe AD patients, the *FLG* mutation carriers showed a greater number of house dust mite Der p1-specific IL-4 producing $CD4^+$ T cells, suggesting that filaggrin mutations predispose to the development of allergen-specific $CD4^+$ Th2 cells. The same result could be seen among HLA-DRB1*1501 (a HLA class II complex which is immunodominant in individuals with AD (Ardern-Jones, et al., 2007)) positive adult individuals with moderate-to-severe AD and *FLG* mutations (McPherson, et al., 2010).

3. Flaky tail mouse as a novel animal model of atopic dermatitis

3.1 Origin of flaky tail mice

The above findings indicate the involvement of filaggrin in the development of AD. Therefore, the impact of filaggrin deficiency on cutaneous biological functions *in vivo* should be analyzed in detail. To address this issue, animal models are of great value.

Flaky tail mice (Flg^{ft}), first introduced in 1958, are spontaneously mutated mice with smaller ears, tail constrictions, and a flaking tail skin appearance (Lane, 1972). Flg^{ft} mice were outcrossed onto B6 mice at Jackson Laboratory (Bar Harbor, ME, USA) (Lane, 1972, Presland, et al., 2000) (Note: Although this strain was crossed with B6, it is not a B6 congenic strain but rather a hybrid stock that is probably semi-inbred). Homozygous Flg^{ft} mice have dry, flaky skin which expresses reduced amounts of profilaggrin mRNA and abnormal profilaggrin protein that is not processed to filaggrin monomers (Fallon, et al., 2009, Presland, et al., 2000).

Recently, it has been revealed that the gene responsible for the characteristic phenotype of Flg^{ft} mice is a single nucleotide deletion at position 5303 in exon 3 (5303delA) of the profilaggrin gene, resulting in a frameshift mutation and premature truncation of the predicted protein product. The copy number of the filaggrin repeat contained within this gene varies depending on the background strain. This mutant occurs in an allele with 16 copies of the filaggrin repeat (Fallon, et al., 2009).

Flg^{ft} mouse carries double gene mutation, *Flg* and matted (*ma*) in which the locations of the mutated genes are within close linkage to one another (Lane, 1972). The *ma* gene characteristic reported by Searle & Spearman (1957) causes the body-hair of affected mice to be brittle and inflexible, which results in longitudinal splitting and breaking due to friction against the cage and other objects. This mutation is a fully penetrant recessive house-mouse mutant which belongs to the "naked" category (i.e., a house-mouse with baldness resulting from the breaking of hairs or from hereditary hairlessness). This mutation can be identified morphologically by (1) erection of hairs, (2) matting of hair in clumps, (3) a tendency towards baldness, (4) a change from black- to brown-colored melanin in old hairs. The age at which this mutant is first identified based on external appearance varies from between two to four weeks (Jarret A, 1957, Searle A.G., 1957).

Recognition of the features of this mouse is more evident between 5 and 14 days of age when constricted, flaking tail skin and thickened short pinna of the ears are observed. In addition, Flg^{ft} mice are often smaller than their normal siblings at this age. Routine histological sections stained with hematoxylin and eosin showed that the stratum granulosum in Flg^{ft} mice at 1, 2, 4, and 8 days of age does not contain as many granular layers as that of non-Flg^{ft} mice (Lane, 1972). Mice of the Flg^{ft} genotype express an abnormal profilaggrin polypeptide that does not form normal keratohyalin F-granules and is not proteolytically processed to filaggrin. Therefore, filaggrin is absent from the cornified layers in the epidermis of the Flg^{ft} mouse (Fallon, et al., 2009, Presland, et al., 2000, Scharschmidt, et al., 2009). Consistently, we and others have described that Flg^{ft} mice express a truncated and smaller profilaggrin protein that is not processed to filaggrin (Fallon, et al., 2009, Moniaga, et al., 2010, Presland, et al., 2000) (Fig.1).

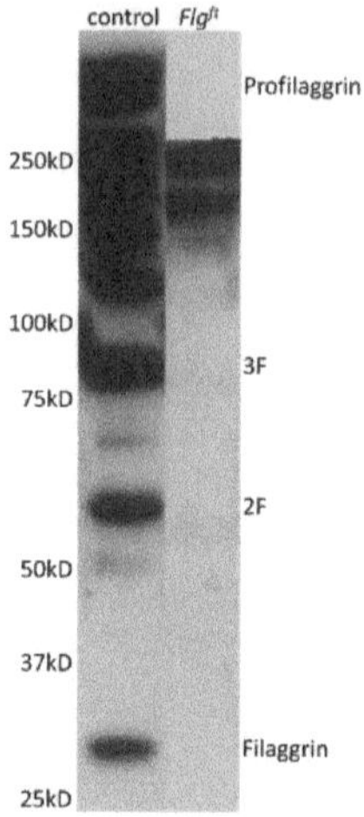

Fig. 1. *Flg^ft^* mouse has a truncated and smaller profilaggin and a lack of filaggrin protein.

3.2 Flaky tail mouse and ichtyosis vulgaris

Ichthyosis vulgaris (IV) is a heterogeneous autosomal skin disease characterized by dry and scaly skin, mild hyperkeratosis, and a decreased or absent granular layer that either lacks, or contains morphologically abnormal, keratohyalin granules (Manabe, et al., 1991). Several lines of evidences point to a genetic defect in a gene encoding *FLG* in IV. Immunoblotting studies showed that filaggrin protein was absent or markedly reduced in the epidermis of individuals with IV (Fleckman, et al., 1987, Sybert, et al., 1985). In line with this, it was proposed that *Flg^ft^* mice could provide insight into the molecular basis of the filaggrin-deficient human skin disorder IV. The epithelia of *Flg^ft^* mice showed defects in tissue organization especially in the tail, an attenuated granular layer, reduced profilaggrin and a lacked of filaggrin granules in SC. In addition, keratinocytes culture from *Flg^ft^* mice synthesized reduced amounts of profilaggrin mRNA and protein (Presland, et al., 2000).

3.3 Flaky tail mouse in a steady state

An early report demonstrated that *Flg^ft^* mice without the *ma* mutation showed flaky skin as early as postnatal day 2, but became normal in appearance by 3 to 4 weeks of age without spontaneous dermatitis except for their slightly smaller ears (Lane, 1972). Later, the lack of filaggrin in the epidermis was proposed in the commercially available strain of *Flg^ft^* mice, which has both *Flg* and *ma* mutations, as a model of IV, and therefore there was no discussion about the cutaneous inflammatory conditions from the perspective of AD (Presland, et al., 2000).

There have been four recent papers of *Flg^ft^* mice as a model of filaggrin deficiency: the first paper used *Flg^ft^* mice from which the *ma* mutation had been eliminated with four additional backcrosses to B6 mice (Fallon, et al., 2009), and the others used the commercially available *Flg^ft^* mice (Moniaga, et al., 2010, Oyoshi, et al., 2009, Scharschmidt, et al., 2009). The first report showed only histological abnormality without clinical manifestation (Fallon, et al., 2009), and the second demonstrated spontaneous eczematous skin lesions after 28 weeks of age (Oyoshi, et al., 2009), and the third contained no notice of any spontaneous dermatitis in Flg^{ft} mice (Scharschmidt, et al., 2009).

The fourth paper by Moniaga et al. have demonstrated that Flg^{ft} mice showed spontaneous dermatitis with skin lesions mimicking human AD as early as 5 weeks of age with mild erythema and fine scales and the cutaneous manifestations advanced with age in a steady state under SPF conditions (Moniaga, et al., 2010) (Fig. 2). The first manifestations to appear when mice were young were erythema and fine scaling; pruritic activity, erosion, and edema followed later (Fig. 3). In contrast, no cutaneous manifestation was observed in either C57BL/6 mice, studied as a control, or heterozygous mice intercrossed with Flg^{ft} and B6 mice kept under SPF conditions. There was no apparent difference in terms of clinical manifestations based on the gender of Flg^{ft} mice throughout the period (Moniaga, et al., 2010).

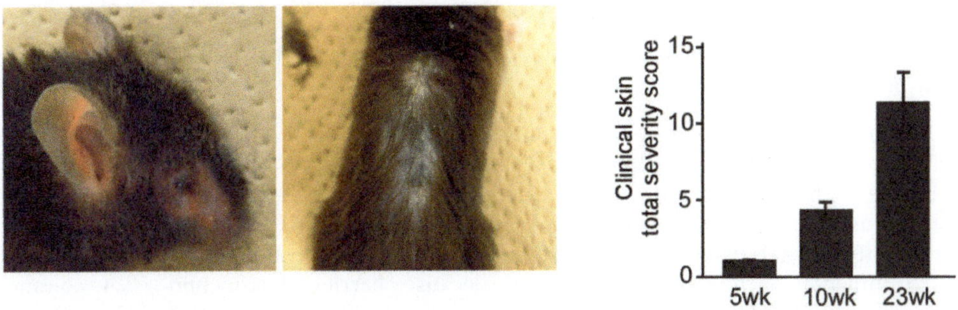

Fig. 2. Clinical photographs of 20-week-old Flg^{ft} mice (left panel) and total clinical severity scores (right panel)

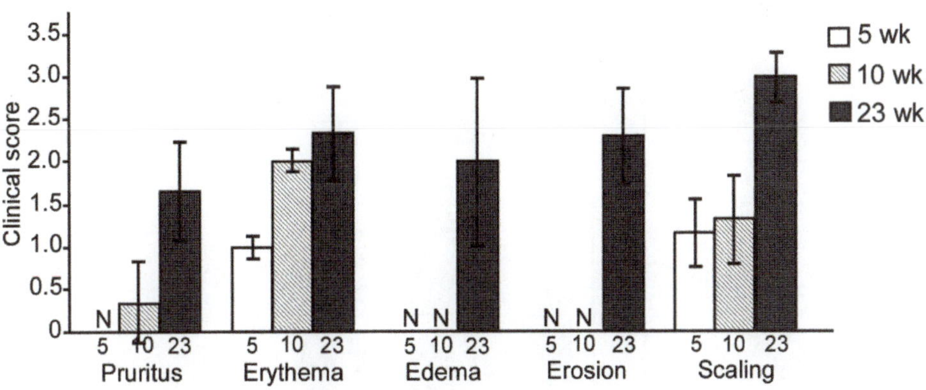

Fig. 3. Characteristics of the clinical skin lesions.

Histological examination of the skin of Flg^{ft} mice stained with H&E revealed epidermal acanthosis, increased lymphocyte and mast cell infiltration and dense fibrous bundles in the dermis, in both younger (8-week-old) and older (18-week-old) Flg^{ft} mice; none of these conditions were observed in B6 mice (Fig. 4) (Moniaga, et al., 2010). These features were also reported in other studies (Fallon, et al., 2009, Oyoshi, et al., 2009) with more total cells, lymphocytes, eosinophils, and mononuclear cells in Flg^{ft} mice compared to control mice. These data support the diagnosis of AD-like dermatitis in Flg^{ft} mice in the steady state under SPF conditions.

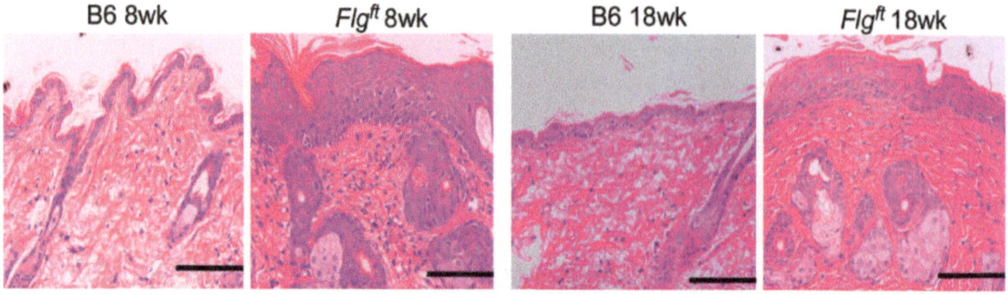

Fig. 4. Hematoxyllin and eosin (H&E)-stained sections in 8- and 18-week old mice. Scale bar, 100μm

Therefore, there exist discrepancies among the results of four recent papers on the cutaneous manifestation in the steady states. It seems to be related to the presence or absence of the *ma* mutation and/or variation in the genetic backgrounds of the different strains used, and to environmental factor. It has been reported that Japan carries a higher morbidity of AD than other countries (1998, Williams, et al., 1999), possibly due to environmental factors such as pollen. Because barrier dysfunction is a common characteristic of AD (Elias, et al., 2008, Nomura, et al., 2007, Palmer, et al., 2006), TEWL is commonly measured as an indicator of barrier function (Gupta, et al., 2008). TEWL was significantly higher in Flg^{ft} mice than in B6 mice from an early age (4 weeks) to an older age (16 weeks) (Fig. 5) (Moniaga, et al., 2010).

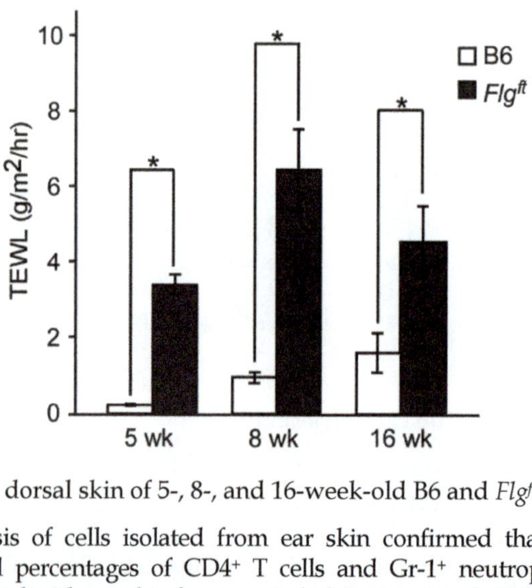

Fig. 5. TEWL through dorsal skin of 5-, 8-, and 16-week-old B6 and Flg^{ft} mice.

Flowcytometry analysis of cells isolated from ear skin confirmed that Flg^{ft} skin contained significantly increased percentages of $CD4^+$ T cells and Gr-1^+ neutrophils, but not $CD11c^+$ dendritic cells, compared with ear skin from controls (Moniaga, et al., 2010, Oyoshi, et al., 2009).

The extent of severity of AD is known to be correlated with elevated serum IgE levels (Novak, 2009). Serum IgE and IgG1 levels in *Flg^ft^* mice were significantly higher than those in control mice in the steady state under SPF conditions (Moniaga, et al., 2010, Oyoshi, et al., 2009). In addition, the numbers of $CD4^+$ and $CD8^+$ cells in the skin draining LNs in *Flg^ft^* mice were significantly higher than those in control mice, but those of the spleen were similar for both groups. Thus, an enhanced cutaneous immune reaction seems to be induced in *Flg^ft^* mice due to the condition of their skin induced by filaggrin and/or matted deficiency.

AD is thought to be mediated by helper T cell subsets, such as Th1, Th2, and Th17 (Bieber, 2008, Hattori, et al., 2010, Koga, et al., 2008). In the steady state, the skin of *Flg^ft^* mice showed no difference of Th1 cytokine IFN-γ and Th2 cytokines IL-4 and IL-13 compared to the control. In contrast, there is a significant increase in mRNA expression of the Th17 cytokine IL-17, IL-17 promoting cytokines IL-6 and IL-23 (p19), and IL-17 inducible neutrophil attractant chemokine CXCL2 in *Flg^ft^* mice (Moniaga, et al., 2010, Oyoshi, et al., 2009).

3.4 Flaky tail mouse showed enhanced percutaneous allergen priming

Since the barrier dysfunction is a key element in the establishment of AD, it is necessary to evaluate outside-to-inside barrier function from the perspective of invasion of external stimuli. Scharschmidt et al. reported increased bidirectional paracellular permeability of water-soluble xenobiotes by ultrastructural visualization in *Flg^ft^* mice suggesting a defect in the outside-to-inside barrier. The ultrastructural visualization of tracer perfusion was analyzed by water-soluble, low molecular weight, electron-dense tracer lanthanum nitrate or fluorophore calcium green with enhanced penetration in *Flg^ft^* mice. The data demonstrated that filaggrin deficiency leads to alterations in basal barrier function through a defect in the SC extracellular matrix and greater permeability through the same paracellular pathway that is used by water itself when exiting the skin (Scharschmidt, et al., 2009).

A new method for evaluating outside-to-inside barrier function quantitatively by measuring the penetrance of fluorescein isothiocyanate isomer 1 (FITC) through the skin has been developed (Moniaga, et al., 2010). The epidermis of *Flg^ft^* mice contained a higher amount of FITC than that of B6 mice did (Fig.6 left panel). Consistently, fluorescence intensities observation in the epidermis of both mice showed stronger fluorescence in *Flg^ft^* mice (Fig.6 right panel). In addition, the *Flg^ft^* embryo was entirely dye permeable to toluidine blue solution compared to its control littermate.

Another AD-like dermatitis model to test allergen priming of the skin in these mice was performed by application of ovalbumin (OVA) (Oyoshi, et al., 2009). Non tape-stripped skin of *Flg^ft^* mice exposed to OVA exhibited significantly increased epidermal thickening, hyperkeratosis, spongiosis, acanthosis, and cellular infiltrates, as well as TEWL compared to control mice. mRNA levels for IL-17, IL-6, IL-23, IL-4, IFN-γ and CXCL2 but not IL-5 and IL-13 in the skin of *Flg^ft^* mice after OVA exposure were significantly higher than those of control mice. The systemic immune response following cutaneous exposure revealed increased specific IgG and IgE to OVA, and splenocytes proliferated and produced OVA-specific Th1, Th2, Th17 and regulatory T cell cytokines (Fallon, et al., 2009, Oyoshi, et al., 2009). These findings demonstrate that *Flg^ft^* mice tend to generate allergen-specific IgE and cytokine following cutaneous allergen challenge to the skin even without additional barrier disruption.

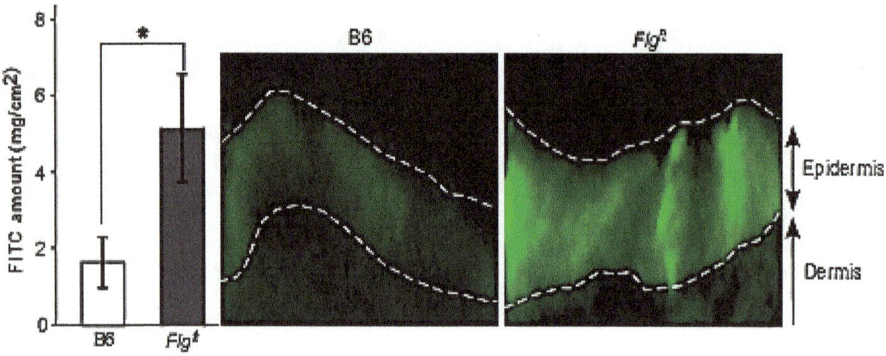

Fig. 6. Amount of FITC in the skin of B6 and *Flg^ft* mice (left panel) and fluorescence intensities of FITC of the skin (right panel) after topical application.

3.5 Altered immunobiology response in flaky tail mouse

The skin abnormality associated with AD is well known to be a predisposing factor to sensitive skin (Farage, et al., 2006, Willis, et al., 2001) and allergic contact dermatitis (Clayton, et al., 2006, Mailhol, et al., 2009). However, children with atopic dermatitis had lower PPD induration size compared to healthy donors, but this was not statistically significant (Gruber, et al., 2001, Yilmaz, et al., 2000). In humans, sensitive skin is defined as reduced tolerance to cutaneous stimulation, with symptoms ranging from visible signs of irritation to subjective neurosensory discomfort (Farage, et al., 2006, Willis, et al., 2001). The question of whether human AD patients are more prone to allergic contact dermatitis than nonatopic individuals is still controversial (Mailhol, et al., 2009).

Using phorbol myristate acetate (PMA) as an irritant, *Flg^ft* mice exhibited an enhanced ear swelling response compared to age-matched B6 mice throughout the experimental period (1 hr to 140 hrs). In addition, *Flg^ft* mice showed an increased skin-sensitized contact hypersensitivity (CHS) reaction to hapten, a form of classic Th1- and Tc1-mediated delayed-type hypersensitivity to haptens, emphasized by increased IFN-γ production, and terminated by regulatory T cells (Honda, et al., 2010, Mori, et al., 2008, Wang, et al., 2001). CHS is induced by epicutaneous sensitization and challenge. The ear thickness change was more prominent in *Flg^ft* mice than in B6 mice. In addition, the relative amount of IFN-γ in the ear of *Flg^ft* mice was higher than that of B6 mice.

To further assess the immune responses of *Flg^ft* mice, we elicited a delayed-type hypersensitivity (DTH) response through non-epicutaneous sensitization and challenge. Mice were immunized intraperitoneally with OVA, and challenged with a subcutaneous injection of OVA into the footpad. In contrast to the CHS response induced epicutaneously, the resulting footpad swelling in *Flg^ft* mice tended to be lower than that in wild-type mice. This finding is consistent with the observation on tuberculin tests in human. The levels of IFN-γ in the spleen were comparable between *Flg^ft* mice and wild-type mice. Thus, Th1/Tc1 immune responses were enhanced in *Flg^ft* mice only when the stimuli operated via the skin, suggesting that the enhanced immune responses seen in *Flg^ft* mice depend on skin barrier dysfunction and skin barrier function regulates cutaneous immune conditions, which hints at a possible mechanism involved in human AD.

A reduced threshold in *Flg^ft* mice for contact dermatitis was also reported. These mice showed enhanced propensity to irritant contact dermatitis via low-dose phorbol ester TPA which provokes only marginal inflammation in wild-type mice, and displayed a reduced threshold for the development of hapten-induced acute allergic contact dermatitis by oxazolone (Ox). Repeated Ox challenges with lower doses of Ox revealed AD-like dermatitis in *Flg^ft^* mice as shown by severe barrier abnormality (enhanced TEWL) and AD-like histological changes (Scharschmidt, et al., 2009).

3.6 Flaky tail mouse denotes human AD

Clinical studies have provided evidence that a house dust mite allergen plays a causative or exacerbating role in human AD (Kimura, et al., 1998), and that a strong correlation exists between *FLG* mutation patients and house dust mite-specific IgE (Henderson, et al., 2008). *Dermatophagoides pteronyssinus* (Dp) is a common mite aeroallergen, which is frequently involved in inducing human AD. Dp exhibits protease activities, and Der p1, Der p3, and Der p9, derived from Dp, are especially capable of activating the PAR-2 in human KC (Jeong, et al., 2008, Vasilopoulos, et al., 2007). A recent report has shown that activation of PAR-2 through Dp application significantly delays barrier recovery rate in barrier function-perturbed skin or otherwise compromised skin (Jeong, et al., 2008). Therefore, Dp may play a dual role in the onset of AD, both as an allergen and proteolytic signal and as a perturbation factor of the barrier function, leading to the persistence of eczematous skin lesions in AD (Jeong, et al., 2008, Roelandt, et al., 2008). It has also been reported that BALB/c and NC/Nga mice develop an allergic cutaneous immune response to mite antigens when they are applied to the skin after vigorous barrier disruption by means of tape-stripping or sodium dodecyl sulfate treatment (Kang, et al., 2006, Yamamoto, et al., 2007). Intriguingly, the application of Dp ointment to the skin without additional barrier disrupt induced dermatitis in *Flg^ft^* mice, while this treatment did not induce any skin inflammation in control C57BL/6 mice (Fig.7). Petrolatum alone, used instead of Dp ointment as a control, induced no skin manifestation (Fig. 7).

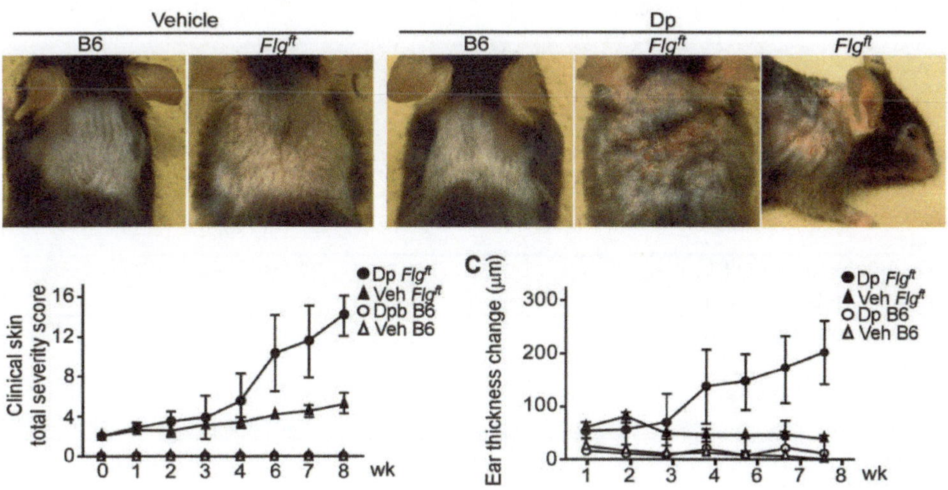

Fig. 7. The mite-induced dermatitis model showed severe eczematous skin lesion after being topically treated with Dp ointment in *Flg^ft^* mice, as well as ear thickness change.

Histological examination of H&E-stained sections of involved *Flg^ft^* skin after 16 applications showed acanthosis, elongation of rete ridges, and dense lymphocyte and neutrophil infiltration in the dermis, accompanied by an increased number of mast cells in the dermis. Consistently, scratching behavior, TEWL, and Dp-specific IgE levels were significantly higher in *Flg^ft^* mice than in B6 mice (Fig.8) (Moniaga, et al., 2010). Thus the treatment of *Flg^ft^* mice with Dp ointment, even without prior barrier disruption, remarkably enhanced both the clinical manifestations and the laboratory findings that correspond to indicators of human AD.

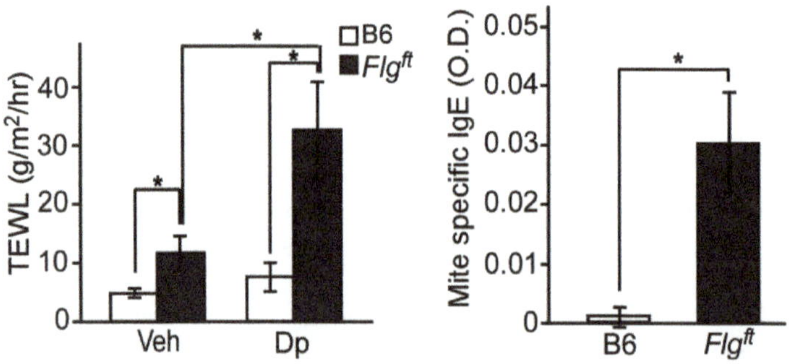

Fig. 8. TEWL and mite-specific serum IgE levels of *Flg^ft^* mice and control mice after the last application.

4. Summary and future direction

We have summarized the findings on *Flg^ft^* mice revealed by four different groups (Table 1). While most of these findings were consistent with each other, there still remain several issues to be solved, for example, the influence of the genetic background and other gene mutations in these mice.

	Fallon et al. (Fallon, et al., 2009)	Oyoshi et al. (Oyoshi, et al., 2009)	Scharschmidt et al. (Scharschmidt, et al., 2009)	Moniaga et al. (Moniaga, et al., 2010)
Spontaneous AD	-	+	n.r.	+
Increased TEWL in steady state	slightly	n.r.	+ (old age)	+
Histopathology AD like skin lesion in steady state	+	+	n.r.	+
Increase total IgE in steady state	n.r.	+	+	+
Enhanced cutaneous antigen ingress	+ (OVA)	+ (OVA)	+ (low dose oxaxolone)	+ (mite, D.p.)
Enhanced non cutaneous antigen (OVA-i.p) response	-	-	n.r	-

Table 1. Summary of the phenotypes of flaky tail mice

Since Flg^{ft} mice are not a homogenous C57BL/6 background, two papers with spontaneous eczematous skin lesion on Flg^{ft} mice compared their outcomes with other mouse strains, such as C57BL6 and BALB/c mice as controls (Oyoshi, et al., 2009); these two strains lie on opposite ends of the spectrum of T helper responses. Nevertheless, the skin inflammation and susceptibility to EC sensitization of non-tape stripped skin observed in Flg^{ft} mice were not observed in other strains. In the second paper, they observed immune responses in mice of other genotypes, such as BALB/c and C3H, as controls, but both of these lines exhibited much less severe CHS responses compared to Flg^{ft} mice (Moniaga, et al., 2010). These data suggested that the enhanced responses seen in Flg^{ft} mice were not solely due to their genetic background. In addition, other studies used the Flg^{ft} mice which were backcrossed four generations to a B6 strain (a background coding sequence showed 99.3% identity between B6 and Flg^{ft}), and similar enhanced responses to OVA-induced AD models were observed (Fallon, et al., 2009).
Furthermore, unlike human AD patients, most of whom are heterozygous for the *FLG* mutation, the heterozygous mice intercrossed with Flg^{ft} mice and B6 mice did not develop spontaneous dermatitis (Moniaga, et al., 2010). Similar results were obtained with the OVA-induced AD model, where homozygous, but not heterozygous (crossed with B6 mice) Flg^{ft} mice, showed enhanced susceptibility to cutaneous exposure to OVA (Fallon, et al., 2009). Not only human studies but also additional mouse studies will be required to clarify these relationships.
Since Flg^{ft} mice express a hair phenotype (matted), one cannot eliminate the possibility that some of the observations could have been influenced by the concurrent *ma* mutation (Scharschmidt, et al., 2009). Nevertheless, one study indeed removed the matted hair allele (*ma*) early in the course of backcrossing with B6 mice, and showed enhanced antigen (OVA) ingress in mice with the same *Flg* mutation, but no *ma* mutation in their background (Fallon, et al., 2009). The effect of the *ma* mutation in relation to the *Flg* mutation in commercially available Flg^{ft} mice in the development of AD-like skin lesions needs to be clarified in future studies.

5. References

(1998). Worldwide variation in prevalence of symptoms of asthma, allergic rhinoconjunctivitis, and atopic eczema: ISAAC. The International Study of Asthma and Allergies in Childhood (ISAAC) Steering Committee. *Lancet,* 351, 9111, (Apr 25), 1225-1232

Aioi, A., et al. (2001). Impairment of skin barrier function in NC/Nga Tnd mice as a possible model for atopic dermatitis. *Br J Dermatol,* 144, 1, (Jan), 12-18

Angelova-Fischer, I., et al. (2011). Distinct barrier integrity phenotypes in filaggrin-related atopic eczema following sequential tape stripping and lipid profiling. *Exp Dermatol,* 20, 4, (Apr), 351-356

Ardern-Jones, M. R., et al. (2007). Bacterial superantigen facilitates epithelial presentation of allergen to T helper 2 cells. *Proc Natl Acad Sci U S A,* 104, 13, (Mar 27), 5557-5562

Bieber, T. (2008). Atopic dermatitis. *N Engl J Med,* 358, 14, (Apr 3), 1483-1494

Briot, A., et al. (2009). Kallikrein 5 induces atopic dermatitis-like lesions through PAR2-mediated thymic stromal lymphopoietin expression in Netherton syndrome. *J Exp Med,* 206, 5, (May 11), 1135-1147

Briot, A., et al. (2010). Par2 inactivation inhibits early production of TSLP, but not cutaneous inflammation, in Netherton syndrome adult mouse model. *J Invest Dermatol,* 130, 12, (Dec), 2736-2742

Brown, S. J., et al. (2011). Loss-of-function variants in the filaggrin gene are a significant risk factor for peanut allergy. *J Allergy Clin Immunol,* 127, 3, (Mar), 661-667

Brown, S. J., et al. (2008). Filaggrin null mutations and childhood atopic eczema: a population-based case-control study. *J Allergy Clin Immunol,* 121, 4, (Apr), 940-946 e943

Brown, S. J., et al. (2008). Prevalent and low-frequency null mutations in the filaggrin gene are associated with early-onset and persistent atopic eczema. *J Invest Dermatol,* 128, 6, (Jun), 1591-1594

Candi, E., et al. (2005). The cornified envelope: a model of cell death in the skin. *Nat Rev Mol Cell Biol,* 6, 4, (Apr), 328-340

Carlsen, B. C., et al. (2011). Association between filaggrin null mutations and concomitant atopic dermatitis and contact allergy. *Clin Exp Dermatol,* (Mar 11),

Clayton, T. H., et al. (2006). Allergic contact dermatitis in children: should pattern of dermatitis determine referral? A retrospective study of 500 children tested between 1995 and 2004 in one U.K. centre. *Br J Dermatol,* 154, 1, (Jan), 114-117

Cork, M. J., et al. (2009). Epidermal barrier dysfunction in atopic dermatitis. *J Invest Dermatol,* 129, 8, (Aug), 1892-1908

Ebner, S., et al. (2007). Thymic stromal lymphopoietin converts human epidermal Langerhans cells into antigen-presenting cells that induce proallergic T cells. *J Allergy Clin Immunol,* 119, 4, (Apr), 982-990

Elias, P. M., et al. (2008). Basis for the barrier abnormality in atopic dermatitis: outside-inside-outside pathogenic mechanisms. *J Allergy Clin Immunol,* 121, 6, (Jun), 1337-1343

Fallon, P. G., et al. (2009). A homozygous frameshift mutation in the mouse Flg gene facilitates enhanced percutaneous allergen priming. *Nat Genet,* 41, 5, (May), 602-608

Farage, M. A., et al. (2006). Sensory, clinical and physiological factors in sensitive skin: a review. *Contact Dermatitis,* 55, 1, (Jul), 1-14

Fleckman, P., et al. (1987). Keratinocytes cultured from subjects with ichthyosis vulgaris are phenotypically abnormal. *J Invest Dermatol,* 88, 5, (May), 640-645

Gan, S. Q., et al. (1990). Organization, structure, and polymorphisms of the human profilaggrin gene. *Biochemistry,* 29, 40, (Oct 9), 9432-9440

Gruber, C., et al. (2001). Delayed hypersensitivity to tuberculin, total immunoglobulin E, specific sensitization, and atopic manifestation in longitudinally followed early Bacille Calmette-Guerin-vaccinated and nonvaccinated children. *Pediatrics,* 107, 3, (Mar), E36

Gupta, J., et al. (2008). Intrinsically defective skin barrier function in children with atopic dermatitis correlates with disease severity. *J Allergy Clin Immunol,* 121, 3, (Mar), 725-730 e722

Hattori, K., et al. (2010). Sustained exogenous expression of therapeutic levels of IFN-gamma ameliorates atopic dermatitis in NC/Nga mice via Th1 polarization. *J Immunol,* 184, 5, (Mar 1), 2729-2735

Henderson, J., et al. (2008). The burden of disease associated with filaggrin mutations: a population-based, longitudinal birth cohort study. *J Allergy Clin Immunol,* 121, 4, (Apr), 872-877 e879

Honda, T., et al. (2010). The role of regulatory T cells in contact hypersensitivity. *Recent Pat Inflamm Allergy Drug Discov,* 4, 2, 85-89

Howell, M. D., et al. (2007). Cytokine modulation of atopic dermatitis filaggrin skin expression. *J Allergy Clin Immunol,* 120, 1, (Jul), 150-155

Hubiche, T., et al. (2007). Analysis of SPINK 5, KLK 7 and FLG genotypes in a French atopic dermatitis cohort. *Acta Derm Venereol,* 87, 6, 499-505

Illi, S., et al. (2004). The natural course of atopic dermatitis from birth to age 7 years and the association with asthma. *J Allergy Clin Immunol,* 113, 5, (May), 925-931

Irvine, A. D. &McLean, W. H. (2006). Breaking the (un)sound barrier: filaggrin is a major gene for atopic dermatitis. *J Invest Dermatol,* 126, 6, (Jun), 1200-1202

Jakasa, I., et al. (2011). Skin barrier function in healthy subjects and patients with atopic dermatitis in relation to filaggrin loss-of-function mutations. *J Invest Dermatol,* 131, 2, (Feb), 540-542

Jarret A, S. R. I. (1957). The keratin defect and hair-cycle of a new mutant (atted) in the house-mouse. *J.Embryol.exp.Morph.,* 5, 103-110

Jeong, S. K., et al. (2008). Mite and cockroach allergens activate protease-activated receptor 2 and delay epidermal permeability barrier recovery. *J Invest Dermatol,* 128, 8, (Aug), 1930-1939

Jin, H., et al. (2009). Animal models of atopic dermatitis. *J Invest Dermatol,* 129, 1, (Jan), 31-40

Jungersted, J. M., et al. (2010). Stratum corneum lipids, skin barrier function and filaggrin mutations in patients with atopic eczema. *Allergy,* 65, 7, (Jul), 911-918

Kang, J. S., et al. (2006). Induction of atopic eczema/dermatitis syndrome-like skin lesions by repeated topical application of a crude extract of Dermatophagoides pteronyssinus in NC/Nga mice. *Int Immunopharmacol,* 6, 10, (Oct), 1616-1622

Kezic, S., et al. (2009). Natural moisturizing factor components in the stratum corneum as biomarkers of filaggrin genotype: evaluation of minimally invasive methods. *Br J Dermatol,* 161, 5, (Nov), 1098-1104

Kezic, S., et al. (2008). Loss-of-function mutations in the filaggrin gene lead to reduced level of natural moisturizing factor in the stratum corneum. *J Invest Dermatol,* 128, 8, (Aug), 2117-2119

Kimura, M., et al. (1998). Correlation of house dust mite-specific lymphocyte proliferation with IL-5 production, eosinophilia, and the severity of symptoms in infants with atopic dermatitis. *J Allergy Clin Immunol,* 101, 1 Pt 1, (Jan), 84-89

Koga, C., et al. (2008). Possible pathogenic role of Th17 cells for atopic dermatitis. *J Invest Dermatol,* 128, 11, (Nov), 2625-2630

Kondo, H., et al. (1998). Percutaneous sensitization with allergens through barrier-disrupted skin elicits a Th2-dominant cytokine response. *Eur J Immunol,* 28, 3, (Mar), 769-779

Lane, P. W. (1972). Two new mutations in linkage group XVI of the house mouse. Flaky tail and varitint-waddler-J. *J Hered,* 63, 3, (May-Jun), 135-140

Lee, K. H., et al. (2011). Filaggrin knockdown and Toll-like receptor 3 (TLR3) stimulation enhanced the production of thymic stromal lymphopoietin (TSLP) from epidermal layers. *Exp Dermatol,* 20, 2, (Feb), 149-151

Leung, D. Y. &Bieber, T. (2003). Atopic dermatitis. *Lancet,* 361, 9352, (Jan 11), 151-160

Listwan, P. &Rothnagel, J. A. (2004). Keratin bundling proteins. *Methods Cell Biol,* 78, 817-827

Mailhol, C., et al. (2009). Prevalence and risk factors for allergic contact dermatitis to topical treatment in atopic dermatitis: a study in 641 children. *Allergy,* 64, 5, (May), 801-806

Manabe, M., et al. (1991). Interaction of filaggrin with keratin filaments during advanced stages of normal human epidermal differentiation and in ichthyosis vulgaris. *Differentiation,* 48, 1, (Sep), 43-50

Marenholz, I., et al. (2006). Filaggrin loss-of-function mutations predispose to phenotypes involved in the atopic march. *J Allergy Clin Immunol,* 118, 4, (Oct), 866-871

Matsuda, H., et al. (1997). Development of atopic dermatitis-like skin lesion with IgE hyperproduction in NC/Nga mice. *Int Immunol,* 9, 3, (Mar), 461-466

McPherson, T., et al. (2010). Frequencies of circulating allergen-specific T cells temporally associate with longitudinal changes in severity of cutaneous atopic disease. *Clin Exp Dermatol,* 35, 7, (Oct), 786-788

McPherson, T., et al. (2010). Filaggrin null mutations associate with increased frequencies of allergen-specific CD4+ T-helper 2 cells in patients with atopic eczema. *Br J Dermatol,* 163, 3, (Sep), 544-549

Mildner, M., et al. (2010). Knockdown of filaggrin impairs diffusion barrier function and increases UV sensitivity in a human skin model. *J Invest Dermatol,* 130, 9, (Sep), 2286-2294

Moniaga, C. S., et al. (2010). Flaky tail mouse denotes human atopic dermatitis in the steady state and by topical application with Dermatophagoides pteronyssinus extract. *Am J Pathol,* 176, 5, (May), 2385-2393

Mori, T., et al. (2010). Comparison of skin barrier function and sensory nerve electric current perception threshold between IgE-high extrinsic and IgE-normal intrinsic types of atopic dermatitis. *Br J Dermatol,* 162, 1, (Jan), 83-90

Mori, T., et al. (2008). Cutaneous hypersensitivities to hapten are controlled by IFN-gamma-upregulated keratinocyte Th1 chemokines and IFN-gamma-downregulated langerhans cell Th2 chemokines. *J Invest Dermatol,* 128, 7, (Jul), 1719-1727

Muller, S., et al. (2009). Association of Filaggrin loss-of-function-mutations with atopic dermatitis and asthma in the Early Treatment of the Atopic Child (ETAC) population. *Pediatr Allergy Immunol,* 20, 4, (Jun), 358-361

Nemoto-Hasebe, I., et al. (2009). Clinical severity correlates with impaired barrier in filaggrin-related eczema. *J Invest Dermatol,* 129, 3, (Mar), 682-689

Nomura, I., et al. (2003). Cytokine milieu of atopic dermatitis, as compared to psoriasis, skin prevents induction of innate immune response genes. *J Immunol,* 171, 6, (Sep 15), 3262-3269

Nomura, T., et al. (2007). Unique mutations in the filaggrin gene in Japanese patients with ichthyosis vulgaris and atopic dermatitis. *J Allergy Clin Immunol,* 119, 2, (Feb), 434-440

Novak, N. (2009). New insights into the mechanism and management of allergic diseases: atopic dermatitis. *Allergy,* 64, 2, (Feb), 265-275

Novak, N., et al. (2008). Loss-of-function mutations in the filaggrin gene and allergic contact sensitization to nickel. *J Invest Dermatol,* 128, 6, (Jun), 1430-1435

O'Regan, G. M., et al. (2010). Chromosome 11q13.5 variant associated with childhood eczema: an effect supplementary to filaggrin mutations. *J Allergy Clin Immunol,* 125, 1, (Jan), 170-174 e171-172

O'Regan, G. M. &Irvine, A. D. (2010). The role of filaggrin in the atopic diathesis. *Clin Exp Allergy,* 40, 7, (Jul), 965-972

O'Regan, G. M., et al. (2009). Filaggrin in atopic dermatitis. *J Allergy Clin Immunol,* 124, 3 Suppl 2, (Sep), R2-6

Onoue, A., et al. (2009). Induction of eosinophil- and Th2-attracting epidermal chemokines and cutaneous late-phase reaction in tape-stripped skin. *Exp Dermatol,* (Jun 23),

Osawa, R., et al. (2011). Filaggrin gene defects and the risk of developing allergic disorders. *Allergol Int,* 60, 1, (Mar), 1-9

Oyoshi, M. K., et al. (2009). Filaggrin-deficient mice exhibit TH17-dominated skin inflammation and permissiveness to epicutaneous sensitization with protein antigen. *J Allergy Clin Immunol,* 124, 3, (Sep), 485-493, 493 e481

Palmer, C. N., et al. (2006). Common loss-of-function variants of the epidermal barrier protein filaggrin are a major predisposing factor for atopic dermatitis. *Nat Genet,* 38, 4, (Apr), 441-446

Poninska, J., et al. (2011). Filaggrin gene defects are independent risk factors for atopic asthma in a Polish population: a study in ECAP cohort. *PLoS One,* 6, 2, e16933

Presland, R. B., et al. (2000). Loss of normal profilaggrin and filaggrin in flaky tail (ft/ft) mice: an animal model for the filaggrin-deficient skin disease ichthyosis vulgaris. *J Invest Dermatol,* 115, 6, (Dec), 1072-1081

Rodriguez, E., et al. (2009). Meta-analysis of filaggrin polymorphisms in eczema and asthma: robust risk factors in atopic disease. *J Allergy Clin Immunol,* 123, 6, (Jun), 1361-1370 e1367

Roelandt, T., et al. (2008). Proteolytically active allergens cause barrier breakdown. *J Invest Dermatol,* 128, 8, (Aug), 1878-1880

Sandilands, A., et al. (2006). Prevalent and rare mutations in the gene encoding filaggrin cause ichthyosis vulgaris and predispose individuals to atopic dermatitis. *J Invest Dermatol,* 126, 8, (Aug), 1770-1775

Sandilands, A., et al. (2007). Comprehensive analysis of the gene encoding filaggrin uncovers prevalent and rare mutations in ichthyosis vulgaris and atopic eczema. *Nat Genet,* 39, 5, (May), 650-654

Scharschmidt, T. C., et al. (2009). Filaggrin deficiency confers a paracellular barrier abnormality that reduces inflammatory thresholds to irritants and haptens. *J Allergy Clin Immunol,* 124, 3, (Sep), 496-506, 506 e491-496

Scharschmidt, T. C. &Segre, J. A. (2008). Modeling atopic dermatitis with increasingly complex mouse models. *J Invest Dermatol,* 128, 5, (May), 1061-1064

Schleimer, R. P., et al. (2007). Epithelium: at the interface of innate and adaptive immune responses. *J Allergy Clin Immunol,* 120, 6, (Dec), 1279-1284

Searle A.G., S. R. I. (1957). `Matted`, a new hair-mutant in the house-mouse: Genetics and morphology. *J.Embryol.exp.Morph.,* 5, 93-102

Sergeant, A., et al. (2009). Heterozygous null alleles in filaggrin contribute to clinical dry skin in young adults and the elderly. *J Invest Dermatol,* 129, 4, (Apr), 1042-1045

Shiohara, T., et al. (2004). Animal models for atopic dermatitis: are they relevant to human disease? *J Dermatol Sci,* 36, 1, (Oct), 1-9

Soumelis, V., et al. (2002). Human epithelial cells trigger dendritic cell mediated allergic inflammation by producing TSLP. *Nat Immunol,* 3, 7, (Jul), 673-680

Sybert, V. P., et al. (1985). Ichthyosis vulgaris: identification of a defect in synthesis of filaggrin correlated with an absence of keratohyaline granules. *J Invest Dermatol,* 84, 3, (Mar), 191-194

Tokura, Y. (2010). Extrinsic and intrinsic types of atopic dermatitis. *J Dermatol Sci,* 58, 1, (Apr), 1-7

Vasilopoulos, Y., et al. (2007). A nonsynonymous substitution of cystatin A, a cysteine protease inhibitor of house dust mite protease, leads to decreased mRNA stability and shows a significant association with atopic dermatitis. *Allergy,* 62, 5, (May), 514-519

Vroling, A. B., et al. (2008). How epithelial cells detect danger: aiding the immune response. *Allergy,* 63, 9, (Sep), 1110-1123

Wang, B., et al. (2001). Insights into molecular mechanisms of contact hypersensitivity gained from gene knockout studies. *J Leukoc Biol,* 70, 2, (Aug), 185-191

Wang, I. J., et al. (2011). Filaggrin polymorphism P478S, IgE level, and atopic phenotypes. *Br J Dermatol,* 164, 4, (Apr), 791-796

Weidinger, S., et al. (2008). Filaggrin mutations, atopic eczema, hay fever, and asthma in children. *J Allergy Clin Immunol,* 121, 5, (May), 1203-1209 e1201

Williams, H., et al. (1999). Worldwide variations in the prevalence of symptoms of atopic eczema in the International Study of Asthma and Allergies in Childhood. *J Allergy Clin Immunol,* 103, 1 Pt 1, (Jan), 125-138

Willis, C. M., et al. (2001). Sensitive skin: an epidemiological study. *Br J Dermatol,* 145, 2, (Aug), 258-263

Wollenberg, A. &Bieber, T. (2000). Atopic dermatitis: from the genes to skin lesions. *Allergy,* 55, 3, (Mar), 205-213

Yamamoto, M., et al. (2007). A novel atopic dermatitis model induced by topical application with dermatophagoides farinae extract in NC/Nga mice. *Allergol Int,* 56, 2, (Jun), 139-148

Yilmaz, M., et al. (2000). Correlation between atopic diseases and tuberculin responses. *Allergy,* 55, 7, (Jul), 664-667

Yoo, J., et al. (2005). Spontaneous atopic dermatitis in mice expressing an inducible thymic stromal lymphopoietin transgene specifically in the skin. *J Exp Med,* 202, 4, (Aug 15), 541-549

Ziegler, S. F. (2010). The role of thymic stromal lymphopoietin (TSLP) in allergic disorders. *Curr Opin Immunol,* 22, 6, (Dec), 795-799

3

Epidermal Serine Proteases and Their Inhibitors in Atopic Dermatitis

Ulf Meyer-Hoffert
University Hospital Schleswig-Holstein, Campus Kiel
Department Dermatology
Germany

1. Introduction

The skin and its appendages protect the body from water loss, chemical and physical damages, UV-radiation and infection by pathogenic as well as non-pathogenic microbes. The protective function of both, the physical and the chemical barrier, is provided from epidermal keratinocytes, which are continuously dividing in the *stratum basale* and differentiating towards the surface (Candi et al. 2005). Cells of the uppermost living epidermis layer, the stratum granulosum, are loosing their nuclei and other organelles at the transition zone to the stratum corneum (SC), forming now flattened polyhedrons, called corneocytes. These corneocytes contain instead of a cell membrane the cornified envelope (CE) consisting of structural proteins, which are crosslinked by glutaminases (Candi et al. 2005). The intercellular space of the corneocytes is filled with lamellar body-derived lipids, which make the SC more hydrophobous. This mechanism protects skin from water loss and other insults.

Finally, in a tightly regulated process termed desquamation that abolishes the cohesion between corneocytes, these cells are shed into the environment by proteolysis of corneodesmosomal proteins. The formation of stratified epithelia requires a specific differentiation program, which includes a timely and spatially well coordinated proteolytic system to detach the corneocytes from each other without any disturbance of the barrier function. During the last years it became evident that this proteolytic balance is not only important for the physical barrier function of the skin but is also paving the way for immunological responses. In this chapter we want to look at the various proteases in the epidermis, their inhibitors and how they might contribute to the pathogenesis of atopic dermatitis (AD).

2. Proteases

A number of different proteases and their inhibitors have been involved in the desquamation process and to contribute to the skin's barrier function. On the basis of the catalytic domain, proteases are classified into aspartate-, cysteine-, glutamate-, metallo-, serine- and threonine proteases. Particularly serine proteases (SP) have a prominent role in epidermal permeability barrier homeostasis, as acute barrier disruption increases SP-activity in skin and inhibition by topical SP-inhibitors accelerated recovery of barrier function after acute abrogation (Hachem et al. 2006).

2.1 Cysteine- and aspartate-proteases

Cysteine peptidases represent phylogenetically ubiquitous enzymes, which can be classified into clans of independent proteins (based on the structural organization of the active site). Two of the major clans in mammal genomes are the "CA" clan, where members share an evolutionary and structural history with papain, and the "CB" clan, which includes the caspases and the legumains.

One of the most skin-relevant caspases is the cysteinyl-aspartate protease caspase-14 (Demerjian et al. 2008). In contrast to other ubiquitously expressed members of the caspase family, caspase-14 is rather specifically expressed within the epidermis, where it is of high importance in the formation of the physical skin barrier. It is expressed in keratinocytes of the uppermost stratum granulosum, where it was found to be associated with the nucleus, the keratohyalin granules and the desmosomes. Although its localization suggested a role for nuclear degradation during cornification, in caspase-14-deficient mice nuclear degradation was not affected. The observation that caspase-14 has only been found in terrestrial mammals but not in birds or reptiles and that profilaggrin is a direct substrate of caspase 14, suggests that it is important for formation of a soft stratum corneum. This could indicate a co-evolution of a soft SC and the caspase-14 gene (Denecker et al. 2007). Caspase-14 is produced as procaspase within the stratum granulosum, where it maturates in cornifying epithelia. Although it is not clear how it maturates, most likely a serine protease with elastase-like properties could be involved (Denecker et al. 2008). Thus, caspase-14 seems to be involved in the correct processing of profilaggrin, preceding its degradation into hygroscopic amino acids as well as the formation of UVB-protective compounds.

Another skin cysteine peptidase is cathepsin C, which represents a lysosomal cysteine peptidase of the papain family CIA, which is important for intracellular degradation and which has a role in the activation of serine proteases in immune cells (Rao et al. 1997). Cathepsin C knockout mice indicated that activation and processing of granzymes A and B, which are important for T-cell-mediated cell-killing, depends on cathepsin C (Pham and Ley 1999). Interestingly, Cathepsin C deficiency in humans leads to a dramatic reduction of both, levels and activities of the neutrophil serine proteases elastase, protease-3 and cathepsin G (Pham et al. 2004), which will be described below.

Cathepsin D represents the main aspartic protease of endolysosomes. It is active at the physiological acidic pH of healthy skin and is of relevance in the desquamation process (Horikoshi et al. 1999). Cathepsin D knockout mice showed reduced levels of involucrin and loricrin and lower transglutaminase 1 activity, which indicates that cathepsin D contributes indirectly to the barrier function of human skin (Egberts et al. 2004).

2.2 Serine proteases

Serine proteases represent a family of enzymes which use a catalytic triad in the substrate-binding pocket (Ser, His, Asp) to cleave peptide bonds. On the basis of their substrate specificity these proteases can be subdivided into trypsin-like enzymes (cleaves C-terminally of Arg and Lys), chymotryptic enzymes (cleave behind aromatic or bulky, hydrophobic amino acids, and the elastase-like enzymes (cleave behind small or medium size non-polar amino acids. These enzymes play an important role in the terminal differentiation process and desquamation.

2.2.1 Matriptase and prostasin

One of the most important players in epidermal barrier function is profilaggrin. It is processed at the stratum granulosum/stratum corneum interphase to filaggrin monomers. These are crosslinked to form macrofibrils and eventually "natural moisturing factors, NMFs), which are important for maintaining the hydration of the SC (reviewed in (Ovaere et al. 2009). The importance of profilaggrin proteolysis to maintain epidermal structure and hydration has been underscored by human genetic studies: These have shown that loss-of-function mutations in profilaggrin cause ichthyosis vulgaris and are strongly predisposing to atopic dermatitis and asthma, possibly due to a disturbed epidermal barrier function, which allows entry of allergens and infectious agents (Sandilands et al. 2006).

Major proteases required for initiating profilaggrin processing are the type II transmembrane serine protease matriptase and prostasin, a glycosylphosphatidylinositol-anchored membrane serine protease. There is now evidence that the autoactivating protease matriptase acts upstream of prostasin in a zymogen activation cascade that regulates terminal epidermal differentiation and is required for prostasin zymogen activation (Netzel-Arnett et al. 2006). A reduced matriptase expression was shown to be associated with incomplete terminal differentiation of epidermis, epidermal appendages, and oral epithelium (Bugge et al. 2007). Matriptase gene mutations lead to ichthyosis as recently reported (Alef et al. 2008). Matriptase is immediately activated by exposure to an acidic pH, as it occurs in skin, suggesting that matriptase activation may be a direct response to proton exposure (Tseng et al. 2010). Recent evidence showed that during epidermal differentiation, the matriptase-prostasin proteolytic cascade is tightly regulated by two mechanisms, either by prostasin activation temporally coupled to matriptase autoactivation or by the hepatocyte growth factor activator-inhibitor-1(HAI-1), which is rapidly inhibiting not only active matriptase but also active prostasin, resulting in an extremely brief window of opportunity for both active matriptase and active prostasin to act on their substrates (Chen et al. 2010). So far these two membrane-bound proteases are thought to be mainly involved in skin homeostasis. However, the ability of matriptase to activate Kallikrein-related proteases in the skin points to a regulatory role of matriptase in inflammatory skin diseases (Sales et al. 2010).

2.2.2 Kallikrein-related peptidases

Kallikrein-related proteases (KLKs) are the largest family of tryptic and chymotryptic serine proteases, which are encoded by 15 genes on chromosome 19q13.4. In skin, KLKs are produced by keratinocytes of the stratum granulosum (SG), where they are released into interstices of the upper SG and lower SC. To date, SC serine protease activity is attributed to human tissue KLKs (Borgono et al. 2007). At least eight KLKs have been reported to be expressed in healthy skin, of which KLK5, KLK7, KLK8, and KLK14 seem to be the most important (reviewed in (Lundwall and Brattsand 2008)). Their putative function has been extensively studied (reviewed in (Eissa and Diamandis 2008; Lundwall and Brattsand 2008). A wealth of literature revealed proteolytic function of the two serine proteases, KLK5 and KLK7, in SC. These proteases, previously termed 'stratum corneum tryptic enzyme, SCTE' (KLK5) and 'stratum corneum chymotryptic enzyme, SCCE' (KLK7), have an important role in the desquamation process, as it was shown that serine protease inhibitors were able to inhibit corneocyte shedding from human plantar skin *ex vivo* (Lundstrom and Egelrud 1988). Both enzymes are maximally expressed in the stratum granulosum, where they are released from lamellar bodies and located within stratum corneum interstices. Here they are

thought to form a proteolytic cascade in which KLK5 activates itself as well as KLK7 (Ovaere et al. 2009). Once active, both enzymes are believed to digest *in vivo* corneodesmosin, DSG1 and desmocollin-1, as these substrates have been shown to be digested *in vitro*. There is now evidence that also other KLKs participate in desquamation: It was recently shown, that KLK14 is responsible for 50% of the total trypsin-like serine protease activity in the stratum corneum. Because KLK14 can activate and be activated by KLK5, it is very likely that it also participates in the cascade pathway.
Apart from these three KLKs also KLK8 seems to be involved in a proteolytic activation cascade regulating skin desquamation: KLK8 is abundantly expressed and co-localized with other KLKs in human epidermis and sweat glands. It is also transported and exocytosed by lamellar bodies into the stratum granulosum/stratum corneum interface and thus may play a role in SC barrier functions. Very recent studies showed that recombinant KLK8 is optimally active at pH 8.5 suggesting that it plays a role in the upper stratum granulosum where the pH is rather neutral (Eissa et al. 2011). Active KLK8 has been found in SC extracts and in sweat, where until recently only KLK1 and kininase II were identified as active serine proteases. This raises its potential functional involvement in skin desquamation, although the physiological substrates need to be identified.

2.3 Proteases of bacterial, fungal and parasite origin

Apart from proteases produced by keratinocytes during differentiation and desquamation, the stratum corneum might also contain extracellular proteases originating from microbes and/or parasites residing at the skin surface. Bacterial proteases are often accessory proteins which are not fundamental for cell growth and division, but are considered to be virulence factors, which are often associated with mobile genetic elements such as plasmids, integrated phages and pathogenic islands. The clustering of bacterial protease genes in operons allows their coordinated expression, which in turn may imply a cooperation of the produced proteins (Wladyka and Pustelny 2008).
Staphylococci produce a number of extracellular proteases, among them epidermolytic toxins, staphylococcal serine proteases like a glutamyl endopeptidase referred to as V8, a cysteine protease in *S. aureus*. Similar and other proteases are produced by skin-relevant bacteria, including commensal *S. epidermidis*, *Streptococcus pyogenes*, *Pseudomonas aeruginosa* and others (Wladyka and Pustelny 2008). Among the proteases, serine proteases, cysteine proteases and metalloproteases represent the most abundant bacterial proteases. These affect the host's innate immune system in a bacterial species-specific manner by targeting phagocytes, cytokines and cytokine receptors, inflammatory signaling pathways, complement, contact activation as well as antimicrobial peptides (Potempa and Pike 2009).
Apart from bacteria also fungi represent an important source of proteases. Upon fungal infections, which are mostly seen at mucosal surfaces, *Candida albicans* represents the most common fungal pathogen. *Candida* species are ubiquitous commensal yeasts that reside as part of the normal mucosa microflora without causing infections. Suitable predisposing conditions will let *C. albicans* change to a 'pathogenic'stage, in which proteases represent major virulence factors. These are exclusively secreted aspartyl proteases (SAPs) (Naglik et al. 2004). It is believed that extracellular proteases of saprophytic microorganisms are primarily secreted to get nutrients from decomposition of complex materials. There is, however, strong evidence, that SAPs are also needed for invasion of the host, thereby interacting with several important host defense functions eventually causing inflammation (Naglik et al. 2004).

Proteolysis is also a vital element for survival of parasites, which enables them to digest resistant structural proteins. E. g. house dust mites (*Dermatophagoides pteronyssinus* and *D. farinae*) produce cysteine proteases and serine proteases (Donnelly et al. 2006), which are well known as 'group 1 house dust mite allergens' to induce allergic reactions. Several reports have shown that these proteases interact with pathways of the innate defense system suggesting that these might be also directly involved in inflammatory skin reactions.

2.4 Neutrophil serine proteases

Upon skin infection or at conditions causing 'neutrophilic dermatoses', the primary cell infiltrate consists of neutrophils. A massive infiltrate in the epidermis can lead to pustule formation. Upon infection, neutrophils phagocytose microbes and then kill these microbes within the phagolysosome by oxygen-radical-generating systems, the alpha-defensins as well as proteases which are released from primary ('azurophilic') as well as secundary ('specific') granules (Faurschou and Borregaard 2003). Only primary granules contain high amounts of the serine proteases human leukocyte elastase (HLE), cathepsin G and protease 3 (PR3). These enzymes are not released upon phagocytosis. But upon 'frustrating phagocytosis' (attempts to phagocytose particles, which are bigger than leukocytes) as well as formation of "neutrophil extracellular traps" (NETs) consisting of neutrophil-derived DNA, where these cationic enzymes are bound (Brinkmann et al. 2004), a release of these enzymes can occur. Indeed, HLE activity is present at the surface of lesional skin of patients with psoriasis, a neutrophilic dermatosis (Wiedow et al. 1992). Neutrophil serine proteases have been identified as important innate immune regulators (Meyer-Hoffert 2009; Meyer-Hoffert and Wiedow 2010). Thus, neutrophil-derived enzymes may further determine the outcome of an inflammatory skin lesion - independent of possible homeostasis of keratinocyte-derived proteases and protease-inhibitors.

3. Protease inhibitors

Proteolytic activity in the skin, which is often restricted to a few target proteins, its tissue localization and its enzymatic activity, needs to be properly controlled in the tissue. Although gene expression and zymogen-activation are important regulatory elements to restrict enzymatic activity, the most important one is the expression of more or less specific protease inhibitors within the skin. These inhibitors regulate more or less protease-specifically in a timely and concentration-dependent fashion the activity of diverse proteases. This review will summarize the current knowledge on the most important epithelial protease-inhibitors.

3.1 Kazal-type-realted protease inhibitors

The 'lympho-epithelial Kazal-type related inhibitor' (LEKTI, today named LEKTI-1) is an effective inhibitor of multiple serine proteases (Roelandt et al. 2009). Processing of this multidomain protease inhibitor into fragments or single domains restricts the inhibitory properties to serine proteases such as trypsin, plasmin, subtilisin A, cathepsin G and human neutrophil elastase. LEKTI-1 consists of 15 complete or incomplete Kazal domains. *In vitro*, recombinant LEKTI-1 fragments or single domains inhibit the keratinocyte-derived serine proteases KLK5, -6, -7, -13 and -14. LEKTI-1 is expressed in various stratified epithelia as three splice variants. In the epidermis LEKTI-1 is expressed in the stratum granulosum, where LEKTI-1 protein is located in lamellar bodies - separate from KLKs, but secreted into the extracellular space together (Ishida-Yamamoto et al. 2004; Ishida-Yamamoto et al. 2005). The 145 kDa form comprises all 15 potential inhibitory Kazal-domains, but it is cleaved rapidly into multidomain fragments, which might be cleaved further to produce single domains and complexes with KLK5 and KLK7 in the SC. These complexes dissociate at acidic pH, which due to a pH gradient within the SC may lead to a controlled homeostatic desquamation. Mutations in *Spink5* (which encodes LEKTI-1) generating premature termination codons, as seen in Netherton Syndrome (Chavanas et al. 2000), result in expression of truncated LEKTI forms lacking several protease-inhibiting domains. This rare ichthyosiform skin disease is characterized by dry skin, increased desquamation, hair abnormalities ('bamboo hair') and atopy. A decreased level of functional LEKTI correlates inversely with serine protease activity in SC, a decrease physical barrier function and severity of the disease.

Another Kazal-type inhibitor is LEKTI-2 (*Spink9*), which has been originally discovered in palmar and plantar SC extracts (Brattsand et al. 2009; Meyer-Hoffert et al. 2009). LEKTI-2/SPINK9 is mainly expressed in palmar and plantar skin, close to KLK5. Apart from skin, expression was seen in the thymus (thus referred as LEKTI-2). All other tissues showed a very low transcription level of *Spink9*. LEKTI-2/SPINK9 selectively inhibited KLK5, but not other proteases including chymotryptic KLK7 and tryptic KLK14 or several serine proteases like trypsin and chymotrypsin. The LEKTI-2/SPINK9 activity differs in this respect from that of LEKTI-1: The K_i of LEKTI-2 was found in the range of 60 – 250 nM. LEKTI-1-domains have been reported to inhibit KLK5 in the range of 3 nM (domain 8-11) to 120 nM (domain 9-15). Further, the LEKTI-1 domains exhibit a more or less broad activity spectrum. It remains to be determined whether LEKTI-2/SPINK9 plays a role in skin diseases. Considering the specific expression of LEKTI-2/SPINK9 at palmar and plantar sites as well as its specific activity to inhibit KLK5, it is intriguing to speculate that it could be a relevant factor in hand and foot eczema.

By following the hypothesis that likely more Kazal-type inhibitors are present in human skin, we identified SPINK6 as a selective inhibitor of KLKs in the skin (Meyer-Hoffert et al. 2010). Unlike LEKTI-1 but similar to LEKTI-2, SPINK6 possesses only one typical Kazal domain. SPINK6 is strongly expressed, unlike LEKTI-2, in skin from various locations and can be purified from human plantar SC extracts. At low levels it is expressed in many other tissues and is induced during keratinocyte differentiation. While immunohistochemical analyses revealed SPINK6 expression in the stratum granulosum of healthy human skin at various anatomical localizations and in the skin appendages, including sebaceous glands and sweat glands, SPINK6 expression was found to be decreased in lesions of atopic dermatitis. Recombinant SPINK6 inhibited KLK4, KLK5, KLK6, KLK7, KLK12, KLK13 and KLK14 but not KLK1, KLK3 and KLK11, suggesting a tissue KLK-selective inhibitory activity, since thrombin, trypsin, plasmin, matriptase, prostasin, mast cell chymase, cathepsin G, neutrophil elastase, and chymotrypsin were not inhibited (Meyer-Hoffert et al. 2010; Kantyka et al. 2011). The finding that SPINK6 inhibited desquamation of human plantar callus in an *ex vivo* model suggests that SPINK6 plays a role in modulating the activity of KLKs in human skin. Interestingly, SPINK6 exhibited some proteolytic inhibitory activity against caspase-14 and is so far the only reversible inhibitor of caspase-14 in human skin (Kantyka et al. 2011).

3.2 Trappins and serpins of human skin

Apart from LEKTIs keratinocytes produce a number of additional protease inhibitors. Members of one group are termed 'trappins' (acronym for transglutaminase substrate,

WAP-domain-containing proteins) (Schalkwijk et al. 1999). Human epidermis contains two, secretory leukocyte protease inhibitor (SLPI) and elafin. Both are efficient inhibitors of neutrophil serine proteases: SLPI inhibits cathepsin G and elastase, elafin inhibits elastase and protease-3. This suggests that these protease inhibitors are important at inflammatory conditions to protect the tissue from damage caused by neutrophil serine proteases. Whereas SLPI is constitutively expressed in the epidermis, elafin is present at a low level in healthy skin, but highly up-regulated at inflammatory conditions such as psoriasis (Wiedow et al. 1990). Elafin is stored in lamellar bodies and thus secreted as precursor at the interphase between stratum granulosum and stratum corneum, where it is crosslinked to proteins of the CE via transglutamination.

Another group of serine protease inhibitors are SERPINs, which encompass nearly 40 members, of which many have been implicated in cancer and inflammation (Meyer-Hoffert 2009). These protease inhibitors have a unique mechanism to inhibit enzymatic activity: SERPINs cause a conformational change of the protease and then covalently bind to it. A few members of the SERPIN family have been reported to be expressed in human skin, among them SERPINB3 (squamous cell carcinoma antigen-1), SERPINB4 (squamous cell carcinoma antigen-2), and SERPINB13 (headpin/hurpin). SERPINs have possibly a role in protecting tissue from proteolysis by bacterial proteases: SERPINB8 and SERPINB9 are inhibiting subtilisin A. SERPINA1 inactivates some microbial proteases including protease K. Further, a C-terminal fragment of SERPINA1 inhibits HIV-1 entry by interaction with the gp41 fusion protein.

3.3 Cystatins

Apart from serine proteases also cysteine protease activity is under the control of inhibitors in skin: These include members of the cystatine gene family (Zeeuwen et al. 2009). Cystatins represent polypeptides which are members of a superfamily of evolutionarily-related proteins that can be divided in three subgroups, and which are widely expressed in several human tissues and secretions. They effectively inhibit various cysteine proteases, such as cathepsins B, L, H, K, and S, at micromolar to picomolar concentration in a competitive and reversible manner. Whereas cystatin A and cystatin C were reported to act as epidermal protease inhibitor with antimicrobial properties - possibly by inhibiting microbial cysteine proteases - cystatin M/E regulates in the epidermis crosslinking of structural proteins by transglutaminase 3 in the cornification process by controlling cathepsin L and legumain activities (Meyer-Hoffert 2009). Cathepsin L has been shown to activate transglutaminase 3, an epidermis-specific enzyme that is important in the cornification process where it is responsible for crosslinking of small proline-rich proteins and loricrin. A deregulation of this pathway by uncontrolled cysteine protease activity leads to abnormal stratum corneum and disturbance of skin barrier function (Zeeuwen et al. 2009).

3.4 Other regulating factors of protease activity

It should not be overlooked that the proteolytic activity of proteinases depends on factors like pH and ion-concentration. All serine proteases including KLKs decrease their proteolytic activity in acidic environments. The physiological pH of around 5.5 already results in more than 90% less active compared to optimal in vitro conditions. Patients with atopic dermatitis often show an elevated pH at the skin surface, which might likely contribute to observed elevated serine protease levels in these patients (Voegeli et al. 2009).

Interestingly, the inhibitory of activity of LEKTI-1 depends on the pH, too, which might enhance proteolytic deregulation, when the epidermal pH is elevated. Moreover, Zn^{2+} inhibits KLK5 (Debela et al. 2007). This might have clinical consequences, when Zink levels are low as in acrodermatits enteropathica. The exfoliation and inflammation observed in this disease might be a result of decreased KLK5 inhibitions.

4. Protease-activated receptors (PARs)

PARs represent seven membrane-spanning G-protein coupled receptors, which are activated by serine proteases, which cleave a 'tethered' receptor-activating ligand at the N-terminus (Steinhoff et al. 2005). To date, four PARs (PAR1-4) have been characterized. PAR-1, PAR-3 and PAR-4 are activated by thrombine, and PAR-2 by trypsin and chymotrypsin. In human skin, PAR-2 is abundantly expressed by keratinocytes (Steinhoff et al. 1999), where it plays a role in regulating permeability barrier homeostasis, inflammation, pruritus, pigmentation, and wound healing upon activation by various endogenous and exogenous serine proteases. Whereas during skin-inflammation, PAR-2 is activated by neutrophil elastase and mast cell tryptase, upon infection or skin barrier defects proteases originating from certain bacteria, house dust mites, cockroaches or parasites can activate this receptor (Shpacovitch et al. 2007). Activation by *Propionibacterium acnes* protease causes induction of certain proinflammatory proteins, matrix metalloproteinases and antimicrobial peptides, including hCAP18/LL-37 (Lee et al. 2010).

5. Epidermal serine proteases and their inhibitors in atopic dermatitis

Our understanding of the pathogenesis of Atopic Dermatitis has increased by the discovery of pro-filaggrin (*FLG*) mutations as the major predisposing factor of AD and the genodermatose Netherthon Syndrom, which shows similarities to AD. *FLG* mutations lead to decreased or missing filaggrin, which leads to dry skin as its cleavage and processing product, the skin moisturizing factor, is decreased. The skin barrier defect leads to increases antigen penetration, which finally leads to specific sensitization and allergic inflammation. Here we have learnt from the ND model that missing LEKT-1 leads to increased KLK activity, which activate PAR-2, thus resulting in increased thymic stromal lymphopoetin (TSLP) (Briot et al. 2009). TSLP finally leads to a Th2 imbalance. Therefore, both events, the Filaggrin defect and the KLK-PAR2-TSLP axis, seem to be crucial for inducing AD.

To date, there is no evident point demonstrating that either intrinsic or extrinsic signals are promoting cutaneous allergic-type inflammation in AD. The fact that only 37–50% of patients with *Ichthyosis vulgaris* develop atopic manifestations (Kuokkanen 1969; Smith et al. 2006), supports the notion that in NS in which all patients develop allergic manifestations, additional mechanisms to primary skin barrier defect have a key role in immune response polarization toward a Th2 response. Since serine protease activity is elevated in AD patients (Voegeli et al. 2009), one might speculate that similar mechanisms are involved in AD as in ND. It was reported recently that KLK11 and KLK7 are elevated in lesions of AD patients (Voegeli et al. 2011). Some genetic studies have suggested that proteases and inhibitors are involved in the genetic predisposition of AD patients. In a case–control study on 103 AD patients and 261 matched controls, a significant association was found between a 4-bp insertion in the 3'-untranslated region of the *KLK7* gene, encoding KLK7 and AD (Vasilopoulos et al. 2004)). This association of the 4-bp insertion mutation with AD could not be confirmed in two independent studies (Hubiche et al. 2007; Weidinger et al. 2008). *SPINK5* gene mutations are linked the with AD, when maternally inherited (Walley et al. 2001; Kato et al. 2003; Nishio et al. 2003; Weidinger et al. 2008). It is worth noting that the association was weaker than in the case of *FLG* mutations, in part, owing to a high prevalence in the control population. In a separate study on a French population, an association between *SPINK5* and AD was not found; however, there was an association between carriers and raised IgE serum levels (Hubiche et al. 2007)). The association of *SPINK5* mutations with raised IgE serum levels and with other atopic conditions, such as asthma, led to the suggestion that they are risk factors for general atopy (Walley et al. 2001; Nishio et al. 2003). In addition to *SPINK5,* a mutation has been identified in the *CSTA* gene encoding the cysteine protease inhibitor, cystatin A, which associates with AD. The cystatin A gene maps to chromosome 3q21, which has been identified as a major susceptibility locus for AD (Lee et al. 2000).

6. Conclusion

Until today the complex pathogenesis of AD is not fully understood. But there is more and more evidence that epidermal proteases and their inhibitors are involved in the pathogenesis of AD. Their expression can be altered by genetic mutations and their activity is influenced by environmental factors like the pH, which is increased in AD patients (Sparavigna et al. 1999). Taken together there seems to exist a feedback regulation system important for skin barrier homeostasis in AD especially for kallikrein activity involving filaggrin mutations, PAR2 and LEKTI expression Tanaka 2011. It will be interesting to see whether inhibition of elevated protease activity will improve severity of AD lesions. Clinical trials are currently on their way with promising preliminary results (http://clinicaltrial.gov).

7. Acknowledgment

Part of this work was supported by grants of Deutsche Forschungsgemeinschaft (Me2037/3-1).

8. References

Alef, T., Torres, S., Hausser, I., Metze, D., Tursen, U., Lestringant, G. G. and Hennies, H. C. (2008). "Ichthyosis, Follicular Atrophoderma, and Hypotrichosis Caused by Mutations in ST14 Is Associated with Impaired Profilaggrin Processing." *J.Invest Dermatol.*

Borgono, C. A., Michael, I. P., Komatsu, N., Jayakumar, A., Kapadia, R., Clayman, G. L., Sotiropoulou, G. and Diamandis, E. P. (2007). "A potential role for multiple tissue kallikrein serine proteases in epidermal desquamation." *J.Biol.Chem.* 282(6): 3640-3652.

Brattsand, M., Stefansson, K., Hubiche, T., Nilsson, S. K. and Egelrud, T. (2009). "SPINK9: A Selective, Skin-Specific Kazal-Type Serine Protease Inhibitor." *J.Invest Dermatol.*

Brinkmann, V., Reichard, U., Goosmann, C., Fauler, B., Uhlemann, Y., Weiss, D. S., Weinrauch, Y. and Zychlinsky, A. (2004). "Neutrophil extracellular traps kill bacteria." *Science* 303(5663): 1532-1535.

Briot, A., Deraison, C., Lacroix, M., Bonnart, C., Robin, A., Besson, C., Dubus, P. and Hovnanian, A. (2009). "Kallikrein 5 induces atopic dermatitis-like lesions through PAR2-mediated thymic stromal lymphopoietin expression in Netherton syndrome." *J Exp.Med.* 206(5): 1135-1147.

Bugge, T. H., List, K. and Szabo, R. (2007). "Matriptase-dependent cell surface proteolysis in epithelial development and pathogenesis." *Front Biosci.* 12: 5060-5070.

Candi, E., Schmidt, R. and Melino, G. (2005). "The cornified envelope: a model of cell death in the skin." *Nat.Rev.Mol.Cell Biol.* 6(4): 328-340.

Chavanas, S., Bodemer, C., Rochat, A., Hamel-Teillac, D., Ali, M., Irvine, A. D., Bonafe, J. L., Wilkinson, J., Taieb, A., Barrandon, Y., Harper, J. I., de Prost, Y. and Hovnanian, A. (2000). "Mutations in SPINK5, encoding a serine protease inhibitor, cause Netherton syndrome." *Nat.Genet.* 25(2): 141-142.

Chen, Y. W., Wang, J. K., Chou, F. P., Chen, C. Y., Rorke, E. A., Chen, L. M., Chai, K. X., Eckert, R. L., Johnson, M. D. and Lin, C. Y. (2010). "Regulation of the matriptase-prostasin cell surface proteolytic cascade by hepatocyte growth factor activator inhibitor-1 during epidermal differentiation." *J Biol.Chem.* 285(41): 31755-31762.

Debela, M., Goettig, P., Magdolen, V., Huber, R., Schechter, N. M. and Bode, W. (2007). "Structural basis of the zinc inhibition of human tissue kallikrein 5." *J.Mol.Biol.* 373(4): 1017-1031.

Demerjian, M., Hachem, J. P., Tschachler, E., Denecker, G., Declercq, W., Vandenabeele, P., Mauro, T., Hupe, M., Crumrine, D., Roelandt, T., Houben, E., Elias, P. M. and Feingold, K. R. (2008). "Acute modulations in permeability barrier function regulate epidermal cornification: role of caspase-14 and the protease-activated receptor type 2." *Am.J.Pathol.* 172(1): 86-97.

Denecker, G., Hoste, E., Gilbert, B., Hochepied, T., Ovaere, P., Lippens, S., Van den, B. C., Van Damme, P., D'Herde, K., Hachem, J. P., Borgonie, G., Presland, R. B., Schoonjans, L., Libert, C., Vandekerckhove, J., Gevaert, K., Vandenabeele, P. and Declercq, W. (2007). "Caspase-14 protects against epidermal UVB photodamage and water loss." *Nat.Cell Biol.* 9(6): 666-674.

Denecker, G., Ovaere, P., Vandenabeele, P. and Declercq, W. (2008). "Caspase-14 reveals its secrets." *J.Cell Biol.* 180(3): 451-458.

Donnelly, S., Dalton, J. P. and Loukas, A. (2006). "Proteases in helminth- and allergen-induced inflammatory responses." *Chem.Immunol.Allergy* 90: 45-64.

Egberts, F., Heinrich, M., Jensen, J. M., Winoto-Morbach, S., Pfeiffer, S., Wickel, M., Schunck, M., Steude, J., Saftig, P., Proksch, E. and Schutze, S. (2004). "Cathepsin D is involved in the regulation of transglutaminase 1 and epidermal differentiation." *J.Cell Sci.* 117(Pt 11): 2295-2307.

Eissa, A., Amodeo, V., Smith, C. R. and Diamandis, E. P. (2011). "Kallikrein-related peptidase-8 (KLK8) is an active serine protease in human epidermis and sweat and is involved in a skin barrier proteolytic cascade." *J Biol.Chem.* 286(1): 687-706.

Eissa, A. and Diamandis, E. P. (2008). "Human tissue kallikreins as promiscuous modulators of homeostatic skin barrier functions." *Biol.Chem.* 389(6): 669-680.

Faurschou, M. and Borregaard, N. (2003). "Neutrophil granules and secretory vesicles in inflammation." *Microbes.Infect.* 5(14): 1317-1327.

Hachem, J. P., Wagberg, F., Schmuth, M., Crumrine, D., Lissens, W., Jayakumar, A., Houben, E., Mauro, T. M., Leonardsson, G., Brattsand, M., Egelrud, T., Roseeuw, D., Clayman, G. L., Feingold, K. R., Williams, M. L. and Elias, P. M. (2006). "Serine protease activity and residual LEKTI expression determine phenotype in Netherton syndrome." *J.Invest Dermatol.* 126(7): 1609-1621.

Horikoshi, T., Igarashi, S., Uchiwa, H., Brysk, H. and Brysk, M. M. (1999). "Role of endogenous cathepsin D-like and chymotrypsin-like proteolysis in human epidermal desquamation." *Br.J.Dermatol.* 141(3): 453-459.

Hubiche, T., Ged, C., Benard, A., Leaute-Labreze, C., McElreavey, K., de Verneuil, H., Taieb, A. and Boralevi, F. (2007). "Analysis of SPINK 5, KLK 7 and FLG genotypes in a French atopic dermatitis cohort." *Acta Derm Venereol* 87(6): 499-505.

Ishida-Yamamoto, A., Deraison, C., Bonnart, C., Bitoun, E., Robinson, R., O'Brien, T. J., Wakamatsu, K., Ohtsubo, S., Takahashi, H., Hashimoto, Y., Dopping-Hepenstal, P. J., McGrath, J. A., Iizuka, H., Richard, G. and Hovnanian, A. (2005). "LEKTI is localized in lamellar granules, separated from KLK5 and KLK7, and is secreted in the extracellular spaces of the superficial stratum granulosum." *J.Invest Dermatol.* 124(2): 360-366.

Ishida-Yamamoto, A., Simon, M., Kishibe, M., Miyauchi, Y., Takahashi, H., Yoshida, S., O'Brien, T. J., Serre, G. and Iizuka, H. (2004). "Epidermal lamellar granules transport different cargoes as distinct aggregates." *J.Invest Dermatol.* 122(5): 1137-1144.

Kantyka, T., Fischer, J., Wu, Z., Declercq, W., Reiss, K., Schroder, J. M. and Meyer-Hoffert, U. (2011). "Inhibition of Kallikrein-related Peptidases by the Serine Protease Inhibitor of Kazal-type 6." *Peptides.*

Kato, A., Fukai, K., Oiso, N., Hosomi, N., Murakami, T. and Ishii, M. (2003). "Association of SPINK5 gene polymorphisms with atopic dermatitis in the Japanese population." *Br.J.Dermatol.* 148(4): 665-669.

Kuokkanen, K. (1969). "Ichthyosis vulgaris. A clinical and histopathological study of patients and their close relatives in the autosomal dominant and sex-linked forms of the disease." *Acta Derm Venereol Suppl (Stockh)* 62: 1-72.

Lee, S. E., Kim, J. M., Jeong, S. K., Jeon, J. E., Yoon, H. J., Jeong, M. K. and Lee, S. H. (2010). "Protease-activated receptor-2 mediates the expression of inflammatory cytokines, antimicrobial peptides, and matrix metalloproteinases in keratinocytes in response to Propionibacterium acnes." *Arch.Dermatol.Res.* 302(10): 745-756.

Lee, Y. A., Wahn, U., Kehrt, R., Tarani, L., Businco, L., Gustafsson, D., Andersson, F., Oranje, A. P., Wolkertstorfer, A., v Berg, A., Hoffmann, U., Kuster, W., Wienker, T., Ruschendorf, F. and Reis, A. (2000). "A major susceptibility locus for atopic dermatitis maps to chromosome 3q21." *Nat Genet* 26(4): 470-473.

Lundstrom, A. and Egelrud, T. (1988). "Cell shedding from human plantar skin in vitro: evidence of its dependence on endogenous proteolysis." *J.Invest Dermatol.* 91(4): 340-343.

Lundwall, A. and Brattsand, M. (2008). "Kallikrein-related peptidases." *Cell Mol.Life Sci.*

Meyer-Hoffert, U. (2009). "Neutrophil-derived serine proteases modulate innate immune responses." *Front Biosci.* 14: 3409-3418.

Meyer-Hoffert, U. (2009). "Reddish, scaly, and itchy: how proteases and their inhibitors contribute to inflammatory skin diseases." *Arch.Immunol.Ther.Exp.(Warsz.)* 57(5): 345-354.

Meyer-Hoffert, U. and Wiedow, O. (2010). "Neutrophil serine proteases: mediators of innate immune responses." *Curr.Opin.Hematol.*

Meyer-Hoffert, U., Wu, Z., Kantyka, T., Fischer, J., Latendorf, T., Hansmann, B., Bartels, J., He, Y., Glaser, R. and Schroder, J. M. (2010). "Isolation of SPINK6 in human skin: selective inhibitor of kallikrein-related peptidases." *J Biol.Chem.* 285(42): 32174-32181.

Meyer-Hoffert, U., Wu, Z. and Schroder, J. M. (2009). "Identification of lympho-epithelial Kazal-type inhibitor 2 in human skin as a kallikrein-related peptidase 5-specific protease inhibitor." *PLoS ONE* 4(2): e4372.

Naglik, J., Albrecht, A., Bader, O. and Hube, B. (2004). "Candida albicans proteinases and host/pathogen interactions." *Cell Microbiol.* 6(10): 915-926.

Netzel-Arnett, S., Currie, B. M., Szabo, R., Lin, C. Y., Chen, L. M., Chai, K. X., Antalis, T. M., Bugge, T. H. and List, K. (2006). "Evidence for a matriptase-prostasin proteolytic cascade regulating terminal epidermal differentiation." *J.Biol.Chem.* 281(44): 32941-32945.

Nishio, Y., Noguchi, E., Shibasaki, M., Kamioka, M., Ichikawa, E., Ichikawa, K., Umebayashi, Y., Otsuka, F. and Arinami, T. (2003). "Association between polymorphisms in the SPINK5 gene and atopic dermatitis in the Japanese." *Genes Immun.* 4(7): 515-517.

Ovaere, P., Lippens, S., Vandenabeele, P. and Declercq, W. (2009). "The emerging roles of serine protease cascades in the epidermis." *Trends Biochem.Sci.* 34(9): 453-463.

Pham, C. T., Ivanovich, J. L., Raptis, S. Z., Zehnbauer, B. and Ley, T. J. (2004). "Papillon-Lefevre syndrome: correlating the molecular, cellular, and clinical consequences of cathepsin C/dipeptidyl peptidase I deficiency in humans." *J.Immunol.* 173(12): 7277-7281.

Pham, C. T. and Ley, T. J. (1999). "Dipeptidyl peptidase I is required for the processing and activation of granzymes A and B in vivo." *Proc.Natl.Acad.Sci.U.S.A* 96(15): 8627-8632.

Potempa, J. and Pike, R. N. (2009). "Corruption of innate immunity by bacterial proteases." *J Innate Immun* 1(2): 70-87.

Rao, N. V., Rao, G. V. and Hoidal, J. R. (1997). "Human dipeptidyl-peptidase I. Gene characterization, localization, and expression." *J.Biol.Chem.* 272(15): 10260-10265.

Roelandt, T., Thys, B., Heughebaert, C., De Vroede, A., De Paepe, K., Roseeuw, D., Rombaut, B. and Hachem, J. P. (2009). "LEKTI-1 in sickness and in health." *Int.J Cosmet.Sci.* 31(4): 247-254.

Sales, K. U., Masedunskas, A., Bey, A. L., Rasmussen, A. L., Weigert, R., List, K., Szabo, R., Overbeek, P. A. and Bugge, T. H. (2010). "Matriptase initiates activation of epidermal pro-kallikrein and disease onset in a mouse model of Netherton syndrome." *Nat.Genet.* 42(8): 676-683.

Sandilands, A., O'Regan, G. M., Liao, H., Zhao, Y., Terron-Kwiatkowski, A., Watson, R. M., Cassidy, A. J., Goudie, D. R., Smith, F. J., McLean, W. H. and Irvine, A. D. (2006). "Prevalent and rare mutations in the gene encoding filaggrin cause ichthyosis vulgaris and predispose individuals to atopic dermatitis." *J.Invest Dermatol.* 126(8): 1770-1775.

Schalkwijk, J., Wiedow, O. and Hirose, S. (1999). "The trappin gene family: proteins defined by an N-terminal transglutaminase substrate domain and a C-terminal four-disulphide core." *Biochem.J* 340 (Pt 3): 569-577.

Shpacovitch, V., Feld, M., Bunnett, N. W. and Steinhoff, M. (2007). "Protease-activated receptors: novel PARtners in innate immunity." *Trends Immunol.* 28(12): 541-550.

Smith, F. J., Irvine, A. D., Terron-Kwiatkowski, A., Sandilands, A., Campbell, L. E., Zhao, Y., Liao, H., Evans, A. T., Goudie, D. R., Lewis-Jones, S., Arseculeratne, G., Munro, C. S., Sergeant, A., O'Regan, G., Bale, S. J., Compton, J. G., DiGiovanna, J. J., Presland, R. B., Fleckman, P. and McLean, W. H. (2006). "Loss-of-function mutations in the gene encoding filaggrin cause ichthyosis vulgaris." *Nat.Genet.* 38(3): 337-342.

Sparavigna, A., Setaro, M. and Gualandri, V. (1999). "Cutaneous pH in children affected by atopic dermatitis and in healthy children: a multicenter study." *Skin Research and Technology* 5(4): 221-227.

Steinhoff, M., Buddenkotte, J., Shpacovitch, V., Rattenholl, A., Moormann, C., Vergnolle, N., Luger, T. A. and Hollenberg, M. D. (2005). "Proteinase-activated receptors: transducers of proteinase-mediated signaling in inflammation and immune response." *Endocr.Rev.* 26(1): 1-43.

Steinhoff, M., Corvera, C. U., Thoma, M. S., Kong, W., McAlpine, B. E., Caughey, G. H., Ansel, J. C. and Bunnett, N. W. (1999). "Proteinase-activated receptor-2 in human skin: tissue distribution and activation of keratinocytes by mast cell tryptase." *Exp.Dermatol.* 8(4): 282-294.

Tseng, I. C., Xu, H., Chou, F. P., Li, G., Vazzano, A. P., Kao, J. P., Johnson, M. D. and Lin, C. Y. (2010). "Matriptase activation, an early cellular response to acidosis." *J Biol.Chem.* 285(5): 3261-3270.

Vasilopoulos, Y., Cork, M. J., Murphy, R., Williams, H. C., Robinson, D. A., Duff, G. W., Ward, S. J. and Tazi-Ahnini, R. (2004). "Genetic association between an AACC insertion in the 3'UTR of the stratum corneum chymotryptic enzyme gene and atopic dermatitis." *J Invest Dermatol* 123(1): 62-66.

Voegeli, R., Doppler, S., Joller, P., Breternitz, M., Fluhr, J. W. and Rawlings, A. V. (2011). "Increased mass levels of certain serine proteases in the stratum corneum in acute eczematous atopic skin." *Int J Cosmet Sci.*

Voegeli, R., Rawlings, A. V., Breternitz, M., Doppler, S., Schreier, T. and Fluhr, J. W. (2009). "Increased stratum corneum serine protease activity in acute eczematous atopic skin." *Br.J Dermatol.*

Walley, A. J., Chavanas, S., Moffatt, M. F., Esnouf, R. M., Ubhi, B., Lawrence, R., Wong, K., Abecasis, G. R., Jones, E. Y., Harper, J. I., Hovnanian, A. and Cookson, W. O. (2001). "Gene polymorphism in Netherton and common atopic disease." *Nat.Genet.* 29(2): 175-178.

Weidinger, S., Baurecht, H., Wagenpfeil, S., Henderson, J., Novak, N., Sandilands, A., Chen, H., Rodriguez, E., O'Regan, G. M., Watson, R., Liao, H., Zhao, Y., Barker, J. N., Allen, M., Reynolds, N., Meggitt, S., Northstone, K., Smith, G. D., Strobl, C., Stahl, C., Kneib, T., Klopp, N., Bieber, T., Behrendt, H., Palmer, C. N., Wichmann, H. E., Ring, J., Illig, T., McLean, W. H. and Irvine, A. D. (2008). "Analysis of the individual and aggregate genetic contributions of previously identified serine peptidase inhibitor Kazal type 5 (SPINK5), kallikrein-related peptidase 7 (KLK7), and filaggrin (FLG) polymorphisms to eczema risk." *J.Allergy Clin.Immunol.* 122(3): 560-568.

Wiedow, O., Schroder, J. M., Gregory, H., Young, J. A. and Christophers, E. (1990). "Elafin: an elastase-specific inhibitor of human skin. Purification, characterization, and complete amino acid sequence." *J.Biol.Chem.* 265(25): 14791-14795.

Wiedow, O., Wiese, F., Streit, V., Kalm, C. and Christophers, E. (1992). "Lesional elastase activity in psoriasis, contact dermatitis, and atopic dermatitis." *J.Invest Dermatol.* 99(3): 306-309.

Wladyka, B. and Pustelny, K. (2008). "Regulation of bacterial protease activity." *Cell Mol.Biol.Lett.* 13(2): 212-229.

Zeeuwen, P. L., Cheng, T. and Schalkwijk, J. (2009). "The biology of cystatin M/E and its cognate target proteases." *J Invest Dermatol.* 129(6): 1327-1338.

4

The Roles of Th2-Type Cytokines in the Pathogenesis of Atopic Dermatitis

Kenji Izuhara[1], Hiroshi Shiraishi[1], Shoichiro Ohta[2], Kazuhiko Arima[1] and Shoichi Suzuki[1]
[1]*Division of Medical Biochemistry, Department of Biomolecular Sciences*
[2]*Department of Laboratory Medicine, Saga Medical School*
Japan

1. Introduction

Atopic dermatitis (AD) is a chronic, relapsing, highly pruritic inflammatory skin disease (1, 2). Analyses of the cytokine expression profile in skin lesions of AD patients show that the Th2-type immune response is dominant in AD inflammation (3, 4). Interleukin-4 (IL-4), IL-5, and IL-13 are signature cytokines of the Th2-type immune response. Expression of IL-4 and IL-13 is significantly high in acute lesions of AD skin; however, it is down-regulated in chronic lesions. In contrast, expression of IL-5 is more elevated in chronic lesions than in acute lesions. High expression of IL-4, IL-5, and IL-13 in AD skins leads to high serum levels of IgE and eosinophilia, typical clinical features of AD. In addition to IL-5, expression of interferon-γ (IFN-γ) and IL-12 is elevated in chronic skin lesions of AD. IFN-γ and IL-12 are signature cytokines of Th1-type immune response. It has remained unclear why this immune milieu change occurs.

Based on observations of the predominant Th2-type immune responses in AD patients, many studies using model mice or involving genetic association have been performed to investigate the role played by Th2-type cytokines in the pathogenesis of AD. It is hoped that Th2-type cytokines will prove to be good targets to develop therapeutic agents for AD. In this chapter, we focus on these topics; we do not review the details of the structures, the signal pathways, or the biological functions of these Th2-type cytokines. Please refer to other articles regarding with these subjects (5-10).

2. Th2-type cytokines in model mice

Animal models are useful to understand the pathogenesis of AD and to develop therapeutic agents for AD. Among various species, mouse models have been primarily used, because genetically manipulated mice are available. Mouse models of AD can be categorized into three groups (2): (1) mice that spontaneously develop AD-like skin lesions, (2) mice epicutaneously sensitized with allergens, and (3) genetically engineered mice. It has been reported that several AD model mice that spontaneously develop AD-like skin lesions such as Nc/Nga mice (11) and DS-Nh mice (12) show a Th2-type–dominant immune milieu, suggesting that Th2-type cytokines are involved in pathogenesis in these mice. However, the situation is more complex, because it has been demonstrated that Nc/Nga mice deficient in STAT6, a common critical transcription factor for IL-4 and IL-13 signals, exhibited skin lesions comparable to those of STAT6-positive littermates (13). Here, we summarize the results of analyses investigating the roles of Th2-type cytokines, using mice epicutaneously sensitized with allergens and genetically engineered mice (Table 1).

Category	Application	Phenotypes	References
Ovalbumin-sensitized mouse	IL-4-deficient mouse	Decreased eosinophils Decreased serum IgE No change in thickness of epidermis and dermis No change in chemokine expression No change in infiltration of CD45+, CD4+, or CD8+ cells	15
	IL-5-deficient mouse	No eosinophil Thinning of epidermis and dermis No change in chemokine expression No change in infiltration of CD45+, CD4+, or CD8+ cells	15
Genetically engineered mouse	IL-4 transgenic mouse	Xerosis Conjunctivitis Pruritis Presence of *Staphylococcus aureus* Spongiosis Acanthosis Infiltration of mononuclear cells and eosinophils in dermis and epidermis Degranulation of mast cells in dermis Increased expression of IL-5, IL-13,IL-12p40, IFN-γ, TNF-α, and IL-1β Increased serum IgE and IgG1 Increased T cell proliferation Increased dendritic cells, macrophages, and NK cells in skin and lymphoid organs	16-19
	IL-13 transgenic mouse	Pruritis Loss of hair Erythema Crusting Excoriation Bacterial pyoderma Erosions Dry lichenified skin lesion Infiltration of macrophages, dendritic cells, eosinophils, CD4+ cells, and mast cells Increased expression of CCL2/MCP-1, CCL5/RANTES, CCL11/Eotaxin, CCL17/TARC, CCL22/MDC, CCL27/CTACK, TSL, and VEGF Increased serum IgE and IgG1 Increased systemic immune responses	20

Table 1. Summary of effects of Th2-type cytokines in model mice

2.1 Ovalbumin (OVA)-sensitized mice

Geha's group established AD model mice by repeated epicutaneous sensitization to OVA (14). These mice manifest AD-like skin lesions including acanthosis, spongiosis, and infiltration of neutrophils, lymphocytes, mast cells, and eosinophils into the dermis. Expression of Th2-type (IL-4, IL-5 and IL-13) cytokines is up-regulated with little or no change of IFN-γ expression (2, 14). Furthermore, serum levels of total or OVA-specific IgE and IgG1 are elevated. This mouse model has been used to investigate involvement of various molecules associated with the pathogenesis of AD.

2.1.1 Application of OVA-sensitized mouse model to IL-4–deficient mice

The role of IL-4 in OVA-sensitized AD model mice is complex (15). The eosinophil numbers decrease in the dermis of OVA-sensitized IL-4–deficient mice showing an important role of IL-4 for infiltration of eosinophils. However, the numbers of $CD45^+$, $CD3^+$, $CD4^+$, and $CD8^+$ cells and expression of MIP-2, MIP-1β, IP-10, and RANTES increase compared to wild type mice, suggesting that IL-4 has an inhibitory role in expression of chemokines to recruit T cells. It is of note that thickness of the epidermis and dermis are not changed compared to wild type mice showing that IL-4 has a subtle effect on skin thickening. In these mice, total or OVA-specific IgE levels significantly decrease, which argues against the roles of IgE in the pathogenesis of this mouse model. Correspondingly, OVA-sensitized IgE-deficient mice show no change in histological views of the skin tissues, infiltration of $CD45^+$, $CD3^+$, $CD4^+$, and $CD8^+$ cells and expression of IL-4, IL-5 and IFN-γ compared to OVA-sensitized wild-type mice (15), suggesting that this mouse model is independent of IgE. Furthermore, the redundancy of IL-4 and IL-13 *in vivo* may be the reason why the effects of IL-4–deficiency on skin thickening are subtle in this mouse model.

2.1.2 Application of OVA-sensitized mouse model to IL-5–deficient mice

IL-5–deficient mice had virtually no eosinophil (15). These mice sensitized with OVA had thinning of the epidermis and dermis compared with wild-type mice. However, infiltration of $CD45^+$, $CD3^+$, $CD4^+$, and $CD8^+$ cells and expression of chemokines were equivalent to wild-type mice. These results may suggest that IL-5 partially contributes to generating AD-like lesions in this mouse model.

2.2 Genetically engineered mice for Th2-type cytokines

Thus far, transgenic mice that express IL-4 or IL-13 specifically in keratinocytes have mainly been generated using keratin promoters. In contrast to the IL-4-deficient mice, these gain-of-function mice manifest overt skin lesions, which indicates topical overexpression of either IL-4 or IL-13 that is sufficient to induce phenotypes similar to AD patients.

2.2.1 IL-4 transgenic mice

Chan's group established and characterized IL-4 transgenic mice in which expression of IL-4 is controlled under the promoter of the keratin 14 gene (16-19). These mice are normal when they are newborn. However, almost four months after birth, they develop AD-like lesions such as xerosis (dry skin), conjunctivitis, and pruritic skin lesions (16). Many skin lesions appear in ears, necks, and eyes. Forty-three percent of the mice develop skin lesions within 12 months. Inflammatory skin lesions show the presence of *Staphylococcus aureus*, a common infectious complication and exacerbating factor in human AD patients. Histological analyses of the lesions in these mice show spongiosis, acanthosis, dermal and epidermal infiltration of mononuclear cells and eosinophils, and degranulating mast cells in the dermis. Expression of Th2-type cytokines (IL-5, IL-13), Th1-type cytokines (IL-12p40, IFN-γ), and inflammatory cytokines (TNF-α, IL-1β) is up-regulated in the skin lesions of these mice. Enhancement of these cytokines except IL-12p40 is even observed in the skin, before the disease onset or in the intact skin (17). Correspondingly, serum levels of IgE and IgG1 are elevated even before the onset, which reflects high expression of IL-4 and IL-13. Afterward, up-regulated serum levels of IgG2a are observed, reflecting high expression of IFN-γ (19). T cells in these mice possess higher proliferating capacity *in vitro* spontaneously or induced by stimulants such as T cell receptor triggering or Staphylococcus enterotoxins A and B compared to T cells in wild-type mice (18). It is of note that the numbers of dendritic cells, macrophages, and NK cells increase in the skin tissues and lymphoid organs of these mice, which suggests that overexpression of IL-4 in skin tissues modulates antigen-presenting activity *in vivo*.

2.2.2 IL-13 transgenic mice

Zhu's group established IL-13 transgenic mice in which withdrawal of doxycycline induces expression of IL-13 under the control of the promoter region of the keratin 5 gene (20). Six to eight weeks after the withdrawal of doxycycline, AD-like skin lesions (i.e. pruritis, loss of hair, erythema, crusting, excoriation, bacterial pyoderma, and erosions, thereafter dry lichenified skin lesion) appear in these mice. All of the mice develop these features within four months. In the skin lesions, F4/80$^+$ cells including macrophages and dendritic cells, eosinophils, CD4$^+$ cells, and mast cells are accumulated. Expression of various chemokines (CCL2/MCP-1, CCL5/RANTES, CCL11/Eotaxin, CCL17/TARC, CCL22/MDC, CCL27/CTACK), TSLP (a critical cytokine correlated with AD at the interface of epidermis and immune cells), and VEGF (a potent cytokine for angiogenesis), is up-regulated in these mice. Serum levels of IgE and IgG1 are elevated. Furthermore, systemic Th2 skewing is enhanced because the lymphocytes in the lymph nodes of these mice produce more IL-4 and IL-13 upon stimulation of anti-CD3/CD28 antibody (Ab) than do those in the wild-type mice.

3. Genetic associations of Th2-type cytokines with AD

An initial linkage analysis in Amish families showed the association of 5q31.1 with serum IgE levels (21). This chromosome region contains a cluster of Th2-type cytokine genes. Therefore, much attention has been paid to the genetic association of Th2-type cytokine genes with atopy (defined as high serum IgE level) or with each specific phenotype of allergic diseases. As a result, several single nucleotide polymorphisms (SNPs) on the *IL4*, *IL5*, and *IL13* genes have been shown to be associated with atopy or AD (Table 2). Furthermore, SNPs located on the *IL4RA* and *IL13RA1* genes encoding the IL-4 receptor α chain (IL-4Rα) and the IL-13R α1 chain (IL-13Rα1) and on the *STAT6* gene encoding STAT6 were also reported to be associated with atopy or AD. IL-4Rα is a component of both type I IL-4R and type II IL-4R/IL-13, whereas IL-13Rα1 is a component of type II IL-4R/IL-13

(Figure 1). STAT6 is a transcriptional factor critical for IL-4 or IL-13 signals. The association of the *IL13, IL4RA,* and *STAT6* genes with IgE is confirmed by recent Genome Wide Association Studies (22, 23).

Gene	Variant	Association	Function	References
IL4	-590C/T	AD	Change in IL-4 production	24-26
IL13	Arg110Gln (Arg130Gln, G4257A)	AD Serum IgE specific anti-allergen IgE	Lower affinity with the IL-13R α2 chain Enhanced stability Transduction of stronger signal via IL-13Rα1	28-36
	-1055C/T ('-1111C/, -1024C/T)	AD Serum IgE specific anti-allergen IgE	Change in IL-13 production	34, 37-40
IL4RA	Gln576Arg (Gln551Arg)	Hyper IgE syndrome AD	Decreased binding to SHP-1 Increased STAT6 activation	41, 42
IL13RA1	1398A/G	Serum IgE		27
STAT6	2964G/A	Serum IgE		43
	in18SNP1C/T	Serum IgE Eosinophil number		44
	GT repeat in exon1	Serum IgE Eosinophil number		44
IL5	-703C/T	Serum IgE Eosinophil number		45

Table 2. Summary of genetic associations in Th2-type cytokines and their related molecules

3.1 IL-4 gene

There exists a SNP in the promoter of the *IL4* gene (-590C/T). This SNP was originally reported to be associated with bronchial asthma (24) and is thought to affect the binding activities to NFAT, resulting in modulating IL-4 production. Transmission disequilibrium testing shows a significantly preferential transmission of the T allele in AD patients (25). Another group confirmed the association of this SNP with AD (26).

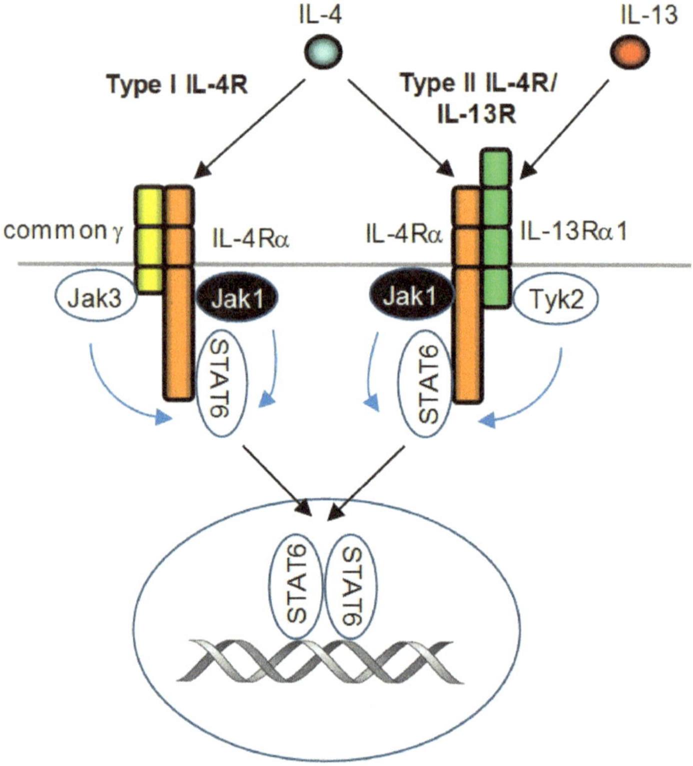

Fig. 1. The receptor structures and signal pathways of IL-4 and IL-13.
IL-4 binds to type I IL-4R or type II IL-4R/IL-13R, and IL-13 binds to type II IL-4R/IL-13R. Type I IL-4R and type II IL-4R/IL-13R are composed of IL-4Rα and the IL-2R γ chain (common γ) or IL-4Rα and IL-13Rα1, respectively. Engagement of the receptors activates Jak kinases followed by activation of STAT6.

3.2 IL-13 gene

There exist several SNPs on the *IL13* gene. Thus far, two of them (Arg110Gln, also referred to as Arg130Gln or G4257A; and -1055C/T, also referred to as -1111C/T or -1024C/T) are reported to be associated with atopy or AD. We and other groups reported the genetic association of Arg110Gln with bronchial asthma (27), serum IgE levels (28, 29), and AD (29). This SNP causes exchange of arginine at the 110 (130) amino acid for glutamine. Several functional differences between the arginine type and the glutamine type have been demonstrated (30-32): (1) The glutamine type has lower affinity with the IL-13R α2 chain, a decoy receptor for IL-13, than the arginine type. (2) The glutamine type has enhanced stability over the arginine type (3). The glutamine type transduces a stronger signal via IL-13Rα1, a functional receptor for IL-13, than the arginine type. All of these results suggest that the glutamine type acts more potently *in vivo* than the arginine type. It has been reproducibly demonstrated that this SNP is genetically associated with serum total IgE levels (33-35), specific anti-allergen IgE (33, 35), or AD (36).

-1055C/T was originally found to be associated with bronchial asthma and positive skin tests (37, 38). This SNP is adjacent to the biding site for NFAT; hence, this variant may affect the complex formation of transcriptional factors. Reproducible genetic associations of this SNP with serum total IgE levels (34, 39), specific anti-allergen IgE (35, 40), or AD (39) have been observed.

3.3 IL-4Rα gene

The type II IL-4R or the IL-13R is composed of IL-4Rα and IL-13Rα1. Both IL-4 and IL-13 bind to this receptor on cell surface, transducing their signals intracellularly (5, 6). Several SNPs on the *IL4RA* gene are known to be genetically associated with atopy or allergic diseases. The genetic association of Gln576Arg, also referred as Gln551Arg, was originally found in hyper IgE syndrome patients, some of who had severe AD (41). Position 576 is adjacent to the tyrosine residue at 575, a binding site for SHP-1, a phosphotyrosine phosphatase. Exchange of glutamine for arginine decreases the binding activities for SHP-1, resulting in up-regulation of STAT6 activation. The genetic association of this SNP with AD was confirmed by another group (42).

3.4 IL-13α1 gene

IL-13Rα1 is another component of type II IL-4R/IL-13R, together with IL-4Rα. A SNP in the coding region of the *IL13RA1* gene, 1398A/G, was reported to be genetically associated with serum IgE levels (27). The function of this SNP is unclear because this SNP is a silent one.

3.5 STAT6 gene

STAT6 is a transcriptional factor, critical for both IL-4 and IL-13 signals (5, 6). Heterodimerization of type I IL-4R or type II IL-4R/IL-13R by binding of IL-4 or IL-13 activates Jak1, Jak3, or Tyk2, tyrosine kinases associated with IL-4Rα, common γ, and IL-13Rα1 respectively, followed by activation of STAT6. Several SNPs on the *STAT6* gene, 2964G/A, in18SNP1C/T, and GT repeat in exon1 were reported to be associated with serum IgE levels or with eosinophil numbers (43, 44).

3.6 IL-5 gene

A SNP on the IL5 gene (-703C/T) was reported to be associated with the numbers of eosinophils in blood and serum IgE levels, but not with AD (45).

4. Th2-type cytokine – Targeted treatment for AD

Because of the importance of Th2-type cytokines in the pathogenesis of AD, it has been thought that Th2-type cytokines have the potential to be targeted to develop novel agents against AD. A clinical trial to administer a humanized anti–IL-5 monoclonal Ab (mepolizumab) to AD patients was performed, with a disappointing result (46). To the best of our knowledge, no trial targeting IL-4 or IL-13 for AD patients has thus far been performed.

4.1 Antagonist of IL-5 for treatment of AD

AD patients received 750 mg of humanized anti–IL-5 monoclonal Abs (mepolizumab) intravenously twice (at day 0 and 7) (46). Efficacy assessed by SCORAD was observed at day 14 but was not statistically significant. There was no difference in pruritis score between mepolizumab- and placebo-administered groups. Even when efficacy was assessed by PGA (the Physician's Global Assessment of Improvement), the numbers showing 'marked improvement' were not statistically significant. However, it is of note that 4 of 18 (22.2%) patients receiving mepolizumab showed 'marked improvement'. These results can be interpreted two ways: one is that the overall efficacy of mepolizumab is not as good as expected. The other is that mepolizumab is effective only for limited patients. The latter is likely when mepolizumab is administered to patients with bronchial asthma. In the first clinical trial, mepolizumab yielded a disappointing result (47, 48). However, it turned out that mepolizumab is quite effective for the patients with sputa containing large numbers of eosinophils (49, 50). It is important to select patients who are sensitive to certain molecular target drugs by so-called 'companion diagnostics': in this case, numbers of eosinophils in sputum. A companion diagnostic should be found to treat AD effectively with mepolizumab.

5. Conclusion

In this chapter, we summarized the studies concerned with Th2-type cytokines in the pathogenesis of AD from the standpoint of the model mice and genetic association. Furthermore, we mentioned a trial in which AD patients were treated by administration of neutralizing Abs against IL-5. We hope the information in this review will be useful in developing new treatments for AD patients in the future.

6. Acknowledgement

We thank Dr. Dovie R. Wylie for critical review of this manuscript. This work was supported in part by Grants-in-Aid for Scientific Research from the Japan Society for the Promotion of Science.

7. References

[1] Leung, D. Y., Boguniewicz, M., Howell, M. D., Nomura, I. & Hamid, Q. A. (2004). New insights into atopic dermatitis. *J Clin Invest,* 113, pp.651-657.

[2] Oyoshi, M. K., He, R., Kumar, L., Yoon, J. & Geha, R. S. (2009). Cellular and molecular mechanisms in atopic dermatitis. *Adv Immunol,* 102, pp.135-226.

[3] Hamid, Q., Boguniewicz, M. & Leung, D. Y. (1994). Differential in situ cytokine gene expression in acute versus chronic atopic dermatitis. *J Clin Invest,* 94, pp.870-876.

[4] Hamid, Q., Naseer, T., Minshall, E. M., Song, Y. L., Boguniewicz, M. & Leung, D. Y. (1996). In vivo expression of IL-12 and IL-13 in atopic dermatitis. *J Allergy Clin Immunol,* 98, pp.225-231.

[5] Izuhara, K., Arima, K. & Yasunaga, S. (2002). IL-4 and IL-13: their pathological roles in allergic diseases and their potential in developing new therapies. *Curr Drug Targets Inflamm Allergy,* 1, pp.263-269.

[6] Izuhara, K., Arima, K., Kanaji, S., Ohta, S. & Kanaji, T. (2006). IL-13: a promising therapeutic target for bronchial asthma. *Curr Med Chem,* 13, pp.2291-2298.

[7] Nelms, K., Keegan, A. D., Zamorano, J., Ryan, J. J. & Paul, W. E. (1999). The IL-4 receptor: signaling mechanisms and biologic functions. *Annu Rev Immunol,* 17, pp.701-738.

[8] Wynn, T. A. (2003). IL-13 effector functions. *Annu Rev Immunol,* 21, pp.425-456.

[9] Takatsu, K., Kouro, T. & Nagai, Y. (2009). Interleukin 5 in the link between the innate and acquired immune response. *Adv Immunol,* 101, pp.191-236.

[10] Martinez-Moczygemba, M. & Huston, D. P. (2003). Biology of common β receptor-signaling cytokines: IL-3, IL-5, and GM-CSF. *J Allergy Clin Immunol,* 112, pp.653-665; quiz 666.

[11] Matsuda, H., Watanabe, N., Geba, G. P., Sperl, J., Tsudzuki, M., Hiroi, J., Matsumoto, M., Ushio, H., Saito, S., Askenase, P. W. & Ra, C. (1997). Development of atopic dermatitis-like skin lesion with IgE hyperproduction in NC/Nga mice. *Int Immunol,* 9, pp.461-466.

[12] Hikita, I., Yoshioka, T., Mizoguchi, T., Tsukahara, K., Tsuru, K., Nagai, H., Hirasawa, T., Tsuruta, Y., Suzuki, R., Ichihashi, M. & Horikawa, T. (2002). Characterization of dermatitis arising spontaneously in DS-Nh mice maintained under conventional conditions: another possible model for atopic dermatitis. *J Dermatol Sci,* 30, pp.142-153.

[13] Yagi, R., Nagai, H., Iigo, Y., Akimoto, T., Arai, T. & Kubo, M. (2002). Development of atopic dermatitis-like skin lesions in STAT6-deficient NC/Nga mice. *J Immunol,* 168, pp.2020-2027.

[14] Spergel, J. M., Mizoguchi, E., Brewer, J. P., Martin, T. R., Bhan, A. K. & Geha, R. S. (1998). Epicutaneous sensitization with protein antigen induces localized allergic dermatitis and hyperresponsiveness to methacholine after single exposure to aerosolized antigen in mice. *J Clin Invest,* 101, pp.1614-1622.

[15] Spergel, J. M., Mizoguchi, E., Oettgen, H., Bhan, A. K. & Geha, R. S. (1999). Roles of TH1 and TH2 cytokines in a murine model of allergic dermatitis. *J Clin Invest,* 103, pp.1103-1111.

[16] Chan, L. S., Robinson, N. & Xu, L. (2001). Expression of interleukin-4 in the epidermis of transgenic mice results in a pruritic inflammatory skin disease: an experimental animal model to study atopic dermatitis. *J Invest Dermatol,* 117, pp.977-983.

[17] Chen, L., Martinez, O., Overbergh, L., Mathieu, C., Prabhakar, B. S. & Chan, L. S. (2004). Early up-regulation of Th2 cytokines and late surge of Th1 cytokines in an atopic dermatitis model. *Clin Exp Immunol,* 138, pp.375-387.

[18] Chen, L., Martinez, O., Venkataramani, P., Lin, S. X., Prabhakar, B. S. & Chan, L. S. (2005). Correlation of disease evolution with progressive inflammatory cell activation and migration in the IL-4 transgenic mouse model of atopic dermatitis. *Clin Exp Immunol,* 139, pp.189-201.

[19] Chen, L., Lin, S. X., Overbergh, L., Mathieu, C. & Chan, L. S. (2005). The disease progression in the keratin 14 IL-4-transgenic mouse model of atopic dermatitis parallels the up-regulation of B cell activation molecules, proliferation and surface and serum IgE. *Clin Exp Immunol,* 142, pp.21-30.

[20] Zheng, T., Oh, M. H., Oh, S. Y., Schroeder, J. T., Glick, A. B. & Zhu, Z. (2009). Transgenic expression of interleukin-13 in the skin induces a pruritic dermatitis and skin remodeling. *J Invest Dermatol,* 129, pp.742-751.

[21] Marsh, D. G., Neely, J. D., Breazeale, D. R., Ghosh, B., Freidhoff, L. R., Ehrlich-Kautzky, E., Schou, C., Krishnaswamy, G. & Beaty, T. H. (1994). Linkage analysis of IL4 and other chromosome 5q31.1 markers and total serum immunoglobulin E concentrations. *Science,* 264, pp.1152-1156.

[22] Moffatt, M. F., Gut, I. G., Demenais, F., Strachan, D. P., Bouzigon, E., Heath, S., von Mutius, E., Farrall, M., Lathrop, M. & Cookson, W. O. (2010). A large-scale, consortium-based genomewide association study of asthma. *N Engl J Med,* 363, pp.1211-1221.

[23] Weidinger, S., Gieger, C., Rodriguez, E., Baurecht, H., Mempel, M., Klopp, N., Gohlke, H., Wagenpfeil, S., Ollert, M., Ring, J., Behrendt, H., Heinrich, J., Novak, N., Bieber, T., Kramer, U., Berdel, D., von Berg, A., Bauer, C. P., Herbarth, O., Koletzko, S., Prokisch, H., Mehta, D., Meitinger, T., Depner, M., von Mutius, E., Liang, L., Moffatt, M., Cookson, W., Kabesch, M., Wichmann, H. E. & Illig, T. (2008). Genome-wide scan on total serum IgE levels identifies FCER1A as novel susceptibility locus. *PLoS Genet,* 4, pp.e1000166.

[24] Rosenwasser, L. J., Klemm, D. J., Dresback, J. K., Inamura, H., Mascali, J. J., Klinnert, M. & Borish, L. (1995). Promoter polymorphisms in the chromosome 5 gene cluster in asthma and atopy. *Clin Exp Allergy,* 25 Suppl 2, pp.74-78; discussion 95-76.

[25] Kawashima, T., Noguchi, E., Arinami, T., Yamakawa-Kobayashi, K., Nakagawa, H., Otsuka, F. & Hamaguchi, H. (1998). Linkage and association of an interleukin 4 gene polymorphism with atopic dermatitis in Japanese families. *J Med Genet,* 35, pp.502-504.

[26] Söderhäll, C., Bradley, M., Kockum, I., Luthman, H., Wahlgren, C. F. & Nordenskjöld, M. (2002). Analysis of association and linkage for the interleukin-4 and interleukin-4 receptor α regions in Swedish atopic dermatitis families. *Clin Exp Allergy,* 32, pp.1199-1202.

[27] Heinzmann, A., Mao, X. Q., Akaiwa, M., Kreomer, R. T., Gao, P. S., Ohshima, K., Umeshita, R., Abe, Y., Braun, S., Yamashita, T., Roberts, M. H., Sugimoto, R., Arima, K., Arinobu, Y., Yu, B., Kruse, S., Enomoto, T., Dake, Y., Kawai, M., Shimazu, S., Sasaki, S., Adra, C. N., Kitaichi, M., Inoue, H., Yamauchi, K., Tomichi, N., Kurimoto, F., Hamasaki, N., Hopkin, J. M., Izuhara, K., Shirakawa, T. & Deichmann, K. A. (2000). Genetic variants of IL-13 signalling and human asthma and atopy. *Hum Mol Genet,* 9, pp.549-559.

[28] Graves, P. E., Kabesch, M., Halonen, M., Holberg, C. J., Baldini, M., Fritzsch, C., Weiland, S. K., Erickson, R. P., von Mutius, E. & Martinez, F. D. (2000). A cluster of seven tightly linked polymorphisms in the IL-13 gene is associated with total serum IgE levels in three populations of white children. *J Allergy Clin Immunol,* 105, pp.506-513.

[29] Liu, X., Nickel, R., Beyer, K., Wahn, U., Ehrlich, E., Freidhoff, L. R., Bjorksten, B., Beaty, T. H. & Huang, S. K. (2000). An *IL13* coding region variant is associated with a high total serum IgE level and atopic dermatitis in the German multicenter atopy study (MAS-90). *J Allergy Clin Immunol,* 106, pp.167-170.

[30] Arima, K., Umeshita-Suyama, R., Sakata, Y., Akaiwa, M., Mao, X. Q., Enomoto, T., Dake, Y., Shimazu, S., Yamashita, T., Sugawara, N., Brodeur, S., Geha, R., Puri, R. K., Sayegh, M. H., Adra, C. N., Hamasaki, N., Hopkin, J. M., Shirakawa, T. & Izuhara, K. (2002). Upregulation of IL-13 concentration in vivo by the *IL13* variant associated with bronchial asthma. *J Allergy Clin Immunol,* 109, pp.980-987.

[31] Chen, W., Ericksen, M. B., Levin, L. S. & Khurana Hershey, G. K. (2004). Functional effect of the R110Q *IL13* genetic variant alone and in combination with *IL4RA* genetic variants. *J Allergy Clin Immunol,* 114, pp.553-560.

[32] Vladich, F. D., Brazille, S. M., Stern, D., Peck, M. L., Ghittoni, R. & Vercelli, D. (2005). IL-13 R130Q, a common variant associated with allergy and asthma, enhances effector mechanisms essential for human allergic inflammation. *J Clin Invest,* 115, pp.747-754.

[33] Leung, T. F., Tang, N. L., Chan, I. H., Li, A. M., Ha, G. & Lam, C. W. (2001). A polymorphism in the coding region of interleukin-13 gene is associated with atopy but not asthma in Chinese children. *Clin Exp Allergy,* 31, pp.1515-1521.

[34] Liu, X., Beaty, T. H., Deindl, P., Huang, S. K., Lau, S., Sommerfeld, C., Fallin, M. D., Kao, W. H., Wahn, U. & Nickel, R. (2003). Associations between total serum IgE levels and the 6 potentially functional variants within the genes *IL4, IL13,* and *IL4RA* in German children: the German Multicenter Atopy Study. *J Allergy Clin Immunol,* 112, pp.382-388.

[35] Zitnik, S. E., Ruschendorf, F., Muller, S., Sengler, C., Lee, Y. A., Griffioen, R. W., Meglio, P., Wahn, U., Witt, H. & Nickel, R. (2009). *IL13* variants are associated with total serum IgE and early sensitization to food allergens in children with atopic dermatitis. *Pediatr Allergy Immunol,* 20, pp.551-555.

[36] Tsunemi, Y., Saeki, H., Nakamura, K., Sekiya, T., Hirai, K., Kakinuma, T., Fujita, H., Asano, N., Tanida, Y., Wakugawa, M., Torii, H. & Tamaki, K. (2002). Interleukin-13 gene polymorphism G4257A is associated with atopic dermatitis in Japanese patients. *J Dermatol Sci,* 30, pp.100-107.

[37] van der Pouw Kraan, T. C., van Veen, A., Boeije, L. C., van Tuyl, S. A., de Groot, E. R., Stapel, S. O., Bakker, A., Verweij, C. L., Aarden, L. A. & van der Zee, J. S. (1999). An IL-13 promoter polymorphism associated with increased risk of allergic asthma. *Genes Immun,* 1, pp.61-65.

[38] Howard, T. D., Whittaker, P. A., Zaiman, A. L., Koppelman, G. H., Xu, J., Hanley, M. T., Meyers, D. A., Postma, D. S. & Bleecker, E. R. (2001). Identification and association of polymorphisms in the interleukin-13 gene with asthma and atopy in a Dutch population. *Am J Respir Cell Mol Biol,* 25, pp.377-384.

[39] Hummelshoj, T., Bodtger, U., Datta, P., Malling, H. J., Oturai, A., Poulsen, L. K., Ryder, L. P., Sorensen, P. S., Svejgaard, E. & Svejgaard, A. (2003). Association between an interleukin-13 promoter polymorphism and atopy. *Eur J Immunogenet,* 30, pp.355-359.

[40] Liu, X., Beaty, T. H., Deindl, P., Huang, S. K., Lau, S., Sommerfeld, C., Fallin, M. D., Kao, W. H., Wahn, U. & Nickel, R. (2004). Associations between specific serum IgE response and 6 variants within the genes *IL4, IL13,* and *IL4RA* in German children: the German Multicenter Atopy Study. *J Allergy Clin Immunol,* 113, pp.489-495.

[41] Hershey, G. K., Friedrich, M. F., Esswein, L. A., Thomas, M. L. & Chatila, T. A. (1997). The association of atopy with a gain-of-function mutation in the α subunit of the interleukin-4 receptor. *N Engl J Med,* 337, pp.1720-1725.

[42] Oiso, N., Fukai, K. & Ishii, M. (2000). Interleukin 4 receptor α chain polymorphism Gln551Arg is associated with adult atopic dermatitis in Japan. *Br J Dermatol,* 142, pp.1003-1006.

[43] Gao, P. S., Mao, X. Q., Roberts, M. H., Arinobu, Y., Akaiwa, M., Enomoto, T., Dake, Y., Kawai, M., Sasaki, S., Hamasaki, N., Izuhara, K., Shirakawa, T. & Hopkin, J. M. (2000). Variants of *STAT6* (signal transducer and activator of transcription 6) in atopic asthma. *J Med Genet,* 37, pp.380-382.

[44] Duetsch, G., Illig, T., Loesgen, S., Rohde, K., Klopp, N., Herbon, N., Gohlke, H., Altmueller, J. & Wjst, M. (2002). *STAT6* as an asthma candidate gene: polymorphism-screening, association and haplotype analysis in a Caucasian sib-pair study. *Hum Mol Genet,* 11, pp.613-621.

[45] Yamamoto, N., Sugiura, H., Tanaka, K. & Uehara, M. (2003). Heterogeneity of interleukin 5 genetic background in atopic dermatitis patients: significant difference between those with blood eosinophilia and normal eosinophil levels. *J Dermatol Sci,* 33, pp.121-126.

[46] Oldhoff, J. M., Darsow, U., Werfel, T., Katzer, K., Wulf, A., Laifaoui, J., Hijnen, D. J., Plotz, S., Knol, E. F., Kapp, A., Bruijnzeel-Koomen, C. A., Ring, J. & de Bruin-Weller, M. S. (2005). Anti-IL-5 recombinant humanized monoclonal antibody (mepolizumab) for the treatment of atopic dermatitis. *Allergy,* 60, pp.693-696.

[47] Leckie, M. J., ten Brinke, A., Khan, J., Diamant, Z., O'Connor, B. J., Walls, C. M., Mathur, A. K., Cowley, H. C., Chung, K. F., Djukanovic, R., Hansel, T. T., Holgate, S. T., Sterk, P. J. & Barnes, P. J. (2000). Effects of an interleukin-5 blocking monoclonal antibody on eosinophils, airway hyper-responsiveness, and the late asthmatic response. *Lancet,* 356, pp.2144-2148.

[48] Kips, J. C., O'Connor, B. J., Langley, S. J., Woodcock, A., Kerstjens, H. A., Postma, D. S., Danzig, M., Cuss, F. & Pauwels, R. A. (2003). Effect of SCH55700, a humanized anti-human interleukin-5 antibody, in severe persistent asthma: a pilot study. *Am J Respir Crit Care Med,* 167, pp.1655-1659.

[49] Haldar, P., Brightling, C. E., Hargadon, B., Gupta, S., Monteiro, W., Sousa, A., Marshall, R. P., Bradding, P., Green, R. H., Wardlaw, A. J. & Pavord, I. D. (2009). Mepolizumab and exacerbations of refractory eosinophilic asthma. *N Engl J Med,* 360, pp.973-984.

[50] Nair, P., Pizzichini, M. M., Kjarsgaard, M., Inman, M. D., Efthimiadis, A., Pizzichini, E., Hargreave, F. E. & O'Byrne, P. M. (2009). Mepolizumab for prednisone-dependent asthma with sputum eosinophilia. *N Engl J Med,* 360, pp.985-993.

5

The Role of Prostanoids in Atopic Dermatitis

Tetsuya Honda and Kenji Kabashima
Department of Dermatology, Kyoto University Graduate School of Medicine, Kyoto
Japan

1. Introduction

Atopic dermatitis (AD) is a common pruritic and chronic inflammatory skin disease, with a prevalence of up to 3% among adults and up to 25% among children (Bieber; Guttman-Yassky et al.; Odhiambo et al., 2009). The clinical features of AD are varied, with patients generally having dry skin, but wet eczematous lesions in the acute stage and lichenification lesions in the chronic stage (Guttman-Yassky et al., 2011). In terms of histology, an increased number of lymphocytes, eosinophils, and mast cells in the dermis are detected. A barrier defect with decreased cornification and epidermal hyperplasia are also characteristic features of AD (Elias and Schmuth, 2009; Guttman-Yassky et al., 2009).

AD is a multi-factorial disease that arises from complex interaction between genetic and environmental factors. As for its pathogenesis, two models have been proposed: the outside-in model and the inside-out model (Bieber, 2008). In the outside-in model, the decreased skin barrier function caused by genetic defects, such as mutations in filaggrin, allows for the penetration of large immunogenic proteins, which subsequently cause T helper type 2 (Th2) deviated immune activation (Elias et al., 2008; Elias and Schmuth, 2009). In the inside-out model, activation of Th2 cells results in reactive epidermal hyperplasia (Nograles et al.; Ong and Leung, 2006). It has been proposed that the lack of environmental antigens during childhood lead to reduced T helper type 1 (Th1) cell-mediated immunity and increased activation of Th2 cells (hygiene hypothesis). In recent reports, involvements of T helper type 17 (Th17) cells and T helper type 22 (Th22) cells have also been proposed (Koga et al., 2008; Nograles et al., 2009).

As for the treatment of AD, various therapies have been employed, and the use of topical steroids plays a major role in therapies (Guttman-Yassky et al.). Although the use of topical corticosteroids is the first-line therapy and provides rapid relief of symptoms, prolonged use can cause severe side effects such as skin atrophy. Therefore, alternative therapies with fewer and less extreme side effects are needed.

2. Characteristics of prostanoids

When tissues are exposed to diverse pathophysiological stimuli, arachidonic acid (AA) is released from membrane phospholipids and converted to lipid mediators, such as prostanoids, leukotrienes (LTs) and hydroxy-eicosatetraenoic acids (HETEs). Prostanoids, including prostaglandins (PG) and thromboxane (TX), are formed by the cyclooxygenase (COX) pathway, whereas LTs and HETEs are formed by the 5-, 12- and 15-lipoxygenase (LO) pathways. COX has two isoforms, COX-1 and COX-2. While COX-1 is constitutively expressed in cells, COX-2 requires specific stimulation by substances such as acetone and the phorbol ester TPA (Narumiya et al., 1999; Scholz et al., 1995). This reaction results in the formation of an unstable endoperoxide intermediate PGH_2, which, in turn, is metabolized to PGD_2, PGE_2, PGF_{2a}, PGI_2, and thromboxane TXA_2 by specific synthases.

Prostanoids are released from cells immediately after their formation. Because they are chemically and metabolically unstable, they usually function only locally through their specific membrane receptors on target cells (Narumiya et al., 1999). Nine types and subtypes of membrane prostanoid receptors are conserved in mammals from mouse to human: two subtypes of the PGD receptor (DP (DP1) and the chemoattractant receptor homologous-molecule expressed on Th2 cells, CRTH2 (DP2)), four subtypes of the PGE receptor (EP1, EP2, EP3, and EP4), the PGF receptor (FP), the PGI receptor (IP), and the TXA receptor (TP) (Figure 1). All are G protein-coupled rhodopsin-type receptors with seven transmembrane domains (Figure 1). The main signal transduction mechanisms of these prostanoid receptors are through the regulation of intracellular cyclic adenosine monophosphate (cAMP) concentration and intracellular free calcium concentration. DP, EP2, EP4 and IP are Gs-coupled receptors and elevate intracellular cAMP concentration, while EP3 and CRTH2 are Gi-coupled receptors and decrease intracellular cAMP. EP1, FP and TP are Gq and other G protein-coupled receptors, which increase intracellular calcium concentration (Narumiya et al., 1999). However, most prostanoid receptors may bind with more than one G protein-coupled receptors via their specific signaling pathway. Recently, individual prostanoid receptor gene-deficient mice have been used as models to dissect out the respective roles of each receptor in combination with the use of compounds that selectively bind to prostanoid

Figure 1

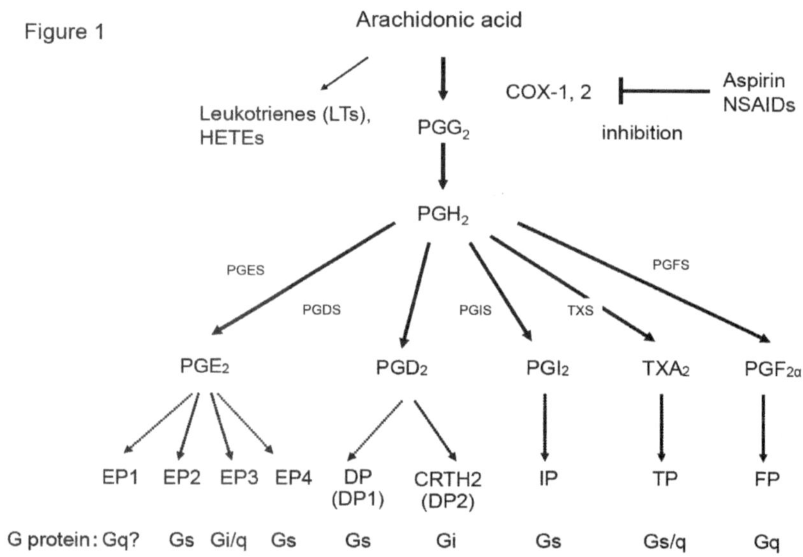

Fig. 1. Biosynthetic pathways of prostanoids. The formation of PGD_2, PGE_2, PGF_{2a}, PGG_2, PGH_2, and PGI_2, and TXA_2 from arachidonic acid is shown. The first two steps of the pathway (i.e., conversion of arachidonic acid to PGG_2 and then to PGH_2) are catalyzed by COX, and the subsequent conversion of PGH_2 to each prostanoid is catalyzed by the respective synthase as shown. All are G protein-coupled rhodopsin-type receptors.

receptors as agonists or antagonists (Narumiya and FitzGerald, 2001). These genetic and pharmacological approaches have revealed new roles for prostanoids and their receptors in allergic and immune diseases (Honda et al., 2010).
In this chapter, we will discuss the recent findings regarding the role of prostanoids in skin immunity, and discuss the possible involvement of prostanoids in the pathogenesis of AD, and also the clinical potential of receptor-selective drugs as a new therapeutic target for AD.

3. Production of prostanoids in skin

Human bodies are exposed to external stimuli continuously. The skin plays an important role in self-defense during exposure to foreign antigens and consists of a vast array of immune cells, such as keratinocytes (KCs), T cells, B cells, mast cells, eosinophils, fibroblasts, and two types of cutaneous dendritic cells (DCs) including epidermal Langerhans cells (LCs) and dermal DCs (dDCs). In the normal human skin, immunohistochemical examinations have revealed that COX-1 is observed throughout the epidermis, whereas COX-2 exists in more differentiated suprabasilar KCs and outer root sheath cells of hair follicles (Leong et al., 1996; Torii et al., 2002). Among prostanoids, PGE_2 is the main COX product in human epidermal homogenates (Hammarstrom et al., 1979). PGD_2 has been detected in human skin (Hammarstrom et al., 1979), and PGD synthase is present predominantly in LCs, dDCs, dermal macrophages and mast cells, but not in KCs (Ruzicka and Aubock, 1987; Ujihara et al., 1988). Among these, mast cells have been found to be one of the major cellular sources of PGD_2. TX synthase activity has been found in keratinocytes (Andoh et al., 2007) and high levels of TXB_2, as a metabolite of TXA_2, were detected in the cultured supernatant of LCs and DCs (Kabashima et al., 2003a). PGI_2 was detected in the skin of the murine AD model (Sugimoto et al., 2006). PGF_{2a}, was observed in skin exudates of nickel allergy patients (Lerche et al., 1989). In biopsy specimens from patients with AD, PGE_2 has been determined in biologically active amounts in both lesional and perilesional skin (Fogh et al., 1989). In contrast, normal levels of eicosanoids were found in the uninvolved skin of these patients. The above findings on the synthesis of prostanoids are summarized in Table 1.

4. Prostanoid receptor expression in skin

Adult human KCs express mRNA for all subtypes of PGE_2 receptors (Konger et al., 1998; Tober et al., 2006) and the expression of all PGE_2 receptors has been detected in mouse KCs by immunohistochemistry (Tober et al., 2007). Mouse LCs and DCs express DP (Angeli et al., 2001), EP1, 2, 3, 4 (Kabashima et al., 2003b), and IP (Huang et al., 2001), and T cells express EP1, 2, 3, 4 (Tilley et al., 2001), IP (Takahashi et al., 2002) and TP (Nataraj et al., 2001). PGE_2 suppresses T cell proliferation and differentiation in the thymus, and interleukin (IL)-1 production by acting at EP2 and EP4 *in vitro* (Nataraj et al., 2001). Mast cells express EP1, 2, 3, 4, DP, and IP (Fedyk and Phipps, 1996; Tilley et al., 2001), and PGE_2 acts at EP3 to suppress their degranulation (Kunikata et al., 2005). Human eosinophils express EP2, EP4, DP, CRTH2 and TP (Nguyen et al., 2002; Schratl et al., 2007), and PGE_2 seems to prolong eosinophil survival (Mita et al., 2002; Peacock et al., 1999). PGE_2 suppresses TNF-a production and enhances IL-6 production from neutrophils stimulated by lipopolysaccharide (LPS) through EP2 and EP4 (Nguyen et al., 2002; Yamane et al., 2000). As summarized in Table 1, prostanoids and their receptors are produced and expressed by a wide variety of cells in the skin. This varied expression pattern of prostanoids maintains the homeostasis of the human body.

	PGDS	PGES	PGFS	PGIS	TXS	DP	CRTH2	EP1	EP2	EP3	EP4	FP	IP	TP
Keratinocytes	m	m, h			m			m, h	m, h	m, h	m, h			m,h
hLangerhans cells	h	m, h			m	m, h		m	m	m	m			
Dendritic cells	h	m, h		m	m, h				m, h		m, h		m	
T cells							m, h(Th2)	m	m	m	m, h		m	m
B cells								m, h	m, h	m, h	m, h		m	
Macrophages	h	m, h		m	m, h		m	m	m	m	m, h			
Eosinophils	h	h	h		h	m	m,h		m, h		h			h
Mast cells, basophils	m, h				h	m, h	m, h	m	m	m	m			
Neutrophils		h			h	h	m		m, h		m			
Blood vessels		h	h	h				m, h	m, h	m, h	m, h		m, h	m, h

PG; prostaglandin, S; synthase, m; mouse, h; human
Modified from the reference by Tilley et al.

Table 1. Expression of prostanoid synthases and prostanoid receptors in the skin

5. Involvement of prostanoids in the pathogenesis of AD: Analysis based on animal models of AD

As mentioned above, there are multiple pathogenetic factors of AD, but the skin barrier dysfunction and Th2 mediated immune response are its general characteristic features.

Mouse ovalbumin (OVA)-induced dermatitis is one of the most frequently used AD models (He et al.; Spergel et al., 1998). In a typical mouse OVA-induced AD model, mice are first sensitized with an OVA patch using a transparent bio-occlusive dressing on a shaved and tape-stripped area of skin for one week. This sensitization to OVA is repeated in two-week intervals. After three to four sensitization cycles, the mice show elevated serum IgE and significant eosinophil and Th2-deviated lymphocyte infiltration in the skin, which is similar to the pathology of AD. In this model, COX-2 deficient mice and the administration of COX-2 inhibitor both showed enhanced eosinophil infiltration and elevated IL-4 expression in the skin lesion with elevated serum IgE and IgG1 (Laouini et al., 2005). These results suggest that COX-2-derived prostanoids play regulatory roles in the development of AD, such as Th differentiation and inflammatory cell infiltration in the skin. In the following sections, we will discuss how prostanoids are involved in Th differentiation, DC function, and inflammatory cell infiltration in skin immunity.

6. Prostanoids as regulatory factors of Th differentiation

In older *in vitro* studies, PGE_2 has been regarded as a suppressant of Th1 cells, because of its suppressive effect on cell proliferation, differentiation and cytokine production from Th1 cells (Betz and Fox, 1991; Goodwin and Ceuppens, 1983). However, recent reports indicate that several PGE_2 receptors are involved in the regulation of Th differentiation in skin immunity via multiple pathways and different directions (Figure 2).

For example, PGE_2-EP1 signaling has been reported to facilitate Th1 differentiation in the sensitization process through the skin (Nagamachi et al., 2007). PGE_2 produced by DCs in draining lymph nodes (dLNs) stimulates EP1 receptors on naïve $CD4^+$ and $CD8^+$ T cells and promotes Th1 and Tc1 differentiation (Nagamachi et al., 2007). PGI_2-IP signaling promotes Th1 and Tc1 differentiation through a cAMP dependent mechanism (Nakajima et al., 2010). Intriguingly, IP deficient mice showed enhanced Th2 response such as elevated IgE concentration in serum in the mouse OVA-induced asthma model (Nagao et al., 2003), suggesting that lack of PGI_2-IP signaling might result in a Th2 biased immune response through the inhibition of Th1 differentiation.

The regulatory mechanism of prostanoid signaling on Th differentiation is complex, because it depends on the context of immune system. For example, PGE_2-EP2/EP4 signaling regulates Th1 and Th17 differentiation (Yao et al., 2009). In a weaker co-stimulation signaling through CD28, PGE_2 suppresses the Th1 differentiation via EP2 and EP4 receptors. In the case of strong co-stimulation signaling, however, stimulation of EP2 and EP4 signaling conversely facilitates the Th1 differentiation through a PI3-kinase-dependent mechanism (Yao et al., 2009). These results suggest that the action of prostanoid receptor signaling can be changed in a context-dependent manner. EP2 and EP4 signaling also regulates the Th17 differentiation. Th17 is a recently identified Th subset, and can be detected in a number of diseases, including AD (Guttman-Yassky et al., 2011; Koga et al., 2008). *In vitro,* Th17 differentiation is induced from naïve T cells in the presence of IL-6 and TGF-b. In this condition, PGE_2 acts on naïve T cells through EP2/EP4 signaling and suppress the Th17 differentiation in a cAMP-dependent manner. However, PGE_2-EP2/EP4 signaling also acts on DCs and increases the IL-23 production from the DCs. Thus, PGE_2 facilitates the expansion of Th17 (Yao et al., 2009). The blockade of EP4 signaling consistently ameliorated the disease progression in a CHS model and an EAE model, which are mediated by Th1 and Th17 cells, respectively (Yao et al., 2009). These results clearly indicate the importance of prostanoid signaling in Th differentiation *in vivo.* The facilitation effect of PGE_2 on Th17 is also reported in human T cells (Boniface et al., 2009).

7. Prostanoids as regulatory factors of DC function

In the initial step of sensitization in AD, allergens which enter the skin are captured by skin DCs and presented to the naïve T cells in the dLNs. Prostanoids can regulate this step by affecting the migration ability or antigen presentation ability of the skin DCs (Figure 2). PGE_2, which is produced by KCs, acts on EP4 on LCs, and stimulates the migration of LCs (Kabashima et al., 2003b). Conversely, stimulation of DP on DCs inhibits the migration of skin DCs. Topical administration of DP inhibits the migration of DCs to dLNs and significantly suppresses the development of the mouse AD model (Angeli et al., 2001; Angeli et al., 2004). Prostanoids also regulate DC-T cell interaction in the priming of naïve T cells (Kabashima et al., 2003a). Cutaneous DCs produce abundant TXA_2, which acts on naïve T cells and increases the motility of T cells, which impairs the stable DC-T cell interaction (Kabashima et al., 2003a). TP-deficient mice or wild-type mice treated with a TP antagonist during the sensitization period show enhanced CHS responses, indicating that TP signaling negatively regulates the priming of T cells *in vivo*.

Although the role of IgE in AD is still controversial (Guttman-Yassky et al., 2011), high serum IgE is one of the hallmarks of AD. Compared to the analysis of T cells and DCs, the reports about the role of prostanoids on B cells are relatively scarce. From the *in vivo* data using COX-2 deficient mice or IP deficient mice, which show increased IgE production in OVA sensitization

(Laouini et al., 2005), it might be possible that some prostanoid signaling regulates the antibody production. *In vitro*, PGE_2 drives Ig class switching to IgE by acting at EP2 and EP4 on B cells under LPS and IL-4 stimulation *in vitro* (Fedyk and Phipps, 1996). Whether such actions occur *in vivo* remains unknown, and this should be clarified in future studies.

8. Prostanoids and Treg induction

T regulatory cells (Treg) make up one of the T cell subsets which has potent suppressive functions in various disease models. There are several reports that analyzed Treg number and function in AD patients, but those results are not necessarily consistent (Brandt et al., 2009; Ou et al., 2004; Schnopp et al., 2007; Verhagen et al., 2006). However, considering the fact that loss of Treg in skin can lead to AD-like skin lesions in both human (Ochs et al., 2005) and mouse (Brunkow et al., 2001), it is very likely that Treg play important roles in the pathogenesis of AD.

It has been well known that ultraviolet (UV) radiation causes immunosuppression, and it is one of the effective treatment options for AD. Although multiple suppression mechanisms have been proposed, induction of Treg is considered one of the central factors for the suppression mechanism. As blocking of prostanoid production by treatment with non-steroidal anti-inflammatory drugs (NSAIDs) treatment can abolish the immunosuppressive effect through UV (Chung et al., 1986; Hart et al., 2002; Walterscheid et al., 2002), it has been suspected that prostanoids play important roles in the UV-induced immunosuppression, especially in Treg induction. By UV radiation, various prostanoids are produced in the skin, with PGE_2 being the most abundant prostanoids (Kuwamoto et al., 2000; Ruzicka et al., 1983; Soontrapa et al., 2011). Recently, it has been revealed that PGE_2-EP4 signaling mediates the induction of Treg by UV irradiation, and regulates UV-induced immunosuppression (Soontrapa et al.). Blockade of EP4 signaling suppresses the increase of Treg in dLNs and abolishes the immunosuppressive effect of UV. Blockade of EP4 signaling also diminishes the RANKL expression on KCs after UV irradiation (Soontrapa et al., 2011). It is known that RANKL expression on UV-irradiated KCs activates LCs, and the RANKL-activated LCs function to induce Treg in dLNs (Loser et al., 2006). These results indicate that PGE_2-EP4 signaling regulates RANKL expression on KCs and controls Treg induction from UV.

Other than PGE_2, it has been reported that PGD_2 induces Treg differentiation through DP in a mouse asthma model (Hammad et al., 2007). Inhalation of a selective DP1 agonist suppressed the cardinal features of asthma by targeting the function of lung DCs. In mice treated with a DP1 agonist or receiving DP1 agonist-treated DCs, there was an increase in Tregs that suppressed inflammation in an IL-10-dependent way (Hammad et al., 2007). These effects of a DP1 agonist on DCs were mediated by cyclic AMP-dependent protein kinase A. Taken together, control of EP4 and/or DP1 signaling could represent a novel immunosuppressive approach.

9. Prostanoids as inflammatory mediators

In an established AD lesion, numerous inflammatory mediators such as cytokines (e.g., IL-4, IL-5, IL-13) and chemokines (e.g., CCL5, CCL11, CCL17) contribute to the development of AD (Guttman-Yassky et al.).

As for the inflammatory mediators in AD lesions, the role of PGD_2-CRTH2 signaling has been the most frequently investigated. In the skin, PGD_2 is the major prostanoid produced by activated mast cells. PGD_2 has two types of receptors, DP and CRTH2. CRTH2 induces chemotaxis in Th2 cells, eosinophils and basophils with enhanced degranulation *in vitro* (Hirai et al., 2001; Yoshimura-Uchiyama et al., 2004). CRTH2 amplifies Th2 responses by preventing apoptosis of Th2 cells and enhancing their capacity to secrete cytokines (Nomiya et al., 2008; Xue et al., 2009). CRTH2 also amplifies eosinophil functions by mobilizing them from the bone marrow, preventing their apoptosis, and promoting their chemokinesis and degranulation (Gervais et al., 2001). CRTH2 mRNA expression is high in peripheral blood mononuclear cells of patients with AD (Hijnen et al., 2005), and circulating eosinophils and T cells in patients with AD have an increased surface expression of CRTH2 (Iwasaki et al., 2002), suggesting the role of CRTH2 in AD.

He et al. have recently reported that lack of CRTH2 signaling ameliorates the inflammation only in newly-challenged skin, while loss of this signaling in chronic challenged areas did not affect the inflammation (He et al., 2011). They used CRTH2 knockout mice in two types of AD models: one that was repeatedly sensitized with OVA for a total of seven weeks, which mimicked the chronic lesions of AD; and one that was challenged with OVA after the repeated sensitization of other skin areas for a total of seven weeks, which was supposed to mimic the acute lesions of AD. In the chronic lesions, the inflammatory cell infiltration and cytokine concentration was similar between wild-type and CRTH2 knockout mice, while in the acute lesions, such factors were significantly decreased in CRTH2 knockout mice compared with wild-type mice (He et al.). Consistently, the concentration of PGD_2 increased significantly in the acute lesions, while the concentration of PGD_2 in the chronic lesions was similar compared with that of non-affected skin. CRTH2 knockout mice also showed comparable levels of IgE production, indicating that CRTH2 signaling had little effect much on the antibody production process. Boehme et al. have previously reported that administration of a CRTH2 antagonist inhibited the development of chronic AD lesions in the same model (Boehme et al., 2009), but the CRTH2 antagonist-treated group also showed reduced IgE production, suggesting the possibility that administration of the CRTH2 antagonist affected the extent of sensitization non-specifically and thus lead to the reduced inflammatory cell infiltration in the skin. Collectively, blockage of PGD_2-CRTH2 signaling might inhibit allergic skin inflammation elicited in patients with AD by re-exposure to antigens to which they have been sensitized (Figure 3).

In contrast, stimulation of EP3-signaling in KCs is reported to play an anti-inflammatory role in skin inflammation by inhibiting chemokine production from KCs (Honda et al., 2009). Administration of an EP3 specific agonist suppressed a CHS response, and EP3 knockout mice showed an enhanced CHS response, suggesting that PGE_2-EP3 signaling works as a negative regulator of allergic cutaneous inflammation. An anti-inflammatory role of EP3 signaling is also reported in other allergic diseases such as mouse asthma and the allergic conjunctivitis model (Kunikata et al., 2005; Ueta et al., 2009).

10. Prostanoids as itch mediators

It is reported that some prostanoids can modulate pruritus, a significant hallmark of AD. In human studies, PGE_2 is a weak pruritogen and prolongs experimentally-induced itch (Hagermark and Strandberg, 1977; Neisius et al., 2002), although injection of PGE_2 alone does not elicit itch-associated response in animal experiments (Andoh and Kuraishi, 1998). TXA_2 is also reported as a mediator of itch (Andoh et al., 2007). Injection of a TP agonist alone elicited itch-associated responses. TP was expressed in both KCs and nerve fibers in skin (Andoh et al., 2007). TX synthase was also expressed in KCs. In some studies, the association of genetic polymorphisms in the TP gene with asthma and atopy has been reported (Shin et al., 2003). TXA_2 may be involved in the pathogenesis of atopic disease not only as an airway constriction factor but also as an itch mediator.

On the other hand, PGD_2 is reported to play anti-pruritic roles in the mouse AD model (Arai et al., 2004). Administration of PGD_2 and a DP1 agonist reduced scratching behaviors in an AD model using NC/Nga mice, while administration of a DP2 agonist did not reduce such behavior (Arai et al., 2004). Inhibition of histamine release from mast cells is proposed as a possible suppression mechanism of the DP signaling (Hashimoto et al., 2005). Blockade of TP signaling or stimulation of DP1 signaling may lead to a new target for the treatment of pruritic disease, including AD.

Figure 2

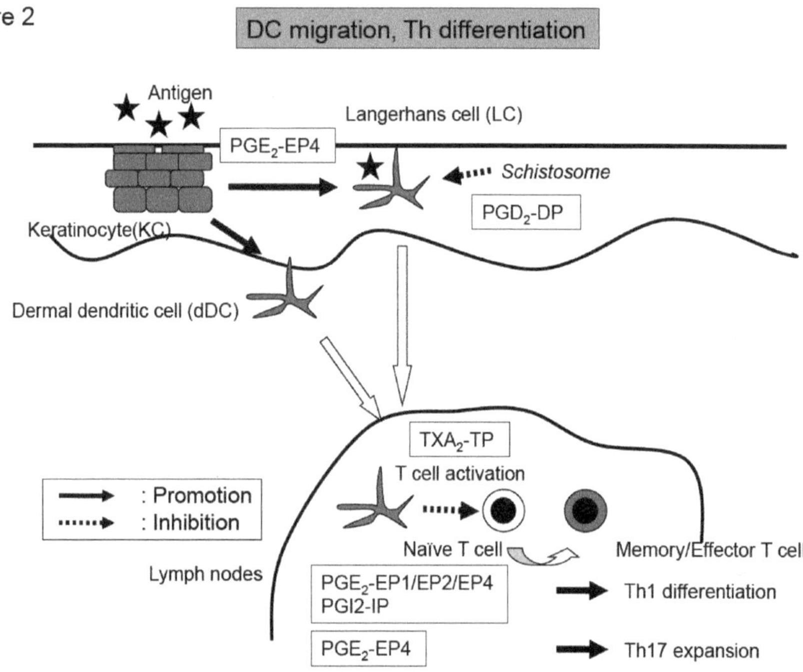

Fig. 2. Regulation of DC migration and Th differentiation by prostanoids

During the sensitization period, antigens induce pro-inflammatory cytokine secretion by KCs, which enhances cutaneous DC (LCs and dDCs) activation and migration to dLNs. In the LNs, cutaneous DCs activate naïve T cells that differentiate into mature memory T cells. During antigen exposure to the skin, KCs produce PGE_2 and mast cells produce PGD_2. Moreover, *schistosomes* produce PGD_2 during a helminthic infection. The PGE_2-EP4 pathway promotes, but PGD_2-DP and PGI_2-IP pathways inhibit cutaneous DC migration and maturation. TXA_2 produced by activated cutaneous DCs seems to act on naïve T cells to disrupt DC-T cell interaction. The PGE_2-EP1/EP2/EP4 pathways promote Th1 cell differentiation, and the PGE_2-EP4 pathway also promotes Th17 cell expansion.

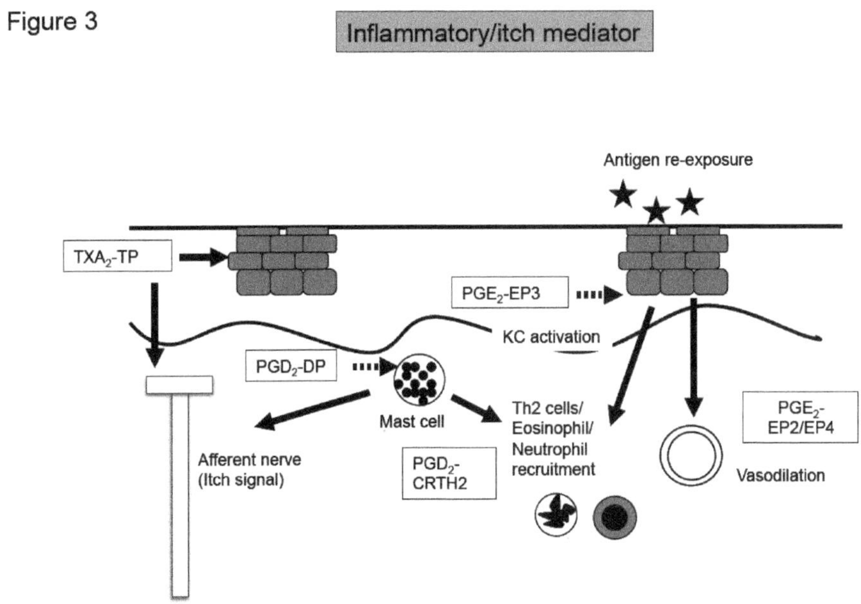

Fig. 3. Prostanoids as inflammatory/itch mediators

Repeated antigen exposure to the skin stimulates KCs to secrete pro-inflammatory cytokines, chemokines and other mediators, which activate the endothelial activation of blood vessels. This activation attracts memory T cell infiltration into the skin. PGE_2 dilates blood vessels possibly through EP2 and EP4. The PGD_2-CRTH2 signaling promotes Th2 cells/eosinophils/neutrophils infiltration in skin. The PGE_2-EP3 signaling inhibits KC activation and plays an anti-inflammatory role in CHS. The TP signaling mediates itch signaling through afferent nerves, while stimulation of DP signaling inhibits itch-associated responses.

11. Summary and future direction

NSAIDs, which block the production of all prostanoids, usually have limited effects on AD (Kabashima and Miyachi, 2004) and therefore have not been given so much attention as a potential therapeutic agent. However, the analysis using the receptor knockout mice and receptor specific drugs has revealed new unexpected roles of prostanoids in the immune systems. In addition, signaling from even the same receptor can produce the opposite effect depending on the context, such as the Th1 modulating effect generated through EP2/EP4 signaling (Yao et al., 2009). Therefore, it would be necessary to reconsider the role of prostanoids in the development of AD. It is also important to correlate these immunomodulatory actions of prostanoids found in mice to their actions in immune diseases of humans. Currently, CRTH2 antagonists are on their way to being used in clinical applications for AD or asthma (Ulven and Kostenis., 2010). Further analysis of the role of each prostanoid receptor has great potential in leading to a new therapeutic target for AD.

12. References

Andoh, T., and Kuraishi, Y. (1998). Intradermal leukotriene B4, but not prostaglandin E2, induces itch-associated responses in mice. Eur J Pharmacol *353*, 93-96.

Andoh, T., Nishikawa, Y., Yamaguchi-Miyamoto, T., Nojima, H., Narumiya, S., and Kuraishi, Y. (2007). Thromboxane A2 induces itch-associated responses through TP receptors in the skin in mice. J Invest Dermatol *127*, 2042-2047.

Angeli, V., Faveeuw, C., Roye, O., Fontaine, J., Teissier, E., Capron, A., Wolowczuk, I., Capron, M., and Trottein, F. (2001). Role of the parasite-derived prostaglandin D2 in the inhibition of epidermal Langerhans cell migration during schistosomiasis infection. J Exp Med *193*, 1135-1147.

Angeli, V., Staumont, D., Charbonnier, A.S., Hammad, H., Gosset, P., Pichavant, M., Lambrecht, B.N., Capron, M., Dombrowicz, D., and Trottein, F. (2004). Activation of the D prostanoid receptor 1 regulates immune and skin allergic responses. J Immunol *172*, 3822-3829.

Arai, I., Takano, N., Hashimoto, Y., Futaki, N., Sugimoto, M., Takahashi, N., Inoue, T., and Nakaike, S. (2004). Prostanoid DP1 receptor agonist inhibits the pruritic activity in NC/Nga mice with atopic dermatitis. Eur J Pharmacol *505*, 229-235.

Betz, M., and Fox, B.S. (1991). Prostaglandin E2 inhibits production of Th1 lymphokines but not of Th2 lymphokines. J Immunol *146*, 108-113.

Bieber, T. Atopic dermatitis. Ann Dermatol *22*, 125-137.

Bieber, T. (2008). Atopic dermatitis. N Engl J Med *358*, 1483-1494.

Boehme, S.A., Chen, E.P., Franz-Bacon, K., Sasik, R., Sprague, L.J., Ly, T.W., Hardiman, G., and Bacon, K.B. (2009). Antagonism of CRTH2 ameliorates chronic epicutaneous sensitization-induced inflammation by multiple mechanisms. Int Immunol *21*, 1-17.

Boniface, K., Bak-Jensen, K.S., Li, Y., Blumenschein, W.M., McGeachy, M.J., McClanahan, T.K., McKenzie, B.S., Kastelein, R.A., Cua, D.J., and de Waal Malefyt, R. (2009). Prostaglandin E2 regulates Th17 cell differentiation and function through cyclic AMP and EP2/EP4 receptor signaling. J Exp Med *206*, 535-548.

Brandt, C., Pavlovic, V., Radbruch, A., Worm, M., and Baumgrass, R. (2009). Low-dose cyclosporine A therapy increases the regulatory T cell population in patients with atopic dermatitis. Allergy *64*, 1588-1596.

Brunkow, M.E., Jeffery, E.W., Hjerrild, K.A., Paeper, B., Clark, L.B., Yasayko, S.A., Wilkinson, J.E., Galas, D., Ziegler, S.F., and Ramsdell, F. (2001). Disruption of a new forkhead/winged-helix protein, scurfin, results in the fatal lymphoproliferative disorder of the scurfy mouse. Nat Genet *27*, 68-73.

Chung, H.T., Burnham, D.K., Robertson, B., Roberts, L.K., and Daynes, R.A. (1986). Involvement of prostaglandins in the immune alterations caused by the exposure of mice to ultraviolet radiation. J Immunol *137*, 2478-2484.

Elias, P.M., Hatano, Y., and Williams, M.L. (2008). Basis for the barrier abnormality in atopic dermatitis: outside-inside-outside pathogenic mechanisms. J Allergy Clin Immunol *121*, 1337-1343.

Elias, P.M., and Schmuth, M. (2009). Abnormal skin barrier in the etiopathogenesis of atopic dermatitis. Curr Opin Allergy Clin Immunol *9*, 437-446.

Fedyk, E.R., and Phipps, R.P. (1996). Prostaglandin E2 receptors of the EP2 and EP4 subtypes regulate activation and differentiation of mouse B lymphocytes to IgE-secreting cells. Proc Natl Acad Sci U S A *93,* 10978-10983.

Fogh, K., Herlin, T., and Kragballe, K. (1989). Eicosanoids in skin of patients with atopic dermatitis: prostaglandin E2 and leukotriene B4 are present in biologically active concentrations. J Allergy Clin Immunol *83,* 450-455.

Gervais, F.G., Cruz, R.P., Chateauneuf, A., Gale, S., Sawyer, N., Nantel, F., Metters, K.M., and O'Neill G, P. (2001). Selective modulation of chemokinesis, degranulation, and apoptosis in eosinophils through the PGD2 receptors CRTH2 and DP. J Allergy Clin Immunol *108,* 982-988.

Goodwin, J.S., and Ceuppens, J. (1983). Regulation of the immune response by prostaglandins. J Clin Immunol *3,* 295-315.

Guttman-Yassky, E., Nograles, K.E., and Krueger, J.G. (2011). Contrasting pathogenesis of atopic dermatitis and psoriasis-Part I: Clinical and pathologic concepts. J Allergy Clin Immunol.

Guttman-Yassky, E., Nograles, K.E., and Krueger, J.G. (2011). Contrasting pathogenesis of atopic dermatitis and psoriasis-Part II: Immune cell subsets and therapeutic concepts. J Allergy Clin Immunol.

Guttman-Yassky, E., Suarez-Farinas, M., Chiricozzi, A., Nograles, K.E., Shemer, A., Fuentes-Duculan, J., Cardinale, I., Lin, P., Bergman, R., Bowcock, A.M., and Krueger, J.G. (2009). Broad defects in epidermal cornification in atopic dermatitis identified through genomic analysis. J Allergy Clin Immunol *124,* 1235-1244 e1258.

Hagermark, O., and Strandberg, K. (1977). Pruritogenic activity of prostaglandin E2. Acta Derm Venereol *57,* 37-43.

Hammad, H., Kool, M., Soullie, T., Narumiya, S., Trottein, F., Hoogsteden, H.C., and Lambrecht, B.N. (2007). Activation of the D prostanoid 1 receptor suppresses asthma by modulation of lung dendritic cell function and induction of regulatory T cells. J Exp Med *204,* 357-367.

Hammarstrom, S., Lindgren, J.A., Marcelo, C., Duell, E.A., Anderson, T.F., and Voorhees, J.J. (1979). Arachidonic acid transformations in normal and psoriatic skin. J Invest Dermatol *73,* 180-183.

Hart, P.H., Townley, S.L., Grimbaldeston, M.A., Khalil, Z., and Finlay-Jones, J.J. (2002). Mast cells, neuropeptides, histamine, and prostaglandins in UV-induced systemic immunosuppression. Methods *28,* 79-89.

Hashimoto, Y., Arai, I., Tanaka, M., and Nakaike, S. (2005). Prostaglandin D2 inhibits IgE-mediated scratching by suppressing histamine release from mast cells. J Pharmacol Sci *98,* 90-93.

He, R., Oyoshi, M.K., Wang, J.Y., Hodge, M.R., Jin, H., and Geha, R.S. (2010). The prostaglandin D receptor CRTH2 is important for allergic skin inflammation after epicutaneous antigen challenge. J Allergy Clin Immunol *126,* 784-790.

Hijnen, D., Nijhuis, E., Bruin-Weller, M., Holstege, F., Koerkamp, M.G., Kok, I., Bruijnzeel-Koomen, C., and Knol, E. (2005). Differential expression of genes involved in skin homing, proliferation, and apoptosis in CD4+ T cells of patients with atopic dermatitis. J Invest Dermatol *125*, 1149-1155.

Hirai, H., Tanaka, K., Yoshie, O., Ogawa, K., Kenmotsu, K., Takamori, Y., Ichimasa, M., Sugamura, K., Nakamura, M., Takano, S., and Nagata, K. (2001). Prostaglandin D2 selectively induces chemotaxis in T helper type 2 cells, eosinophils, and basophils via seven-transmembrane receptor CRTH2. J Exp Med *193*, 255-261.

Honda, T., Matsuoka, T., Ueta, M., Kabashima, K., Miyachi, Y., and Narumiya, S. (2009). Prostaglandin E(2)-EP(3) signaling suppresses skin inflammation in murine contact hypersensitivity. J Allergy Clin Immunol *124*, 809-818 e802.

Honda, T., Tokura, Y., Miyachi, Y., and Kabashima, K. Prostanoid (2010). receptors as possible targets for anti-allergic drugs: recent advances in prostanoids on allergy and immunology. Curr Drug Targets *11*, 1605-1613.

Huang, Q., Liu, D., Majewski, P., Schulte, L.C., Korn, J.M., Young, R.A., Lander, E.S., and Hacohen, N. (2001). The plasticity of dendritic cell responses to pathogens and their components. Science *294*, 870-875.

Iwasaki, M., Nagata, K., Takano, S., Takahashi, K., Ishii, N., and Ikezawa, Z. (2002). Association of a new-type prostaglandin D2 receptor CRTH2 with circulating T helper 2 cells in patients with atopic dermatitis. J Invest Dermatol *119*, 609-616.

Kabashima, K., and Miyachi, Y. (2004). Prostanoids in the cutaneous immune response. J Dermatol Sci *34*, 177-184.

Kabashima, K., Murata, T., Tanaka, H., Matsuoka, T., Sakata, D., Yoshida, N., Katagiri, K., Kinashi, T., Tanaka, T., Miyasaka, M., *et al.* (2003a). Thromboxane A2 modulates interaction of dendritic cells and T cells and regulates acquired immunity. Nat Immunol *4*, 694-701.

Kabashima, K., Sakata, D., Nagamachi, M., Miyachi, Y., Inaba, K., and Narumiya, S. (2003b). Prostaglandin E2-EP4 signaling initiates skin immune responses by promoting migration and maturation of Langerhans cells. Nat Med *9*, 744-749.

Koga, C., Kabashima, K., Shiraishi, N., Kobayashi, M., and Tokura, Y. (2008). Possible pathogenic role of Th17 cells for atopic dermatitis. J Invest Dermatol *128*, 2625-2630.

Konger, R.L., Malaviya, R., and Pentland, A.P. (1998). Growth regulation of primary human keratinocytes by prostaglandin E receptor EP2 and EP3 subtypes. Biochim Biophys Acta *1401*, 221-234.

Kunikata, T., Yamane, H., Segi, E., Matsuoka, T., Sugimoto, Y., Tanaka, S., Tanaka, H., Nagai, H., Ichikawa, A., and Narumiya, S. (2005). Suppression of allergic inflammation by the prostaglandin E receptor subtype EP3. Nat Immunol *6*, 524-531.

Kuwamoto, K., Miyauchi-Hashimoto, H., Tanaka, K., Eguchi, N., Inui, T., Urade, Y., and Horio, T. (2000). Possible involvement of enhanced prostaglandin E2 production in the photosensitivity in xeroderma pigmentosum group A model mice. J Invest Dermatol *114*, 241-246.

Laouini, D., Elkhal, A., Yalcindag, A., Kawamoto, S., Oettgen, H., and Geha, R.S. (2005). COX-2 inhibition enhances the TH2 immune response to epicutaneous sensitization. J Allergy Clin Immunol *116*, 390-396.

Leong, J., Hughes-Fulford, M., Rakhlin, N., Habib, A., Maclouf, J., and Goldyne, M.E. (1996). Cyclooxygenases in human and mouse skin and cultured human keratinocytes: association of COX-2 expression with human keratinocyte differentiation. Exp Cell Res *224*, 79-87.

Lerche, A., Bisgaard, H., Kassis, V., Christensen, J.D., and Sondergaard, J. (1989). Prostaglandin E1 and prostaglandin F2 alpha in exudate in nickel allergy. Acta Derm Venereol *69*, 253-256.

Loser, K., Mehling, A., Loeser, S., Apelt, J., Kuhn, A., Grabbe, S., Schwarz, T., Penninger, J.M., and Beissert, S. (2006). Epidermal RANKL controls regulatory T-cell numbers via activation of dendritic cells. Nat Med *12*, 1372-1379.

Mita, H., Hasegawa, M., Higashi, N., and Akiyama, K. (2002). Characterization of PGE2 receptor subtypes in human eosinophils. J Allergy Clin Immunol *110*, 457-459.

Nagamachi, M., Sakata, D., Kabashima, K., Furuyashiki, T., Murata, T., Segi-Nishida, E., Soontrapa, K., Matsuoka, T., Miyachi, Y., and Narumiya, S. (2007). Facilitation of Th1-mediated immune response by prostaglandin E receptor EP1. J Exp Med *204*, 2865-2874.

Nagao, K., Tanaka, H., Komai, M., Masuda, T., Narumiya, S., and Nagai, H. (2003). Role of prostaglandin I2 in airway remodeling induced by repeated allergen challenge in mice. Am J Respir Cell Mol Biol *29*, 314-320.

Nakajima, S., Honda, T., Sakata, D., Egawa, G., Tanizaki, H., Otsuka, A., Moniaga, C.S., Watanabe, T., Miyachi, Y., Narumiya, S., and Kabashima, K. Prostaglandin I2-IP signaling promotes Th1 differentiation in a mouse model of contact hypersensitivity. J Immunol *184*, 5595-5603.

Narumiya, S., and FitzGerald, G.A. (2001). Genetic and pharmacological analysis of prostanoid receptor function. J Clin Invest *108*, 25-30.

Narumiya, S., Sugimoto, Y., and Ushikubi, F. (1999). Prostanoid receptors: structures, properties, and functions. Physiol Rev *79*, 1193-1226.

Nataraj, C., Thomas, D.W., Tilley, S.L., Nguyen, M.T., Mannon, R., Koller, B.H., and Coffman, T.M. (2001). Receptors for prostaglandin E(2) that regulate cellular immune responses in the mouse. J Clin Invest *108*, 1229-1235.

Neisius, U., Olsson, R., Rukwied, R., Lischetzki, G., and Schmelz, M. (2002). Prostaglandin E2 induces vasodilation and pruritus, but no protein extravasation in atopic dermatitis and controls. J Am Acad Dermatol *47*, 28-32.

Nguyen, M., Solle, M., Audoly, L.P., Tilley, S.L., Stock, J.L., McNeish, J.D., Coffman, T.M., Dombrowicz, D., and Koller, B.H. (2002). Receptors and signaling mechanisms required for prostaglandin E2-mediated regulation of mast cell degranulation and IL-6 production. J Immunol *169*, 4586-4593.

Nograles, K.E., Suarez-Farinas, M., Shemer, A., Fuentes-Duculan, J., Chiricozzi, A., Cardinale, I., Zaba, L.C., Kikuchi, T., Ramon, M., Bergman, R., *et al.* Atopic dermatitis keratinocytes exhibit normal T(H)17 cytokine responses. J Allergy Clin Immunol *125*, 744-746, 746 e741-746 e742.

Nograles, K.E., Zaba, L.C., Shemer, A., Fuentes-Duculan, J., Cardinale, I., Kikuchi, T., Ramon, M., Bergman, R., Krueger, J.G., and Guttman-Yassky, E. (2009). IL-22-producing "T22" T cells account for upregulated IL-22 in atopic dermatitis despite reduced IL-17-producing TH17 T cells. J Allergy Clin Immunol *123,* 1244-1252 e1242.

Nomiya, R., Okano, M., Fujiwara, T., Maeda, M., Kimura, Y., Kino, K., Yokoyama, M., Hirai, H., Nagata, K., Hara, T., *et al.* (2008). CRTH2 plays an essential role in the pathophysiology of Cry j 1-induced pollinosis in mice. J Immunol *180,* 5680-5688.

Ochs, H.D., Ziegler, S.F., and Torgerson, T.R. (2005). FOXP3 acts as a rheostat of the immune response. Immunol Rev *203,* 156-164.

Odhiambo, J.A., Williams, H.C., Clayton, T.O., Robertson, C.F., and Asher, M.I. (2009). Global variations in prevalence of eczema symptoms in children from ISAAC Phase Three. J Allergy Clin Immunol *124,* 1251-1258 e1223.

Ong, P.Y., and Leung, D.Y. (2006). Immune dysregulation in atopic dermatitis. Curr Allergy Asthma Rep *6,* 384-389.

Ou, L.S., Goleva, E., Hall, C., and Leung, D.Y. (2004). T regulatory cells in atopic dermatitis and subversion of their activity by superantigens. J Allergy Clin Immunol *113,* 756-763.

Peacock, C.D., Misso, N.L., Watkins, D.N., and Thompson, P.J. (1999). PGE 2 and dibutyryl cyclic adenosine monophosphate prolong eosinophil survival in vitro. J Allergy Clin Immunol *104,* 153-162.

Ruzicka, T., and Aubock, J. (1987). Arachidonic acid metabolism in guinea pig Langerhans cells: studies on cyclooxygenase and lipoxygenase pathways. J Immunol *138,* 539-543.

Ruzicka, T., Walter, J.F., and Printz, M.P. (1983). Changes in arachidonic acid metabolism in UV-irradiated hairless mouse skin. J Invest Dermatol *81,* 300-303.

Schnopp, C., Rad, R., Weidinger, A., Weidinger, S., Ring, J., Eberlein, B., Ollert, M., and Mempel, M. (2007). Fox-P3-positive regulatory T cells are present in the skin of generalized atopic eczema patients and are not particularly affected by medium-dose UVA1 therapy. Photodermatol Photoimmunol Photomed *23,* 81-85.

Scholz, K., Furstenberger, G., Muller-Decker, K., and Marks, F. (1995). Differential expression of prostaglandin-H synthase isoenzymes in normal and activated keratinocytes in vivo and in vitro. Biochem J *309 (Pt 1),* 263-269.

Schratl, P., Royer, J.F., Kostenis, E., Ulven, T., Sturm, E.M., Waldhoer, M., Hoefler, G., Schuligoi, R., Lippe, I.T., Peskar, B.A., and Heinemann, A. (2007). The role of the prostaglandin D2 receptor, DP, in eosinophil trafficking. J Immunol *179,* 4792-4799.

Shin, H.D., Park, B.L., Jung, J.H., Wang, H.J., Park, H.S., Choi, B.W., Hong, S.J., Lee, Y.M., Kim, Y.H., and Park, C.S. (2003). Association of thromboxane A2 receptor (TBXA2R) with atopy and asthma. J Allergy Clin Immunol *112,* 454-457.

Soontrapa, K., Honda, T., Sakata, D., Yao, C., Hirata, T., Hori, S., Matsuoka, T., Kita, Y., Shimizu, T., Kabashima, K., and Narumiya, S. Prostaglandin E2-prostoglandin E receptor subtype 4 (EP4) signaling mediates UV irradiation-induced systemic immunosuppression. Proc Natl Acad Sci U S A.

Spergel, J.M., Mizoguchi, E., Brewer, J.P., Martin, T.R., Bhan, A.K., and Geha, R.S. (1998). Epicutaneous sensitization with protein antigen induces localized allergic dermatitis and hyperresponsiveness to methacholine after single exposure to aerosolized antigen in mice. J Clin Invest *101*, 1614-1622.

Sugimoto, M., Arai, I., Futaki, N., Hashimoto, Y., Sakurai, T., Honma, Y., and Nakaike, S. (2006). Time course changes of scratching counts, dermatitis symptoms, and levels of cutaneous prostaglandins in NC/Nga mice. Exp Dermatol *15*, 875-882.

Takahashi, Y., Tokuoka, S., Masuda, T., Hirano, Y., Nagao, M., Tanaka, H., Inagaki, N., Narumiya, S., and Nagai, H. (2002). Augmentation of allergic inflammation in prostanoid IP receptor deficient mice. Br J Pharmacol *137*, 315-322.

Tilley, S.L., Coffman, T.M., and Koller, B.H. (2001). Mixed messages: modulation of inflammation and immune responses by prostaglandins and thromboxanes. J Clin Invest *108*, 15-23.

Tober, K.L., Thomas-Ahner, J.M., Kusewitt, D.F., and Oberyszyn, T.M. (2007). Effects of UVB on E prostanoid receptor expression in murine skin. J Invest Dermatol *127*, 214-221.

Tober, K.L., Wilgus, T.A., Kusewitt, D.F., Thomas-Ahner, J.M., Maruyama, T., and Oberyszyn, T.M. (2006). Importance of the EP(1) receptor in cutaneous UVB-induced inflammation and tumor development. J Invest Dermatol *126*, 205-211.

Torii, E., Segi, E., Sugimoto, Y., Takahashi, K., Kabashima, K., Ikai, K., and Ichikawa, A. (2002). Expression of prostaglandin E(2) receptor subtypes in mouse hair follicles. Biochem Biophys Res Commun *290*, 696-700.

Ueta, M., Matsuoka, T., Narumiya, S., and Kinoshita, S. (2009). Prostaglandin E receptor subtype EP3 in conjunctival epithelium regulates late-phase reaction of experimental allergic conjunctivitis. J Allergy Clin Immunol *123*, 466-471.

Ujihara, M., Horiguchi, Y., Ikai, K., and Urade, Y. (1988). Characterization and distribution of prostaglandin D synthetase in rat skin. J Invest Dermatol *90*, 448-451.

Ulven, T., and Kostenis, E. Novel CRTH2 antagonists: a review of patents from 2006 to 2009. Expert Opin Ther Pat *20*, 1505-1530.

Verhagen, J., Akdis, M., Traidl-Hoffmann, C., Schmid-Grendelmeier, P., Hijnen, D., Knol, E.F., Behrendt, H., Blaser, K., and Akdis, C.A. (2006). Absence of T-regulatory cell expression and function in atopic dermatitis skin. J Allergy Clin Immunol *117*, 176-183.

Walterscheid, J.P., Ullrich, S.E., and Nghiem, D.X. (2002). Platelet-activating factor, a molecular sensor for cellular damage, activates systemic immune suppression. J Exp Med *195*, 171-179.

Xue, L., Barrow, A., and Pettipher, R. (2009). Novel function of CRTH2 in preventing apoptosis of human Th2 cells through activation of the phosphatidylinositol 3-kinase pathway. J Immunol *182*, 7580-7586.

Yamane, H., Sugimoto, Y., Tanaka, S., and Ichikawa, A. (2000). Prostaglandin E(2) receptors, EP2 and EP4, differentially modulate TNF-alpha and IL-6 production induced by lipopolysaccharide in mouse peritoneal neutrophils. Biochem Biophys Res Commun *278*, 224-228.

Yao, C., Sakata, D., Esaki, Y., Li, Y., Matsuoka, T., Kuroiwa, K., Sugimoto, Y., and Narumiya, S. (2009). Prostaglandin E2-EP4 signaling promotes immune inflammation through Th1 cell differentiation and Th17 cell expansion. Nat Med *15*, 633-640.

Yoshimura-Uchiyama, C., Iikura, M., Yamaguchi, M., Nagase, H., Ishii, A., Matsushima, K., Yamamoto, K., Shichijo, M., Bacon, K.B., and Hirai, K. (2004). Differential modulation of human basophil functions through prostaglandin D2 receptors DP and chemoattractant receptor-homologous molecule expressed on Th2 cells/DP2. Clin Exp Allergy *34*, 1283-1290.

6

Expression and Function of CCL17 in Atopic Dermatitis

Susanne Stutte[1], Nancy Gerbitzki[2], Natalija Novak[3] and Irmgard Förster[2]
[1]*Department of Microbiology and Immunobiology*
Division of Immunology, Harvard Medical School, Boston
[2]*Molecular Immunology, IUF – Leibniz Research Institute for Environmental Medicine, Düsseldorf*
[3]*Department of Dermatology and Allergy*
University of Bonn Medical Center, Bonn
[1]*USA*
[2,3]*Germany*

1. Introduction

Chemokines are a superfamily of potent leukocyte chemoattractant cytokines with a molecular weight of 8-12 kDa. Historically, many chemokines had more than one name until the 1999 Keystone Symposium on Chemokines, when a new nomenclature was introduced (Zlotnik & Yoshie, 2000). Chemokines have been subdivided into four subfamilies on the basis of the position of either one or two cysteine residues located near the N-terminus of the protein and an L (ligand) was added (CXCL, CCL, CL and CXXXCL) to designate all chemokines as ligands of their respective receptors (R). The chemokine network comprises about 50 chemokines, as well as 20 classical (10 CCRs, 7 CXCRs, two XCR and a single CX3CR) and 3 atypical chemokine receptors (Duffy antigen receptor for chemokines = DARC, CC-X-chemokine receptor (CCX-CKR), and the D6 molecule) (Cyster, 2005; Comerford & McColl, 2011; Hansell & Nibbs, 2007; Ransohoff, 2009; Sallusto & Baggiolini, 2008). Many ligands bind multiple receptors, although each of them bind in a slightly different way, thereby inducing distinct downstream responses. The timing and venue of specific ligand-receptor interactions determines the nature of various biological processes. Although their best known function is the regulation of leukocyte migration, chemokines also enhance cell adhesion or costimulation, and stimulate myelopoiesis, tumor growth or angiogenesis (Ransohoff, 2009; Sallusto & Baggiolini, 2008; Viola & Luster, 2008). In addition, chemokines participate in the organization of the microenvironmental architecture of primary and secondary lymphoid organs during physiological and pathological conditions (Cyster, 2005). Importantly, a defined subset of chemokines and their receptors drive certain inflammatory immune responses to protect the body against microbial and environmental pathogens. Dysregulation of such chemokines may contribute to the pathogenesis of inflammatory diseases, like acute respiratory distress syndrome, multiple sclerosis, inflammatory bowel diseases, atherosclerosis, or rheumatoid arthritis (Charo & Ransohoff, 2006). Furthermore, chemokines produced in barrier organs are known to substantially contribute to the pathogenesis of atopic diseases, like asthma, rhinitis and atopic dermatitis (D'Ambrosio, 2005; Homey et al., 2006; Pease, 2011).

1.1 Chemokine signaling

Chemokine receptors are pertussis toxin-sensitive heterotrimeric (αβγ) G-protein coupled receptors (GPCR) with seven helical membrane-spanning regions connected by extra-membranous loops. Ligand binding induces a series of intracellular signalling pathways, leading to changes in actin cytoskeleton, activation of integrins, cell migration and alterations of the cellular activation status. For detailed information on chemokine receptor signaling pathways we refer the reader to other review articles covering this topic specifically (Randolph et al., 2008; Thelen & Stein, 2008; Wu, 2005). Briefly, chemokine ligand binding induces activation of the G proteins associated with the chemokine receptor causing the dissociation of Gα-GTP from the receptor and from the Gβγ heterodimer. Whereas the Gα subunit inhibits adenylyl cyclases, the Gβγ subunit is able to activate several effectors, including phosphatidylinositol-3-OH-kinase (PI3K) and members of the phospholipase C family. In addition, chemokine receptor signaling leads to activation of small GTPases of the Rho and Ras families.

1.2 Regulation of chemokine receptor expression

Many chemokine receptor genes are constitutively expressed and their cell surface expression ranges from as few as around 1000/cell in the case of CXCR4 to around 40,000/cell in the case of CXCR2 on neutrophils (Holmes et al., 1991; Loetscher et al., 1994). Chemokine receptor expression can be regulated by two major mechanisms: enhanced/reduced gene expression and/or desensitization. Altered gene expression of chemokine receptors is evident in naïve T lymphocytes expressing high levels of homeostatic receptors that mediate circulation through secondary lymphoid organs. Once activated, homeostatic receptors are down-regulated, and inflammatory chemokine receptors are up-regulated on effector cells (Ebert & McColl, 2002; Sallusto et al., 1998a). This allows effector cells to migrate into tissues where the ligands for the inflammatory receptors are being expressed. This mechanism also regulates DC trafficking into tissues, within tissues and from tissues into draining LN. Chemokine receptors may also undergo transient homologous or heterologous desensitization (Aragay et al., 1998; Mashikian et al., 1999). Binding of the ligand leads to phosphorylation-dependent internalization of the receptor and abolishes further chemokine stimulation. This is called homologous desensitization. In contrast, heterologous desensitization happens when molecules other than those that bind directly can desensitize chemokine receptors, for example by utilization of common intracellular signalling pathways, or by alterations in the phosphorylation status of the receptor.

2. Chemokine and chemokine receptor expression in AD

AD represents a chronic relapsing skin disease induced by epidermal barrier dysfunctions, sensitization to environmental allergens, microbial stimulation, and genetic predisposition (Bieber, 2008). The lesional skin contains many signs of leukocytic inflammation, resulting from enhanced production of proinflammatory cytokines and chemokines (Gros et al., 2009; Homey et al., 2006; Pastore et al., 2004). One of the initial events in the pathogenesis of AD is a disturbance of the epidermal barrier and subsequent activation of keratinocytes by penetrating microbial and environmental pathogens or allergens. Release of pro-inflammatory cytokines, such as thymic stromal lymphopoetin (TSLP), IL-25 and IL-33 initially leads to the activation and/or attraction of innate immune cells, including cutaneous DC, and induction of a Th2-biased immune response (Carmi-Levy et al., 2011). During this phase a panel of homeostatic and inflammatory chemokines are upregulated in the affected skin areas, promoting the attraction of pro-allergic effector cells, like mast cells, eosinophils, inflammatory DC and cutaneous lymphocyte antigen $(CLA)^{+}CCR4^{+}$ skin-homing Th cells. Chemokines associated with an AD phenotype comprise CCL1, CCL2, CCL3, CCL5, CCL11, CCL13, CCL17, CCL18, CCL20, CCL22, CCL26, CCL27 and CX3CL1, and serum levels of CCL11, CCL17, CCL22, CCL26, CCL27 and CX3CL1 correlate with disease activity (Homey et al., 2006).

CCL1, CCL11 and CCL26 have been shown to interact with CCR8 and CCR3 on endothelial cells in AD, thereby inducing angiogenesis and tissue remodelling (Owczarek et al., 2010; Salcedo et al., 2001; Yawalkar et al., 1999). CCL1-CCR8 interactions also lead to recruitment of T cells and LC-like DC to the inflamed skin (Gombert et al., 2005), and have been associated with emigration of LC to the draining LN (Qu et al., 2004).

CCL27 is already expressed under homeostatic conditions and is further induced under inflammatory conditions in epidermal keratinocytes. In addition, CCL27 binds to the extracellular matrix and is displayed on endothelial cells in inflamed skin (Homey et al., 2002). CCR10, the receptor of CCL27, is preferentially expressed by $CLA^{+}CD4^{+}$ or $CD8^{+}$ memory T cells (Hudak et al., 2002). Neutralization of CCL27 significantly inhibited inflammatory skin responses in mouse models that mimic allergic contact dermatitis and AD (Homey et al., 2002; Hudak et al., 2002). In addition to CCR10, the skin-homing CLA^{+} memory T cells express CCR4 on their cell surface. As further discussed below, CCR4 and CCR10 ligands cooperate in the recruitment of memory T cells to sites of skin inflammation (Mirshahpanah et al., 2008; Reiss et al., 2001).

The human chemokine CCL18 is one of the most highly expressed chemokines produced by DC in lesional skin of AD patients but not in psoriasis (Fujita et al., 2011; Gros et al., 2009; Pivarcsi et al., 2004). Pivarcsi et al. showed that allergen exposure, as well as staphylococcal products induced its expression *in vitro* and *in vivo*. Although the receptor of CCL18 is still unknown, this chemokine has been shown to attract CLA+ memory T cells (Günther et al., 2005).

3. Function and expression of CCL17

3.1 Classification of CCL17 as an inflammatory chemokine

The β-chemokine CCL17 formerly known as Thymus- and Activation Regulated Chemokine (TARC), was first identified as a T cell chemoattractant by the group of O. Yoshie in human thymus, and phytohemagglutin stimulated peripheral blood mononuclear cells (Imai et al., 1996). Later on, the murine homologue was identified in murine bone marrow derived DC (BMDC) (Lieberam & Förster, 1999) and anti-CD40 stimulated splenic B cells (Schaniel et al., 1999). CCL17 shares the highest homology (32% amino acid identity) with CCL22 (macrophage-derived chemokine (MDC) and both chemokines signal through CCR4. CCR4 is expressed on T helper (Th)-1 and Th2 cells (D'Ambrosio et al., 1998; Sallusto et al., 1998a) but also on Th17 cells (Acosta-Rodriguez et al., 2007; Annunziato et al., 2007), $CD8^{+}$ T cells (Kondo & Takiguchi, 2009; Semmling et al., 2010), regulatory T cells (Treg) (Iellem et al.,

2001), natural killer T (NKT) cells (Kim et al., 2002), NK cells (Inngjerdingen et al., 2000), platelets (Clemetson et al., 2000), eosinophils and monocytes (Bochner et al., 1999). Despite the broad expression pattern of CCR4, CCL17 has been mainly associated with Th2 type immune reactions and is implicated in the pathogenesis of several Th2-mediated diseases like atopic dermatitis (Sallusto et al., 1998a; Imai et al., 1999; Saeki & Tamaki, 2006). Besides attraction of Th2 cells, however, CCL17 may also induce chemotaxis of memory T cells, Treg and Th1 cells (Iellem et al., 2001; Lieberam & Förster, 1999). In addition, other CCR4-expressing cell types like $CD8^+$ T cells, NK cells, basophils, eosinophils and DC may also respond to CCL17. As an inflammatory chemokine CCL17 is strongly upregulated in immature DC after stimulation with TLR ligands (Alferink et al., 2003; Lieberam & Förster, 1999). In addition, it can be upregulated following stimulation with various pro-inflammatory cytokines, as detailed below.

3.1.1 Transcriptional regulation of CCL17 expression

Whereas most CC chemokine genes are clustered on human chromosome 17 (mouse chromosome 11), *ccl17* is located downstream of *ccl22* and *cx3cl1* on the human chromosome 16q13 and mouse chromosome 8q (Hiroyama et al., 2001). The promoter region of *ccl17* contains several transcriptional regulation sites, like signal transducer and activator of transcription (STAT)6 binding sites and a nuclear factor kappa B (NF-κB) site (Liddiard et al., 2006; Liu et al., 2007; Monick et al., 2007; Nakayama et al., 2004; Wirnsberger et al., 2006). Expression of CCL17 is induced by the Th2 cytokines interleukin (IL)-4 and IL-13 via STAT6, and NF-κB activation occurs in response to TLR signaling. In the case of CCL17 expression, both pathways appear to act synergistically (Monick et al., 2007). In addition, other cytokines, like tumor necrosis factor (TNF)-α, granulocyte/macrophage colony stimulating factor (GM-CSF), and TSLP have also been shown to upregulate CCL17 expression (Heijink et al., 2007; Imai et al., 1999; Liu et al., 2007; Soumelis et al., 2002; Wirnsberger et al., 2006; Xiao et al., 2003). TSLP is an IL-7-like cytokine produced mainly by keratinocytes in an inflammatory environment. TSLP induces maturation of myeloid DC, which in turn produce CCL17 and CCL22. In contrast, Interferon gamma (IFN-γ) has been shown to act as a counter regulator of CCL17 production (Fujita et al., 2005; Xiao et al., 2003), although this cytokine enhances CCL17 expression in conjunction with TNF-α in the HaCaT keratinocyte cell line (Vestergaard et al., 2001). A unique feature of murine CCL17 is that additionally to its own promoter, transcription in brain and kidney may be initiated from the promoter of the closely linked CX3CL1 (fractalkine) gene, resulting in expression of a protein containing the CX3CL1 signal sequence and the CCL17 coding region (Hiroyama et al., 2001).

3.2 Cell-type specificity of CCL17 expression in human and mouse

In mice, mature $CD11c^+CD8^-CD11b^+$ myeloid DC represent the predominant source of CCL17 production. Under steady state conditions, CCL17 is highly expressed in DC of the thymus, peripheral and mesenteric LN, small intestine, colon, and lung (Alferink et al., 2003). Apart from the thymus, all of these organs are associated with environmental barriers. The expression pattern of CCL17 emphasizes its importance in mediating the attraction of immune cells to sites, which are frequently exposed to environmental pathogens or allergens. Interestingly, CCL17 expression is normally not found in the spleen, even after systemic LPS challenge (Alferink et al., 2003). The only agent identified so far, which is able to strongly induce CCL17 in splenic DC, is the synthetic glycolipid α–galactosylceramide, a well known CD1d-dependent inducer of NKT cell activation (Semmling et al., 2010). After licensing by activated NKT cells, cross-priming CD8+ DC produce CCL17 and attract naïve cytotoxic T cells expressing CCR4. Based on the analysis of CCL17/EGFP reporter mice, expression of CCL17 is fairly restricted to DC and has not been observed in keratinocytes, B cells, endothelial or epithelial cells. Dermal DC (dDC) and LC in normal, untreated skin of mice are also CCL17-negative but turn on CCL17 expression following irritation or injury of the skin (Stutte et al., 2010).

Although healthy human skin is devoid of CCL17 expression as well, human keratinocytes were shown to express CCL17 in inflamed skin, such as lesional skin of AD patients (Kakinuma et al., 2001; Vestergaard et al., 2000). *In vitro*, CCL17 expression is also found constitutively in HaCaT cells and is further inducible by cytokine stimulation (Vestergaard et al., 2001), whereas normal human keratinocytes did not express CCL17 protein *in vitro*, even after cytokine stimulation (Tsuda et al., 2003; Saeki & Tamaki, 2006). In contrast, human LC, Inflammatory Dendritic Epidermal Cells (IDEC) and dDC strongly express CCL17 (and CCL22) in inflammatory environments, particularly in lesional skin of AD patients, as do LPS stimulated human monocyte-derived DC (D'Ambrosio et al., 2002; Fujita et al., 2011; Kang et al., 2010; Soumelis et al., 2002). In addition, non-haematopoietic cells, such as bronchial epithelial cells, endothelial cells, fibroblasts, as well as smooth muscle cells can be a source of inducible CCL17 in humans (D'Ambrosio et al., 2002; Faffe et al., 2003; Sekiya et al., 2003; Yu et al., 2002). Taken together, under inflammatory conditions CCL17 appears much more widely expressed in different cell-types in human as opposed to mice, where CCL17 expression is quite restricted to DC subsets. However, detection of CCL17 protein expression by immunohistology as it has frequently been performed in human studies, may also pick up CCL17 that is passively absorbed to the cell membrane, for example by adhesion to surface glycosaminoglycans, and may not necessarily reflect transcription of the *ccl17* gene in the same cell-type.

3.3 Clearance of CCL17

CCL17 interacts with two chemokine decoy receptors, the Duffy antigen (DARC) and the D6 receptor. The Duffy antigen is found on red blood cells and binds both CC and CXC chemokines. In contrast, D6 is expressed on lymphatic endothelial cells in skin, gut and lung and interacts with inflammatory CC chemokines only. Although D6 is structurally similar to other chemokine receptors, it is most homologous to CCR4 and CCR5. Ligand binding induces rapid internalization of the ligand-receptor complexes, which facilitates regulation of inflammatory immune responses and enables the final return to homeostatic levels. Interestingly, the homeostatic chemokines CCL19 and CCL21 cannot efficiently bind D6 (Bonecchi et al., 2004). Instead, CCL19, CCL21 and CCL25 are able to bind with high affinity to another hepta-helical surface protein, termed CCX-CKR, which also acts as a chemokine scavenger (Comerford et al., 2006; Gosling et al., 2000).

4. CCL17 in atopic dermatitis

AD is one of the most frequent chronic inflammatory skin diseases in children and adults and is characterized by pruritic skin lesions in typical body areas such as the flexural folds on dry skin (Bieber, 2008). Various exogenous and endogenous factors, including allergens

and microbial antigens have been identified as triggers of acute flare ups of the disease as well as risk factors for severe persistent courses (Novak & Simon, 2011). In addition, a multitude of genetic modifications impact on disease manifestation, including a partially genetically predetermined disturbed skin barrier (Barnes, 2010; O'Regan & Irvine, 2010). Not only lesional AD skin, but also clinically non-lesional skin of AD patients displays multiple histologic as well as immunologic differences as compared to the skin of healthy individuals (Suárez-Fariñas et al., 2011). One of those differences is the expression of the high affinity receptor for IgE (FcεRI) on the surface of skin DC. While FcεRI$^+$ LC are present in non-lesional AD skin, development of skin lesions goes along with the infiltration of the epidermis by another CD1a$^+$ myeloid DC subpopulation, highly expressing FcεRI but negative for Birbeck granules and respective Langerin expression, which have been characterized as IDEC (Novak & Bieber, 2005; Wollenberg et al., 1995).
As mentioned above, a large number of chemokines have been found to be upregulated in lesional skin and serum of AD patients and several chemokine-chemokine receptor pairs have been linked to the pathogenesis of AD, in particular CCL1-CCR8, CCL17/CCL22-CCR4, CCL18, CCL20-CCR6, and CCL27-CCR10 (Gros et al., 2009; Homey et al., 2006; Pastore et al., 2004; Pease & Williams, 2006). In AD, chemokines regulate the emigration of DC to the draining LN as well as the attraction of activated T cells, eosinophils, basophils and mast cells to the site of inflammation. In the following, we will focus on the role of the two CCR4 ligands CCL17 (TARC) and CCL22 (MDC) as biomarkers of disease severity in AD, and the functional influence of these chemokines on the pathogenesis of AD.

4.1 CCL17 as a biomarker for disease severity in AD

The first indication that CCL17 is upregulated in lesional AD skin came from the analysis of inflamed skin from NC/Nga mice, which spontaneously develop AD-like skin lesions (Vestergaard et al., 1999). Soon after that, enhanced frequencies of CLA$^+$CCR4$^+$ T lymphocytes were detected in the blood of AD patients, as well as a localized upregulation of CCL17 in the basal layers of the epidermis in lesional skin, presumably in keratinocytes (Vestergaard et al., 2000). Later on, numerous clinical studies demonstrated that CCL17 levels in serum of AD patients and the presence of CCL17 in lesional skin correlate with disease activity (for review see (Saeki & Tamaki, 2006)). As shown recently, expression of both, CCL17 as well as CCL22 is higher in LC and IDEC of patients with AD as compared to LC in healthy skin or epidermal DC isolated from the epidermis of patients with other chronic inflammatory skin diseases such as psoriasis (Fujita et al., 2011). Moreover, even dermal DC in AD express higher levels of CCL17 and CCL22. The selective upregulation of those chemokines in DC in AD skin further supports the concept of CCL17 and CCL22 being crucial for the recruitment of Th2 cells, which predominate in particular in the acute phase of the disease (Grewe et al., 1998). Sequential biopsies taken from the same individuals during atopy patch testing revealed more detailed insights into the kinetics and nature of chemokine upregulation in the skin during early and late phases of eczema development. For this diagnostic test, allergens are applied to the skin occlusively for 24 hours and eczema develops within 24-72 hours in the region of allergen application in sensitized individuals (Darsow et al., 1996). Expression of CCL17 and CCL22 is among other chemokines rapidly upregulated on the mRNA level already 24 hours later and increases further during the following 48 hours. In parallel, the number of inflammatory DC subtypes in the epidermis as well as T cells in the dermis increases

(Gros et al., 2009). The intensity of chemokine upregulation as well as the pattern of chemokines induced seem to be decisive for the development of eczematous skin lesions. Consequently, it is very likely that improvement of the skin lesions will occur in parallel with the reduction in amount of particular chemokines in the skin, leading to the discontinuation of the recruitment of inflammatory cell subtypes. In line with this, treatment of AD patients by immunotherapy (Bussmann et al., 2007; Kwon et al., 2010), or culture of PBMC with antihistamines (Furukawa et al., 2004; Shoji et al., 2011) leads to a significant reduction of CCL17 expression. Recently, immunofluorescence detection of CCL17 in the skin of AD patients showed that CCL17 expression levels in the stratum corneum correlate with disease activity as well (Morita et al., 2010). As for CCL17, similar findings have been obtained for the other CCR4 ligand CCL22 (Goebeler et al., 2001; Shimada et al., 2004), although CCL17 or CCL22 appear to be expressed by different cell types in the skin as determined by immunohistology (Vestergaard et al., 1999). Whereas CCL17 expression was mostly located to the basal layers of the epidermis, CCL22 expression was predominantly found in dermal cells. In addition, Hashimoto et al. described CCL22 to be more strongly upregulated in human monocyte-derived DC isolated from AD patients than CCL17, when compared to expression levels in healthy controls (Hashimoto et al., 2006).

Interestingly, the keratinocyte-derived cytokine TSLP, which is strongly upregulated in the epidermis of AD lesional skin specifically induces CCL17 and CCL22 expression in human peripheral blood CD11c^{+} DC (Soumelis et al., 2002) as well as human epidermal LC (Ebner et al., 2007). TSLP expression levels in the skin also correlated with enhanced migratory activity of LC (Guttman-Yassky et al., 2007; Soumelis et al., 2002). A possible link between skin barrier dysfunction and CCL17 was recently reported by Nakahigashi et al., who showed that CCL17 was able to induce aquaporin-3 in human keratinocytes, which in turn promoted keratinocyte proliferation and disturbed barrier function (Nakahigashi et al., 2010).

Whereas elevated levels of CCL17 and CCL22 have also been observed in allergic contact dermatitis (Bäumer et al., 2004; Goebeler et al., 2001; Kamsteeg et al., 2010; Martín et al., 2002;), CCL17/CCL22 expression is not significantly increased in Psoriasis vulgaris (Gros et al., 2009; Kakinuma et al., 2002; Kamsteeg et al., 2010; Saeki & Tamaki, 2006; Uchida et al., 2002). This correlates with the fact that psoriasis is a Th1 dominated disease, whereas Th2-type cytokines and chemokines dominate the initial phase of AD, with a shift to Th1-type cytokines in the chronic phase (Grewe et al., 1998; Fujita et al., 2011). In psoriasis, Th17 cells act together with Th1 cells in disease pathogenesis (Lowes et al., 2008; Nograles et al., 2009). The Th17 T cell subset has also been detected at enhanced frequencies in lesional skin and peripheral blood of AD patients, mainly in the acute phase of the disease (Koga et al., 2008; Toda et al., 2003). In addition, IL-17 was found to be produced by T cells infiltrating the skin of filaggrin-deficient mice (Oyoshi et al., 2009). In another study, however, T22 cells, which produce IL-22 but not IL-17, rather than Th17 cells were reported to be especially increased in AD as opposed to psoriasis (Nograles et al., 2009). In line with this, Hayashida et al. reported that the presence of Th17 cells negatively correlated with CCL17 and IgE levels in AD patients, whereas serum IL-22 levels positively correlated with those of CCL17 (Hayashida et al., 2011a; 2011b). Whereas IL-17 has proinflammatory and anti-microbial effects, IL-22 inhibits terminal differentiation of keratinocytes and enhances epidermal hyperplasia (Nograles et al., 2008).

4.2 Pathogenic role of CCL17 in mouse models of AD

To study the mechanism of action of CCL17 in the pathogenesis of AD several mouse models have been employed. In general, mouse models of AD can be classified into spontaneous or intentional genetic mutants, and AD models induced by chronic treatment of wild-type or genetically modified mouse strains with epicutaneous allergens (for review see (Jin et al., 2009a)). There are two major spontaneous mouse models of AD, the NC/Nga (Matsuda et al., 1997) and the flaky tail mice (Fallon et al., 2009; Moniaga et al., 2010). In NC/Nga mice, dermatitis occurs only when the animals are kept under conventional breeding conditions but not under specified pathogen free conditions (Vestergaard et al., 1999), indicating that both genetic and environmental factors contribute to disease pathogenesis. In this mouse strain upregulation of CCL17 and CCL22 in lesional skin was first described (Vestergaard et al., 1999). Flaky tail mice harbor a single base pair nonsense mutation in the filaggrin gene, mimicking similar mutations found in AD patients (Fallon et al., 2009; Moniaga et al., 2010). Filaggrin deficiency results in an outside-to-inside skin barrier dysfunction and development of AD symptoms. In a modification of the original AD mouse model induced by chronic epicutaneous application of ovalbumin (OVA) as a model allergen (Spergel et al., 1998), a skin barrier dysfunction is induced by repeated tape-stripping of the skin, which disrupts the upper layers of the epidermis (Wang et al., 2007). Using our CCL17/EGFP reporter mice we could show that such mechanical irritation of the skin already leads to upregulation of CCL17 expression in cutaneous DC, as does epicutaneous treatment with DNFB, whereas CCL17 is not expressed in untreated skin (Alferink et al., 2003; Stutte et al., 2010). Upregulated expression of CCL17 in the skin was also observed in a transgenic mouse model of AD based on inducible expression of TSLP in keratinocytes. In this model only *ccl17* but not *ccl22* mRNA was increased in the skin (Yoo et al., 2005). To directly study the pathogenic effects of constitutive CCL17 expression in the skin, Tamaki and colleagues generated transgenic mice, in which *ccl17* is expressed under control of the human keratin 14 promoter. Expression of CCL17 in keratinocytes did not induce skin inflammation as such, whereas contact hypersensitivity (CHS) responses were differentially modulated by CCL17 depending on the contact sensitizer. In addition, increased numbers of Th2 cells and mast cells were recruited to the skin, and serum IgE levels were elevated (Tsunemi et al., 2006). Thus, when inflammation was induced by allergic sensitizers or irritants, CCL17 modified the inflammatory response and enhanced AD-like symptoms.

To obtain further insight into the pathogenic role of CCL17 in AD, we analyzed the development of AD-like symptoms in wild-type, CCL17/EGFP-reporter and CCL17-knockout mice after tape-stripping of the skin and chronic application of OVA (Stutte et al., 2010). In this model, a small area of the back skin was tape-stripped and a patch soaked with OVA was applied to the skin for three consecutive periods of one week, separated by two week breaks. Sham treated mice showed no signs of AD, whereas OVA treatment lead to acanthosis and thickening of the dermal layer. We found that CCL17-deficiency significantly diminished dermal infiltration with mast cells, eosinophils and CD4 T cells, whereas the development of acanthosis was unaffected. OVA-specific IgG and IgE antibody production was decreased and levels of inflammatory cytokines in the draining LN and in the skin were significantly reduced. Taken together, the majority of AD symptoms were strongly ameliorated in CCL17-deficient mice (Stutte et al., 2010). In addition, we made the unexpected and interesting observation that LC of CCL17-deficient mice failed to emigrate from the affected skin area, despite the presence of acanthosis, which is indicative of an ongoing inflammatory process. This finding was also supported by the fact that OVA-treated CCL17-knockout mice had reduced total numbers of skin-derived DC in the draining LN. Furthermore, we tested the ability of LC to emigrate from the skin using epidermal sheets of DNFB sensitized ear skin. As already observed in the AD model, CCL17-deficient LC were strongly impaired in emigration from the epidermis in this short-term assay. In contrast, LC emigration could be restored when recombinant (r) CCL17 was injected into the ear skin prior to DNFB treatment (Stutte et al., 2010). Thus, we could show that CCL17 is instrumental for the emigration of LC from the skin to the draining LN. Based on the reduced numbers of skin-derived DC in draining LN of OVA-treated CCL17-deficient mice, it might be possible that the migration of dDC is also affected by CCL17. The main conclusion from these experiments is that CCL17 contributes to the pathogenesis of AD in two different ways: i) upregulation of the inflammatory chemokine CCL17 in cutaneous DC is essential for LC emigration from the skin and thus for priming of immune responses in the draining LN, and ii) CCL17 (together with other chemokines, such as CCL22 and CCL27) enhances the attraction of activated T cells from the circulation to the inflamed skin. Our finding on the role of CCL17 in the induction of LC emigration is in line with histological observations in the skin of AD patients that expression of TSLP, a major inducer of CCL17, correlates with enhanced migratory activity of LC (Guttman-Yassky et al., 2007; Soumelis et al., 2002). Already in 2001, Katou et al. reported that about 50% of LC in inflamed skin but not dermal DC express the CCR4 receptor, suggesting that CCR4 ligands also influence LC migration (Katou et al., 2001).

4.2.1 Molecular processes involved in emigration of DC from the skin

To access non-lymphoid peripheral tissues, immature DC utilize specific chemokine receptor-ligand interactions, such as CCR2-CCL2, CCR5-CCL5 and CCR6-CCL20. In the periphery they are mostly sessile and constantly scan for antigens. Once stimulated, peripheral DC mature and actively migrate to the draining LN, where they act as professional antigen-presenting cells to prime naïve T cells and initiate antigen-specific responses. LC are located in between the basal keratinocyte layers of the epidermis and sample antigens that penetrated through the outer skin barrier - the stratum corneum. In the presence of danger signals induced by recognition of chemical or microbial antigens, or by physical stress, the sequential process of LC emigration from the skin to the draining LN is initiated. This process can be divided into the phases of mobilization, detachment, penetration of the basal membrane, interstitial migration within the dermis, traversing of the afferent lymphatic endothelium and transit to the LN within the lymphatic vessel (for review see (Alvarez et al., 2008)). Mobilization of LC is initiated by the pro-inflammatory cytokines TNF-α and IL-1β, and passage through the basal membrane depends on the presence of matrix metalloproteinases (MMP), like MMP-2 and MMP-9 (Ratzinger et al., 2002). Epicutaneous sensitization increases CXCR4 and CCR7 expression on cutaneous DC (Dieu et al., 1998; Sallusto et al., 1998b; Sozzani et al., 1998). Blocking experiments with CXCR4 antagonists showed that CXCL12-CXCR4 interactions are required for transit of LC from the epidermis to the dermis (Kabashima et al., 2007), whereas CCR7 appears not to be essential for this step but rather for entry of the cells into the afferent lymphatics from the dermis (Ohl et al., 2004). In addition, CCL1-CCR8 interactions may also be involved in the migration of DC from the skin to the LN (Qu et al., 2004).

Because of the impaired emigration of LC from the skin of CCL17-deficient mice in models of AD and CHS, we analyzed the responsiveness of CCL17-deficient BMDC to the CCR7 ligands CCL19 and CCL21, and the CXCR4 ligand CXCL12 in *in vitro* migration assays. In a transwell assay as well as a 3D migration assay in collagen gels, migration of CCL17-deficient BMDC was partially impaired as compared to heterozygous control cells (Stutte et al., 2010). This migratory deficiency could be fully restored by addition of rCCL17 or rCCL22 to the cultures in a time- and concentration dependent manner. Because we did not detect major differences in the level of CCR7 expression, we hypothesized that CCL17 sensitizes CCR7 and CXCR4 for optimal responsiveness to their ligands, as previously reported for prostaglandin E_2 (PGE_2) in the case of CCR7 (Sánchez-Sánchez et al., 2006; Scandella et al., 2004). In this context, it is interesting that histamine and PGE_2 were shown to upregulate CCL17 and CCL22 production in human myeloid DC (McIlroy et al., 2006). In addition to the observed changes in chemokine responsiveness of CCL17-deficient BMDC, a potential influence of CCL17 on the initial steps of LC emigration from the epidermis, like mobilization and detachment, as well as the production of MMP and penetration of the basal membrane still need to be investigated. Enzymatic activity of MMP-2 in epidermal and dermal cell suspensions was shown to be increased by IL-21 in wild-type but not IL-21 receptor (IL-21R)-deficient mice. Of note, AD-like symptoms, *ccl17* mRNA expression in OVA-treated skin, and migration of cutaneous DC to CCR7 ligands were also reduced in IL-21RKO mice (Jin et al., 2009b).

4.2.2 Phenotypic differences of CCL17- and CCR4-deficient mice

Because both CCL17 and CCL22 bind to CCR4 and thus may have redundant functions, one might anticipate that the amelioration of AD symptoms would be even more pronounced in CCR4-deficient mice compared to CCL17-deficient mice. Surprisingly, CCR4 knockout mice were not protected from the development of AD-like symptoms and exhibited normal emigration of DC from the skin after epicutaneous treatment with a contact sensitizer (Stutte et al., 2010). Similar findings were also reported by another group, showing that deficiency of CCR4 had no phenotype in the AD model, whereas absence of CCL8-CCR8 interactions diminished AD pathology (Islam et al., 2011). One possible explanation for this finding is the existence of an additional, as yet unknown receptor for CCL17. Inngjerdingen et al. demonstrated that CCL17 binding completely desensitized a calcium flux induced by CCL22, whereas CCL22 only partially reduced the calcium release to CCL17 (Inngjerdingen et al., 2000), indicating a different receptor binding activity of the two chemokines, or the presence of a second receptor for CCL17. In some studies, CCR8 was reported to function as a receptor for CCL17 (Bernardini et al., 1998; Inngjerdingen et al., 2000), but this finding is controversial and was disproven by others (Garlisi et al., 1999). For unknown reasons, genetic ablation of CCR4 also resulted in a deficiency of splenocytes to migrate to CCL3 (MIP-1α) (Chvatchko et al., 2000), which may also affect the phenotype of CCR4 knockout mice.

Another explanation for the different phenotype of CCL17- and CCR4-knockout mice may lie in differential expression patterns (Hashimoto et al., 2006; Vestergaard et al., 1999; 2000) and partially opposing functions of CCL17 and CCL22. In particular, CCL22-CCR4 interactions have been associated with enhanced recruitment of Treg (Curiel et al., 2004), whereas CCL17 appears to restrict the expansion of Treg in a mouse model of artherosclerosis (Weber et al., 2011). Furthermore, CCL22 is more potent in inducing integrin-dependent adhesion of CCR4+ Th cells (D'Ambrosio et al., 2002) and very rapidly induces CCR4 desensitization and receptor internalization from the cell surface. Thus, treatment of human Th2 cells with 1000 ng/ml CCL22 was sufficient to induce 90% internalization of CCR4, whereas no more than 20% CCR4 internalization was triggered by the same amount of CCL17 (Mariani et al., 2004). D'Ambrosio et al. also suggested that CCL17 and CCL22 may act sequentially in the course of T cell extravasation into the skin, because only CCL17 is presented by endothelial cells in skin vessel, whereas CCL22 is more dominantly expressed in interstitial DC (D'Ambrosio et al., 2002). Another difference between CCL17 and CCL22 was reported regarding their ability to bind to the decoy receptor D6. Full length CCL22 had a much higher affinity to D6 than CCL17, and cleavage of CCL22 by the dipeptidyl-peptidase IV completely prevented binding to D6 (Bonecchi et al., 2004).

Taken together, CCL17 and CCL22 appear to be non-redundant in many aspects and differential, cell-type specific expression of these two chemokines may additionally account for the fact that genetic deficiency of CCL17 cannot be compensated by CCL22 *in vivo* (Stutte et al., 2010). On the other hand, targeting of CCR4 may have opposing effects on the immune response, as CCR4 is involved in both the attraction of pro-inflammatory T cells and of immunosuppressive Treg.

5. Implication of CCL17, CCL22 and CCR4 in other diseases

In addition to AD, enhanced expression of CCL17 and CCL22, as well as elevated frequencies of CCR4+ T cells have been observed in asthma (Panina-Bordignon et al., 2001; Vijayanand et al., 2010) and rhinitis (Takeuchi et al., 2005; Terada et al., 2001), the two other forms of atopic diseases. In the case of asthma the pathogenic role of the CCL17/CCL22-CCR4 axis is still controversial (Pease, 2006), as some reports demonstrate efficient improvement of disease symptoms after CCR4 or CCL17 blockade (Kawasaki et al., 2001; Perros et al., 2009; Vijayanand et al., 2010), whereas others do not (Chvatchko et al., 2000; Conroy et al., 2003). As already mentioned above, enhanced expression of CCL17 and CCL22 has also been observed in allergic contact dermatitis (Bäumer et al., 2004; Goebeler et al., 2001; Kamsteeg et al., 2010; Martín et al., 2002), and contact hypersensitivity responses were significantly inhibited in CCL17-deficient mice (Alferink et al., 2003). Regarding non-allergic diseases, CCL17 has recently been shown to enhance the formation of artherosclerotic lesions in mice by inhibition of Treg cell expansion (Weber et al., 2011). Furthermore, deficiency in CCL17 or CCR4 prolongs graft survival in mouse models of cardiac allograft rejection (Alferink et al., 2003; Hüser et al., 2005).

As CCL17 expression is strongly upregulated in response to TLR stimulation (Lieberam & Förster, 1999; Alferink et al., 2003), it is possible that this chemokine is also involved in the defence against microbial infections. After cutaneous infection with the murine filaria *Litomosoides sigmodontis*, CCL17 was shown to control filarial worm load as a consequence of reduced mast cell dependent larval entry (Specht et al., 2011). In contrast, blockade of CCL17 but not CCL22 enhanced protection from murine pulmonary aspergillosis, and CCR4-deficient mice were similarly protected (Carpenter & Hogaboam, 2005). CCL17 production induced by NKT cell activation licensed splenic DC for efficient cross-presentation of OVA and stimulation of CTL responses (Semmling et al., 2010). Thus, CCL17 may also be involved in the defence against viral infections, although this has not been directly assessed so far.

6. Perspectives on chemokines and chemokine receptors as therapeutic targets in AD

Because of the crucial role of chemokine/chemokine-receptor interactions in the pathogenesis of allergic responses, it seems very attractive to use specific inhibitors, like neutralizing antibodies or small molecule antagonists, as therapeutic drugs to prevent or dampen the inflammatory reaction. Many inhibitors of chemokines and their receptors have already been developed and are currently tested in various disease models and in clinical studies (for recent reviews see (Garin & Proudfoot, 2011; Mackay, 2008; Pease, 2011)) However, the pleiotropic action of many chemokines and the frequent redundancies in the system hamper the development of efficient drugs and their approval for clinical use. Nevertheless, there is still optimism that chemokines and their receptors are promising targets for treatment of inflammatory diseases.

In the case of CCR4 at least four different small molecule inhibitors have been developed and successfully tested *in vitro* as well as in T cell migration models in mice (Nakagami et al., 2010; Pease, 2011; Sato et al., 2009). As indicated by the fact that CCR4 knockout mice develop AD-like symptoms (Islam et al., 2011; Stutte et al., 2010) and OVA-induced lung inflammation (Chvatchko et al., 2000) comparable to wild-type mice, blockade of CCR4 alone may not be sufficient to prevent these allergic reactions. In two studies addressing skin inflammation, simultaneous blockade of CCR4- and CCR10-ligands, or of CCR4 and the CCR10 ligand CCL27 was shown to be required for efficient inhibition of contact hypersensitivity at the time of challenge, or for homing of allergen-specific T cells to the skin (Mirshahpanah et al., 2008; Reiss et al., 2001). In another study, however, treatment with anti-CCL27 alone led to a significant inhibition of CHS and development of AD-like symptoms (Homey et al., 2002). As discussed above the amelioration of AD symptoms in CCL17-deficient mice but not CCR4-deficient mice indicates the presence of an additional receptor for CCL17, in particular with relevance for the emigration of LC from the skin. In addition, differences in the function of CCL17 and CCL22 regarding the attraction of Treg versus T helper cells may limit the usefulness of CCR4 antagonists in the treatment of allergic reactions. In fact, CCR4 blockade has also been proposed as a means to reduce attraction of tumor infiltrating Treg in cancer therapy (Yang et al., 2011). Therefore, it may be reasonable to also consider neutralization of certain chemokine ligands like CCL17 and CCL27 for therapy of AD, as an alternative to the blockade of chemokine receptors.

7. Acknowledgment

We are grateful to Heike Weighardt, Sonja Didovic and Theresa Globisch for comments on the manuscript. This work was supported by the Deutsche Forschungsgemeinschaft through SFB 704.

8. References

Acosta-Rodriguez, E. V., Rivino, L., Geginat, J., Jarrossay, D., Gattorno, M., Lanzavecchia, A., Sallusto, F., & Napolitani, G. (2007). Surface phenotype and antigenic specificity of human interleukin 17-producing T helper memory cells. *Nat. Immunol.* 8, 639-646.

Alferink, J., Lieberam, I., Reindl, W., Behrens, A., Weiss, S., Hüser, N., Gerauer, K., Ross, R., Reske-Kunz, A. B., Ahmad-Nejad, P., et al. (2003). Compartmentalized production of CCL17 in vivo: strong inducibility in peripheral dendritic cells contrasts selective absence from the spleen. *J. Exp. Med.* 197, 585–599.

Alvarez, D., Vollmann, E. H., & Andrian, von, U. H. (2008). Mechanisms and consequences of dendritic cell migration. *Immunity* 29, 325–342.

Annunziato, F., Cosmi, L., Santarlasci, V., Maggi, L., Liotta, F., Mazzinghi, B., Parente, E., Fili, L., Ferri, S., Frosali, F., et al. (2007). Phenotypic and functional features of human Th17 cells. *J. Exp. Med.* 204, 1849–1861.

Aragay, A. M., Mellado, M., Frade, J. M., Martin, A. M., Jimenez-Sainz, M. C., Martinez-A, C., & Mayor, F. (1998). Monocyte chemoattractant protein-1-induced CCR2B receptor desensitization mediated by the G protein-coupled receptor kinase 2. *Proc. Natl. Acad. Sci. U.S.A.* 95, 2985–2990.

Barnes, K. C. (2010). An update on the genetics of atopic dermatitis: scratching the surface in 2009. *J. Allergy Clin. Immunol.* 125, 16–29.

Bäumer, W., Seegers, U., Braun, M., Tschernig, T., & Kietzmann, M. (2004). TARC and RANTES, but not CTACK, are induced in two models of allergic contact dermatitis. Effects of cilomilast and diflorasone diacetate on T-cell-attracting chemokines. *Br. J. Dermatol.* 151, 823–830.

Bernardini, G., Hedrick, J., Sozzani, S., Luini, W., Spinetti, G., Weiss, M., Menon, S., Zlotnik, A., Mantovani, A., Santoni, A., et al. (1998). Identification of the CC chemokines TARC and macrophage inflammatory protein-1 beta as novel functional ligands for the CCR8 receptor. *Eur. J. Immunol.* 28, 582–588.

Bieber, T. (2008). Atopic dermatitis. *N. Engl. J. Med.* 358, 1483–1494.

Bochner, B. S., Bickel, C. A., Taylor, M. L., MacGlashan, D. W., Gray, P. W., Raport, C. J., & Godiska, R. (1999). Macrophage-derived chemokine induces human eosinophil chemotaxis in a CC chemokine receptor 3- and CC chemokine receptor 4-independent manner. *J. Allergy Clin. Immunol.* 103, 527–532.

Bonecchi, R., Locati, M., Galliera, E., Vulcano, M., Sironi, M., Fra, A. M., Gobbi, M., Vecchi, A., Sozzani, S., Haribabu, B., et al. (2004). Differential recognition and scavenging of native and truncated macrophage-derived chemokine (macrophage-derived chemokine/CC chemokine ligand 22) by the D6 decoy receptor. *J. Immunol.* 172, 4972–4976.

Bussmann, C., Maintz, L., Hart, J., Allam, J.-P., Vrtala, S., Chen, K.-W., Bieber, T., Thomas, W. R., Valenta, R., Zuberbier, T., et al. (2007). Clinical improvement and immunological changes in atopic dermatitis patients undergoing subcutaneous immunotherapy with a house dust mite allergoid: a pilot study. *Clin. Exp. Allergy* 37, 1277–1285.

Carmi-Levy, I., Homey, B., & Soumelis, V. (2011). A Modular View of Cytokine Networks in Atopic Dermatitis. *Clin Rev Allergy Immunol.*, in press.

Carpenter, K. J., & Hogaboam, C. M. (2005). Immunosuppressive effects of CCL17 on pulmonary antifungal responses during pulmonary invasive aspergillosis. *Infect. Immun.* 73, 7198–7207.

Charo, I. F., & Ransohoff, R. M. (2006). The many roles of chemokines and chemokine receptors in inflammation. *N. Engl. J. Med.* 354, 610–621.

Chvatchko, Y., Hoogewerf, A. J., Meyer, A., Alouani, S., Juillard, P., Buser, R., Conquet, F., Proudfoot, A. E., Wells, T. N., & Power, C. A. (2000). A key role for CC chemokine receptor 4 in lipopolysaccharide-induced endotoxic shock. *J. Exp. Med.* 191, 1755–1764.

Clemetson, K. J., Clemetson, J. M., Proudfoot, A. E., Power, C. A., Baggiolini, M., & Wells, T. N. (2000). Functional expression of CCR1, CCR3, CCR4, and CXCR4 chemokine receptors on human platelets. *Blood* 96, 4046–4054.

Comerford, I., Milasta, S., Morrow, V., Milligan, G., & Nibbs, R. (2006). The chemokine receptor CCX-CKR mediates effective scavenging of CCL19 in vitro. *Eur. J. Immunol.* 36, 1904–1916.

Comerford, I., & McColl, S. R. (2011). Mini-review series: focus on chemokines. Immunol Cell Biol *89*, 183–184.

Conroy, D. M., Jopling, L. A., Lloyd, C. M., Hodge, M. R., Andrew, D. P., Williams, T. J., Pease, J. E., and Sabroe, I. (2003). CCR4 blockade does not inhibit allergic airways inflammation. *J. Leukoc. Biol.* 74, 558–563.

Curiel, T. J., Coukos, G., Zou, L., Alvarez, X., Cheng, P., Mottram, P., Evdemon-Hogan, M., Conejo-Garcia, J. R., Zhang, L., Burow, M., et al. (2004). Specific recruitment of regulatory T cells in ovarian carcinoma fosters immune privilege and predicts reduced survival. *Nat. Med.* 10, 942–949.

Cyster, J. G. (2005). Chemokines, sphingosine-1-phosphate, and cell migration in secondary lymphoid organs. *Annu. Rev. Immunol.* 23, 127–159.

D'Ambrosio, D. (2005). Targeting chemoattractant receptors in allergic inflammation. *Curr Drug Targets Inflamm Allergy* 4, 163–167.

D'Ambrosio, D., Albanesi, C., Lang, R., Girolomoni, G., Sinigaglia, F.,& Laudanna, C. (2002). Quantitative differences in chemokine receptor engagement generate diversity in integrin-dependent lymphocyte adhesion. *J. Immunol.* 169, 2303–2312.

D'Ambrosio, D., Iellem, A., Bonecchi, R., Mazzeo, D., Sozzani, S., Mantovani, A., & Sinigaglia, F. (1998). Selective up-regulation of chemokine receptors CCR4 and CCR8 upon activation of polarized human type 2 Th cells. *J. Immunol.* 161, 5111–5115.

Darsow, U., Vieluf, D., & Ring, J. (1996). The atopy patch test: an increased rate of reactivity in patients who have an air-exposed pattern of atopic eczema. *Br. J. Dermatol.* 135, 182–186.

Dieu, M. C., Vanbervliet, B., Vicari, A., Bridon, J. M., Oldham, E., Aït-Yahia, S., Brière, F., Zlotnik, A., Lebecque, S., & Caux, C. (1998). Selective recruitment of immature and mature dendritic cells by distinct chemokines expressed in different anatomic sites. *J. Exp. Med.* 188, 373–386.

Ebert, L. M., & McColl, S. R. (2002). Up-regulation of CCR5 and CCR6 on distinct subpopulations of antigen-activated CD4+ T lymphocytes. *J. Immunol.* 168, 65–72.

Ebner, S., Nguyen, V. A., Forstner, M., Wang, Y.-H., Wolfram, D., Liu, Y.-J., & Romani, N. (2007). Thymic stromal lymphopoietin converts human epidermal Langerhans cells into antigen-presenting cells that induce proallergic T cells. *J. Allergy Clin. Immunol.* 119, 982–990.

Faffe, D. S., Whitehead, T., Moore, P. E., Baraldo, S., Flynt, L., Bourgeois, K., Panettieri, R. A., & Shore, S. A. (2003). IL-13 and IL-4 promote TARC release in human airway smooth muscle cells: role of IL-4 receptor genotype. *Am. J. Physiol. Lung Cell Mol. Physiol.* 285, L907–14.

Fallon, P. G., Sasaki, T., Sandilands, A., Campbell, L. E., Saunders, S. P., Mangan, N. E., Callanan, J. J., Kawasaki, H., Shiohama, A., Kubo, A., et al. (2009). A homozygous frameshift mutation in the mouse Flg gene facilitates enhanced percutaneous allergen priming. *Nat. Genet.* 41, 602–608.

Fujita, H., Asahina, A., Sugaya, M., Nakamura, K., Gao, P., Fujiwara, H., & Tamaki, K. (2005). Differential production of Th1- and Th2-type chemokines by mouse Langerhans cells and splenic dendritic cells. *J. Invest. Dermatol.* 124, 343–350.

Fujita, H., Shemer, A., Suárez-Fariñas, M., Johnson-Huang, L. M., Tintle, S., Cardinale, I., Fuentes-Duculan, J., Novitskaya, I., Carucci, J. A., Krueger, J. G., et al. (2011). Lesional dendritic cells in patients with chronic atopic dermatitis and psoriasis exhibit parallel ability to activate T-cell subsets. *J. Allergy Clin. Immunol.*, 128, 574-582.

Furukawa, H., Takahashi, M., Nakamura, K., & Kaneko, F. (2004). Effect of an antiallergic drug (Olopatadine hydrochloride) on TARC/CCL17 and MDC/CCL22 production by PBMCs from patients with atopic dermatitis. *J. Dermatol. Sci.* 36, 165–172.

Garin, A., & Proudfoot, A. E. I. (2011). Chemokines as targets for therapy. *Ex.l Cell Research* 317, 602–612.

Garlisi, C. G., Xiao, H., Tian, F., Hedrick, J. A., Billah, M. M., Egan, R. W., & Umland, S. P. (1999). The assignment of chemokine-chemokine receptor pairs: TARC and MIP-1 beta are not ligands for human CC-chemokine receptor 8. *Eur. J. Immunol.* 29, 3210–3215.

Goebeler, M., Trautmann, A., Voss, A., Bröcker, E. V., Toksoy, A., & Gillitzer, R. (2001). Differential and sequential expression of multiple chemokines during elicitation of allergic contact hypersensitivity. *Am. J. Pathol.* 158, 431–440.

Gombert, M., Dieu-Nosjean, M.-C., Winterberg, F., Bünemann, E., Kubitza, R. C., Da Cunha, L., Haahtela, A., Lehtimäki, S., Müller, A., Rieker, J., et al. (2005). CCL1-CCR8 interactions: an axis mediating the recruitment of T cells and Langerhans-type dendritic cells to sites of atopic skin inflammation. *J. Immunol.* 174, 5082–5091.

Gosling, J., Dairaghi, D. J., Wang, Y., Hanley, M., Talbot, D., Miao, Z., & Schall, T. J. (2000). Cutting edge: identification of a novel chemokine receptor that binds dendritic cell- and T cell-active chemokines including ELC, SLC, and TECK. *J. Immunol.* 164, 2851–2856.

Grewe, M., Bruijnzeel-Koomen, C. A., Schöpf, E., Thepen, T., Langeveld-Wildschut, A. G., Ruzicka, T., & Krutmann, J. (1998). A role for Th1 and Th2 cells in the immunopathogenesis of atopic dermatitis. *Immunol. Today* 19, 359–361.

Gros, E., Bussmann, C., Bieber, T., Förster, I., & Novak, N. (2009). Expression of chemokines and chemokine receptors in lesional and nonlesional upper skin of patients with atopic dermatitis. *J. Allergy Clin. Immunol.* 124, 753–60.

Guttman-Yassky, E., Lowes, M. A., Fuentes-Duculan, J., Whynot, J., Novitskaya, I., Cardinale, I., Haider, A., Khatcherian, A., Carucci, J. A., Bergman, R., et al. (2007). Major differences in inflammatory dendritic cells and their products distinguish atopic dermatitis from psoriasis. *J. Allergy Clin. Immunol.* 119, 1210–1217.

Günther, C., Bello-Fernandez, C., Kopp, T., Kund, J., Carballido-Perrig, N., Hinteregger, S., Fassl, S., Schwärzler, C., Lametschwandtner, G., Stingl, G., et al. (2005). CCL18 is expressed in atopic dermatitis and mediates skin homing of human memory T cells. *J. Immunol.* 174, 1723–1728.

Hansell, C., & Nibbs, R. (2007). Professional and part-time chemokine decoys in the resolution of inflammation. *Sci. STKE* 2007, pe18.

Hashimoto, S., Nakamura, K., Oyama, N., Kaneko, F., Tsunemi, Y., Saeki, H., & Tamaki, K. (2006). Macrophage-derived chemokine (MDC)/CCL22 produced by monocyte derived dendritic cells reflects the disease activity in patients with atopic dermatitis. *J. Dermatol. Sci.* 44, 93–99.

Hayashida, S., Uchi, H., Moroi, Y., & Furue, M. (2011a). Decrease in circulating Th17 cells correlates with increased levels of CCL17, IgE and eosinophils in atopic dermatitis. *J. Dermatol. Sci.* 61, 180–186.

Hayashida, S., Uchi, H., Takeuchi, S., Esaki, H., Moroi, Y., & Furue, M. (2011b). Significant correlation of serum IL-22 levels with CCL17 levels in atopic dermatitis. *J. Dermatol. Sci.* 61, 78–79.

Heijink, I. H., Marcel Kies, P., van Oosterhout, A. J. M., Postma, D. S., Kauffman, H. F.,& Vellenga, E. (2007). Der p, IL-4, and TGF-beta cooperatively induce EGFR-dependent TARC expression in airway epithelium. *Am. J. Respir. Cell Mol. Biol.* 36, 351–359.

Hiroyama, T., Iwama, A., Nakamura, Y., &Nakauchi, H. (2001). Fractalkine shares signal sequence with TARC: gene structures and expression profiles of two chemokine genes. *Genomics* 75, 3–5.

Holmes, W. E., Lee, J., Kuang, W. J., Rice, G. C., & Wood, W. I. (1991). Structure and functional expression of a human interleukin-8 receptor. *Science* 253, 1278–1280.

Homey, B., Alenius, H., Müller, A., Soto, H., Bowman, E. P., Yuan, W., McEvoy, L., Lauerma, A. I., Assmann, T., Bünemann, E., et al. (2002). CCL27-CCR10 interactions regulate T cell-mediated skin inflammation. *Nat. Med.* 8, 157–165.

Homey, B., Steinhoff, M., Ruzicka, T., & Leung, D. Y. M. (2006). Cytokines and chemokines orchestrate atopic skin inflammation. *J. Allergy Clin. Immunol.* 118, 178–189.

Hudak, S., Hagen, M., Liu, Y., Catron, D., Oldham, E., McEvoy, L. M., & Bowman, E. P. (2002). Immune surveillance and effector functions of CCR10(+) skin homing T cells. *J. Immunol.* 169, 1189–1196.

Hüser, N., Tertilt, C., Gerauer, K., Maier, S., Traeger, T., Assfalg, V., Reiter, R., Heidecke, C.-D.,& Pfeffer, K. (2005). CCR4-deficient mice show prolonged graft survival in a chronic cardiac transplant rejection model. *Eur. J. Immunol.* 35, 128–138.

Iellem, A., Mariani, M., Lang, R., Recalde, H., Panina-Bordignon, P., Simigaglia, F., & D'Ambrosio, D. (2001). Unique chemotactic response profile and specific expression of chemokine receptors CCR4 and CCR8 by CD4(+)CD25(+) regulatory T cells. *J. Exp. Med.* 194, 847–853.

Imai, T., Yoshida, T., Baba, M., Nishimura, M., Kakizaki, M., & Yoshie, O. (1996). Molecular cloning of a novel T cell-directed CC chemokine expressed in thymus by signal sequence trap using Epstein-Barr virus vector. *J. Biol. Chem.* 271, 21514-21521.

Imai, T., Nagira, M., Takagi, S., Kakizaki, M., Nishimura, M., Wang, J., Gray, P. W., Matsushima, K., & Yoshie, O. (1999). Selective recruitment of CCR4-bearing Th2 cells toward antigen-presenting cells by the CC chemokines thymus and activation-regulated chemokine and macrophage-derived chemokine. *Int. Immunol.* 11, 81–88.

Inngjerdingen, M., Damaj, B., & Maghazachi, A. A. (2000). Human NK cells express CC chemokine receptors 4 and 8 and respond to thymus and activation-regulated chemokine, macrophage-derived chemokine, and I-309. *J. Immunol.* 164, 4048–4054.

Islam, S. A., Chang, D. S., Colvin, R. A., Byrne, M. H., McCully, M. L., Moser, B., Lira, S. A., Charo, I. F., & Luster, A. D. (2011). Mouse CCL8, a CCR8 agonist, promotes atopic dermatitis by recruiting IL-5+ T(H)2 cells. *Nat. Immunol.* 12, 167–177.

Jin, H., He, R., Oyoshi, M., & Geha, R. S. (2009a). Animal models of atopic dermatitis. *J. Invest. Dermatol.* 129, 31–40.

Jin, H., Oyoshi, M. K., Le, Y., Bianchi, T., Koduru, S., Mathias, C. B., Kumar, L., Le Bras, S., Young, D., Collins, M., et al. (2009b). IL-21R is essential for epicutaneous sensitization and allergic skin inflammation in humans and mice. *J. Clin. Invest.* 119, 47–60.

Kabashima, K., Shiraishi, N., Sugita, K., Mori, T., Onoue, A., Kobayashi, M., Sakabe, J.-I., Yoshiki, R., Tamamura, H., Fujii, N., et al. (2007). CXCL12-CXCR4 engagement is required for migration of cutaneous dendritic cells. *Am. J. Pathol.* 171, 1249–1257.

Kakinuma, T., Nakamura, K., Wakugawa, M., Mitsui, H., Tada, Y., Saeki, H., Torii, H., Komine, M., Asahina, A., & Tamaki, K. (2002). Serum macrophage-derived chemokine (MDC) levels are closely related with the disease activity of atopic dermatitis. *Clin. Exp. Immunol.* 127, 270–273.

Kakinuma, T., Nakamura, K., Wakugawa, M., Mitsui, H., Tada, Y., Saeki, H., Torii, H., Asahina, A., Onai, N., Matsushima, K., et al. (2001). Thymus and activation-regulated chemokine in atopic dermatitis: Serum thymus and activation-regulated chemokine level is closely related with disease activity. *J. Allergy Clin. Immunol.* 107, 535–541.

Kamsteeg, M., Jansen, P. A. M., van Vlijmen-Willems, I. M. J. J., van Erp, P. E. J., Rodijk-Olthuis, D., van der Valk, P. G., Feuth, T., Zeeuwen, P. L. J. M., & Schalkwijk, J. (2010). Molecular diagnostics of psoriasis, atopic dermatitis, allergic contact dermatitis and irritant contact dermatitis. *Br. J. Dermatol.* 162, 568–578.

Kang, S., Xie, J., Ma, S., Liao, W., Zhang, J., & Luo, R. (2010). Targeted knock down of CCL22 and CCL17 by siRNA during DC differentiation and maturation affects the recruitment of T subsets. *Immunobiology* 215, 153–162.

Katou, F., Ohtani, H., Nakayama, T., Ono, K., Matsushima, K., Saaristo, A., Nagura, H., Yoshie, O., & Motegi, K. (2001). Macrophage-derived chemokine (MDC/CCL22) and CCR4 are involved in the formation of T lymphocyte-dendritic cell clusters in human inflamed skin and secondary lymphoid tissue. *Am. J. Pathol.* 158, 1263–1270.

Kawasaki, S., Takizawa, H., Yoneyama, H., Nakayama, T., Fujisawa, R., Izumizaki, M., Imai, T., Yoshie, O., Homma, I., Yamamoto, K., et al. (2001). Intervention of thymus and activation-regulated chemokine attenuates the development of allergic airway inflammation and hyperresponsiveness in mice. *J. Immunol.* 166, 2055-2062.

Kim, C. H., Johnston, B., & Butcher, E. C. (2002). Trafficking machinery of NKT cells: shared and differential chemokine receptor expression among V alpha 24(+)V beta 11(+) NKT cell subsets with distinct cytokine-producing capacity. *Blood* 100, 11-16.

Koga, C., Kabashima, K., Shiraishi, N., Kobayashi, M., & Tokura, Y. (2008). Possible Pathogenic Role of Th17 Cells for Atopic Dermatitis. *J. Investig. Dermatol.* 128, 2625-2630.

Kondo, T., & Takiguchi, M. (2009). Human memory CCR4+CD8+ T cell subset has the ability to produce multiple cytokines. *Int. Immunol.* 21, 523-532.

Kwon, Y. S., Oh, S. H., Wu, W. H., Bae, B. G., Lee, H. J., Lee, M.-G., & Lee, K. H. (2010). CC chemokines as potential immunologic markers correlated with clinical improvement of atopic dermatitis patients by immunotherapy. *Exp. Dermatol.* 19, 246-251.

Liddiard, K., Welch, J. S., Lozach, J., Heinz, S., Glass, C. K., & Greaves, D. R. (2006). Interleukin-4 induction of the CC chemokine TARC (CCL17) in murine macrophages is mediated by multiple STAT6 sites in the TARC gene promoter. *BMC Mol. Bio.l* 7, 45.

Lieberam, I., & Förster, I. (1999). The murine beta-chemokine TARC is expressed by subsets of dendritic cells and attracts primed CD4+ T cells. *Eur. J. Immunol.* 29, 2684-2694.

Liu, L. Y., Bates, M. E., Jarjour, N. N., Busse, W. W., Bertics, P. J., & Kelly, E. A. B. (2007). Generation of Th1 and Th2 chemokines by human eosinophils: evidence for a critical role of TNF-alpha. *J. Immunol.* 179, 4840-4848.

Loetscher, M., Geiser, T., O'Reilly, T., Zwahlen, R., Baggiolini, M., & Moser, B. (1994). Cloning of a human seven-transmembrane domain receptor, LESTR, that is highly expressed in leukocytes. *J. Biol. Chem.* 269, 232-237.

Lowes, M. A., Kikuchi, T., Fuentes-Duculan, J., Cardinale, I., Zaba, L. C., Haider, A. S., Bowman, E. P., & Krueger, J. G. (2008). Psoriasis vulgaris lesions contain discrete populations of Th1 and Th17 T cells. *J. Invest. Dermatol.* 128, 1207-1211.

Mackay, C. R. (2008). Moving targets: cell migration inhibitors as new anti-inflammatory therapies. *Nat. Immunol.* 9, 988-998.

Mariani, M., Lang, R., Binda, E., Panina-Bordignon, P., & D'Ambrosio, D. (2004). Dominance of CCL22 over CCL17 in induction of chemokine receptor CCR4 desensitization and internalization on human Th2 cells. *Eur. J. Immunol.* 34, 231-240.

Martín, A., Gallino, N., Gagliardi, J., Ortiz, S., Lascano, A. R., Diller, A., Daraio, M. C., Kahn, A., Mariani, A. L., & Serra, H. M. (2002). Early inflammatory markers in elicitation of allergic contact dermatitis. *BMC Dermatol.* 2, 9-17.

Mashikian, M. V., Ryan, T. C., Seman, A., Brazer, W., Center, D. M., & Cruikshank, W. W. (1999). Reciprocal desensitization of CCR5 and CD4 is mediated by IL-16 and macrophage-inflammatory protein-1 beta, respectively. *J. Immunol.* 163, 3123-3130.

Matsuda, H., Watanabe, N., Geba, G. P., Sperl, J., Tsudzuki, M., Hiroi, J., Matsumoto, M., Ushio, H., Saito, S., Askenase, P. W., et al. (1997). Development of atopic dermatitis-like skin lesion with IgE hyperproduction in NC/Nga mice. *Int. Immunol.* 9, 461–466.

McIlroy, A., Caron, G., Blanchard, S., Frémaux, I., Duluc, D., Delneste, Y., Chevailler, A., & Jeannin, P. (2006). Histamine and prostaglandin E up-regulate the production of Th2-attracting chemokines (CCL17 and CCL22) and down-regulate IFN-gamma-induced CXCL10 production by immature human dendritic cells. *Immunology* 117, 507–516.

Mirshahpanah, P., Li, Y.-Y. Y., Burkhardt, N., Asadullah, K., & Zollner, T. M. (2008). CCR4 and CCR10 ligands play additive roles in mouse contact hypersensitivity. *Exp. Dermatol.* 17, 30–34.

Moniaga, C. S., Egawa, G., Kawasaki, H., Hara-Chikuma, M., Honda, T., Tanizaki, H., Nakajima, S., Otsuka, A., Matsuoka, H., Kubo, A., et al. (2010). Flaky tail mouse denotes human atopic dermatitis in the steady state and by topical application with Dermatophagoides pteronyssinus extract. *Am. J. Pathol.* 176, 2385–2393.

Monick, M. M., Powers, L. S., Hassan, I., Groskreutz, D., Yarovinsky, T. O., Barrett, C. W., Castilow, E. M., Tifrea, D., Varga, S. M., & Hunninghake, G. W. (2007). Respiratory syncytial virus synergizes with Th2 cytokines to induce optimal levels of TARC/CCL17. *J. Immunol.* 179, 1648–1658.

Morita, E., Takahashi, H., Niihara, H., Dekio, I., Sumikawa, Y., Murakami, Y., & Matsunaka, H. (2010). Stratum corneum TARC level is a new indicator of lesional skin inflammation in atopic dermatitis. *Allergy* 65, 1166–1172.

Nakagami, Y., Kawashima, K., Etori, M., Yonekubo, K., Suzuki, C., Jojima, T., Kuribayashi, T., Nara, F., & Yamashita, M. (2010). A Novel CC Chemokine Receptor 4 Antagonist RS-1269 Inhibits Ovalbumin-Induced Ear Swelling and Lipopolysaccharide-Induced Endotoxic Shock in Mice. *Basic & Clinical Pharmacology & Toxicology* 107, 793–797.

Nakahigashi, K., Kabashima, K., Ikoma, A., Verkman, A. S., Miyachi, Y., & Hara-Chikuma, M. (2010). Upregulation of Aquaporin-3 Is Involved in Keratinocyte Proliferation and Epidermal Hyperplasia. *J. Invest. Dermatol.* 131, 865–873.

Nakayama, T., Hieshima, K., Nagakubo, D., Sato, E., Nakayama, M., Kawa, K.,& Yoshie, O. (2004). Selective induction of Th2-attracting chemokines CCL17 and CCL22 in human B cells by latent membrane protein 1 of Epstein-Barr virus. *J. Virol.* 78, 1665-1674.

Nograles, K. E., Zaba, L. C., Shemer, A., Fuentes-Duculan, J., Cardinale, I., Kikuchi, T., Ramon, M., Bergman, R., Krueger, J. G., & Guttman-Yassky, E. (2009). IL-22-producing "T22" T cells account for upregulated IL-22 in atopic dermatitis despite reduced IL-17-producing TH17 T cells. *J. Allergy Clin. Immunol.* 123, 1244–1252.

Nograles, K. E., Zaba, L. C., Guttman-Yassky, E., Fuentes-Duculan, J., Suárez-Fariñas, M., Cardinale, I., Khatcherian, A., Gonzalez, J., Pierson, K. C., White, T. R., et al. (2008). Th17 cytokines interleukin (IL)-17 and IL-22 modulate distinct inflammatory and keratinocyte-response pathways. *Br. J. Dermatol.* 159, 1092–1102.

Novak, N., & Bieber, T. (2005). The role of dendritic cell subtypes in the pathophysiology of atopic dermatitis. *J. Am. Acad. Dermatol.* 53, S171–6.

Novak, N., & Simon, D. (2011). Atopic dermatitis - from new pathophysiologic insights to individualized therapy. *Allergy* 66, 830–839.

O'Regan, G. M., & Irvine, A. D. (2010). The role of filaggrin in the atopic diathesis. *Clin. Exp. Allergy* 40, 965–972.

Ohl, L., Mohaupt, M., Czeloth, N., Hintzen, G., Kiafard, Z., Zwirner, J., Blankenstein, T., Henning, G., & Förster, R. (2004). CCR7 governs skin dendritic cell migration under inflammatory and steady-state conditions. *Immunity* 21, 279–288.

Owczarek, W., Paplinska, M., Targowski, T., Jahnz-Rozyk, K., Paluchowska, E., Kucharczyk, A., & Kasztalewicz, B. (2010). Analysis of eotaxin 1/CCL11, eotaxin 2/CCL24 and eotaxin 3/CCL26 expression in lesional and non-lesional skin of patients with atopic dermatitis. *Cytokine* 50, 181–185.

Oyoshi, M. K., Murphy, G. F., & Geha, R. S. (2009). Filaggrin-deficient mice exhibit TH17-dominated skin inflammation and permissiveness to epicutaneous sensitization with protein antigen. *J. Allergy Clin. Immunol.* 124, 485–93, 493.e1.

Panina-Bordignon, P., Papi, A., Mariani, M., Di Lucia, P., Casoni, G., Bellettato, C., Buonsanti, C., Miotto, D., Mapp, C., Villa, A., et al. (2001). The C-C chemokine receptors CCR4 and CCR8 identify airway T cells of allergen-challenged atopic asthmatics. *J. Clin. Invest.* 107, 1357–1364.

Pastore, S., Mascia, F., Mariotti, F., Dattilo, C., & Girolomoni, G. (2004). Chemokine networks in inflammatory skin diseases. *Eur. J. Dermatol.* 14, 203–208.

Pease, J. E. (2006). Asthma, allergy and chemokines. *Curr Drug Targets* 7, 3–12.

Pease, J. E. (2011). Targeting chemokine receptors in allergic disease. *Biochem. J.* 434, 11–24.

Pease, J. E., & Williams, T. J. (2006). Chemokines and their receptors in allergic disease. *J. Allergy Clin. Immunol.* 118, 305–18; quiz 319–20.

Perros, F., Hoogsteden, H. C., Coyle, A. J., Lambrecht, B. N., & Hammad, H. (2009). Blockade of CCR4 in a humanized model of asthma reveals a critical role for DC-derived CCL17 and CCL22 in attracting Th2 cells and inducing airway inflammation. *Allergy* 64, 995–1002.

Pivarcsi, A., Gombert, M., Dieu-Nosjean, M.-C., Lauerma, A., Kubitza, R., Meller, S., Rieker, J., Müller, A., Da Cunha, L., Haahtela, A., et al. (2004). CC chemokine ligand 18, an atopic dermatitis-associated and dendritic cell-derived chemokine, is regulated by staphylococcal products and allergen exposure. *J. Immunol.* 173, 5810–5817.

Qu, C., Edwards, E. W., Tacke, F., Angeli, V., Llodrá, J., Sanchez-Schmitz, G., Garin, A., Haque, N. S., Peters, W., van Rooijen, N., et al. (2004). Role of CCR8 and other chemokine pathways in the migration of monocyte-derived dendritic cells to lymph nodes. *J. Exp. Med.* 200, 1231–1241.

Randolph, G. J., Ochando, J., & Partida-Sánchez, S. (2008). Migration of dendritic cell subsets and their precursors. *Annu. Rev. Immunol.* 26, 293–316.

Ransohoff, R. M. (2009). Chemokines and chemokine receptors: standing at the crossroads of immunobiology and neurobiology. *Immunity* 31, 711–721.

Ratzinger, G., Stoitzner, P., Ebner, S., Lutz, M. B., Layton, G. T., Rainer, C., Senior, R. M., Shipley, J. M., Fritsch, P., Schuler, G., et al. (2002). Matrix metalloproteinases 9 and 2 are necessary for the migration of Langerhans cells and dermal dendritic cells from human and murine skin. *J. Immunol.* 168, 4361–4371.

Reiss, Y., Proudfoot, A. E., Power, C. A., Campbell, J. J., & Butcher, E. C. (2001). CC chemokine receptor (CCR)4 and the CCR10 ligand cutaneous T cell-attracting chemokine (CTACK) in lymphocyte trafficking to inflamed skin. *J. Exp. Med.* 194, 1541–1547.

Saeki, H., & Tamaki, K. (2006). Thymus and activation regulated chemokine (TARC)/CCL17 and skin diseases. *J. Dermato.l Sci.* 43, 75–84.

Salcedo, R., Young, H. A., Ponce, M. L., Ward, J. M., Kleinman, H. K., Murphy, W. J., &Oppenheim, J. J. (2001). Eotaxin (CCL11) induces in vivo angiogenic responses by human CCR3+ endothelial cells. *J. Immunol.* 166, 7571–7578.

Sallusto, F., Lanzavecchia, A., & Mackay, C. R. (1998a). Chemokines and chemokine receptors in T-cell priming and Th1/Th2-mediated responses. *Immunol. Today* 19, 568–574.

Sallusto, F., Schaerli, P., Loetscher, P., Schaniel, C., Lenig, D., Mackay, C. R., Qin, S., & Lanzavecchia, A. (1998b). Rapid and coordinated switch in chemokine receptor expression during dendritic cell maturation. *Eur. J. Immunol.* 28, 2760–2769.

Sallusto, F., & Baggiolini, M. (2008). Chemokines and leukocyte traffic. *Nat. Immunol.* 9, 949–952.

Sato, T., Komai, M., Iwase, M., Kobayashi, K., Tahara, H., Ohshima, E., Arai, H.,& Miki, I. (2009). Inhibitory effect of the new orally active CCR4 antagonist K327 on CCR4+CD4+ T cell migration into the lung of mice with ovalbumin-induced lung allergic inflammation. *Pharmacology* 84, 171–182.

Sánchez-Sánchez, N., Riol-Blanco, L., & Rodríguez-Fernández, J. L. (2006). The multiple personalities of the chemokine receptor CCR7 in dendritic cells. *J. Immunol.* 176, 5153–5159.

Scandella, E., Men, Y., Legler, D. F., Gillessen, S., Prikler, L., Ludewig, B.,& Groettrup, M. (2004). CCL19/CCL21-triggered signal transduction and migration of dendritic cells requires prostaglandin E2. *Blood* 103, 1595–1601.

Schaniel, C., Sallusto, F., Ruedl, C., Sideras, P., Melchers, F., & Rolink, A. G. (1999). Three chemokines with potential functions in T lymphocyte-independent and -dependent B lymphocyte stimulation. *Eur. J. Immunol.* 29, 2934–2947.

Sekiya, T., Tsunemi, Y., Miyamasu, M., Ohta, K., Morita, A., Saeki, H., Matsushima, K., Yoshie, O., Tsuchiya, N., Yamaguchi, M., et al. (2003). Variations in the human Th2-specific chemokine TARC gene. *Immunogenetics* 54, 742–745.

Semmling, V., Lukacs-Kornek, V., Thaiss, C. A., Quast, T., Hochheiser, K., Panzer, U., Rossjohn, J., Perlmutter, P., Cao, J., Godfrey, D. I., et al. (2010). Alternative cross-priming through CCL17-CCR4-mediated attraction of CTLs toward NKT cell-licensed DCs. *Nat. Immunol.* 11, 313–320.

Shimada, Y., Takehara, K., & Sato, S. (2004). Both Th2 and Th1 chemokines (TARC/CCL17, MDC/CCL22, and Mig/CXCL9) are elevated in sera from patients with atopic dermatitis. *J. Dermatol. Sci.* 34, 201–208.

Shoji, N., Asano, K., Furuta, A., Hirano, K., & Suzaki, H. (2011). Effect of histamine H1 receptor antagonists on TARC/CCL17 and MDC/CCL22 production from CD14+ cells induced by antigenic stimulation in vitro. *Int. Arch. Allergy Immunol.* 155, 38–51.

Soumelis, V., Reche, P. A., Kanzler, H., Yuan, W., Edward, G., Homey, B., Gilliet, M., Ho, S., Antonenko, S., Lauerma, A., et al. (2002). Human epithelial cells trigger dendritic cell mediated allergic inflammation by producing TSLP. *Nat. Immunol.* 3, 673–680.

Sozzani, S., Allavena, P., D'Amico, G., Luini, W., Bianchi, G., Kataura, M., Imai, T., Yoshie, O., Bonecchi, R., & Mantovani, A. (1998). Differential regulation of chemokine receptors during dendritic cell maturation: a model for their trafficking properties. *J. Immunol.* 161, 1083–1086.

Specht, S., Frank, J. K., Alferink, J., Dubben, B., Layland, L. E., Denece, G., Bain, O., Förster, I., Kirschning, C. J., Martin, C., et al. (2011). CCL17 Controls Mast Cells for the Defense against Filarial Larval Entry. *J. Immunol.* 186, 4845–4852.

Spergel, J. M., Mizoguchi, E., Brewer, J. P., Martin, T. R., Bhan, A. K., & Geha, R. S. (1998). Epicutaneous sensitization with protein antigen induces localized allergic dermatitis and hyperresponsiveness to methacholine after single exposure to aerosolized antigen in mice. *J. Clin. Invest.* 101, 1614–1622.

Stutte, S., Quast, T., Gerbitzki, N., Savinko, T., Novak, N., Reifenberger, J., Homey, B., Kolanus, W., Alenius, H., & Förster, I. (2010). Requirement of CCL17 for CCR7- and CXCR4-dependent migration of cutaneous dendritic cells. *Proc. Natl. Acad. Sci. U.S.A.* 107, 8736–8741.

Suárez-Fariñas, M., Tintle, S. J., Shemer, A., Chiricozzi, A., Nograles, K., Cardinale, I., Duan, S., Bowcock, A. M., Krueger, J. G., and Guttman-Yassky, E. (2011). Nonlesional atopic dermatitis skin is characterized by broad terminal differentiation defects and variable immune abnormalities. *J. Allergy Clin. Immunol.* 127, 954–64.e1-4.

Takeuchi, H., Yamamoto, Y., Kitano, H.,& Enomoto, T. (2005). Changes in thymus- and activation-regulated chemokine (TARC) associated with allergen immunotherapy in patients with perennial allergic rhinitis. *J. Investig. Allergo.l Clin. Immunol.* 15, 172–176.

Terada, N., Nomura, T., Kim, W. J., Otsuka, Y., Takahashi, R., Kishi, H., Yamashita, T., Sugawara, N., Fukuda, S., Ikeda-Ito, T., et al. (2001). Expression of C-C chemokine TARC in human nasal mucosa and its regulation by cytokines. *Clin. Exp. Allergy* 31, 1923–1931.

Thelen, M.,& Stein, J. V. (2008). How chemokines invite leukocytes to dance. *Nat. Immunol.* 9, 953–959.

Toda, M., Leung, D. Y. M., Molet, S., Boguniewicz, M., Taha, R., Christodoulopoulos, P., Fukuda, T., Elias, J. A., & Hamid, Q. A. (2003). Polarized in vivo expression of IL-11 and IL-17 between acute and chronic skin lesions☆. *J. Allergy Clin. Immunol.* 111, 875–881.

Tsuda, T., Tohyama, M., Yamasaki, K., Shirakata, Y., Yahata, Y., Tokumaru, S., Sayama, K., & Hashimoto, K. (2003). Lack of evidence for TARC/CCL17 production by normal human keratinocytes in vitro. *J. Dermatol. Sci.* 31, 37–42.

Tsunemi, Y., Saeki, H., Nakamura, K., Nagakubo, D., Nakayama, T., Yoshie, O., Kagami, S., Shimazu, K., Kadono, T., Sugaya, M., et al. (2006). CCL17 transgenic mice show an enhanced Th2-type response to both allergic and non-allergic stimuli. *Eur. J. Immunol.* 36, 2116–2127.

Uchida, T., Suto, H., Ra, C., Ogawa, H., Kobata, T., & Okumura, K. (2002). Preferential expression of T(h)2-type chemokine and its receptor in atopic dermatitis. *Int. Immunol.* 14, 1431–1438.

Vestergaard, C., Bang, K., Gesser, B., Yoneyama, H., Matsushima, K., & Larsen, C. G. (2000). A Th2 chemokine, TARC, produced by keratinocytes may recruit CLA+CCR4+ lymphocytes into lesional atopic dermatitis skin. *J. Invest. Dermatol.* 115, 640–646.

Vestergaard, C., Kirstejn, N., Gesser, B., Mortensen, J. T., Matsushima, K., & Larsen, C. G. (2001). IL-10 augments the IFN-gamma and TNF-alpha induced TARC production in HaCaT cells: a possible mechanism in the inflammatory reaction of atopic dermatitis. *J. Dermatol. Sci.* 26, 46–54.

Vestergaard, C., Yoneyama, H., Murai, M., Nakamura, K., Tamaki, K., Terashima, Y., Imai, T., Yoshie, O., Irimura, T., Mizutani, H., et al. (1999). Overproduction of Th2-specific chemokines in NC/Nga mice exhibiting atopic dermatitis-like lesions. *J. Clin. Invest.* 104, 1097–1105.

Vijayanand, P., Durkin, K., Hartmann, G., Morjaria, J., Seumois, G., Staples, K. J., Hall, D., Bessant, C., Bartholomew, M., Howarth, P. H., et al. (2010). Chemokine receptor 4 plays a key role in T cell recruitment into the airways of asthmatic patients. *J. Immunol.* 184, 4568–4574.

Viola, A. & Luster, A. D. (2008). Chemokines and their receptors: drug targets in immunity and inflammation. *Annu. Rev. Pharmacol. Toxicol.* 48, 171–197.

Wang, G., Savinko, T., Wolff, H., Dieu-Nosjean, M. C., Kemeny, L., Homey, B., Lauerma, A. I., & Alenius, H. (2007). Repeated epicutaneous exposures to ovalbumin progressively induce atopic dermatitis-like skin lesions in mice. *Clin. Exp. Allergy* 37, 151–161.

Weber, C., Meiler, S., Döring, Y., Koch, M., Drechsler, M., Megens, R. T. A., Rowinska, Z., Bidzhekov, K., Fecher, C., Ribechini, E., et al. (2011). CCL17-expressing dendritic cells drive atherosclerosis by restraining regulatory T cell homeostasis in mice. *J. Clin. Invest.* 121, 2898-910.

Wirnsberger, G., Hebenstreit, D., Posselt, G., Horejs-Hoeck, J., & Duschl, A. (2006). IL-4 induces expression of TARC/CCL17 via two STAT6 binding sites. *Eur. J. Immunol.* 36, 1882–1891.

Wollenberg, A., Wen, S.,& Bieber, T. (1995). Langerhans cell phenotyping: a new tool for differential diagnosis of inflammatory skin diseases. *Lancet* 346, 1626–1627.

Wu, D. (2005). Signaling mechanisms for regulation of chemotaxis. *Cell Res* 15, 52–56.

Xiao, T., Fujita, H., Saeki, H., Mitsui, H., Sugaya, M., Tada, Y., Kakinuma, T., Torii, H., Nakamura, K., Asahina, A., et al. (2003). Thymus and activation-regulated chemokine (TARC/CCL17) produced by mouse epidermal Langerhans cells is upregulated by TNF-alpha and IL-4 and downregulated by IFN-gamma. *Cytokine* 23, 126–132.

Yang, Y.-M., Feng, A.-L., Zhou, C.-J., Liang, X.-H., Mao, H.-T., Deng, B.-P., Yan, S., Sun, J.-T., Du, L.-T., Liu, J., et al. (2011). Aberrant expression of chemokine receptor CCR4 in human gastric cancer contributes to tumor-induced immunosuppression. *Cancer Sci* , 1264–1271.

Yawalkar, N., Uguccioni, M., Schärer, J., Braunwalder, J., Karlen, S., Dewald, B., Braathen, L. R., & Baggiolini, M. (1999). Enhanced expression of eotaxin and CCR3 in atopic dermatitis. *J. Invest. Dermatol.* 113, 43–48.

Yoo, J., Omori, M., Gyarmati, D., Zhou, B., Aye, T., Brewer, A., Comeau, M. R., Campbell, D. J.,& Ziegler, S. F. (2005). Spontaneous atopic dermatitis in mice expressing an inducible thymic stromal lymphopoietin transgene specifically in the skin. *J. Exp. Med.* 202, 541-549.

Yu, B., Koga, T., Urabe, K., Moroi, Y., Maeda, S., Yanagihara, Y., & Furue, M. (2002). Differential regulation of thymus- and activation-regulated chemokine induced by IL-4, IL-13, TNF-alpha and IFN-gamma in human keratinocyte and fibroblast. *J. Dermatol. Sci.* 30, 29–36.

Zlotnik, A., & Yoshie, O. (2000). Chemokines: a new classification system and their role in immunity. *Immunity* 12, 121–127.

Part 2

Microorganisms in Atopic Dermatits

7

Microorganisms and Atopic Dermatitis

Itaru Dekio
Department of Dermatology, Faculty of Medicine, Shimane University, Izumo
Japan

1. Introduction

The relationship between microorganisms and human skin is complex. Some microorganisms are friendly residents, while others are harmful pathogens. Human skin has a variety of mechanisms for interacting with microorganisms, which promote the propagation of certain organisms while attacking others. Each of the different microorganisms discussed in this chapter has a unique relationship with humans. Their stories are not simple but are quite interesting.

To make the stories easier to understand, this chapter is divided into two sections. One section is devoted to the characteristics of the resident microbiota (microflora) of patients with atopic dermatitis (AD), while the other covers secondary infections that frequently occur in AD patients which are sometimes life-threatening. The microbiota of AD patients is significantly different from that of the normal population, and the relationship of microbiota with AD is widely accepted.

2. The microbiota (microflora) and atopic dermatitis

Human skin harbours many bacterial and fungal species, which are not apparently harmful. The total population of such residential microorganisms is known as the 'microbiota' (microflora). The microbiota is well balanced with the effect of natural human immunity, and the microorganisms have mechanisms to balance their population as a part of this community. Thus, it is appropriate to consider the microbiota as a 'microbial community'. It is generally accepted that the microbiota become stabilised at different points of balance in AD patients. This altered balance relates to the pathogenesis of AD as will be discussed below.

2.1 Ecology of skin microbiota

The microbiota of human skin differs largely according to skin sites. This is probably due to the fact that the structure and physiology of the surface of the skin differs at different sites of the body. This leads to the natural selection of certain species for particular sites. Thus, facial skin may be considered as a 'swamp' of sebum, soles could be considered as a 'pond' of sweat, axillae could be analogous to a 'rain forest', and forearms are 'deserts' which generally lack water and lipid.

As a reflection of this, for example, healthy facial skin harbours about 10^8 microbial cells per square centimetre, which comprises up to 2 g of microorganisms per face. On the other hand, healthy forearm skin harbours only 10^3 microbes per square centimetre. Therefore, in some body sites, the population is large enough to consider that the microbiota has a certain physiological effects on the microecology of the skin. The scalp, face, neck, axilla, external genitalia, groin, and soles are examples of such sites. On the other hand, the microbiota seems to have little effect on the skin physiology at other sites with smaller populations, such as arms, hands, and legs.

2.2 Members of the normal skin microbiota

Because the skin microbiota differs considerably across different sites of the human body, it is not possible to describe the microbiota of the entire body in a single entity. In general terms, however, the major population of the normal microbiota consists of coagulase-negative *Staphylococcus* species, *Propionibacterium acnes*, and *Malassezia* species. Coagulase-negative *Staphylococcus* species are aerobic bacteria, *P. acnes* is a facultative anaerobic bacterium, and *Malassezia* species are yeasts (a single-cell form of fungus). All of these microorganisms live on the surface of the skin and in the hair follicles (Fig. 1). No other human organ has such a unique composition of microbiota. These three groups of microorganisms are retained in a balance between human immunity and each other.

2.2.1 Bacteria

Coagulase-negative *Staphylococcus* species are Gram-positive cocci. This group comprises *Staphylococcus* species other than *Staphylococcus aureus* and includes more than 10 species as *Staphylococcus epidermidis*. These bacteria grow under the aerobic condition and live in the colonisable layers of the skin. The term 'colonisable layers' here includes stratum corneum, the outermost barrier layer of the epidermis, and the outer thin section of viable layers of epidermis underneath the stratum corneum. These species can also grow under strict anaerobic conditions. This allows them to grow not only on the very surface of the skin but also deeper within skin layers where they compete for oxygen with other species. They are known to form grape-like clumps when cultured and normally also exist as clumps in skin layers.

Propionibacterium acnes is a Gram-positive bacillus, and is the most abundant in the human skin. Although this species is known to be an anaerobe, most strains also grow well in aerobic conditions (that is, facultative anaerobe). They live in the 'colonisable layers', in hair follicles, and in sebaceous glands. The genome analysis has revealed that they possess a lipase gene that enables them to degrade and metabolise lipids produced from sebaceous glands (Brüggemann et al., 2004). This species prospers in humans in the skin, conjunctiva, and prostate, but strangely, it is rarely found in other host species. This species usually forms a two-cell structure similar to the shape of eyeglasses when cultured, and they also take this form in human skin.

At certain skin sites, other species are the major species. For example, *Micrococcus* species, *Streptococcus* species, *Aerobacter* species, and *Proteus* species are cultured sometimes from the axilla and groin.

During the last decade, research on unculturable microorganisms using culture-independent molecular techniques has been carried out on various human organs. The results were surprising; the microbiota of some organs such as the oral cavity and gut are dominated mainly by unculturable or difficult-to-culture species. With regard to the skin, Dekio et al. first reported such an analysis of the skin microbiota including a large number of unculturable species in 2005 (Dekio et al., 2005). The microbiota included 22 species that remained unidentified on the skin, in addition to the 11 known skin bacteria (Table 1).

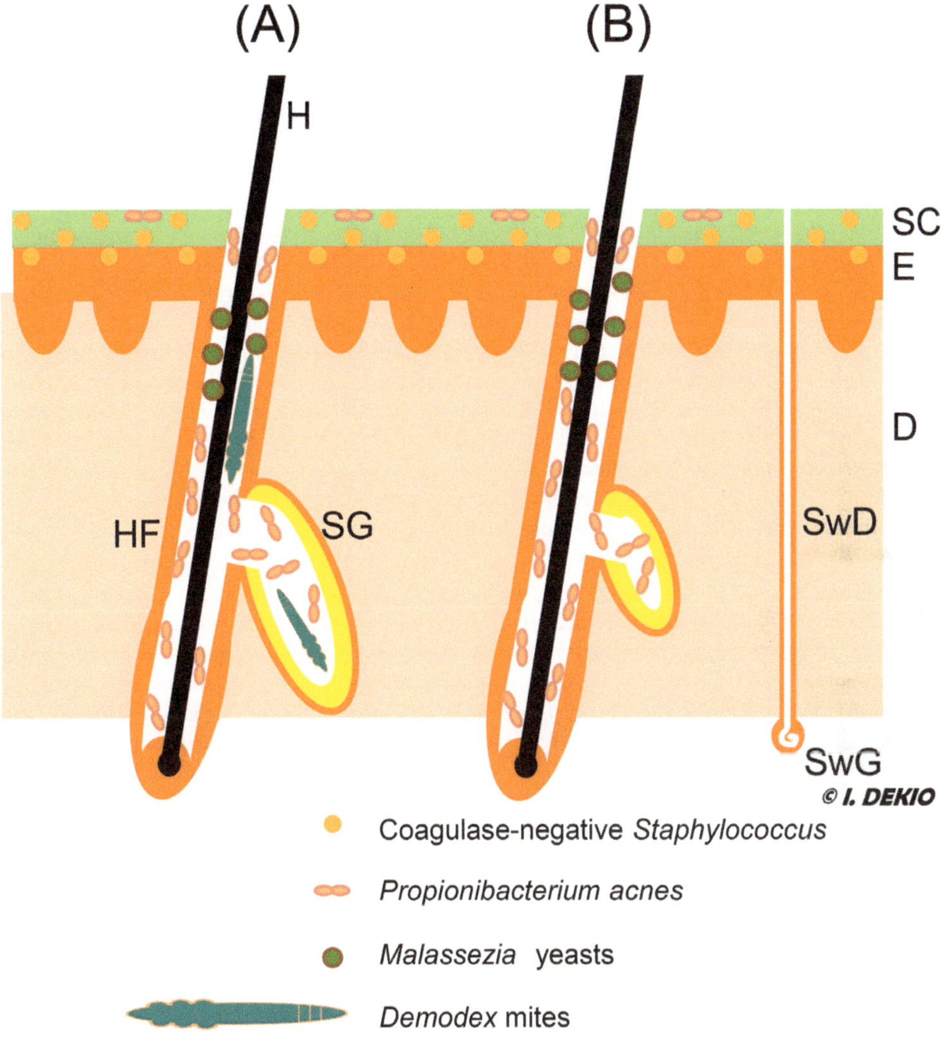

Fig. 1. Distribution of well-known skin inhabitants. (A) Typical hair follicle of the face. (B) Typical hair follicle of the trunk. SC, stratum corneum (a part of epidermis); E, viable portion of epidermis; D, dermis; H, hair; HF, hair follicle; SG, sebaceous gland; SwD, sweat duct; SwG, sweat gland. Note that the sweat duct and the sweat gland are considered to be sterile.

After this report, additional reports employing similar methods were published and a more complete picture of skin microbiota is emerging (Bek-Thomsen et al., 2008, Costello et al., 2009, Grice et al., 2009).

Known species	Unknown (uncultured) species
Stenotrophomonas maltophilia	Species close to *Methylophilus methylotrophus*
Acidovorax temperans	Species close to *Ideonella dechloratans*
Corynebacterium species	Species close to *Ammoniphilus oxalaticus*
Dietzia maris	Species close to *Anabaena cylindrica*
Bacillus species	Species close to *Aquaspirillum autotrophicum*

Table 1. Example of novel bacterial species identified in facial skin by molecular methods (Dekio et al., 2005)

2.2.2 Fungi

Malassezia species are fungal species that usually exist as yeasts in the healthy human skin. The major fungal members of human skin are *M. restricta* and *M. globosa* (Sugita et al., 2004). These fungi are aerobic and live only within the superficial portion of the hair follicle and the surface of the stratum corneum. The yeast forms are believed to be harmless to humans, but can change their shapes to form filaments if an unknown shift in the host-parasite relationship occurs. This shape change is associated with a disease known as tinea versicolor, a common infectious disease of the skin.

In addition, *Candida* species are detected in the skin less frequently. *Candida* species are well-known members of microbiota of the gut, but also colonise on the skin.

2.2.3 Viruses

It remains controversial whether viruses exist on the skin as members of the microbiota. The classical idea is that viruses do not exist on the healthy human skin. However, in a small percentage of healthy humans, there exists a phage PA6, which infects *P. acnes* cells. It is classified as a member of *Siphoviridae* family (Farrar et al., 2007). It is thought that the presence of this virus may explain why the resident bacteria cannot be cultured from certain skin samples.

In addition, there are some conditions that viruses lurk below the skin. Herpes simplex virus (HSV), which causes herpes simplex, becomes latent deep within the sensory ganglions after the first infection. Nearly 100% of adult humans are believed to have this virus somewhere in the ganglions. Certain healthy adults develop recurrent herpes simplex around the mouth or the genitalia, when exhausted. Under such conditions, HSV invades the skin from the ganglions via sensory nerves. Varicella-zoster virus (VZV) first invades humans from the throat when varicella, a febrile condition with small pustules also called chickenpox, appears. After relief from this condition, VZV remains in some of the sensory ganglions in 70% of the population, and after decades, it may appear via sensory nerves as herpes zoster. Both are categorised as members of the *Herpesviridae* (herpesvirus) family.

2.2.4 Arthropods

Surprisingly, mites also live within the hair follicle structures. *Demodex folliculorum* and *Demodex brevis* are such arthropods. Nearly 100% of the humans have these mites as a part of their microbiota. *D. folliculorum,* which has a long body, is believed to live in the follicles. *D. brevis* has a shorter body and lives in the sebaceous glands. These mites usually live in some but not all of the follicles of the facial skin without causing any harm. However, in some cases, the mites cause severe acne (demodex folliculitis), rosacea (rosacea-like demodicidosis [demodicosis]), or perioral dermatitis (Burns et al., 2010).

2.2.5 Possible interactions between a human host and microorganisms

Interactions of humans and members of the microbiota or among the members themselves (Fig. 2) are difficult to investigate because the phenomenon is often quite complex. Research is under way despite such difficulties.

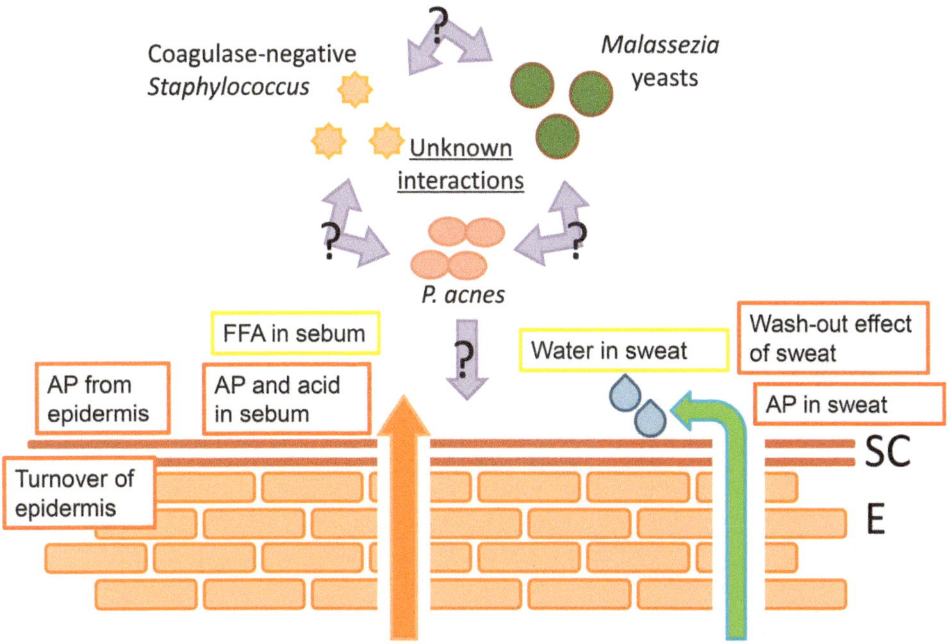

Fig. 2. Scheme of interactions between a human host and microorganisms. SC, stratum corneum; E, viable part of epidermis; AP, antimicrobial peptide; FFA, free fatty acid. The text encased in red rectangles indicates adverse effects towards microorganisms, and the text encased in yellow rectangles implies beneficial effects for them.

2.3 Characteristics of the microbiota in the skin of atopic dermatitis patients and its implications

Unlike the skin of healthy humans, the skin of AD patients is a 'rough ground' with less natural immunity. In a typical population of AD patients, the mutation in filaggrin gene (Palmer et al., 2006; Sasaki et al., 2008) results in impairment of the barrier function, and it allows the water content to evaporate. In addition, the sweat production is decreased because of the atrophy of the sweat glands. The resulting dry and rough surface allows easy colonisation of environmental bacteria. Moreover, a decrease in the amount of antimicrobial peptides in the sweat exaggerates the lack of immune function.

2.3.1 Bacteria in AD

The major outcome of AD is the presence of *Staphylococcus* species in very high numbers. The staphylococcal population in AD patients is about 10-100 times larger than that of normal individuals (Gloor et al., 1982). The *Staphylococcus* species here includes both coagulase-negative *Staphylococcus*, a major member of normal microbiota, and *S. aureus*, a harmful enemy from the environment that irritates the skin. In the skin of AD patients, the former is higher than usual while the latter also increases.

Coagulase-negative *Staphylococcus* provides a protective function to the skin by producing antimicrobial peptides against *S. aureus* (Cogen et al., 2010). Therefore, the growth of *S. aureus* leads to their production of exotoxins which exaggerate AD while the coagulase-negative *Staphylococcus* tries to eliminate them by they produce. The skin of AD patients is a battlefield of outnumbered 'the good' and growing 'the evil'.

Furthermore, *Stenotrophomonas maltophilia*, a previously unidentified bacterium on the skin and occasionally causes opportunistic sepsis in immunodeficient patients, was detected on the skin of patients with AD at a high frequency (Dekio et al., 2007). This species is closely related to *Pseudomonas* species and is considered to have high pathogenicity. This bacterial species may thus plays a specific role in development of AD.

2.3.2 Fungus in AD

In addition to bacteria, fungal species also contribute to the pathogenesis of AD. Although there is no convincing report that the *Malassezia* species in patients with AD differs from the *Malassezia* species of healthy humans, Sugita et al. (2004) reported that the genome sequence of the intergenic spacer (IGS) of *M. restricta*, one of the major members of the microbiota, differs between AD patients and healthy humans. Possessing a certain group of strains of *M. restricta* may be a worsening factor of AD.

Moreover, 10-20% of patients with AD have specific IgE against *Malassezia* species in the serum and show a positive result to the prick test of the fungus. Such AD patients tend to present a diffuse erythema on the face and neck (Darabi et al., 2008). This condition is often observed in adult humans and is improved by frequent washing, unlike most symptoms of AD.

2.3.3 Conclusion

A complete picture of the skin microbiota has not yet been attained. Therefore, its distinction in AD patients is also underinvestigated. However, biochemical and genomic techniques focused on specific molecules should lead to a total understanding in the near future.

3. Infections in atopic dermatitis

The skin of patients with AD often causes a variety of secondary infections. This may be due to dryness, impairment of natural immunity, scratching behaviour, and application of topical drugs. The dryness attracts pathogens because the rough surface yields a high point of scaling that easily captures environmental pathogens and deep crevices that make the pathogens accessible to deeper tissues. The presence of *S. aureus* in high numbers irritates the skin and results in aggravation of dryness. The decrease of antimicrobial peptides in the sweat exaggerates the possibility of the pathogen growing at the site. Extensive scratching by the patient enlarges the area of infection and also helps the pathogen to degrade the skin and invade it further. Topical drugs commonly used for treatment of AD, such as steroids and pimecrolimus/tacrolimus, suppress the immune function of the host and allows infectious microorganisms to grow at the site. In such cases, the diagnosis becomes difficult because it is not easy to ascertain that the lesion is caused by a secondary infection or by AD itself.

3.1 Colonisation and infection

Colonisation is a condition wherein parasitic organisms become attached to the skin and multiply without an apparent reaction of the host. Colonization is clinically invisible but may be detected in a culture test. When a microorganism colonises a host, there is a possibility that the microorganism will only harm the host incrementally. It may therefore become a hidden pathogen.

On the other hand, infection accompanies apparent host reaction in addition to colonisation. A host reaction is a kind of defence mechanism, and at the skin it is expressed as inflammation or oozing. Inflammation is a cytokine-mediated complex mechanism. Oozing is also a defensive reaction, because serum prevents microorganisms from multiplying. Therefore, when human skin is infected, a mixed reaction of inflammation and oozing occur. The clinical expression of this is redness, oozing, itching, and pain.

The colonisation may change to infection. This is due to a shift of the host defence mechanism (Table 2) and when it occurs, hidden pathogens increase in number and become infectious to do apparent harm; *Streptococcus* species is such an example in AD to develop impetigo. Therefore, doctors should be aware of this phenomenon and instruct patients to avoid activities that may cause such infections.

Possible triggers converting colonisation to infection
- Application of an anti-inflammatory ointment that is too strong for the site
- Oral administration of steroids or immunodepressants
- Scratching
- Flare-up of AD due to other allergic disease or failure to perform appropriate skin care
- Infrequent bathing

Table 2. Triggers to potentially causing a decline in the host defence mechanisms in the skin of AD patients

3.2 Impetigo

Impetigo is a bacterial infection caused by *S. aureus* or *Streptococcus* species. The former causes bullous impetigo and the latter causes non-bullous (or crusted) impetigo. This condition is typically seen in children but adult patients with AD are also affected and sometimes pre-sepsis occurs with high fever. In children without AD, the pathogen is considered to originate from the environment, but in patients with AD, it may also originate from their own colonising microbiota.

As these pathogens often reside on the skin of AD patients as members of the microbiota, they may not originate directly come from the outer environment, as they do for impetigo patients without AD. It is impossible to assess whether the pathogen originates from a patient's own microbiota or the environment, but it is meaningful to evaluate the patient's microbiota by using culture analysis after a successful treatment.

The clinical appearance of impetigo in AD patients includes sudden oozing, crust, and itching (Fig. 3). Culture tests using a scrubbed swab usually show the presence of pathogenic Gram-positive cocci. However, culture results require 2-3 days, so treatment should be administered before identification of the pathogen. Therefore, diagnosis by professional observation is needed. Otherwise, Gram stain may be used to visualise the pathogen at the point of consultation. Treatment should include a combination of oral and topical antibiotics. Usually treatment fails when only topical antibiotics are prescribed. Washing helps improvement of the healing process.

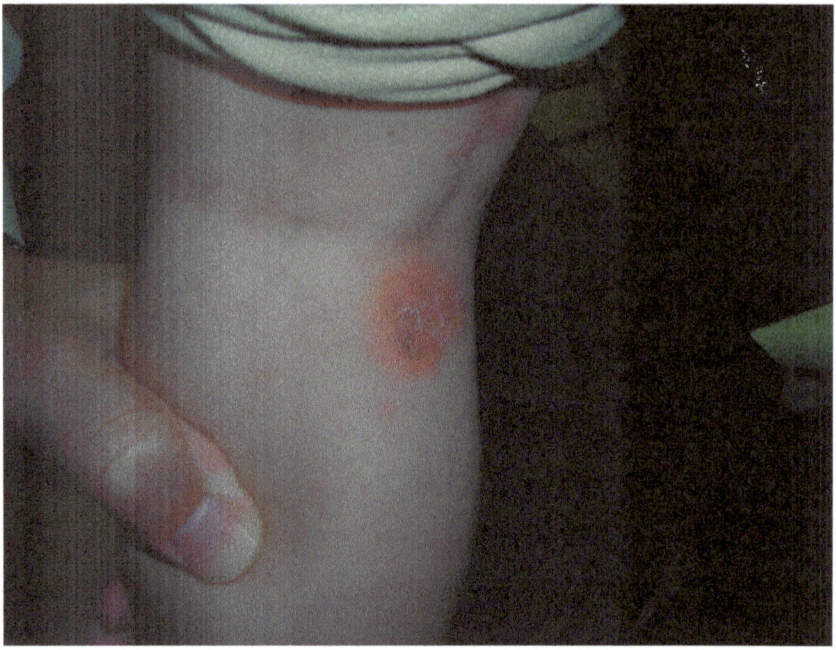

Fig. 3. Mild impetigo in a child with AD exhibiting erythema and crust.

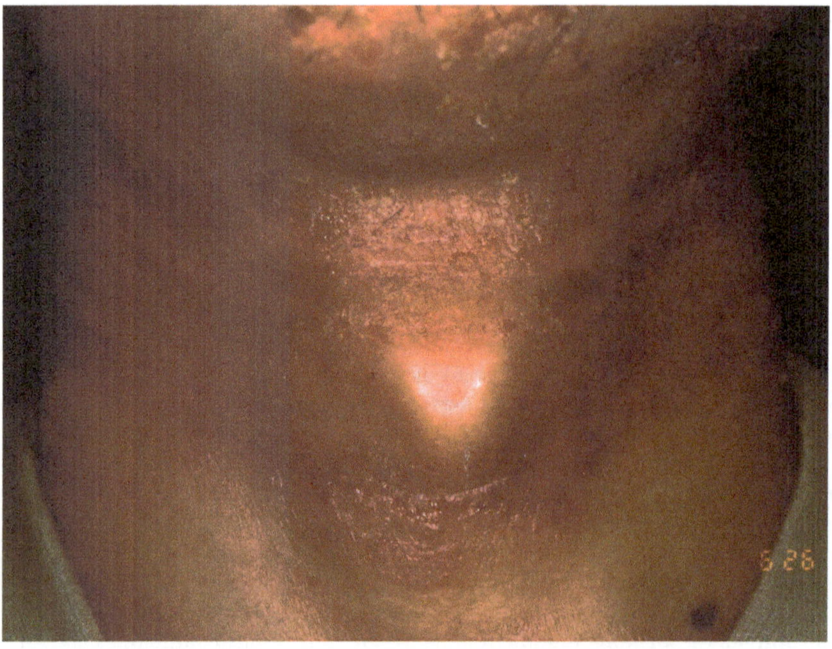

Fig. 4. Severe impetigo in an adult patient with AD. Erythema, oozing, and crust are visible.

The impetigo sites of AD patients are often very itchy and patients tend to scratch too much and exaggerate the infection. Scratching not only worsens the site but also inoculates the pathogen at other sites and other individuals. Doctors should advise the patient not to touch the site. Covering with a gauze or a sticking plaster helps to do this. The site should be kept dry beneath the covering.
In adult patients, it sometimes worsens at the neck (Fig. 4). This is because skin of the site is fragile and easy to scratch. A severe condition at this site causes difficulties in rotating the head because of the pain at the skin. This lowers activities of daily living of the patients.

3.3 Tinea corporis

Tinea corporis is a fungal infection caused by ringworm-forming fungi, such as *Trichophyton rubrum*. The pathogen is not contained in the microbiota and is thus considered to originate from patients with tinea pedis (athlete's foot) or from the outer environment.
The symptom is an erythema with a margin and slightly raised edge (Fig. 5). The erythema grows daily. In patients without AD, a strong itch is a hallmark, but patients with AD tend to suppress the itchy sensation with the use of ointments. This has the effect of masking this hallmark. Attention is needed to diagnose this infectious condition and careful examination with a microscope is required.
The filamentous fungus is easily seen in microscopic observation of the scales using the KOH technique (Fig. 6). Usually there is no need to perform a culture test, but it should be done if the patient is involved in close contact sports such as wrestling. This is because *Trichophyton tonsurans*, one of the pathogens transmitted by close contact, is difficult to observe using KOH technique. In most cases, the recommended treatment is a topical antifungal drug combined with discontinuance of topical application of drugs for AD. Oral antifungals should be administered in severe cases.

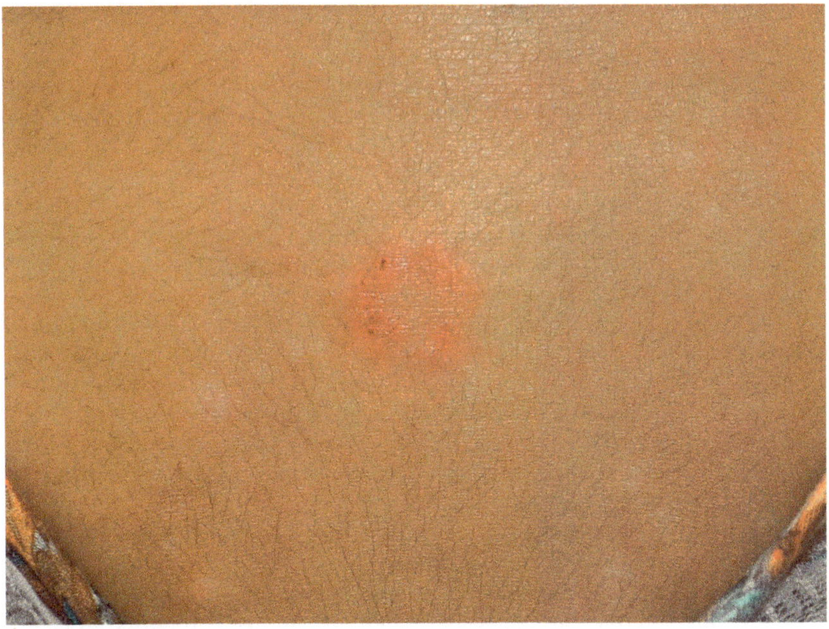

Fig. 5. Ring-like erythema on the back of a patient with AD.

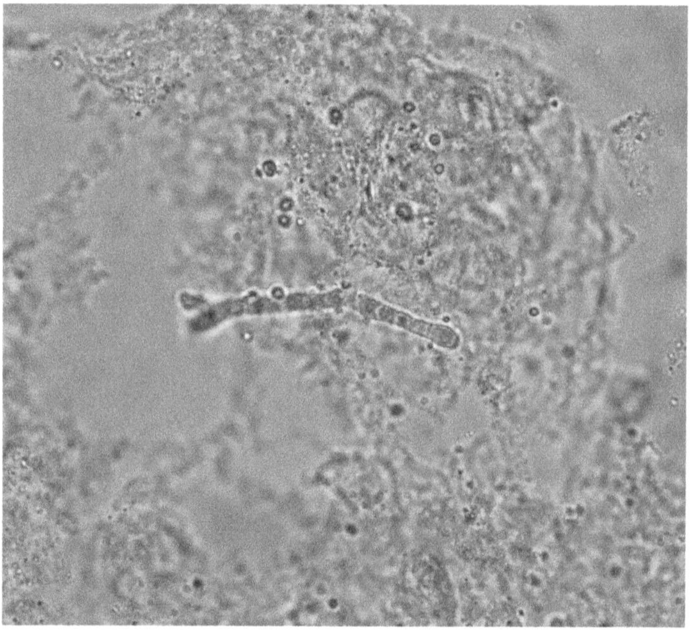

Fig. 6. Observation of a scale of the patient by KOH technique.

3.4 Kaposi's varicelliform eruption

Kaposi's varicelliform eruption (KVE) is an infection caused by herpes simplex virus (HSV). It rarely occurs in individuals without AD, but occurs often in patients with severe AD. HSV is also a pathogen of herpes simplex, a common latent infection of skin, and has life-long persistence in the ganglia of the sensory nerve. Regarding the aetiology of KVE, both persistent HSV in the ganglia and environmental HSV can be the possible cause of the disease. If the patient has a history of developing herpes simplex near the KVE site, it is natural to consider that the pathogen originated from the ganglia via sensory nerve, but otherwise it is impossible to determine the origin of the virus.

Once HSV begins to multiply on the surface of the skin, a varicella-like pustule with an erythematous surrounding appears. The number of the pustules increases and they become crusted. The formation of a crust usually reflects a secondary bacterial infection. Within a couple of days, the area of the lesion exceeds the size of a hand and a high fever develops (Fig. 7). Treatment must include a systemic antiviral drug for HSV (such as aciclovir or valaciclovir) and an antibacterial drug to treat the secondary bacterial infection with Gram-positive cocci.

In some rare cases, KVE recurs and it becomes difficult to manage. In such cases, preventive antivirals are efficient. Administration of topical acyclovir once in two days, in addition to the usual topical treatment of AD, is effective in many cases. In cases where this treatment is not effective, oral valaciclovir at a low dosage is reported to be effective (Dekio et al., 2011).

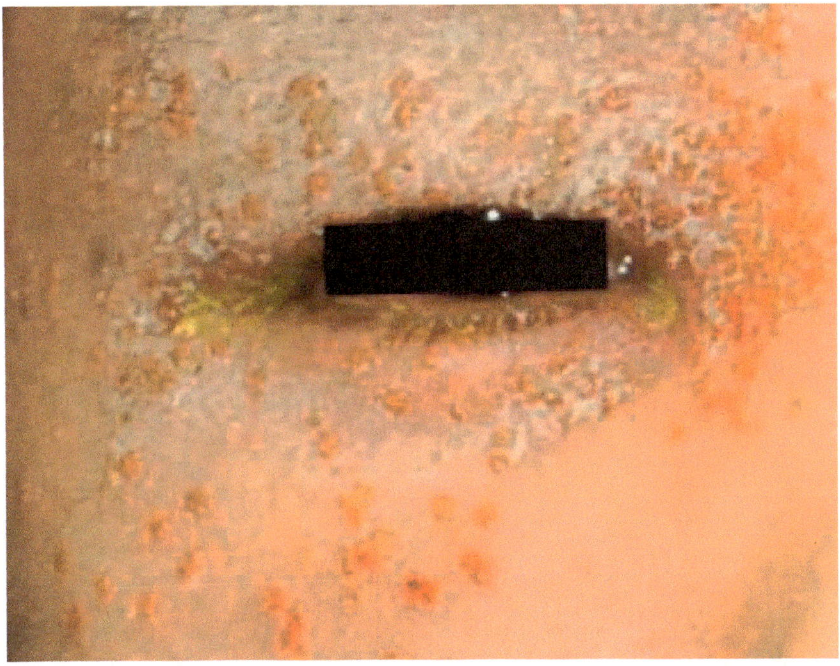

Fig. 7. Kaposi's varicelliform eruption. Crusted lesions around an eye of a patients with AD.

3.5 Molluscum contagiosum

Molluscum contagiosum is an infection caused by molluscum contagiosum virus (MCV). The condition is frequent in healthy children and also in patients (children and adults) with AD. The pathogen is not a member of the microbiota in AD skin so its presence reflects a simple infection from other patients or the environment. Because the clinical picture is far more severe in patients with AD and management strategy is different, it warrants a discussion in this chapter.

The skin lesions are whitish papules with diameters of 1 mm to 4 mm (Fig. 8). Scratching causes breakage of the surface of the papule and releases the viral ingredients. This leads to spreading of the lesions (Koebner phenomenon). In patients without AD, itch is not severe and often insensible, but patients with AD usually feel itch within the area of scattered lesion and scratching behaviour worsens the disease (Fig. 9).

In healthy children, the lesions disappear within months, but in patients with AD, the lesions may persist for years. The reason for this may be impairment of skin barrier and the use of topical anti-inflammatory drugs for the treatment. Molluscum contagiosum is not harmful to humans, but to prevent transmission to others, extirpation using tweezers is highly recommended.

Fig. 8. Molluscum contagiosum on the chest of a patient with AD.

3.6 Verruca vulgaris (viral wart)

Verruca vulgaris is an infection caused by human papilloma virus (HPV). There are more than 70 types of HPV which are identified by type numbers, and types that infect the human skin are different from those that infect the mucous of the oropharynx and genitalia. Therefore, doctors should inform the patients that the disease is not sexually transmitted. The pathogen is not included in the microbiota of AD skin, so it is a simple infection from other patients or the environment. The condition is frequent in healthy children and also in patients (children and adults) with AD. The clinical picture is different in patients with AD and the management strategy is also different, so it is discussed in this chapter.

The lesions are slightly elevated papules with obvious margins. Sometimes the lesions grow like cauliflower with a rough surface. The colour is more yellowish-white than the uninfected skin (Fig. 10). HPV promotes the growth of capillaries for their survival. Therefore, small black dots are often seen within a lesion. HPV is observed in piles within the lesion by electron microscopy.

When the skin of the face and the neck is affected in AD patients, the lesions often become itchy, and scratching releases HPV into the nearby skin. It results in an assembled manner of the lesions (Koebner phenomenon). The itching of the lesions is often ignored because the lesions are not itchy in patients without AD. Patients often apply topical anti-inflammatory drug to the lesion but it should be avoided because it promotes the proliferation of HPV. Therefore, the treatment for such HPV is often complex and difficult.
The first step of treatment should include cryotherapy using liquid nitrogen. When the lesion successfully drops off as a consequence, it is appropriate to apply topical anti-inflammatory ointment immediately.

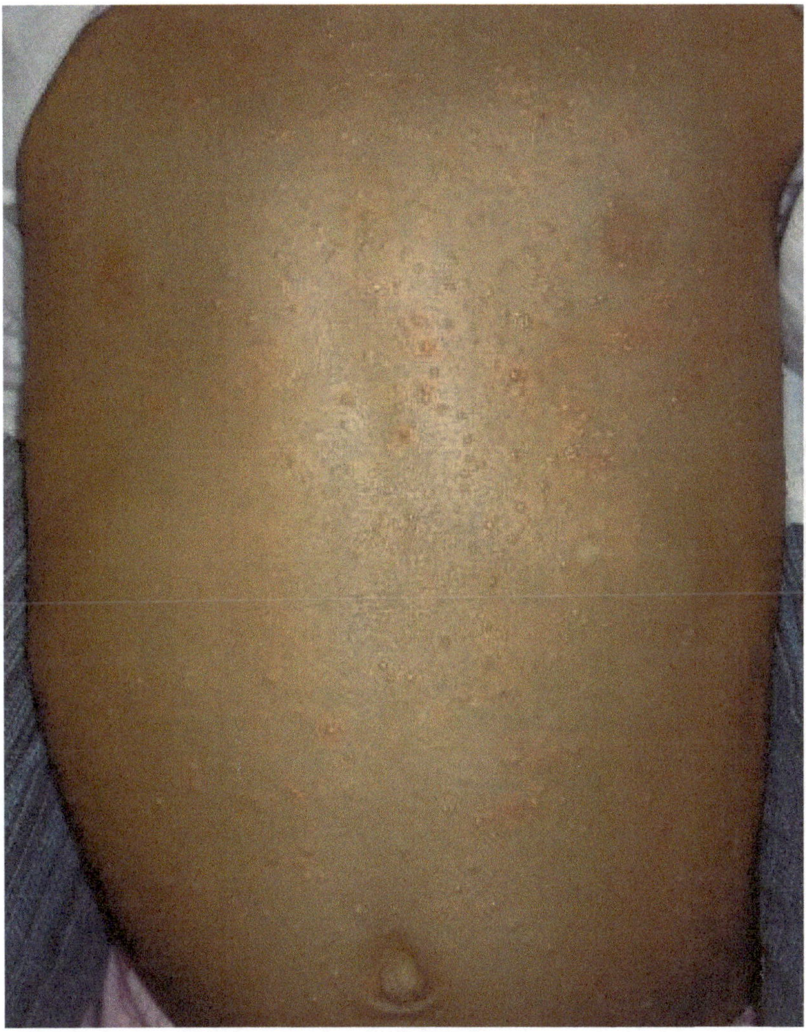

Fig. 9. Severe molluscum contagiosum in an infant with AD.

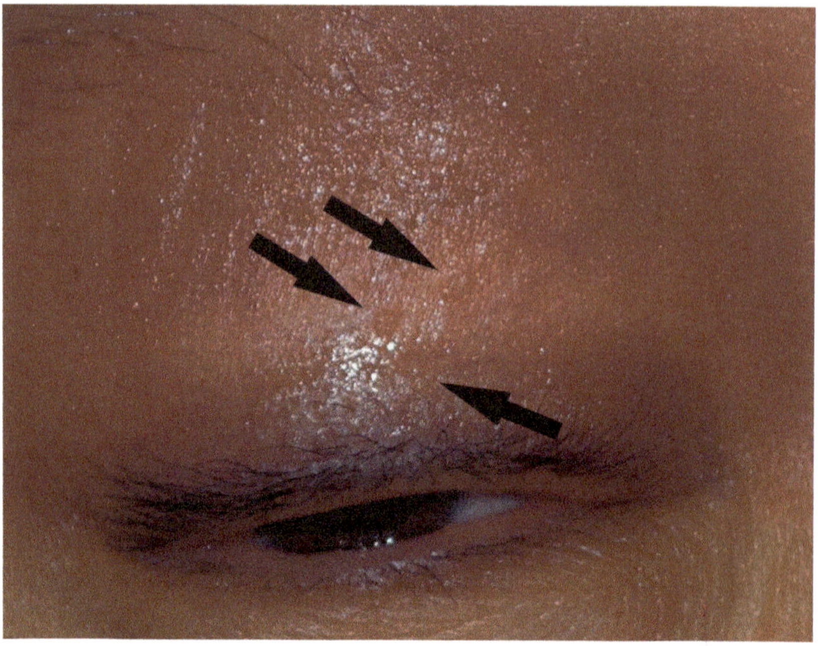

Fig. 10. Multiple verruca vulgaris on the eyelid of an adult patient with AD.

4. Conclusion

As microorganisms have close and complex relationships with human skin, doctors and scientists should be aware of the presence of good and harmful species in the skin. Human skin has mechanisms to allow microbes to reside on the skin, and good microbes may help humans.

On the other hand, certain microbes may trigger AD under certain conditions and others are consistent pathogens. When considering microorganisms as exacerbating factors, research should be performed in order to clarify their roles. Such research may lead to advances in the treatment and prevention of AD.

In treatment of various infectious conditions in AD patients, careful and well-considered strategy by dermatologists is necessary.

5. Acknowledgment

I thank Prof. Haroun N. Shah, London for the insightful comments on this manuscript.

This work is partly supported by Grant-in-Aid 22791073 from the Ministry of Education, Culture, Sports, Science and Technology (MEXT) of Japan.

6. References

Bek-Thomsen, M., Lomholt, H.B., & Kilian, M. (2008). Acne is not associated with yet-uncultured bacteria. *Journal of Clinical Microbiology* Vol. 46, No. 10, pp. 3355-3360

Brüggemann, H., Henne, A., Hoster, F., Liesegang, H., Wiezer, A., Strittmatter, A., Hujer, S., Dürre, P., & Gottschalk, G. (2004). The complete genome sequence of *Propionibacterium acnes*, a commensal of human skin. *Science* Vol. 305, pp. 671-673

Burns, T., Breathnach, S., Cox, N., & Griffiths, C. (Eds.) (2010). *Rook's Textbook of Dermatology 8th ed.* Wiley-Blackwell, ISBN: 9781405161695

Cogen, A.L., Yamasaki, K., Sanchez, K.M., Dorschner, R.A., Lai, Y., MacLeod, D.T., Torpey, J.W., Otto, M., Nizet, V., Kim, J.E., Gallo, R.L. (2010). Selective antimicrobial action is provided by phenol-soluble modulins derived from *Staphylococcus epidermidis*, a normal resident of the skin. *Journal of Investigative Dermatology* Vol. 130, No. 1, pp. 192-200

Costello, E.K., Lauber, C.L., Hamady, M., Fierer, N., Gordon, J.I., Knight, R. (2009). Bacterial community variation in human body habitats across space and time. *Science* Vol. 326, No. 5960, pp. 1694-1697

Darabi, K., Hostetler, S. G., Bechtel, M.A., & Zirwas, M. (2009). The role of Malassezia in atopic dermatitis affecting the head and neck of adults. *Journal of American Academy of Dermatology* Vol. 60, No. 1, pp. 125-136

Dekio, I., Hayashi, H., Sakamoto, M., Kitahara, M., Nishikawa, T., Suematsu, M., & Benno, Y. (2005). Detection of potentially novel bacterial components of the human skin microbiota using culture-independent molecular profiling. *Journal of Medical Microbiology* Vol. 54, No.12, pp. 1231-1238

Dekio, I., Sakamoto, M., Hayashi, H., Amagai, M., Suematsu, M., & Benno, Y. (2007). Characterization of skin microbiota in patients with atopic dermatitis and normal subjects using 16S rRNA gene-based comprehensive analysis. *Journal of Medical Microbiology* Vol.56, No.12, pp. 1675-1683

Dekio, I., Chinuki, Y., Furumura, M., & Morita, E. (2011). Recurrent Kaposi's varicelliform eruption successfully controlled by low-dose oral valaciclovir. *The Journal of Dermatology* Epub Apr 2011, DOI: 10.1111/j.1346-8138.2011.01245.x

Gloor, M., Peters, G., & Stoika, D. (1982). On the resident aerobic bacterial skin flora in unaffected skin of patients with atopic dermatitis and in healthy controls. *Dermatologica* Vol. 164, No. 4, pp. 258-265

Farrar, M.D., Howson, K.M., Bojar, R.A., West, D., Towler, J.C., Parry, J., Pelton, K., & Holland, K.T. (2007). Genome Sequence and Analysis of a *Propionibacterium acnes* Bacteriophage. *The Journal of Bacteriology* Vol. 189, No. 11, pp. 4161–4167

Grice, E.A., Kong, H.H., Conlan, S., Deming, C.B., Davis, J., Young, A.C., NISC Comparative Sequencing Program, Bouffard, G.G., Blakesley, R.W., Murray, P.R., Green, E.D., Turner, M.L., Segre, J.A. Topographical and temporal diversity of the human skin microbiome. (2009). *Science* Vol. 324, No. 5931, pp. 1190-1192

Palmer, C.N., Irvine, A.D., Terron-Kwiatkowski, A., et al. (2006). Common loss-of-function variants of the epidermal barrier protein filaggrin are a major predisposing factor for atopic dermatitis. *Nature Genetics* Vol. 38, No. 4, pp. 441-446

Sasaki, T., Kudoh, J., Ebihara, T., Shiohama, A., Asakawa, S., Shimizu, A., Takayanagi, A., Dekio, I., Sadahira, C., Amagai, M., Shimizu, N. (2008). Sequence analysis of filaggrin gene by novel shotgun method in Japanese atopic dermatitis. *Journal of Dermatological Science* Vol. 51, No. 2, pp. 113-120

Sugita, T., Tajima, M., Amaya, M., Tsuboi, R., & Nishikawa, A. (2004). Genotype analysis of *Malassezia restricta* as the major cutaneous flora in patients with atopic dermatitis and healthy subjects. *Microbiology and Immunology* Vol. 48, No. 10, pp.755-759

8

Fungus as an Exacerbating Factor of Atopic Dermatitis, and Control of Fungi for the Remission of the Disease

Takuji Nakashima and Yoshimi Niwano
Kitasato University, Tohoku University
Japan

1. Introduction

Atopic dermatitis (AD) is a common, chronic fluctuating skin disease with prevalence in children (Williams, 2000; Williams & Wüthrich, 2000). The disease is an inflammatory skin disorder characterized by itching, and chronically relapsing course. Moreover, it also produces vulnerablity to surface infections caused by pathogenic bacteria, fungi and viruses. The most common skin infections in AD patients are caused by *Staphylococcus aureus* and herpes simplex virus (Ong & Leung, 2010). *S. aureus* is frequently detected in AD patients (Abeck & Mempel, 1998; Katsarou & Armenaka, 2011) and becomes an aggravating factor. In addition, toxins, such as staphylococcal enterotoxins and toxic shock syndrome toxin-1 (McFadden et al., 1993; Bunikowski et al., 1999), generated from *S. aureus* may act as superantigens (Herz et al., 1999; Niebuhr et al., 2011; Yeung et al., 2011). In AD patients, viral infection is most often caused by herpes simplex virus (HSV) (Wollenberg et al., 2003). Eczema herpeticum is a potentially life-threatening disseminated HSV type 1 or type 2 infection that occurs in 10% to 20% of AD patients (Peng et al., 2007). However, not only bacteria and viruses but also fungi, such as *Malassezia* species and *Candida* species, may play an important role as aggravation factors in AD patients. It has been reported that antifungal therapy is beneficial in the treatment of some AD patients (Bäck et al. 1995; Svejgaard et al. 2004; Broberg et al. 1995; Mayser et al., 2006). In addition, several candidate *Malassezia* antigens have been implicated in the pathogenesis of AD. In this chapter, the involvement of fungi in the pathogenesis of AD is discussed.

2. Fungi isolated from AD patients and treatment

The genus *Malassezia* has recently been shown to consist of fifteen species based on the database of National Center for Biotechnology Information (2011), one lipid-independent species, *M. pachydermatis* and fourteen lipid-dependent species, *M. sympodialis, M. furfur, M. globosa, M. obtusa, M. restricta, M. slooffiae, M. caprae, M. equine, M. dermatis, M. equi, M. japonica, M. nana, M. yamatoensis* and *M. cuniculi*. *Malassezia* species have been recognized as members of the microbiological flora of human and animal skin. *M. globosa* and *M. restricta* are frequently isolated from the skin scales of human AD (Sugita et al., 2001; Tajima et al., 2008; Kaga et al., 2009) and *M. pachydermatis* and *M. nana* are isolated from some animals (Aizawa et al., 2001; Hirai et al., 2004). Antifungal drugs, e.g. ketoconazole and itraconazole, are used in AD patients with signs of a fungal infection (Sugita et al., 2005; Bäck et al., 1995). Antifungal therapy may remit the severity of AD by controlling these *Malassezia* yeasts.

2.1 Related pathogenic fungi

The yeasts of the genus *Malassezia* are members of the normal cutaneous flora. However, *Malassezia* colonization on the skin of AD patients shows a different pattern from that on healthy skin (Faergemann, 2002; Gupta et al., 2001; Nakabayashi et al., 2000; Sandström et al., 2005; Sugita et al., 2004, 2006) and may aggravate AD due to an allergic reaction, especially on the head and neck area in adults (Brehler & Luger, 2001; Broberg et al., 1992; Faergemann, 1999; Huang et al., 1995; Jensen-Jarolim et al., 1992; Lintu et al., 1997; Rokugo et al., 1990; Schmidt et al., 1997; Nakabayashi et al., 2000; Savolainen et al., 2001; Scalabrin et al., 1999). Scalabrin et al. (1999) measured total IgE and specific IgE to *Malassezia furfur* in 73 AD patients. In the AD patients, specific IgE to *M. furfur* was observed more frequently in adults than children. The reaction of specific IgE to *M. furfur* was 132 times higher than that in healthy subjects. This result suggests that *Malassezia* yeast is associated with IgE-mediated skin inflammation in AD.

Culture-dependent methods have been used for the detection of *Malassezia* species from AD patients (Nakabayashi et al., 2000; Sandström et al., 2005). However, in recent years, many researchers have attempted the detection of *Malassezia* species from AD patients by means of a molecular-based culture-independent method that is not affected by the isolation medium, sampling method, or incubation period. Table 1 summarizes the three major studies applying molecular based PCR assay to detect *Malassezia* species from AD patients and healthy subjects, indicating that the number of detected *Malassetia* species was similar to AD patients and healthy subjects (Sugita et al., 2001; Tajima et al., 2008; Kaga et al., 2009).

Species	Sugita et al.		Tajima et al.		Kaga et al.	
	AD (32)*	HS (18)	AD (36)	HS (30)	AD (56)	HS(32)
M. globosa	93.8**	44.4	100	86.7	100	100
M. restricta	87.5	61.1	97.2	83.3	100	100
M. furfur	40.6	11.1	33.3	26.7	16.1	12.5
M. sympodialis	40.6	50.0	58.3	36.7	65.2	62.5
M. slooffiae	6.3	0	30.6	16.7	17.9	6.3
M. obtuse	0	0	27.8	10	14.3	12.5
M. pachydermatis	0	0	-	-	-	-
M. yamatoensis	-	-	13.9	6.7	21.4	15.6
M. japonicum	-	-	33.3	10	10.7	12.5
M. dermatis	-	-	30.6	30	37.5	34.4

* Number of cases. ** Percentage of the number of patients. AD, atopic detmatitis; HS, healthy subjects. -, not detected.

Table 1. Comparison of published research on *Malassezia* colonization in AD patients and healthy subjects.

In both AD patients and healthy subjects, the predominant species were *M. globosa* and *M. restricta*. However, the study by Kaga et al. (2009), who applied real-time PCR to determine the number of rDNA copies of *M. globosa* and *M. restricta*, revealed that *Malassezia* colonization in severe AD patients was approximately two to five times higher than that in other AD patients (mild and moderate) and healthy subjects. Since the species-specific DNA of *M. globosa* and *M. restricta* were frequently and massively detected, the two *Malassezia* species may be related to the severity of AD.

Besides the *Malassezia* species, *Candida* species and dermatophytes are also involved in the pathogenesis of AD, and especially *C. albicans* may play a role in the alimentary canal of AD patients, becuase *Candida* species have been cultured more frequently from the gastrointestinal tract in AD patients than healthy subjects (Arzumanyan et al., 2000; Savolainen et al., 2003). Moreover, the possible involvement of dermatophytes, especially *Trichophyton rubrum*, in the inflammation in AD patients was reported (Klein et al., 1999).

2.2 Control of fungi in AD patients

Ketoconazole and itraconazole, azole antimycotics, have been the most frequently studied therapeutic agents for AD. The antimycotics showed strong antifungal activities against *Malassezia* species isolated from AD patients *in vitro* (Sugita et al. 2005). In clinical studies, ketoconazole and itraconazole have shown a significant therapeutic effect on AD patients. Bäck et al. (1995) assessed the efficacy of oral ketoconazole treatment on 20 AD patients using a positive radioallergosorbent test. The AD patients were treated with ketoconazole 200 mg daily for 2 months and 200 mg twice a week for another 3 months. Of the 20 patients, 18 completed the ketoconazole treatment regimen for 5 months and most patients showed a good to moderate response for ketoconazole 200 mg daily during the 2 months but no further improvement after the administration of ketoconazole 200 mg twice a week for another 3 months. Svejgaard et al. (2004) evaluated the efficacy of oral itraconazole in the treatment of AD patients with head and neck dermatitis in a randomized, double-blind, placebo-controlled study. The AD patients were treated daily with itraconazole 200 mg, 400 mg or placebo for 7 days. The treatment with 200 mg and 400 mg of itraconazole exerted a remarkable therapeutic effect on AD patients. Therefore, the systemic antimycotic administration is expected to be highly effective in treating AD patients.

Meanwhile, the application of topical antimycotics could decrease *Malassezia* colonization and the severity of eczematous lesions in AD patients. For instance, as reported by Broberg et al. (1995), the treatment of AD patients who had head and neck dermatitis with twice-daily miconazole-hydrocortisone cream and twice weekly ketoconazole shampoo for 4 weeks resulted in decreased *Malassezia* colonization although clinical scores were not greatly improved. In addition, they confirmed the effect of ciclopiroxolamine on AD patients with moderate to severe head and neck dermatitis, which is often difficult to be treated, in a double-blind, placebo-controlled study.

3. Fungal infection in animals with AD

Fungal infection in animals with AD has been reported mainly in canines and felines. For instance, Morris et al. (2002) reported that cell-mediated and humoral reactivities to *M. pachydermatis* contribute to the pathogenesis of AD in dogs but are not directly correlated. They investigated whether the potential cell-mediated immune response of atopic dogs to the yeast *M. pachydermatis* is correlated with the type-1 hypersensitivity (humoral) response of the same population of dogs. Atopic dogs with cytologic evidence of *Malassezia* dermatitis had an increased lymphocyte blastogenic response to crude *M. pachydermatis* extract, compared with clinically normal dogs and dogs with *Malassezia* otitis. The blastogenic responses in atopic control dogs (without *Malassezia* dermatitis or otitis) did not differ significantly from those in atopic dogs with *Malassezia* dermatitis. No significant correlation was found between the lymphocyte blastogenic response and the type-1 hypersensitivity response to *M. pachydermatis* within any of the groups, suggesting that modification of the dysregulated immune response toward *M. pachydermatis* may assist in the reduction of pathologic changes associated with an AD phenotype in dogs. In another study, Chen et al. (2002) compared IgE responses to separated proteins of *M. pachydermatis* in atopic dogs with *Malassezia* dermatitis and clinically normal dogs. The results of their study showed that the majority of atopic dogs with *Malassezia* dermatitis have a greater IgE response than normal dogs, suggesting an IgE-mediated immune response may be clinically important in the pathogenesis of the disease. In felines, *Malassezia* spp. have been more frequently isolated from healthy ear canals and skin in feline leukaemia (FeLV)- or feline immunodeficiency virus (FIV)-infected cats than in those noninfected (Sierra et al., 2000). In addition, *Malassezia* spp. overgrowth has been described in feline localized benign exfoliative skin diseases, such as chin acne and the idiopathic facial dermatitis of Persian cats (Jazic et al., 2006; Bond et al., 2000). Based on these findings, Ordeix et al. (2007) conducted a multicentre, retrospective and descriptive study to document *Malassezia* spp. overgrowth in allergic cats. Their results suggested that *Malassezia* spp. overgrowth may represent a secondary cutaneous problem in allergic cats particularly in those with greasy adherent brownish scales on their skin. The favorable response to treatment with antifungal agent alone suggests that, as in dogs, *Malassezia* spp. may be partly responsible for both pruritus and cutaneous lesions in allergic cats.

4. Mechanisms by which fungi act as an exacerbating factor for atopic dermatitis

4.1 Antigen-specific inflammation caused via activation of antigen-specific T cells

Allergy to fungi such as *Candida* spp. and *Malassezia* spp. has been implicated as an exacerbating or intractable factor in the symptoms of AD (Savolainen et al., 1993; Tanaka et al., 1994; Kitamura et al., 1997; Morita et al., 1999; Linder et al., 2000; Faergemann 2002; Kanda et al., 2002; Svejgaard et al., 2004). *Candida* spp. are indigenous fungi inhabiting the oral cavity, digestive tract and vagina. Healthy people are thought to acquire the Th1 type immunity against *Candida* spp. (Tanaka et al., 1994; Romani et al., 1995). For instance, the activation of Th1-type CD4+ cell induces phagocyte-dependent immunity, which apparently represents an important mechanism of anti-*Candida* resistance, and it was demonstrated that healthy subjects with a normal immune response show high peripheral blood lymphocyte proliferative responses as well as positive scarification patch tests to *C. albicans* antigen, suggesting the dominant presence of Thl type T cells specific to *C. albicans* antigen. It is well known that Thl clones secrete IL-2 and IFN-γ and preferentially induce delayed type hypersensitivity (Stout & Bottomly, 1989), while Th2 clones produce IL-4, IL-5 (Mosmann et al., 1986) and IL-10 (Fiorentino et al., 1989) and help to promote IgE production (Boom et al., 1988; Killar et al., 1987). In AD patients, Th1-type immunity has been shown to shift to Th2-type (Fig. 1) since the patients immediately react to skin testing using *Candida*-antigen (Tanaka et al., 1994; Kitamura et al., 1997), and *Candida*-specific IgE increases with the severity of the symptoms of AD (Tanaka et al., 1994). Specifically, AD patients displayed a significantly lower incidence of positive patch test reactions to *C. albicans* allergen than the healthy control subjects, and the patients with negative *C. albicans* patch tests tended to have higher levels of total serum IgE including anti-*C. albicans* IgE antibody. In other words, the delayed-type hypersensitivity to *C. albicans* antigen, which is highly prevalent in atopics without dermatitis as well as non-atopics, was reduced in most of the AD patients.

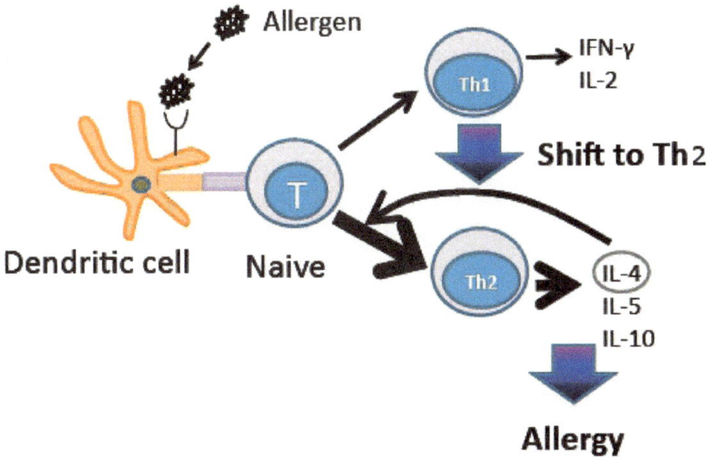

Fig. 1. Shift of Th1-type immunity to Th2-type immunity in allergic diseases including atopic dermatitis (AD). In healthy individuals, dendritic cells present fungal antigen to naive T cells which in turn differentiate to Th1 type cells, resulting in the cellular immune response. In AD patients, Th1-type immunity shifts to Th2-type immunity in which Th2 clones produce IL-4, IL-5 and IL-10 and induce IgE production.

The lipophilic fungus *M. furfur* indigenously inhabits the seborrheic region of the body, such as head, neck and upper part of the back. It was also reported that the fungus may be implicated in rosacea-like dermatitis and edematous erythema, which are chromic and intractable symptoms characteristic to the face with adult-type AD (Mukai et al., 1997), and that *Malassezia*-specific IgE level is high in the head and neck of AD patients (Bayrou et al., 2005; Darabi et al., 2009). Regarding the 11 currently recognized *Malassezia* species as an exacerbating factor in AD, *M. globosa* and *M. restricta* are found to frequently colonize the skin of AD patients. For instance, specific IgE antibodies against eight *Malassezia* species (*M. dermatitis, M. furfur, M. globosa, M. obtusa, M. pachydermatis, M. slooffiae, M. sympodialis*, and *M. restricta*) in sera from AD patients were examined using an enzyme-linked immunosorbent assay, and it was found that the specific IgE value against *M. restricta* was greater than those against the other *Malassezia* species (Kato et al., 2006).

4.2 *Candida albicans* gut colonization

It has been hypothesized that excessive colonization by *C. albicans* in the gastrointestinal tract may constitute an aggravating factor in AD, but this remains controversial (Faergemann et al., 2002; Lacour et al., 2002; Nikkels & Pierard, 2003). To date, laboratory and clinical investigations have demonstrated that IgE mediated food allergy plays a pathogenic role in a subset of AD patients (Eigenmann et al., 1998; Lever et al., 1998; van Reijsen et al., 1998). Some reports have shown increased gastrointestinal permeability in

AD patients (Jackson et al., 1981; Majamaa et al., 1996; Pike et al., 1986). Hyperpermeability of the gastrointestinal mucosal barrier results in enhanced transport of intact and degraded antigens across the gastrointestinal mucosal barrier, which could induce food protein sensitization and food allergy in susceptible individuals (Farhadi et al., 2003) (Fig. 2). Yamaguchi et al. (2006) therefore hypothesized that gastrointestinal colonization by *C albicans* may be involved in aggravation of AD by affecting the mucosal barrier in a manner that results in increased permeation of food allergens and subsequent manifestation of a food allergy. Using mice, they examined whether gastrointestinal colonization by *C. albicans* contributes to the aggravation of AD. *Candida* colonization was establised by intragastric inoculation with *C. albicans*, and then mice were intragastrically administered ovalbumin every other day for nine weeks. As a result, ovalbumin specific IgG and IgE titres were higher in BALB/c mice with *Candida* colonization than in normal mice, suggesting that gastrointestinal permeation of ovalbumin was enhanced by colonization in the mice. Histological examination showed that colonization promoted infiltration and degranulation of mast cells.

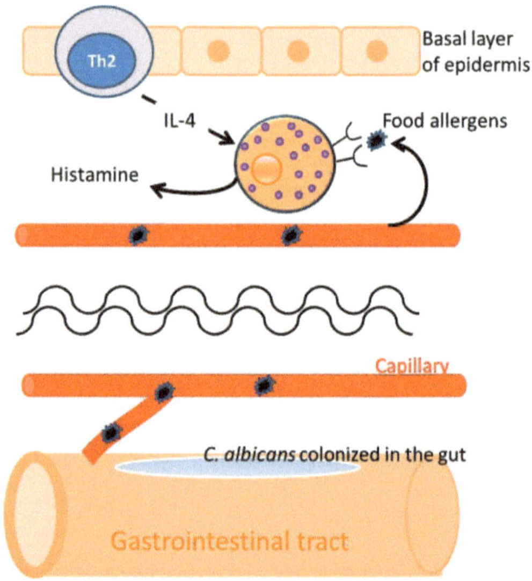

Fig. 2. *Candida albicans* gut colonization as an aggravating factor in atopic dermatitis. Excessive colonization by *C. albicans* in the gastrointestinal tract induces hyperpermeability of the gastrointestinal mucosal barrier, resulting in enhanced transport of intact and degraded antigens across the gastrointestinal mucosal barrier. This induces food protein sensitization and food allergy in susceptible individuals.

Candida colonization did not enhance ovalbumin permeation in mast cell deficient W/Wv mice but did in congenic littermate control +/+ mice. Reconstitution of mast cells in W/Wv mice by transplantation of bone marrow-derived mast cells restored the ability to increase ovalbumin permeation in response to *Candida* colonization. These results suggest that gastrointestinal *Candida* colonization promotes sensitization against food antigens, at least partly due to mast cell-mediated hyperpermeability in the gastrointestinal mucosa of mice. To confirm that gut colonization of *C. albicans* aggravates atopic dermatitis, Sonoyama et al.

(2011) examined whether *C. albicans* gut colonization aggravates immune diseases in mice. Mice were inoculated intragastrically with *C. albicans* to establish chronic and latent *C. albicans* gut colonization. Allergic diarrhea was induced by repeated intragastric administration of ovalbumin in BALB/c mice. Contact hypersensitivity was evaluated by measuring ear swelling after topical application of 2, 4-dinitrofluorobenzene in NC/Nga mice, which are often used as a mouse model of AD (Jin et al., 2011; Orita et al., 2010). Arthritis was induced by intradermal injection of bovine type-II collagen emulsified with complete Freund's adjuvant in DBA/1J mice. *C. albicans* gut colonization increased the incidence of allergic diarrhea, which was accompanied by gut hyperpermeability, as well as increased infiltration of inflammatory cells in the colon. Contact hypersensitivity was also exacerbated by *C. albicans* gut colonization, as demonstrated by increased swelling, myeloperoxidase activity, and proinflammatory cytokines in ear auricles. Furthermore, *C. albicans* gut colonization promoted limb joint inflammation in collagen-induced arthritis in an animal model of rheumatoid arthritis (Setoguchi et al., 2010; Takagi et al., 2009). These findings suggest that *C. albicans* gut colonization in mice aggravates inflammation in allergic and autoimmune diseases, and evokes the necessity of investigating the pathogenic role of *C. albicans* gut colonization in immune diseases in humans.

4.3 Skin barrier dysfunction

Skin barrier dysfunction (Ogawa et al., 1993; Cork et al., 2006 & 2009; Elias et al., 2008; Palmer et al., 2006) has emerged as a critical driving force in the initiation and exacerbation of AD with a recent major breakthrough in the genetics of AD (O'Regan et al., 2009; Hudson et al., 2006; Brown SJ, McLean, 2009). For instance, as addressed by Ogawa et al. (1993), dryness of the skin is an important component of the atopic diathesis, thereby reflecting possible skin barrier dysfunction. When the two abnormalities, dry skin/barrier dysfunction and allergy/immunological dysfunction, are considered as the major underlying defects of AD, the wide range of clinical manifestations seen in AD can be more easily comprehended. A defect of the mucocutaneous barrier readily allows penetration of multiple antigens or haptens, which enhances allergic inflammation. On the other hand, an allergic inflammation derived from the immunological abnormalities damages barrier functions. This sequence cycle could answer the question as to why AD patients show IgE production against, and contact hypersensitivity to, various antigens or haptens. A set of protective/defensive functions generated in the epidermis is likely mediated by its unique differentiation end product, the stratum corneum (Elias 2005; Elias & Choi, 2005). Basically, a markedly increased transepidermal water loss and a markedly decreased water holding capacity of the stratum corneum were reported in AD patients (Watanabe et al., 1991). In addition, since the patients showed a higher transepidermal water loss following irritant exposure, the susceptibility to irritants in AD patients seemed to be closely related with a breakdown in the barrier function of the stratum corneum (Tupker et al., 1990). More recently, it has been proposed that AD is a multifactorial, heterogenous disease that arises as a result of the interaction between both environmental and genetic factors (Cork et al., 2009). Changes in at least three groups of genes encoding structural proteins, epidermal proteases, and protease inhibitors make AD patients prone to a defective epidermal barrier, resulting in increased risk of developing AD. Loss-of-function mutations found within the FLG gene, which encodes the structural protein, filaggrin, could be the most significant genetic factor toward AD. In addition, enhanced protease activity and decreased synthesis of the lipid lamellae lead to exacerbated breakdown of the epidermal barrier. It can be summarized that these functions include the permeability barrier, which prevents transcutaneous evaporative water loss, and an antimicrobial barrier, which simultaneously encourages colonization by nonpathogenic "normal" flora (Elias, 2007). According to the report by Selander et al. (2009), approximately 50% of adult AD patients have allergen-specific IgE reactivity to the skin commensal yeast *Malassezia* spp. Due to the ruptured skin barrier in AD, it is likely that *Malassezia* come into contact with mast cells, which are known to be involved in AD. Since mast cells are located in the superficial dermis close to blood vessels, they are advantageously positioned to react with allergens diffusing through a ruptured epidermis. They are, therefore, recognized as key effector cells during IgE-associated Th2-type immune responses (Galli et al., 2005), and cross-linking of the high-affinity IgE receptor (FcεRI) leads to release of potent inflammatory mediators (Turner & Kinet, 1999) such as histamine, proteases, chemotactic factors, cytokines, and metabolites of arachidonic acid (Henz et al., 2001). Mast cells have a wide variety of cell surface receptors that can interact directly with pathogens, including Toll-like receptors (TLRs), which are involved in innate immune recognition of invading microorganisms (Qiao et al., 2006). Fungal products such as zymosan can activate mast cells through TLR2 (Marshall, 2004). It has recently been reported that a synergistic activation between TLR2 and FcεRI can occur in mast cells, resulting in increased production of inflammatory cytokines (Qiao et al., 2006) (Fig. 3). Although both a defective epidermal permeability (Sugarman et al., 2003; Seidenari & Giusti, 1995; Proksch et al., 2006; Chamlin et al., 2002; Eberlein-Konig et al., 2000) and a propensity to secondary infection (Boguniewicz et al., 2006; Baker, 2006) are well-recognized features of AD, these abnormalities have been widely assumed to reflect downstream consequences of a primary immunologic abnormality.

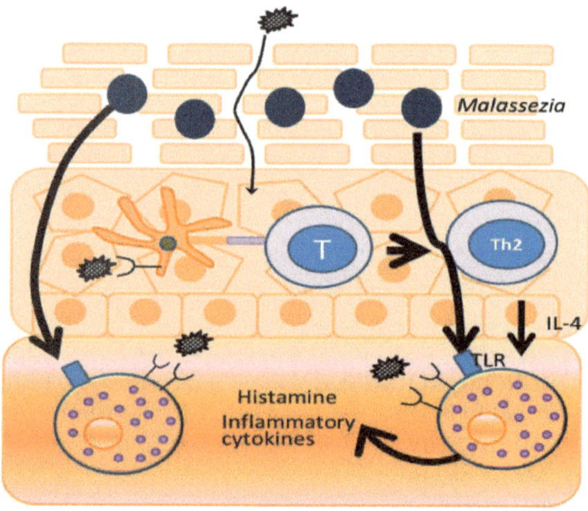

Fig. 3. Skin barrier dysfunction in combination with skin indigenous *Malassezia* as an exacerbating factor in atopic dermatitis (AD). Due to the ruptured skin barrier in AD, it is likely that *Malassezia* and/or its products come into contact with mast cells which have a wide variety of cell surface receptors that interact directly with pathogens, including Toll-like receptors (TLRs). A synergistic activation between TLR and IgE receptor (Fcε RI) can occur in mast cells, resulting in increased production of inflammatory cytokines.

5. Conclusion

Well-known representative fungi that exacerbate AD are the resident fungi in the skin, *Malassezia* spp. such as *M. furfur*, *M. globosa* and *M. restricta*, and the resident fungus in the intestinal tract, *C. albicans*. The lipophilic fungus *M. furfur* indigenously inhabits the seborrheic region of the body such as the face, cervical part, and upper part of back. It was also reported that the fungus may be implicated in rosacea-like dermatitis and edematous erythema, which are chronic and intractable symptoms characteristic to the face in adult-type AD. Regarding the underlying mechanism by which clinical manifestation of AD is affected in the presence of *M. furfur*, the following points have been proposed: 1) antigen-specific inflammation caused via activation of antigen-specific T cells, and 2) dysfunction of skin barrier. A defect of skin barrier readily allows penetration of multiple antigens or haptens, which enhances allergic inflammation, and vice versa. That is, an allergic inflammation derived from the immunological abnormalities damages barrier functions. This sequence cycle could answer the question as to why AD patients show IgE production against, and contact hypersensitivity to, various antigens or haptens. Gut colonization of *C. albicans* is also regarded as the other fungal factor exacerbating AD by promoting sensitization against food antigens, at least partly due to mast cell-mediated hyperpermeability in the gastrointestinal mucosa.

6. References

Abeck, D. & Mempel, M. (1998). *Staphylococcus aureus* colonization in atopic dermatitis and its therapeutic implications. *British Journal of Dermatology*, Vol.139, Supplement 53, (December 1998), pp.13–16. ISSN 0007-0963

Aizawa, T., Kano, R., Nakamura, Y., Watanabe, S. & Hasegawa, A. (2001). The genetic diversity of clinical isolates of Malassezia pachydermatis from dogs and cats. *Medical Mycology*. Vol.39, No.4, (August 2001), pp.329-334, ISSN 1369-3786

Arzumanyan, G., Magarshak, O. & Semenov, B. (2000). Yeast fungi in patients with allergic diseases: species variety and sensitivity to antifungal drugs. *Bulletin of Experimental Biology and Medicine*, Vol.129, No.6, (June 2000) pp.601–604, ISSN 0007-4888

Bäck, O., Scheynius, A. & Johansson, G. (1995). Ketoconazole in atopic dermatitis: therapeutic response is correlated with decrease in serum IgE. *Archives of dermatological research*, Vol.287, No.5, (May 1995) pp.448-451, ISSN 0340-3696

Baker, S. (2006). The role of microorganisms in atopic dermatitis. *Clinical and Experimental Immunology*, Vol.144, No.1, (April 2006), pp.1-9, (ISSN 0009-9104)

Bayrou, O., Pecquet, C., Flahault, A., Artigou, C., Abuaf, N. & Leynadier, F. (2005). Head and neck atopic dermatitis and *Malassezia-furfur*-specific IgE antibodies. *Dermatology* Vol.211, No.2, (August 2005), pp.107-113, ISSN 1018-8665

Boguniewicz, M., Schmid-Grendelmeier, P. & Leung, Y. Atopic dermatitis. *The Journal of Allergy and Clinical Immunology*, Vol.118, No.1, (July 2006), pp.40-43, ISSN 0091-6749

Bond, R., Curtis, F., Ferguson, A., Mason, S. & Rest, J. (2000). An idiopathic facial dermatitis of Persian cats. *Veterinary Dermatolog,* Vol.11, No.1, (March 2000), pp.35-41, ISSN 0959-4493

Boom, H., Liano, D. & Abbas, K. (1998). Heterogeneity of helper/inducer T lymphocytes. II. Effects of interleukin 4- and interleukin 2-producing T cell clones on resting B lymphocytes. *The Journal of Experimental Medicine,* Vol.167, No.4, (April 1998), pp.1350-1363, ISSN 0022-1007

Brehler, S., & Luger, T. (2001). Atopic dermatitis: the role of *Pityrosporum ovale. Journal of the European Academy of Dermatology and Venereology,* Vol.15, No.1, (January 2001), PP.5–6, ISSN 0926-9959

Broberg, A., Faergemann, J., Johansson, S., Johansson, S. & Strannegard, I. (1992). *Pityrosporum ovale* and atopic dermatitis in children and young adults. *Acta Dermato-Venereologica,* Vol.72, No.3, (March 1992), pp.187–192, ISSN 0001-5555

Broberg, A. & Faergemann, J. (1995). Topical antimycotic treatment of atopic dermatitis in the head/neck area. A double-blind randomized study. *Acta Dermato-Venereologica,* Vol.75, No.1, (January 1995), pp.46–49, ISSN 0001-5555

Brown, J. & McLean, H. (2009). Eczema genetics: current state of knowledge and future goals. *The Journal of Investigative Dermatology,* Vol.129, No.3, (March 2009), pp.543-552, ISSN 0022-202X

Bunikowski, R., Mielke, M., Skarabis, H., Herz, U., Bergmann, L., Wahn, U. & Renz, H. (1999). Prevalence and role of serum IgE antibodies to the *Staphylococcus aureus-*derived superantigens SEA and SEB in children with atopic dermatitis. *Journal of Allergy and Clinical Immunology,* Vol.103, No.1, (January 1999), pp.119–124, ISSN 0091-6749

Buslau, M., Menzel, I. & Holzmann, H. (1990). Fungal flora of human feces in psoriasis and atopic dermatitis. *Mycoses,* Vol.33, No.2, (February 1990), pp.90-94, ISSN: 1439-0507

Chamlin, L., Kao, J., Frieden, J., Sheu, Y., Fowler, J., Fluhr, W., Williams, L. & Elias, M. (2002). Ceramide-dominant barrier repair lipids alleviate childhood atopic dermatitis: changes in barrier function provide a sensitive indicator of disease activity. *Journal of the American Academy of Dermatology,* Vol.47, No.2, (August 2002), pp.198-208, ISSN 0190-9622

Chen, A., Halliwell, E., Pemberton, D. & Hill, B. (2002). Identification of major allergens of *Malassezia pachydermatis* in dogs with atopic dermatitis and *Malassezia* overgrowth. *Veterinary Dermatology,* Vol.13, No.3, (June 2002), pp.141-150, ISSN 0959-4493

Cork, J., Danby, G., Vasilopoulos, Y., Hadgraft, J., Lane, E., Moustafa, M., Guy, H., Macgowan, L., Tazi-Ahnini, R. & Ward, J. (2009). Epidermal barrier dysfunction in atopic dermatitis. *The Journal of Investigative Dermatology,* Vol.129, No.8, (August 2009), 1892-1908, ISSN 0022-202X

Cork, J., Robinson, A., Vasilopoulos, Y., Ferguson, A., Moustafa, M., MacGowan, A., Duff, W., Ward, J. & Tazi-Ahnini R. (2006). New perspectives on epidermal barrier dysfunction in atopic dermatitis: gene-environment interactions. *The Journal of*

Allergy and Clinical Immunology, Vol.118, No.1, (July 2006), pp.3-21, ISSN 0091-6749

Darabi, K., Hostetler, G., Bechtel, A. & Zirwas, M. (2009). The role of *Malassezia* in atopic dermatitis affecting the head and neck of adults. *Journal of the American Academy of Dermatology*, Vol.60, No.1, (January 2009), pp.125-136, ISSN 0190-9622

Eberlein-Konig, B., Schafer, T., Huss-Marp, J., Darsow, U., Mohrenschlager, M., Herbert, O., Abeck, D., Kramer, U., Behrendt, H. & Ring, J. (2000). Skin surface pH, stratum corneum hydration, trans-epidermal water loss and skin roughness related to atopic eczema and skin dryness in a population of primary school children. *Acta Dermato-Venereologica*, Vol.80, No.3, (May 2000), pp.188-191, ISSN 0001-5555

Eigenmann, A., Sicherer, H., Borkowski, A., Cohen, A. & Sampson, A. (1998). Prevalence of IgE-mediated food allergy among children with atopic dermatitis. *Pediatrics*, Vol.101, No.3, (March 1998), p.E8, ISSN 0031-4005

Elias, M. (2005). Stratum corneum defensive functions: an integrated view. *The Journal of Investigative Dermatology*, Vol.125, No.2, (August 2005), pp.183-200, ISSN 0022-202X

Elias, M. & Choi, H. (2005). Interactions among stratum corneum defensive functions. *Experimental Dermatology*, Vol.14, No.10, (October 2005), pp.719-726, ISSN 0906-6705

Elias, M. (2007). The skin barrier as an innate immune element. *Seminars in Immunopathology*, Vol.29, No.1, (April 2007), pp.3-14, ISSN 1863-2297

Elias, M., Hatano, Y. & Williams, L. (2008). Basis for the barrier abnormality in atopic dermatitis: outside-inside-outside pathogenic mechanisms. *The Journal of Allergy and Clinical Immunology*, Vol.121, No.6, (June 2006), pp.1337-1343, ISSN 0091-6749

Faergemann, J. (1999). *Pityrosporum* species as a cause of allergy and infection. *Allergy*, Vol.54, No.5, (May 1999), pp.413–419, ISSN 1398-9995

Faergemann, J. (2002). Atopic dermatitis and fungi. *Clinical Microbiology Reviews*, Vol.15, No.4, (October 2002), pp.545-563, ISSN 0893-8512

Farhadi, A., Banan, A., Fields, J. & Keshavarzian A. (2003). Intestinal barrier: an interface between health and disease. *Journal of Gastroenterology and Hepatology*, Vol.18, No.5, (May 2003), pp.479-497, ISSN 0815-9319

Fiorentino, F., Bond, W. & Mosmann, R. (1989). Two types of mouse T helper cell. IV. Th2 clones secrete a factor that inhibits cytokine production by Th1 clones. *The Journal of Experimental Medicine*, Vol.170, No.6, (December 1989), pp.2081-2095, ISSN 0022-1007

Galli, J., Nakae, S. & Tsai, M. (2005). Mast cells in the development of adaptive immune responses. *Nature Immunology*, Vol.6, No.2, (February 2005), pp.135-142, ISSN 1529-2908

Gupta, K., Batra, R., Bluhm, R., Boekhout, T. & Dawson, L, Jr. (2004). Skin diseases associated with *Malassezia* species. *Journal of the American Academy of Dermatology*, Vol.51, No.5, (November 2004), pp.785-98, ISSN 0190-9622

Gupta, K., Kohli, Y., Summerbell, C., & Faergemann, J. (2001). Quantitative culture of *Malassezia* species from different body sites of individuals with or without dermatoses. *Medical mycology*, Vol.39, No.3, (Jun 2001), pp.243-251, ISSN 1369-3786

Henz, M., Maurer, M., Lippert, U., Worm, M. & Babina, M. (2001). Mast cells as initiators of immunity and host defense. *Experimental Dermatology*, Vol.10, No.1, (February 2001), pp.1-10, ISSN 0906-6705

Herz, U., Bunikowski, R., Mielke, M. & Renz, H. (1999). Contribution of bacterial superantigens to stopic dermatitis. *International Archives of Allergy and Immunology*, Vol.118, No.2-4, (February-April 1999), pp.240–241, ISSN 1018-2438

Hirai, A., Kano, R., Makimura, K., Duarte, R., Hamdan, S., Lachance, A., Yamaguchi, H. & Hasegawa, A. (2004). *Malassezia* nana sp. nov., a novel lipid-dependent yeast species isolated from animals. *International Journal of Systematic and Evolutionary Microbiology*. Vol.54, No.2, (March 2004), pp.623-627, ISSN 1466-5026

Huang, X., Johansson, G., Zargari, A. & Nordvall, L. (1995). Allergen cross-reactivity between *Pityrosporum orbiculare* and *Candida albicans*. *Allergy*, Vol.50, No.8, (August 1995), pp.648–656, ISSN 1398-9995

Hudson, J. (2006). Skin barrier function and allergic risk. *Nature Genetics*, Vol.38, No.4, (April 2006), pp.399-400, ISSN, 1061-4036

Jackson, G., Lessof, H., Baker, W., Ferrett, J. & MacDonald, M. (1981). Intestinal permeability in patients with eczema and food allergy. *Lancet*, Vol.317, No.8233, (June 1981), pp.1285-1286, ISSN 0140-6736

Jazic, E., Coyner, S., Loeffler, G. & Lewis, P. (2006). An evaluation of the clinical, cytological, infectious and histopathological features of feline acne. *Veterinary Dermatology*, Vol.17, No.2, (April 2006), pp.134-140, ISSN 0959-4493

Jensen-Jarolim, E., Poulsen, K., With, H., Kieffer, M., Ottevanger, V., Stahl Skov, P. (1992). Atopic dermatitis of the face, scalp and neck: type I reaction to the yeast *Pityrosporum ovale*? *The Journal of Allergy and Clinical Immunology*, Vol.89, No.1, (January 1992), pp.44–50, ISSN 0091-6749

Jin, J.H., Ngoc, T.M., Bae K, Kim, Y.S., & Kim, H.P. (2011). Inhibition of experimental atopic dermatitis by rhubarb (rhizomes of *Rheum tanguticum*) and 5-lipoxygenase inhibition of its major constituent, emodin. *Phytotherpy Research*, Vol.25, No.5, (May 2011), pp.755-759, ISSN 0951-418X

Kaga, M., Sugita, T., Nishikawa, A., Wada, Y., Hiruma, M. & Ikeda, S. (2009). Molecular analysis of the cutaneous *Malassezia microbiota* from the skin of patients with atopic dermatitis of different severities. *Mycoses*. Article first published online: 11 December 2009, ISSN: 1439-0507

Kanda, N., Tani, K., Enomoto, U., Nakai, K. & Watanabe, S. (2002). The skin fungus-induced Th1- and Th2-related cytokine, chemokine and prostaglandin E2 production in peripheral blood mononuclear cells from patients with atopic dermatitis and psoriasis vulgaris. *Clinical and Experimental Allergy*, Vol.32, No.8, (August 2002), pp.1243-1250, ISSN 0954-7894

Kato, H., Sugita, T., Ishibashi, Y. & Nishikawa, A. (2006). Detection and quantification of specific IgE antibodies against eight *Malassezia* species in sera of patients with atopic dermatitis by using an enzyme-linked immunosorbent assay. *Microbiology and Immunology*, Vol.50, No.11, (November 2006), pp.851-856, ISSN 1348-0421

Katsarou, A. & Armenaka, M. (2011). Atopic dermatitis in older patients: particular points. *Journal of the European Academy of Dermatology and Venereology*, Vol.25, No.1, (January 2011), pp.12-18, ISSN 0926-9959

Killar, L., MacDonald, G., West, J., Woods, A. & Bottomly, K. (1987). Cloned, Ia-restricted T cells that do not produce interleukin 4(IL 4)/B cell stimulatory factor 1(BSF-1) fail to help antigen-specific B cells. *The Journal of Immunology*, Vol.138, No.6, (March 1987), pp.1674-1679, ISSN 0022-1767

Kitamura, K., Suga, C., Onuma, S., Kawaguchi, T., Yamazaki, F., Suguro, H. & Ikezawa, Z. (1997). Efficacy of oral amphotericin B for refractory atopic dermatitis with specific IgE to *Candida albicans* and food allergens in sera. *Allergology International*, Vol.46, No.2, (June 1997), pp.125-133, ISSN 1323-8930

Klein, A., Clark, A. & Nicol, H. (1999). Acute infection with *Trichophyton rubrum* associated with flares of atopic dermatitis. *Cutis*, Vol.63, No.3, (March 1999), pp.171-172, ISSN 0011-4162

Lacour M, Zunder T, Huber R, Sander A, Daschner F, Frank U. (2002). The pathogenetic significance of intestinal *Candida* colonization--a systematic review from an interdisciplinary and environmental medical point of view. *International Journal of Hygiene and Environmental Health*, Vol.205, No.4, (May 2002), pp.257-268, ISSN 1438-4639

Lever, R., MacDonald, C., Waugh, P. & Aitchison, T. (1998). Randomised controlled trial of advice on an egg exclusion diet in young children with atopic eczema and sensitivity to eggs. *Pediatric Allergy and Immunology*, Vol.9, No.1, (February 1998), pp.13-19, ISSN 0905-6157

Linder, M., Johansson, C., Scheynius, A. & Wahlgren, C. (2000). Positive atopy patch test reactions to *Pityrosporum orbiculare* in atopic dermatitis patients. *Clinical and Experimental Allergy*, Vol.30, No.1, (January 2000), pp.122-131, ISSN 0954-7894

Lintu, P., Savolainen, J. & Kalimo, K. (1997). IgE antibodies tp protein and mannan antigens of *Pityrosporum ovale* in atopic dermatitis patients. *Clinical and Experimental Allergy*, Vol.27, No.1, (January 1997), pp.87–95, ISSN 0954-7894

Mayser, P., Kupfer, J., Nemetz, D., Schäfer, U., Nilles, M., Hort, W. & Gieler, U. (2006). Treatment of head and neck dermatitis with ciclopiroxolamine cream--results of a double-blind, placebo-controlled study. *Skin Pharmacology and Physiology*, Vol.19, No.3, (June 2006), pp.153-158, ISSN 1660-5527

Majamaa, H. & Isolauri, E. (1996). Evaluation of the gut mucosal barrier: evidence for increased antigen transfer in children with atopic eczema. *The Journal of allergy and clinical immunology*, Vol.97, No.4, (April 1996), pp.985-990, ISSN 0091-6749

Marshall, S. (2004). Mast-cell responses to pathogens. *Nature Reviews Immunology*, Vol.4, No.10, (October 2004), pp.787-799, ISSN 1474-1733

McFadden, P., Noble, C. & Camp, R. (1993). Superantigenic exotoxin secreting potential of staphylococci isolated from atopic eczematous skin. *British Journal of Dermatology*, Vol.128, No.6, (January 1993), pp.631–632, ISSN 0007-0963

Morita, E., Hide, M., Yoneya, Y., Kannbe, M., Tanaka, A. & Yamamoto S. (1999). An assessment of the role of *Candida albicans* antigen in atopic dermatitis. *The Journal of dermatology*, Vol.26, No.5, (May 1999), pp.282-287, ISSN 0385-2407

Morris, O., Clayton, J., Drobatz, J. & Felsburg, J. (2002). Response to *Malassezia pachydermatis* by peripheral blood mononuclear cells from clinically normal and atopic dogs. *American Journal of Veterinary Research,* Vol.63, No.3, (March 2002), pp.358-362, ISSN 0002-9645

Mosmann, R., Cherwinski, H., Bond, W., Giedlin, A. & Coffman, L. (1986). Two types of murine helper T cell clone. I. Definition according to profiles of lymphokine activities and secreted proteins. *The Journal of Immunology,* Vol.136, No.7, (April 1987), pp.2348-2357, ISSN 0022-1767

Mukai, H., Kaneko, S., Saito, N., Nagase, A., Arai, S. & Hiramatsu M. (1997). Clinical significance of *Malassezia furfur* specific IgE antibody in atopic dermatitis. *Arerugi,* Vo.46, No.1, (January 1997), pp.26-33, ISSN 0021-4884

Nakabayashi, A., Sei, Y. & Guillot, J. (2000). Identification of *Malassezia* species isolated from patients with seborrheic dermatitis, atopic dermatitis, pityriasis versicolor and normal subjects. *Medical Mycology,* Vol.38, No.5, (May 2000), pp.337-341, ISSN:1369-3786

National Center for Biotechnology Information, http://www.ncbi.nlm.nih.gov/taxonomy, May, 2011.

Niebuhr, M., Gathmann, M., Scharonow, H., Mamerow, D., Mommert, S., Balaji, H. & Werfel, T. (2011). Staphylococcal alpha-toxin is a strong inducer of interleukin-17 in humans. *Infection and Immunity,* Vol.79, No.4, (April 2011), pp.1615-1622, ISSN 1098-5522

Nikkels, F. & Pierard, E. (2003). Framing the future of antifungals in atopic dermatitis. *Dermatology,* Vol.206, No.4, (June 2003), pp.398-400, ISSN 1018-8665

Nikkels, F. & Pierard, E. (2003). Framing the future of antifungals in atopic dermatitis. *Dermatology,* Vol.206, No.4, (May 2003), pp.398-400, ISSN 1018-8665

Ogawa, H. & Yoshiike, T. (1993) A speculative view of atopic dermatitis: barrier dysfunction in pathogenesis. *Journal of Dermatological Science,* Vol.5, No.3, (June 1993), pp.197-204, ISSN 0923-1811

Ong, Y. & Leung, Y. (2010). The infectious aspects of atopic dermatitis. *Immunology and Allergy Clinics of North America,* Vol.30, No.3, (August 2010), pp.309-321, 0889-8561

Ordeix, L., Galeotti, F., Scarampella, F., Dedola, C., Bardagi, M., Romano, E. & Fondati, A. (2007). *Malassezia* spp. overgrowth in allergic cats. *Veterinary Dermatology,* Vol.18, No.5, (October 2007), pp.316-323, ISSN 0959-4493

O'Regan, M., Sandilands, A., McLean, H. & Irvine, D. (2009). Filaggrin in atopic dermatitis. *The Journal of Allergy and Clinical Immunology,* Vol.124, No.3, Supplement 2, (September 2009), pp.R2-6, ISSN 0091-6749

Orita, K., Hiramoto, K., Inoue, R., Sato, E.F., Kobayashi, H., Ishii, M., & Inoue, M. (2010). Strong exercise stress exacerbates dermatitis in atopic model mice, NC/Nga mice, while proper exercise reduces it. *Experimental Dermatology,* Vol.19, No.12, (December 2010), pp.1067- 1072, ISSN 0906-6705

Palmer, N., Irvine, D., Terron-Kwiatkowski, A., Zhao, Y., Liao, H., Lee, P., Goudie, R., Sandilands, A., Campbell, E., Smith, J., O'Regan, M., Watson, M., Cecil, E., Bale, J., Compton, G., DiGiovanna, J., Fleckman, P., Lewis-Jones, S., Arseculeratne, G.,

Sergeant, A., Munro, S., El Houate, B., McElreavey, K., Halkjaer, B., Bisgaard, H., Mukhopadhyay, S. & McLean, H. (2006). Common loss-of-function variants of the epidermal barrier protein filaggrin are a major predisposing factor for atopic dermatitis. *Nature Genetics*, Vol.38, No.4, (April 2006), pp.441-446, ISSN 1061-4036

Peng, M., Jenneck, C., Bussmann, C., Bogdanow, M., Hart, J., Leung, Y., Bieber, T., Eis-Hübinger, M. & Novak, N. (2007). Risk factors of atopic dermatitis patients for eczema herpeticum. *Journal of Investigative Dermatology*, Vol.127, No.5, (May 2007), pp.1261-1263. ISSN: 0022-202X

Pike, G., Heddle, J., Boulton, P., Turner, W. & Atherton, J. (1986). Increased intestinal permeability in atopic eczema. *The Journal of Investigative Dermatology*, 1986;Vol.86, No.2, (February 1986), pp.101-104, ISSN 0022-202X

Proksch, E., Folster-Holst, R. & Jensen, M. (2006). Skin barrier function, epidermal proliferation and differentiation in eczema. *Journal of Dermatological Science*, 2006;Vol.43, No.3, (September 2006), pp.159-169, ISSN 0923-1811

Qiao, H., Andrade, V., Lisboa, A., Morgan, K. & Beaven, A. FcepsilonR1 and toll-like receptors mediate synergistic signals to markedly augment production of inflammatory cytokines in murine mast cells. *Blood* 2006;Vol.107, No.2, (January 2006), pp.610-618, ISSN 0006-4971

Rokugo, M., Tagami, H., Usuba, Y. & Tomota, Y. (1990). Contact sensitivity to *Pityrosporum ovale* in patients with atopic dermatitis. *Archives of Dermatology*, Vol.126, No.5, (May 1990), pp.627–632, ISSN 0003-987X

Romani, L., Cenci, E., Menacci, A., Bistoni, F. & Puccetti, P. (1995). T helper cell dichotomy to *Candida albicans*: implications for pathology, therapy, and vaccine design. *Immunologic Research*, Vol.14, No.2, (June 1995), pp.148-162, ISSN 0257-277X

Sandström, H., Tengvall, M., Johansson, C., Bartosik, J., Bäck, O., Särnhult, T., Wahlgren, F., Scheynius, A. & Faergemann, J. (2005). The prevalence of *Malassezia* yeasts in patients with atopic dermatitis, seborrheic dermatitis and healthy controls. *Acta Dermato-Venereologica*, Vol.85, No.1, (January 2005), pp.17-23, ISSN 0001-5555

Savolainen, J. Lammintausta, K., Kalimo, K. & Viander, M. (1993). *Candida albicans* and atopic dermatitis. *Clinical and Experimental Allergy*, Vol.23, No.4, (April 1993), pp.332–339, ISSN 0954-7894

Savolainen, J., Lintu, P., Kosonen, J., Kortekangas-Savolainen, O., Viander, M., Pene, J., Kalimo, K., Terho, E. & Bousquet, J. (2001). *Pityrosporum* and *Candida* specific and non-specific humoral, cellular and cytokine responses in atopic dermatitis patients. *Clinical and Experimental Allergy*, Vol.31, No.1, (January 2001), pp.125–134, ISSN 0954-7894

Scalabrin, M., Bavbek, S., Perzanowski, S., Wilson, B., Platts-Mills, A. & Wheatley, M. (1999). Use of specific IgE in assessing the relevance of fungal and dust mite allergens to atopic dermatitis: a comparison with asthmatic and nonasthmatic control subjects. *The Journal of Allergy and Clinical Immunology*, Vol.104, No.6, (December 1999), pp.1273-1279, ISSN 0091-6749

Schmidt, M., Zargari, A., Holt, P., Lindbom, L., Hellman, U., Whitley, P., van der Ploeg, I., Härfast, B. & Scheynius, A. (1997). The complete cDNA sequence and expression of the first major allergenic protein of *Malassezia furfur*, Mal f 1. *European Journal of Biochemistry*, Vol.246, No.1, (May 1997), pp.181–185, ISSN 0014-2956

Seidenari, S. & Giusti, G. (1995). Objective assessment of the skin of children affected by atopic dermatitis: a study of pH, capacitance and TEWL in eczematous and clinically uninvolved skin. *Acta Dermato-Venereologica*, Vol.75, No.6, (November 1995), pp.429-433, ISSN 0001-5555

Selander, C., Engblom, C., Nilsson, G., Scheynius, A. & Andersson, L. TLR2/MyD88-dependent and -independent activation of mast cell IgE responses by the skin commensal yeast *Malassezia sympodialis*. *The Journal of Immunology*, Vol.182, No.7, (April 2009), pp.4208-4216, ISSN 0022-1767

Setoguchi, C., Tsuji, F., Katsuta, O., Okamoto, M. & Aono, H. (2010). Combined effects of bucillamine and etanercept on a rat type II collagen-induced arthritis model. *Modern Rheumatology*, Vol.20, No.4, (August 2010), pp.381-388, ISSN 1439-7595

Sierra, P., Guillot, J., Jacob, H., Bussieras, S. & Chermette, R. (2000). Fungal flora on cutaneous and mucosal surfaces of cats infected with feline immunodeficiency virus or feline leukemia virus. *American Journal of Veterinary Research*, Vol.61, No.2, (February 2000), pp.158-161, ISSN 0002-9645

Sonoyama, K., Miki, A., Sugita, R., Goto, H., Nakata, M. & Yamaguchi, N. (2011). Gut colonization by *Candida albicans* aggravates inflammation in the gut and extra-gut tissues in mice. *Medical Mycology*, Vol.49, No.3, (April 2011), pp.237-247, ISSN 1369-3786

Stout, D. & Bottomly, K. (1989). Antigen-specific activation of effector macrophages by IFN-gamma producing (TH1) T cell clones. Failure of IL-4-producing (TH2) T cell clones to activate effector function in macrophages. *The Journal of Immunology*, Vol.142, No.3, (February 1989), pp.760-765, ISSN 0022-1767

Sugarman, L., Fluhr, W., Fowler, J., Bruckner, T., Diepgen, L. & Williams, L. (2003). The objective severity assessment of atopic dermatitis score: an objective measure using permeability barrier function and stratum corneum hydration with computer-assisted estimates for extent of disease. *Archives of Dermatology*, Vol.139, No.11, (November 2003), pp.1417-1422, ISSN 0003-987X

Sugita, T., Suto, H., Unno, T., Tsuboi, R., Ogawa, H., Shinoda, T. & Nishikawa, A. (2001). Molecular analysis of *Malassezia* microflora on the skin of atopic dermatitis patients and healthy subjects. *Journal of Clinical Microbiology*, Vol.39, No.10, (October 2001), pp.3486-3490, ISSN 0095-1137

Sugita, T., Tajima, M., Amaya, M., Tsuboi, R. & Nishikawa, A. (2004). Genotype analysis of *Malassezia restricta* as the major cutaneous flora in patients with atopic dermatitis and healthy subjects. *Microbiology and Immunology*, Vol.48, No.10, (October 2004), 755-759, ISSN 1348-0421

Sugita, T., Tajima, M., Tsubuku, H., Tsuboi, R. & Nishikawa, A. (2006). Quantitative analysis of cutaneous *Malassezia* in atopic dermatitis patients using real-time PCR. *Microbiology and Immunology*, Vol.50, No.7, (July 2006), pp.549-552, ISSN 1348-0421

Svejgaard, E., Larsen, Ø., Deleuran, M., Ternowitz, T., Roed-Petersen, J. & Nilsson, J. (2004). Treatment of head and neck dermatitis comparing itraconazole 200 mg and 400 mg daily for 1 week with placebo. *Journal of the European Academy of Dermatology and Venereology*, Vol.18, No.4, (July 2004), pp.445-449, ISSN 0926-9959

Tajima, M., Sugita, T., Nishikawa, A. & Tsuboi, R. (2008). Molecular analysis of *Malassezia* microflora in seborrheic dermatitis patients: comparison with other diseases and healthy subjects. *The Journal of Investigative Dermatology*, Vol.128, No.2, (February 2008), pp.345-351, ISSN 0022-202X

Takagi, T., Naito, Y., Inoue, M., Akagiri, S., Mizushima, K., Handa, O., Kokura, S., Ichikawa, H. & Yoshikawa, T. (2009). Inhalation of carbon monoxide ameliorates collagen-induced arthritis in mice and regulates the articular expression of IL-1beta and MCP-1. *Inflammation*, Vol.32, No.2, (April 2009), pp.83-88, ISSN 0360-3997

Tanaka, M., Aiba, S., Matsumura, N., Aoyama, H., Tabata, N., Sekita, Y. & Tagami, H. (1994). IgE-mediated hypersensitivity and contact sensitivity to multiple environmental allergens in atopic dermatitis. *Archives of Dermatology*, Vol.130, No.11, (November 1994), pp.1393-1401, ISSN 0365-6020

Tupker, A., Pinnagoda, J., Coenraads, J. & Nater, P. (1990). Susceptibility to irritants: role of barrier function, skin dryness and history of atopic dermatitis. *The British Journal of Dermatology*, Vol.123, No.2, (August 1990), pp.199-205, ISSN 0007-0963

Turner, H. & Kinet, P. (1999). Signalling through the high-affinity IgE receptor Fc epsilonRI. *Nature*, 1999;Vol.402, No.6760, Supplement :B24-30, ISSN: 0028-0836

van Reijsen, C., Felius, A., Wauters, A., Bruijnzeel-Koomen, A. & Koppelman, J. (1998). T-cell reactivity for a peanut-derived epitope in the skin of a young infant with atopic dermatitis. *The Journal of Allergy and Clinical Immunology*, Vol.101, No.2, Part1, (February 1998), 207-209, ISSN 0091-6749

Watanabe, M., Tagami, H., Horii, I., Takahashi, M. & Kligman, M. (1991). Functional analyses of the superficial stratum corneum in atopic xerosis. *Archives of Dermatology*, 1991;Vol.127, No.11, (November 1991), pp.1689-1692, ISSN 0003-987X

Williams, C. (2000). Epidemiology of atopic dermatitis. *Clinical and Experimental Dermatology*, Vol.25, No.7, (October 2000), pp. 522–529. ISSN 0307-6938

Williams, C., & Wüthrich, B. (2000). The natural history of atopic dermatitis, In Atopic dermatitis, H.C. Williams (Ed.), 41–59, Cambridge University Press, ISBN 0-521-57075-1, Cambridge, United Kingdom.

Wollenberg, A., Wetzel, S., Burgdorf, H. & Haas, J. (2003). Viral infections in atopic dermatitis: pathogenic aspects and clinical management. *Journal of Allergy and Clinical Immunology*, Vol.112, No.4, (October 2003), pp.667-674, ISSN 0091-6749

Yamaguchi, N., Sugita, R., Miki, A., Takemura, N., Kawabata, J., Watanabe, J. & Sonoyama, K. (2006). Gastrointestinal Candida colonisation promotes sensitisation against food antigens by affecting the mucosal barrier in mice. *Gut*, Vol.55, No.7, (July 2006), pp.954-960, ISSN 0017-5749

Yeung, M., Balma-Mena, A., Shear, N., Simor, A., Pope, E., Walsh, S. & McGavin, J. (2011). Identification of major clonal complexes and toxin producing strains among *Staphylococcus aureus* associated with atopic dermatitis. *Microbes and Infection*, Vol.13, No.2, (February 2011), pp.189-197, ISSN 1286-4579

Yim, M., Kim, Y., Ko, H., Lee, W., Choe, B. & Ahn, J. (2010). Molecular analysis of *Malassezia* microflora on the skin of the patients with atopic dermatitis. *Annals of Dermatology*, Vol.22, No.1, (February 2010), pp.41-47, ISSN 1013-9087

9

Atopic Dermatitis and Skin Fungal Microorganisms

Takashi Sugita[1], Enshi Zhang[3], Takafumi Tanaka[1], Mami Tajima[3], Ryoji Tsuboi[3], Yoshio Ishibashi[2], Akemi Nishikawa[2]
[1]*Department of Microbiology, Meiji Pharmaceutical University, Kiyose, Tokyo*
[2]*Department of Immunobiology, Meiji Pharmaceutical University, Kiyose, Tokyo*
[3]*Department of Dermatology, Tokyo Medical University, Shinjuku, Tokyo*
Japan

1. Introduction

A wide variety of bacteria and fungi are found on the human skin. Although some skin microorganisms produce antibacterial peptides that inhibit invasion by pathogens or promote the integrity of cutaneous defenses by eliciting host immune responses, the normal microbiome can also cause several skin diseases.

Atopic dermatitis (AD) is a chronic disease that causes pruritus and involves cycles of remission and deterioration. AD is the result of dry hypersensitive skin. When the skin is dry, the protective barrier function of the cutaneous surface horny layer is compromised, and the skin readily develops dermatitis in response to various external stimuli, including skin microorganisms. Serum from almost all AD patients contains IgE antibodies against some skin microorganisms. For example, staphylococcal superantigen-specific IgE is present in the serum of AD patients, but not in the serum of healthy individuals. Normally, the weakly acidic condition of healthy skin prevents colonization by *Staphylococcus aureus*. However, in patients with AD, the skin pH is shifted toward neutrality, allowing *S. aureus* to grow and exacerbate AD.

In the cutaneous fungal microbiome, lipophilic yeasts of the genus *Malassezia* are the predominant species on human skin. As *Malassezia* species require lipids for growth, they preferentially colonize sebum-rich areas such as the head, face, and neck, as opposed to the limbs or trunk. Specific IgE antibody against *Malassezia* species is found in the serum of AD patients. Antifungal therapy improves the symptoms of AD by decreasing the level of *Malassezia* colonization, suggesting that these microorganisms also exacerbate AD. *Malassezia* species, unlike *S. aureus*, colonize both AD patients and healthy subjects. Currently, the genus *Malassezia* consists of 14 species. Of these, *M. globosa* and *M. restricta* have been detected in almost all AD patients, suggesting that these two *Malassezia* species play a significant role in AD. The level of specific IgE antibody against both species is greater than that against other *Malassezia* species.

This chapter discusses cutaneous fungi as an exacerbating factor in AD, focusing on:

- the fungal microbiome in patients with AD.
- immunological aspects of fungal colonization, and
- treatment with antifungal agents.

2. The fungal microbiome in patients with atopic dermatitis

2.1 Colonization by the fungus *Malassezia* in patients with atopic dermatitis

The lipophilic yeast *Malassezia* is the predominant fungus on human skin. Morphologically, these microorganisms are ovoid, elongate, and cylindrical (Fig. 1). Their genome is smaller than that of other fungi (Xu *et al.* 2007). As *Malassezia* species require lipids for growth, they preferentially colonize sebum-rich areas such as the head, face, or neck, rather than the limbs or trunk. Specific IgE antibodies against *Malassezia* are present in the serum of patients with AD, and antifungal therapy can improve the symptoms of AD by decreasing the degree of colonization by *Malassezia*; thus, this fungus is believed to be an exacerbating factor in AD (more details are provided in a later chapter). In contrast to *S. aureus*, *Malassezia* species colonize both AD patients and healthy individuals. In addition to AD, *Malassezia* species are responsible for seborrheic dermatitis, folliculitis, and ptiryasis versicolor (Gupta *et al.* 2004; Ashbee 2007). Currently, 14 species are recognized within the genus *Malassezia* (Table 1), and five of these (*M. caprae, M. cuniculi, M. equina, M. nana,* and *M. pachydermatis*) show affinity for nonhuman animals.

Host	Species	Species implicated in skin disease in human
Human associated species	*Malassezia dermatis*	AD
	Malassezia furfur	SI
	Malassezia globosa	AD, SD, PV
	Malassezia japonica	
	Malassezia obtusa	
	Malassezia slooffiae	
	Malassezia sympodialis	AD, SD
	Malassezia restricta	AD, SD, PV
	Malassezia yamatoensis	
Nonhuman animal associated species	*Malassezia caprae*	
	Malassezia cuniculi	
	Malassezia equina	
	Malassezia nana	
	Malassezia pachydermatis	

AD, atopic dermatitis; SD, seborrheic dermatitis; SI, systemic infection; PV, pityriasis versicolor

Table 1. Currently accepted *Malassezia* species

A number of epidemiological studies have been conducted during the past decade to elucidate the role of *Malassezia* as an exacerbating factor in AD. The first was carried out by Nakabayashi *et al.* (2000) in Japan and detected *M. furfur, M. globosa, M. sympodialis,* and *M.*

slooffiae in 21.4, 14.3, 7.1, and 3.6% of samples from Japanese AD patients, respectively. A study conducted in Sweden in 2005 produced similar results (Sandström *et al.* 2005). However, a Canadian study by Gupta *et al.* (2001) reported the predominant species to be *M. sympodialis,* which was detected in 51.3% of the samples from AD patients. All of these studies were performed using culture-dependent methods. In all cases, scale samples were collected by an appropriate method, e.g., swabbing, scratching, or stripping, and were incubated in medium containing several types of fatty acids. The recovered microorganisms were identified based on biochemical or physiological characteristics, including assimilation of Tween compounds and esculin, catalase reaction, and maximum growth temperature (Guého-Kellermann 2010; Kaneko *et al.* 2007). However, culture-dependent methods may not provide accurate and reliable results for *Malassezia*. The efficiency of culturing *Malassezia* strains depends on the isolation medium used, and the growth of some species, such *M. obtusa* and *M. restricta,* is slower than that of others.

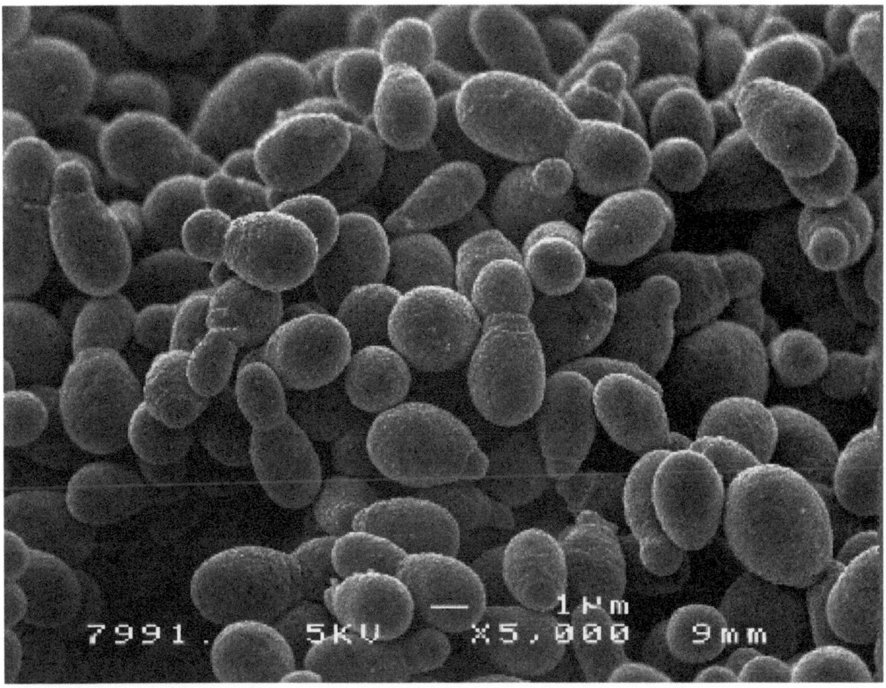

Magnification is x5,000.

Fig. 1. Morphology of *Malassezia restricta* by scanning electron microscope

To overcome the difficulties of culture-dependent methods, including scale sampling methods, culturing conditions, and isolation techniques, Sugita *et al.* (2001) developed the first molecular analytical method for *Malassezia*. For this method, scale samples are collected by stripping with medical transparent dressing, and skin *Malassezia* DNA is directly extracted from the dressing. The *Malassezia* microbiota is then analyzed by real-time PCR, specific detection by PCR with a species-specific primer, or an rRNA clone method (Sugita *et al.* 2011). Although more expensive than culture-dependent methods, a molecular-based, non-culture approach appears to be the most reliable and appropriate for analysis of the skin *Malassezia* microbiota (Sugita *et al.* 2001; Morishita *et al.* 2006; Takahata *et al.* 2007a, 2007b; Tajima *et al.* 2008; Amaya *et al.* 2007). In all scale samples from AD patients, both *M. globosa* and *M. restricta* were detected by the molecular-based method, with the level of colonization by *M. restricta* being approximately 1.6 times that of *M. globosa* (Sugita *et al.* 2006a). *Malassezia sympodialis* was the second most predominant species (detected in 58% of the cases), and *M. dermatitis, M. furfur, M. obtusa,* and *M. slooffiae* were detected in less than 30% of the cases (Fig. 2). These results suggest that both *M. globosa* and *M. restricta* may significantly exacerbate AD.

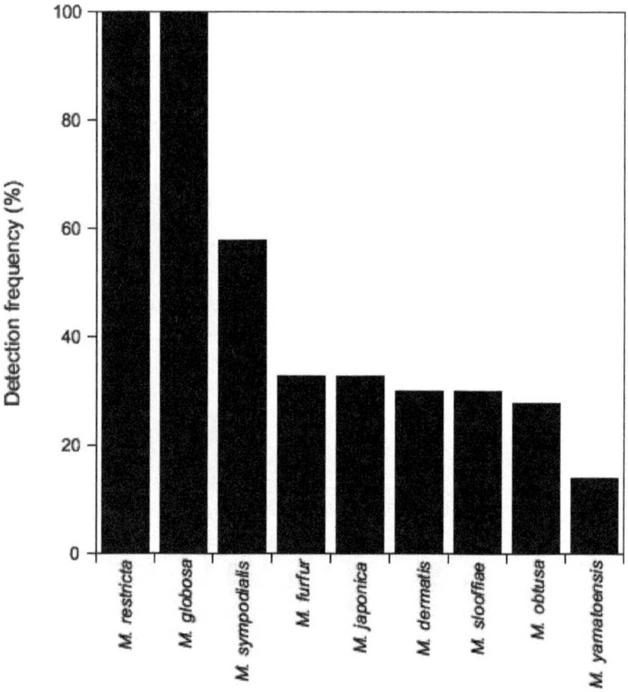

Malassezia DNA was detected by nested PCR assay with species-specific primers

Fig. 2. Colonization frequency of *Malassezia* in the scale of patient with atopic dermatitis

Given that *M. globosa* and *M. restricta* commonly colonize both AD patients and healthy individuals, specific genotypes of these microorganisms may play a role in AD (Sugita *et al.* 2003, 2004, 2010). The fungal rRNA gene consists of four subunits: 5S, 5.8S, 18S (small), and 26S (large). Located between the subunits are an internal transcribed spacer (ITS) and an intergenic spacer (IGS). In *M. globosa,* the IGS is 444 to 454 bp long and has four short sequence repeats (SSRs), $(CT1)_n$, $(CT2)_n$, $(CT3)_n$, and $(GT)_n$, which occur at positions 29–49, 278–291, 380–485, and 242–267, respectively, in the IGS sequence of *M. globosa* strain CBS 7996. Alignments of IGS 1 sequences of two *M. globosa* strains are shown in Fig. 3. The number of $(CT)_n$ SSRs in the IGS 1 region is more variable in samples from healthy individuals than in those from AD patients. In samples from AD patients, the number of sequence repeats in the IGS 1 region ranged from 4 to 11 for $(CT1)_n$, 3 to 10 for $(CT2)_n$, and 3 to 11 for $(CT3)_n$, with 4 $(CT1)_n$ repeats in 50% of the samples, 8 $(CT2)_n$ in 60%, and 9–11 $(CT3)_n$ in 80%. For $(GT)_n$, the respective numbers of repeats in 70–80% of the SSRs in the IGS 1 region were 9–11 in samples from AD patients and 15–19 in samples from healthy individuals. A phylogenetic tree constructed from 52 IGS 1 sequences is shown in Fig. 4. The tree consists of four major groups, which correspond to the sources of the samples (AD patients or healthy individuals). Two groups are from AD patients, and one is from healthy individuals. The remaining group included samples from both AD patients and healthy individuals. The IGS 1 sequences were more diverse in the samples from healthy individuals compared with AD patients. The IGS 1 sequence similarity was 94.5 ± 3.5% among the AD patient samples and 89.9 ± 3.5% among the samples from healthy individuals. The IGS 1 sequences of *M. restricta* are divided into two major groups, corresponding to AD patients and healthy individuals.

GTGCATACCACACTCGAGCGCTT**CTCTCTCTCTCTCTCT**
CT1
CTCTCTGTGAGCGAGGCAATGGAGGTGTGTACCTCCAAC

ACACCATCGCCCCAGGTACAGCCAATGGAGGTGTGTGTG

CGCGCTCCGGTTCCGCTCTCTTCTCGTACGCTTGGCTTC

GGATTCTCTCTCTCCTACGTACT**GTGTGTGTGTGTGTGT**
GT
GTGTGTGTGTGTGTGTGTGTGGATCTATG**TCTCTCTCTC**
CT2
TTTCTCCTTCAAATGGAGGTGTGTGTGCACCCTCACCCT

CGCCCTCGCTCACCCCCTCCTTTCCCATTCCCTTTTCCC

TATACCC**CTCTCTCTCTCTCT**
CT3

Fig. 3. DNA sequences of the IGS 1 region of *M. globosa*.

2.2 *Malassezia* colonization and severity of AD

The *Malassezia* microbiota of the skin is also associated with the severity of AD. Fifty-six adult neck and head AD patients (21 mild, 18 moderate, and 17 severe cases) and 32 healthy individuals were examined for skin *Malassezia* microbiota, using a real-time PCR assay (Kaga *et al.* 2011). The level of colonization by *Malassezia* was almost identical among the mild and moderate AD patients and the healthy individuals, while *Malassezia* colonization in the severe AD cases was approximately 2- to 5-fold that in the mild and moderate AD patients and healthy individuals (Fig. 5A). Two major species, *M. globosa* and *M. restricta,* accounted for more than 80% of all *Malassezia* colonization in AD patients of all severities, but their proportions differed with severity. In the mild and moderate cases, *M. restricta* predominated over *M. globosa* ($p < 0.05$), whereas the proportions of *M. globosa* and *M. restricta* were almost identical ($p > 0.05$) in the severe patients (Fig. 5B).

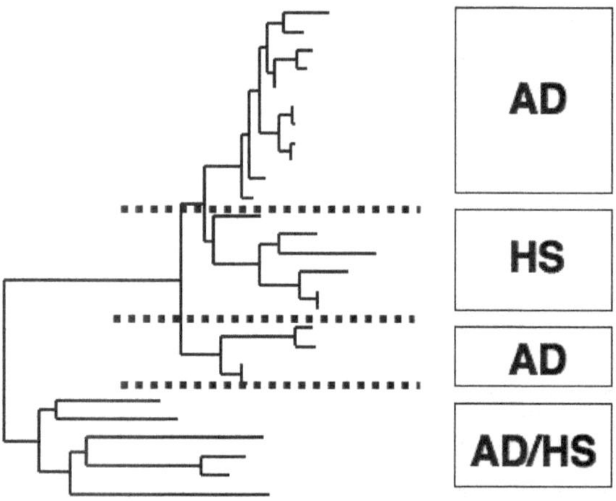

AD, patients with atopic dermatitis; HS, healthy subjects.

Fig. 4. Phylogenetic tree of *M. globosa* colonizing the skin surface of AD patients and healthy subjects based on DNA sequences of the IGS 1 region

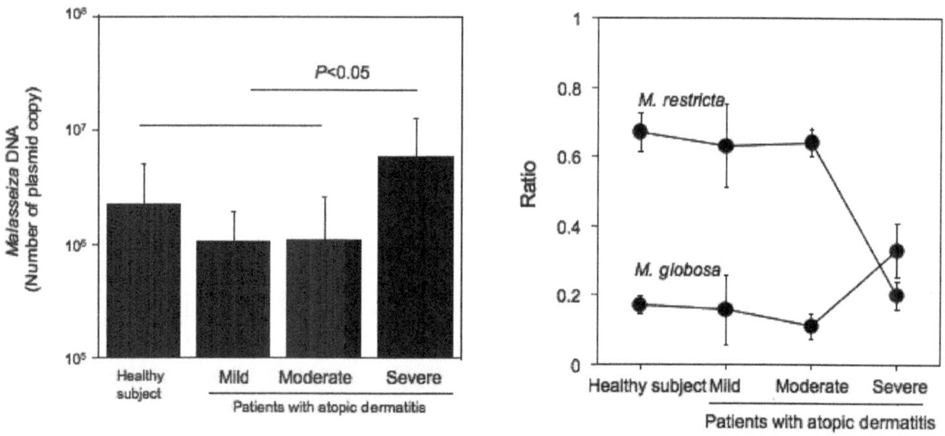

Fig. 5. Level of *Malassezia* colonization in patients with atopic dermatitis and in healthy individuals (A). Ratio of the two major *Malassezia* species, *M. globosa* and *M. restricta*, in patients with atopic dermatitis and in healthy individuals (B)

In a comprehensive analysis using an rRNA gene clone library method, Zhang *et al.* (2011) found that not only *Malassezia* but also the overall fungal microbiota differed according to AD severity. Their analysis of 3,647 clones of the fungal rRNA gene in scale samples from nine AD patients (3 mild, 3 moderate, and 3 severe cases) and 10 healthy individuals revealed 58 fungi and seven unknown phylotypes. *Malassezia* predominated, representing 63–86% of the clones identified from each subject. The number of clones had no noticeable relationship to disease severity, with the mild, moderate, and severe cases accounting for 67.8 ± 2.2, 70.7 ± 2.8, and 64.9 ± 1.8% of the clones, respectively. The study also confirmed that both *M. globosa* and *M. restricta* were the predominant species regardless of disease severity, with a detection rate of 57.5–70.4% in all clones analyzed. However, the ratio of *M. globosa* to *M. restricta* in the mild and moderate cases (*M. restricta/M. globosa*: 3.1–3.4 in mild and 2.1–4.1 in moderate cases) differed from that in the severe cases (1.1–1.4). Figure 6 shows the phylogenetic distribution between AD patients and healthy individuals, based on principal coordinates analysis. Patients with mild or moderate symptoms of AD constituted a single cluster, and patients with severe disease formed a separate cluster. Similarly, the healthy individuals clustered independently.

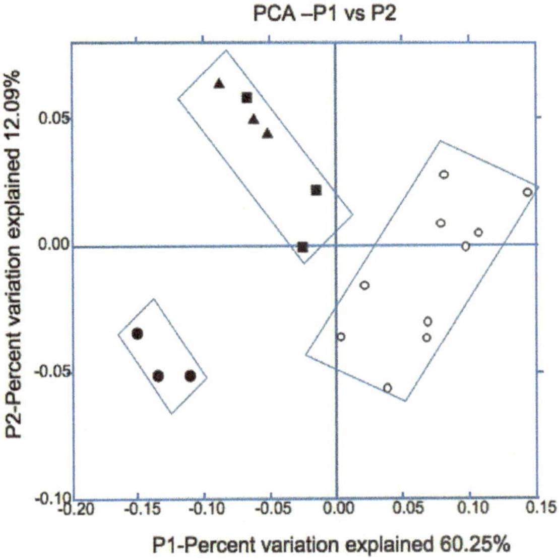

Closed triangle, patients with mild symptoms; closed square, patient with moderate symptoms; closed circle, patients with severe symptoms; open circle, healthy individuals

Fig. 6. Principal coordinates analysis (PCA) score plot of the sequence profiles for the predominant skin fungi

Differences in microbiota are thought to be attributable to differences in the physiological condition of the skin between patients with AD and healthy subjects. For example, skin pH may change skin microbiota (Seidenari and Giusti, 1995). *Staphylococcus epidermidis* is present in the skin microbiota of healthy individuals, whereas *S. aureus* is not. The level of colonization by *S. aureus* increases according to the severity of AD. In contrast, the level of colonization by *S. epidermidis* decreases gradually with increasing AD severity. Healthy skin is weakly acidic, whereas the skin pH in patients with AD is near neutral, which facilitates invasion by exogenous microorganisms, including *S. aureus* (Higaki *et al.* 1999; Hoeger *et al.* 1992). The expression levels of antimicrobial peptides may also affect the fungal microbiota (Howell 2007). The antimicrobial peptides known as defensins and cathelicidins are deficient in the skin of AD patients, and thus the fungal microbiota should be different between AD patients and healthy individuals. Sebum is a growth medium for skin microorganisms and consists of squalene, cholesterol esters, wax esters, triglycerides, free fatty acids, cholesterol, ceramides, cholesterol sulfate, and phospholipids. Of these, the proportion of ceramide 1, which is a carrier of linoleate and responsible for the water-barrier function of the skin, is significantly lower in patients with AD (Yamamoto *et al.* 1991). Therefore, the composition of sebum may also affect the fungal microbiota.

3. Immunological aspects of *Malassezia* colonizaiton

3.1 *Malassezia* specific IgE antibody

Specific IgE antibodies against skin *Malassezia* are present in the serum of AD patients whereas no anti-*Malassezia* specific IgE antibody is found in the serum of healthy individuals (Sugita *et al.* 2001). Many studies have reported on anti-*Malassezia* specific IgE antibodies in AD patients (Zargari *et al.* 2003; Kato *et al.* 2006). Using an enzyme-linked immunosorbent assay (ELISA), Kato *et al.* (2006) quantified specific IgE antibodies against soluble proteins of eight *Malassezia* species in mechanically disrupted extracts of serum samples from AD patients. The level of IgE specific for *M. restricta* was greater than that against other *Malassezia* species (*M. dermatis, M. furfur, M. globosa, M. obtusa, M. pachydermatis, M. slooffiae,* and *M. sympodialis*) (Fig. 7); however, a competitive inhibition ELISA revealed that *M. restricta* contained species-specific as well as shared antigens.

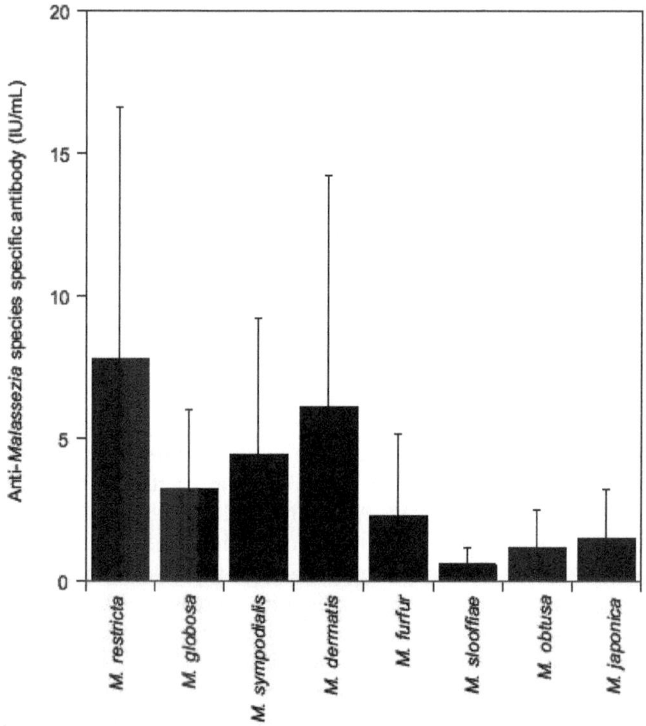

N=24

Fig. 7. The species-specific IgE values of eight *Malassezia* species in sera from patients with atopic dermatitis determined using an ELISA.

The precise mechanisms by which *Malassezia* colonization induces IgE antibody production and the inflammatory cascades that lead to AD remain unclear. The presence of IgE antibodies has been implicated in the production of Th2-type cytokines such as interleukins (IL)-4, -5, -6, -10, and -13, the promotion of IgE antibody production, the differentiation of mast cells, and the growth, migration, and activation of eosinophils (Hamid *et al.* 1994; Leung *et al.* 2000; Chen *et al.* 2004). Keratinocytes, the major cell type in the epidermis, have roles in both skin structural and immunological defense (Esche *et al.* 2004; Albanesi *et al.* 2005). Keratinocytes produce a range of proinflammatory and immune cytokines in response to microorganisms and/or skin damage (Grone *et al.* 2002; Watanabe *et al.* 2001). A recent study has demonstrated that keratinocytes secrete several Th2-type cytokines that are critical in the pathogenesis of AD (Ishibashi *et al.* 2006). Cytokine secretion profiling by antibody array analysis has revealed that *M. globosa* and *M. restricta* induce the secretion of distinct Th2-type cytokines by human keratinocytes: *M. globosa* induces IL-5, IL-10, and IL-13 secretion, while *M. restricta* induces IL-4 secretion. These findings have been confirmed by cDNA microarray analysis showing that *M. globosa* and *M. restricta* upregulate the transcription of the *IL-5* and *IL-4* genes, respectively, in keratinocytes. These observations provide evidence of a possible relationship between *Malassezia* colonization and increased IgE production in AD. It is possible that *M. globosa* and *M. restricta* play a synergistic role in triggering a Th2-shifted humoral immune response in AD. Another important connection between *Malassezia* colonization and AD relates to the increased secretion of granulocyte-macrophage colony-stimulating factor (GM-CSF) and cutaneous T-cell-attracting chemokine (CTACK) by keratinocytes (Ishibashi *et al.* 2006). *Malassezia globosa* is capable of stimulating keratinocytes to secrete GM-CSF, which primarily contributes to the maintenance of the chronic inflammatory process in AD by enhancing the antigen-presenting capacity of Langerhans cells and dendritic cells (Witmer-Pack *et al.* 1987). *Malassezia restricta* induces the secretion of CTACK by keratinocytes. CTACK selectively attracts cutaneous lymphocyte antigen-positive memory T cells to inflammatory sites (Morales *et al.* 1999) and is upregulated in AD patients (Kakinuma *et al.* 2003). The above findings suggest the following possible mechanism by which *Malassezia* species induce an IgE-immune response in patients with AD: a skin barrier dysfunction facilitates skin penetration by colonized *Malassezia*, allowing interactions between *Malassezia* and epidermal Langerhans cells, dendritic cells, and keratinocytes, which subsequently present *Malassezia* antigens, thereby inducing an immune response. This may be augmented by keratinocyte-derived GM-CSF. *Malassezia*-stimulated keratinocytes produce Th2 cytokines, including IL-4 and IL-13, which may in turn stimulate B cells to undergo IgE class switching and produce *Malassezia*-specific IgE. In addition, keratinocyte-derived IL-5 may attract and locally activate eosinophils in lesions of AD.

3.2 *Malassezia* allergens

Many *Malassezia* allergens have been identified, including Mala f2-4, Mala s1, and Mala s5-13. Several researchers have attempted to produce recombinant *Malassezia* allergens (rMala s1 and rMala s5–11) for diagnostic purposes (Schmidt *et al.* 1997; Schmid-Grendelmeier *et al.* 2005, 2006; Limacher *et al.* 2007) (Table 2). Recently, proteomics analysis has been applied to identify major allergens of *M. globosa* (Ishibashi *et al.* 2009). The IgE-reactive component of *M. globosa*, with a molecular mass of 42 kDa and designated as MGp42, has been identified by two-dimensional immunoblotting and partially sequenced by matrix-assisted laser desorption ionization time of flight mass spectrometry with post-source decay of the peptide digest. The full-length cDNA encoding MGp42 has been cloned and sequenced by the rapid amplification of cDNA ends method. MGp42 exhibits properties similar to those of heat shock protein (hsp) family members, and evidence indicates that MGp42 may be a cleavage product of intact HSP70. However, no IgE cross-reactivity has been observed between MGp42 and recombinant human HSP70, suggesting that the epitopes of MGp42 recognized by serum IgE of AD patients are masked by steric hindrance in the presence of intact HSP70 and become exposed as a result of conformational changes during HSP70 cleavage.

Allergens	Function	Species	Reference
Mala s1	Unknown	*M. sympodialis*	Schmidt et al. 1997
Mala f2	peroxisomal protein	*M. furfur*	Yasueda et al. 1998
Mala f3	peroxisomal protein	*M. furfur*	Yasueda et al. 1998
Mala f4	Malate dehydrogenase	*M. furfur*	Onishi et al. 1999
Mala s5	peroxisomal protein	*M. sympodialis*	Hemmann et al. 1997
Mala s6	Cyclophilin	*M. sympodialis*	Hemmann et al. 1997
Mala s7	Unknown	*M. sympodialis*	Weichel et al. 2002
Mala s8	Unknown	*M. sympodialis*	Weichel et al. 2002
Mala s9	Unknown	*M. sympodialis*	Weichel et al. 2002
Mala s10	Heat shock protein	*M. sympodialis*	Lindborg et al. 1999
Mala s11	MnSOD	*M. sympodialis*	Lindborg et al. 1999
Mala s12	GMC oxidoreductase	*M. sympodialis*	Rasool et al. 2000
Mala s13	Thioredoxin	*M. sympodialis*	Limacher et al. 2007
MGp42	Heat shock protein	*M. globosa*	Ishibashi et al. 2009

Table 2. *Malassezia* allergens

4. Treatment with antifungal agents

4.1 Anti-*Malassezia* IgE in the serum of AD patients

Skin prick tests positive for *Malassezia* antigen and specific IgE antibodies have been demonstrated in head and neck AD (HANAD) patients. A delayed-type hypersensitivity to *Malassezia* antigen also seems to play a role. Of 33 HANAD patients, 79% were prick-test positive for *Malassezia* antigen, but only 44% of 22 AD patients without head and neck involvement were prick-test positive (Kieffer *et al.* 1990). Rokugo *et al.* (1990) found that 71% of 35 AD patients who were prick-test positive for *Malassezia* antigen also demonstrated delayed hypersensitivity to *Malassezia* antigen in 64% of 118 AD patients. The presence of anti-*Malassezia* IgE antibody has been demonstrated in several studies (Table 3). The frequency of *Malassezia* specific IgE antibody in serum was higher in AD patients with head and neck dermatitis than without. For example, Bayrou *et al.* (2005) found IgE antibodies against *Malassezia* antigen in 100% of 106 HANAD patients, but in only 28% of 25 AD patients without head and neck involvement. Total IgE levels were also significantly higher in the AD group with head and neck dermatitis (mean, 2,823 kU/L) than without (546 kU/L).

Authors	Patients	Production of anti-*Malassezia* specific IgE antibodies
Devos and Valk, 2000	HANAD	100% (n=22)
	Non-HANAD	14% (n=22)
Johansson et al. 2003	HANAD	55% (n=98)
	Non-HANAD	19% (n=33)
Jensen-Jarolim et al. 1992	HANAD	68% (n=80)

Table 3. *Malassezia* IgE antibodies in sera of patient with atopic dermatitis

There was also a significant correlation between the level of *Malassezia* specific IgE antibody and clinical severity criteria, as reflected by the SCORAD index ($p < 0.0001$, $r^2 = 0.55$), whereas total IgE showed only a slight correlation with severity criteria ($p < 0.001$, $r^2=0.29$). No correlation was found between age or gender, and specific or total IgE. Based on prick-test results and specific IgE antibody levels, treatment of HANAD patients with antifungal agents has been recommended for the previous two decades.

4.2 Susceptibility of *Malassezia* to drug treatment

Compared with the plethora of antibacterial agents, only a small number of antifungal agents are available, which limits the treatment options for HANAD. Ketoconazole and itraconazole are highly effective *in vitro* (Sugita *et al.* 2005, Miranda *et al.* 2007, Sancak *et al.* 2005, Velegraki *et al.* 2004). In a large-scale study using 125 strains of 11 *Malassezia* species, all of the *Malassezia* species were highly susceptible to both itraconazole and ketoconazole, with minimum inhibitory concentrations (MICs) ranging from 0.016 to 0.25 mg/ml; approximately 80% of the strains had a MIC of ≤0.03 mg/ml (Sugita *et al.* (2005). This efficacy is not specific to these species, but applies to all members of the genus *Malassezia*. To our knowledge, no resistant strain has been detected. Ketoconazole and itraconazole are chemically classified as azole compounds, but other azole agents, fluconazole, voriconazole, and terbinafine, cannot inhibit the growth of *Malassezia*.

A calcineurin inhibitor, topical tacrolimus, is widely used to treat AD. This compound had antifungal activity against half of the known *Malassezia* strains, with MICs of 16-32 mg/mL (Sugita *et al.* 2005). The immunosuppressive drugs cyclosporine and tacrolimus target calcineurin and are also toxic to *Candida albicans* and *Cryptococcus neoformans* (Cruz *et al.* 2001). A combination of either ketoconazole or itraconazole and tacrolimus had a synergistic effect against *Malassezia* strains, based on a fractional inhibitory index of 0.245 to 0.378. These observations follow earlier reports on the effectiveness of a combination of tacrolimus and fluconazole against *C. albicans* and *C. neoformans* strains. The combination of topical tacrolimus and an azole agent can simultaneously treat AD and reduce the number of exacerbating *Malassezia* cells colonizing the skin surface. Although the synergistic mechanism of this combination is not known, Maesaki *et al.* (1998) demonstrated that tacrolimus increases the intracellular concentration of the azole agent in *C. albicans*. This observation may provide the basis for future clinical trials of these agents aimed at reducing the number of *Malassezia* cells colonizing the skin of AD patients (more details are provided in the following section).

Authors	Drug	Study design	Number of patients	Dosage
Bäck et al. 1995	Ketoconazole	Open-label study	20 AD patients with positive RAST to *Malassezia*	200 mg daily for 2 months and 200 mg twice weekly for further 3 months.
Broberg and Faergemann, 1995	Ketoconazole shampoo	Randomized double-blind placebo-controlled study	53 HANAD patients	Group A: miconazole-hydrocortisone cream and ketoconazole shampoo for 6 weeks
				Group B: hydrocortisone cream and placebo shampoo for 6 weeks
Bäck and Bartosik, 2001	Ketoconazole	Randomized double-blind placebo-controlled study	29 HANAD patients with specific IgE antibodies to *Malassezia*	Group A: 200 mg ketoconazole daily for 3 months
				Group B: placebo for 3 months
Ikezawa et al. 2004	Itraconazole	Randomized double-blind crossover study	34 AD patients with positive RAST to *Malassezia*	Group A: 100 mg daily of itraconazole and lactobacillus preparation for 8 weeks and lactobacillus preparation alone for further 8 weeks
				Group B: Lactobacillus preparation alone for 8 weeks and 100 mg daily of itraconazole and lactobacillus preparation for additionally 8 weeks
Svejgaard et al. 2005	Itraconazole	Randomized double-blind placebo-controlled study	53 HANAD patients	Group A: 200 mg itraconazole for 7 days
				Group B: 400 mg itraconazole for 7 days
				Group C: placebo

Table 4. Treatment for ketoconazole or itraconazole in HANAD patients

4.3 Ketoconazole and itraconazole in AD treatment (Table 4)

A relationship between *Malassezia* and AD was first suggested by Clemmensen and Hjorth (1983), who demonstrated that oral ketoconazole was efficacious in adult HANAD patients with positive prick tests for *Malassezia*. A study of 20 AD patients with positive radioallergosorbent test results for *Malassezia* showed that treatment with oral ketoconazole improved clinical scores and reduced the levels of *Malassezia* specific IgE, particularly in the head and neck area (Bäck *et al.* 1995). However, in a double-blind study with 53 HANAD patients, no difference in the clinical score was detected between those treated with miconazole-hydrocortisone cream and ketoconazole shampoo and those treated with hydrocortisone cream and placebo shampoo, although the ketoconazole group showed decreased *Malassezia* colonization (Broberg and Faergemann 1995). In another randomized double-blind placebo-controlled study comparing treatment with 200 mg ketoconazole daily *versus* placebo for 3 months in 29 HANAD patients with specific IgE antibodies to *Malassezia*, the clinical score decreased in both groups, and the improvement was correlated with the use of topical steroids in the control group, but not in the ketoconazole group (Bäck and Bartosik 2001).

A number of studies have also been conducted with itraconazole. In one study, 53 HANAD patients were divided into three groups that received 200 mg itraconazole, 400 mg itraconazole, or placebo daily (Svejgaard *et al.* 2004). The study included a 7-day treatment period and a follow-up period of 105 days. At days 7 and 14, a significant improvement was observed in the SCORAD of the head and neck area in the groups given 400 and 200 mg itraconazole daily. At day 14, a comparison among all three groups showed a significant improvement in the SCORAD of the head and neck area in the 200 mg itraconazole group compared with the placebo group. A randomized double-blind crossover study was also conducted (Ikezawa *et al.* 2004). One group was treated with a combination of itraconazole (100 mg daily) plus a conventional *Lactobacillus* preparation for 8 weeks, followed by the *Lactobacillus* preparation alone for 8 weeks. The other group received the *Lactobacillus* preparation alone for 8 weeks, followed by itraconazole (100 mg daily) plus *Lactobacillus* for 8 weeks. In both groups, a decrease in the dose or strength of concomitant topical steroids was observed at the end of the treatment course with itraconazole, and improvements in the eosinophil count, serum IgE, and fungi-specific IgE were found after the administration of itraconazole.

Itraconazole appears to be a promising treatment option for HANAD patients who do not respond to conventional therapeutic approaches. To optimize the selection of patients most likely to respond to itraconazole treatment, the levels of *Malassezia* colonization of the skin and specific IgE antibody should be evaluated.

5. Acknowledgment

This study was supported in part by a research grant from the Japan Society for the Promotion of Science (TS), a research grant for "High-Tech Research Center Project" from the Ministry of Education, Culture, Sports, Science, and Technology (TS).

6. References

Albanesi C, Scarponi C, Giustizieri ML, Girolomoni G. 2005, Keratinocytes in inflammatory skin diseases. *Curr Drug Targets Inflamm Allergy.* 4, 329-334.

Amaya M, Tajima M, Okubo Y, Sugita T, Nishikawa A, Tsuboi R. 2007, Molecular analysis of *Malassezia* microflora in the lesional skin of psoriasis patients. *J Dermatol.* 34, 619-624.

Ashbee HR. 2007, Update on the genus Malassezia. *Med Mycol.* 45, 287-303.

Bäck O, Scheynius A, Johansson SG. 1995, Ketoconazole in atopic dermatitis: therapeutic response is correlated with decrease in serum IgE. *Arch Dermatol Res.* 287, 448-451.

Bäck O, Bartosik J. 2001, Systemic ketoconazole for yeast allergic patients with atopic dermatitis. *J Eur Acad Dermatol Venereol* 15, 34-38.

Bayrou O, Pecquet C, Flahault A, Artigou C, Abuaf N, Leynadier F. 2005, Head and neck atopic dermatitis and malassezia-furfur-specific IgE antibodies. *Dermatology* 211, 107-113.

Broberg A, Faergemann J. 1995, Topical antimycotic treatment of atopic dermatitis in the head/neck area. A double-blind randomised study. *Acta Derm Venereol.* 75, 46-49.

Chen L, Martinez O, Overbergh L, Mathieu C, Prabhakar BS, Chan LS. 2004, Early up-regulation of Th2 cytokines and late surge of Th1 cytokines in an atopic dermatitis model. *Clin Exp Immunol.* 138, 375-387.

Clemmensen OJ, Hjorth N. 1983, Treatment of dermatitis of head and neck with ketoconazole in patients with type 1 sensitivity to *Pityrosporum orbiculare. Semin. Dermatol.* 2, 26-29.

Cruz M C, A L Goldstein, J Blankenship, M Del Poeta, J R Perfect, J H McCusker, Y L Bennani, M E Cardenas, J Heitman. 2001. Rapamycin and less immunosuppressive analogs are toxic to *Candida albicans* and *Cryptococcus neoformans* via FKBP12-dependent inhibition of TOR. *Antimicrob. Agents Chemother.* 45, 3162-3170.

Devos SA, van der Valk PG. 2000, The relevance of skin prick tests for *Pityrosporum ovale* in patients with head and neck dermatitis. Allergy. 55, 1056-1058.

Esche C, de Benedetto A, Beck LA. 2004, Keratinocytes in atopic dermatitis. inflammatory signals. *Curr Allergy Asthma Rep.* 4, 276-284.

Grone, A. 2002, Keratinocytes and cytokines. *Vet Immunol Immunopathol.* 88, 1-12.

Guého-Kellermann E, Boekhout T, Begerow D. 2010, Biodiversity, Phylogeny and Ultrastructure. *In Malassezia* and the skin. Edited by Boekhout, Guého-Kellermann E, Mayser P, and Velegraki A, pp. 17-64, Springer, 2010.

Gupta AK, Kohli Y, Summerbell RC, Faergemann J. 2001, Quantitative culture of *Malassezia* species from different body sites of individuals with or without dermatoses. *Med Mycol.* 39, 243-251.

Gupta AK, Batra R, Bluhm R, Boekhout T, Dawson TL Jr. 2004, Skin diseases associated with *Malassezia* species. *J Am Acad Dermatol.* 51, 785-798.

Hamid Q, Boguniewicz M, Leung DY. 1994, Differential *in situ* cytokine gene expression in acute versus chronic atopic dermatitis. *J Clin Invest.* 94, 870-876.

Hemmann S, Blaser K, Crameri R. 1997, Allergens of *Aspergillus fumigatus* and *Candida boidinii* share IgE-binding epitopes. Am J Respir Crit Care Med. 156, 1956-1962.

Higaki S, Morohashi M, Yamagishi T, Hasegawa Y. 1999, Comparative study of staphylococci from the skin of atopic dermatitis patients and from healthy subjects. *Int J Dermatol.* 38, 265-269.

Hoeger PH, Lenz W, Boutonnier A, Fournier JM. 1992, Staphylococcal skin colonization in children with atopic dermatitis: prevalence, persistence, and transmission of toxigenic and nontoxigenic strains. *J Infect Dis.* 165, 1064-1068.

Howell MD. 2007, The role of human beta defensins and cathelicidins in atopic dermatitis. *Curr Opin Allergy Clin Immunol.* 7, 413-417.

Ikezawa Z, Kondo M, Okajima M, Nishimura Y, Kono M. 2004, Clinical usefulness of oral itraconazole, an antimycotic drug, for refractory atopic dermatitis. *Eur J Dermatol.* 14, 400-406.

Ishibashi Y Sugita T Nishikawa A. 2006, Cytokine secretion profile of human keratinocytes exposed to Malassezia yeasts. *FEMS Immunol Med Microbiol.* 48, 400-409.

Ishibashi Y, Kato H, Asahi Y, Sugita T, Nishikawa A. 2009, Identification of the major allergen of *Malassezia globosa* relevant for atopic dermatitis. *J Dermatol. Sci.* 55, 185-192.

Jensen-Jarolim E, Poulsen LK, With H, Kieffer M, Ottevanger V, Stahl Skov P. 1992, Atopic dermatitis of the face, scalp, and neck: type I reaction to the yeast *Pityrosporum ovale*? J Allergy Clin Immunol. 89, 44-51.

Johansson C, Sandström MH, Bartosik J, Särnhult T, Christiansen J, Zargari A, Bäck O, Wahlgren CF, Faergemann J, Scheynius A, Tengvall Linder M. 2003, Atopy patch test reactions to *Malassezia* allergens differentiate subgroups of atopic dermatitis patients. *Br J Dermatol* 148, 479-488.

Kaga M, Sugita T, Nishikawa A, Wada Y, Hiruma M, Ikeda S. 2011, Molecular analysis of the cutaneous *Malassezia* microbiota from the skin of patients with atopic dermatitis of different severities. *Mycoses* 54, e24-28.

Kakinuma T, Saeki H, Tsunemi Y, Fujita H, Asano N, Mitsui H, Tada Y, Wakugawa M, Watanabe T, Torii H, Komine M, Asahina A, Nakamura K, Tamaki K. 2003, Increased serum cutaneous T cell-attracting chemokine (CCL27) levels in patients with atopic dermatitis and psoriasis vulgaris. *J Allergy Clin Immunol.* 111, 592-597.

Kaneko T, Makimura K, Abe M, Shiota R, Nakamura Y, Kano R, Hasegawa A, Sugita T, Shibuya S, Watanabe S, Yamaguchi H, Abe S, Okamura N. 2007, Revised culture-based system for identification of *Malassezia* species. *J Clin Microbiol.* 45, 3737-3742.

Kato H, Sugita T, Ishibashi Y, Nishikawa A. 2006, Detection and quantification of specific IgE antibodies against eight *Malassezia* species in sera of patients with atopic dermatitis by using an enzyme-linked immunosorbent assay. *Microbiol Immunol.* 50, 851-856.

Kieffer M, Bergbrant I-M, Faergeman J, Jemec GBE, Ottevanger V, Skov PS, Svejgaard E. 1990, Immune reactions to Pityrosporum ovale in adult patients with atopic and seborrhoeic dermatitis. *J. Am. Acad. Dermatol.* 22, 739-742.

Leung DY. 2000, Atopic dermatitis. new insights and opportunities for therapeutic intervention. *J Allergy Clin Immunol.* 105, 860-876.

Limacher A, Glaser AG, Meier C, Schmid-Grendelmeier P, Zeller S, Scapozza L, Crameri R. 2007, Cross-reactivity and 1.4-A crystal structure of *Malassezia sympodialis* thioredoxin (Mala s 13), a member of a new pan-allergen family. *J Immunol* 178, 389-396.

Lindborg M, Magnusson CG, Zargari A, Schmidt M, Scheynius A, Crameri R, Whitley P. 1999, Selective cloning of allergens from the skin colonizing yeast *Malassezia furfur* by phage surface display technology. *J Invest Dermatol* 113, 156-161.

Maesaki S, P Marichal, M A Hossain, D Sanglard, H Vanden Bossche, S Kohno. 1998, Synergic effects of tactolimus and azole antifungal agents against azole-resistant *Candida albican* strains. *J. Antimicrob. Chemother.* 42, 747-753.

Miranda KC, de Araujo CR, Costa CR, Passos XS, de Fátima Lisboa Fernandes O, do Rosário Rodrigues Silva M. 2007, Antifungal activities of azole agents against the Malassezia species. *Int J Antimicrob Agents.* 29, 281-284.

Morales J, Homey B, Vicari AP, Hudak S, Oldham E, Hedrick J, Orozco R, Copeland NG, Jenkins NA, McEvoy LM, Zlotnik A. 1999, CTACK, a skin-associated chemokine that preferentially attracts skin-homing memory T cells. *Proc Natl Acad Sci USA* 96, 14470-14475.

Morishita N, Sei Y, Sugita T. 2006, Molecular analysis of malassezia microflora from patients with pityriasis versicolor. *Mycopathologia* 161, 61-65.

Nakabayashi A, Sei Y, Guillot J. 2000, Identification of *Malassezia* species isolated from patients with seborrhoeic dermatitis, atopic dermatitis, pityriasis versicolor and normal subjects. *Med Mycol.* 38, 337-341.

Onishi Y, Kuroda M, Yasueda H, Saito A, Sono-Koyama E, Tunasawa S, Hashida-Okado T, Yagihara T, Uchida K, Yamaguchi H, Akiyama K, Kato I, Takesako K. 1999, Two-dimensional electrophoresis of *Malassezia* allergens for atopic dermatitis and isolation of Mal f 4 homologs with mitochondrial malate dehydrogenase. Eur J Biochem. 261, 148-154.

Rasool O, Zargari A, Almqvist J, Eshaghi H, Whitley P, Scheynius A. 2000, Cloning, characterization and expression of complete coding sequences of three IgE binding *Malassezia furfur* allergens, Mal f 7, Mal f 8 and Mal f 9. *Eur J Biochem* 267, 4355-4361.

Rokugo M, Tagami H, Usuba Y, Tomita Y. 1990, Contact sensitivity to *Pityrosporum ovale* in patients with an atopic dermatitis. *Arch. Dermatol.* 126, 627-634.

Sancak B, Ayhan M, Karaduman A, Arikan S. 2005, In vitro activity of ketoconazole, itraconazole and terbinafine against *Malassezia* strains isolated from neonates. *Mikrobiyol Bul.* 39, 301-308. Turkish.

Sandström Falk MH, Tengvall Linder M, Johansson C, Bartosik J, Bäck O, Särnhult T, Wahlgren CF, Scheynius A, Faergemann J. 2005, The prevalence of *Malassezia* yeasts in patients with atopic dermatitis, seborrhoeic dermatitis and healthy controls. *Acta Derm Venereol.* 85, 17-23.

Schmidt M, Zargari A, Holt P, Lindbom L, Hellman U, Whitley P, van der Ploeg I, Härfast B, Scheynius A. 1997, The complete cDNA sequence and expression of the first major allergenic protein of *Malassezia furfur*, Mal f 1. *Eur J Biochem* 246, 181-185.

Schmid-Grendelmeier P, Flückiger S, Disch R, Trautmann A, Wüthrich B, Blaser K, Scheynius A, Crameri R. 2005, IgE-mediated and T cell-mediated autoimmunity against manganese superoxide dismutase in atopic dermatitis. *J Allergy Clin Immunol* 115, 1068-1075.

Schmid-Grendelmeier P, Scheynius A, Crameri R. 2006, The role of sensitization to *Malassezia sympodialis* in atopic eczema. *Chem Immunol Allergy* 91, 98-109.

Seidenari S, Giusti G. 1995, Objective assessment of the skin of children affected by atopic dermatitis: a study of pH, capacitance and TEWL in eczematous and clinically uninvolved skin. *Acta Derm Venereol.* 75, 429-433.

Sugita T, Suto H, Unno T, Tsuboi R, Ogawa H, Shinoda T, Nishikawa A. 2001, Molecular analysis of *Malassezia* microflora on the skin of atopic dermatitis patients and healthy subjects. *J Clin Microbiol.* 39, 3486-3490.

Sugita T, Kodama M, Saito M, Ito T, Kato Y, Tsuboi R, Nishikawa A. 2003, Sequence diversity of the intergenic spacer region of the rRNA gene of *Malassezia globosa* colonizing the skin of patients with atopic dermatitis and healthy individuals. *J Clin Microbiol.* 41, 3022-3027.

Sugita T, Tajima M, Amaya M, Tsuboi R, Nishikawa A. 2004, Genotype analysis of *Malassezia restricta* as the major cutaneous flora in patients with atopic dermatitis and healthy subjects. *Microbiol Immunol.* 48, 755-759.

Sugita T, Tajima M, Ito T, Saito M, Tsuboi R, Nishikawa A. 2005, Antifungal activities of tacrolimus and azole agents against the eleven currently accepted *Malassezia* species. *J Clin Microbiol.* 43, 2824-2829.

Sugita T, Tajima M, Tsubuku H, Tsuboi R, Nishikawa A. 2006a, Quantitative analysis of cutaneous *Malassezia* in atopic dermatitis patients using real-time PCR. *Microbiol Immunol.* 50, 549-552.

Sugita T, Boekhout T, Velegraki A, Guillot J, Hadina S, Cabanes FJ. 2010, Epidemiology of *Malassezia*-related skin diseases. *In Malassezia* and the skin. Edited by Boekhout, Guého-Kellermann E, Mayser P, and Velegraki A, pp. 65-120, Springer, 2010.

Sugita T, Zhang E, Miyamoto M, Tajima M, Tsuboi R, Nishikawa A. 2011, Chapter 73 *Malassezia, In* Molecular Detection of Human Fungal Pathogens. Edited by Dongyou Liu, Taylor & Francis Group. 631-638.

Svejgaard E, Larsen PØ, Deleuran M, Ternowitz T, Roed-Petersen J, Nilsson J. 2004, Treatment of head and neck dermatitis comparing itraconazole 200 mg and 400 mg daily for 1 week with placebo. *J Eur Acad Dermatol Venereol.* 18, 445-449.

Tajima M, Sugita T, Nishikawa A, Tsuboi R. 2008, Molecular analysis of *Malassezia* microflora in seborrheic dermatitis patients: comparison with other diseases and healthy subjects. *J Invest Dermatol.* 128, 345-351.

Takahata Y, Sugita T, Hiruma M, Muto M. 2007a, Quantitative analysis of *Malassezia* in the scale of patients with psoriasis using a real-time polymerase chain reaction assay. *Br J Dermatol.* 157, 670-673.

Takahata Y, Sugita T, Kato H, Nishikawa A, Hiruma M, Muto M. 2007b, Cutaneous *Malassezia* flora in atopic dermatitis differs between adults and children. *Br J Dermatol.* 157, 1178-1182.

Velegraki A, Alexopoulos EC, Kritikou S, Gaitanis G. 2004, Use of fatty acid RPMI 1640 media for testing susceptibilities of eight *Malassezia* species to the new triazole posaconazole and to six established antifungal agents by a modified NCCLS M27-A2 microdilution method and Etest. *J Clin Microbiol.* 42, 3589-3593.

Watanabe S, Kano R, Sato H, Nakamura Y, Hasegawa A. 2001, The effects of *Malassezia* yeasts on cytokine production by human keratinocytes. *J Invest Dermatol.* 116, 769-773.

Weichel M, Fluckiger S, Crameri R. 2002. Molecular characterization of mould allergens involved in respiratory complications. Rencet Res devel Resp Critical Care Med. 2, 29-45.

Witmer-Pack MD, Olivier W, Vaiinsky J. 1987, Granulocyte-macrophage colony-stimulating factor is essential for the viability and function of cultured murine epidermal Langerhans cells. *J Exp Med.* 166, 1484-1498.

Xu J, Saunders CW, Hu P, Grant RA, Boekhout T, Kuramae EE, Kronstad JW, Deangelis YM, Reeder NL, Johnstone KR, Leland M, Fieno AM, Begley WM, Sun Y, Lacey MP, Chaudhary T, Keough T, Chu L, Sears R, Yuan B, Dawson TL Jr. 2007, Dandruff-associated *Malassezia* genomes reveal convergent and divergent virulence traits shared with plant and human fungal pathogens. *Proc Natl Acad Sci* U S A. 104, 18730-18735.

Yamamoto A, Serizawa S, Ito M, Sato Y. 1991, Stratum corneum lipid abnormalities in atopic dermatitis. *Arch Dermatol Res.* 283, 219-223.

Yasueda H, Hashida-Okado T, Saito A, Uchida K, Kuroda M, Onishi Y, Takahashi K, Yamaguchi H, Takesako K, Akiyama K. 1998. Identification and cloning of two novel allergens from the lipophilic yeast, *Malassezia furfur*. Biochem Biophys Res Commun. 248, 240-244.

Zargari A, Midgley G, Bäck O, Johansson SG, Scheynius A. 2003, IgE-reactivity to seven *Malassezia* species. *Allergy* 58, 306-311.

Zhang E, Tanaka T, Tajima M, Tsuboi R, Nishikawa A, Sugita T. 2011, Characterization of the skin fungal microbiota in patients with atopic dermatitis and healthy subjects. *Microbiol Immunol* Jun 24. doi: 10.1111/j.1348-0421.2011.00364.x. [Epub ahead of print]

Part 3

Diagnosis and Clinical Management

10

Atopic Dermatitis: From Pathophysiology to Diagnostic Approach

Nicola Fuiano[1] and Cristoforo Incorvaia[2]
[1]*Paediatric Allergy Service, ASL Fg, Torremaggiore*
[2]*Allergy/Pulmonary rehabilitation, ICP Hospital, Milan*
Italy

1. Introduction

Atopic eczema/dermatitis syndrome (AEDS) is a chronic inflammatory skin disease, very common in childhood (1). The prevalence of AEDS is estimated to 15–30% in children and 2–10% in adults while the incidence has shown a 2- to 3-fold increase in the past 3 decades in developed countries (2). This results in a significant socio-economic impact, that in the United States was estimated in a range from $364 million to $3.8 billion US dollars per year, usually considering only the direct but not the indirect costs (3). The disease is sustained by a complex interaction between genetic and environmental factors and is characterized by a skin barrier dysfunction resulting in epidermal damage and altered permeability to allergens and microbes (4). Depending on the association or not to IgE sensitization, AEDS may be defined as atopic or nonatopic. The two forms are clinically similar but show some differences regarding the histology, the kind of cells involved, and the cytokine pattern (5).

2. Pathophysiology of AEDS

The pathophysiologic mechanisms leading to AEDS originate from an initial skin defect at epidermal level, above all in the *stratum corneum*, which is the first of the four epidermal layers. The *stratum corneum* (from the Latin words for horned layer) is composed of large, flat cells containing keratin, a protein that helps keep the skin hydrated by preventing water evaporation, and surrounded by lamellae sheets rich in hydrophobic lipids, including ceramides, sphyngosynes and free fatty acids. Keratin is produced by the keratinocytes of the basal layer, which also keep the Langerhans cells and the intradermal lymphocytes in position with the epidermis. They also work to modulate the immune response by secreting cytokines such as TGF-beta and alpha, and a number of interleukins (6). A major advance in the understanding of epidermal barrier dysfunction which occurs in AEDS was the identification of the fundamental role of filaggrin (7). Filaggrin, which derives from the highly phosphorylated polypeptide profilaggrin, the main constituent of the keratohyalin substance in the granular layer, is a structural protein associated to filaments which are bound to keratin fibres in epidermal cells. Recent studies found that loss-of-function mutations in the gene encoding filaggrin, particularly the R501X and 2282de14 mutation, are associated with the development of atopic dermatitis (8-10).

The alteration of the epidermal structure due to filaggrin mutation induces a significant reduction of the lipidic component, particularly of ceramide levels (11) that leads to the well known phenomenon of trans-epidermal water loss (TEWL) resulting in dry skin and itching, while the impaired skin barrier associated with filaggrin deficiency favours the penetration of foreign noxae, especially allergens and microbes (12).

Concerning allergens, it is conceivable that their facilitated access favours the sensitization process, especially for house dust mites, the protease activity of their major allergen being a further enhancing factor (13). Once entered, allergens are captured by dendritic cells (14) that activate an initially local Th2 but a later Th1 response along with a systemic Th2 response inducing the Ig isotype switching to IgE synthesis and the involvement of eosinophils (2). In this kind of response an important factor seems to be thymic stromal lymphopoietin (TSLP), an IL-7-like cytokine expressed by barrier epithelial cells able to activate myeloid-derived dendritic cells, macrophages and mast cells (15). The ongoing inflammatory process is then sustained by the Th2-related cytokine such as IL-5, IL-13, TNF-alpha, IL-17, and IL-31, the latter being primarily expressed in skin-homing Th2 cells (16). An important clinical aspect of the allergen-caused AEDS is the frequent evolution of manifestations to respiratory symptoms such as asthma and rhinitis. This process has been defined as the "atopic march" (17). Also in this case, filaggrin null mutation were found to be associated with the development of asthma (18). However, more than one model of atopic march was reported, because in a significant number of children asthma precedes AEDS as the onset manifestation of the atopic disease (19). Of note, in subjects with AEDS and no filaggrin gene mutations, the cytokines IL-4 and IL-13 (typical of the Th2 profile) are able to inhibit the expression of filaggrin (20). This suggests that if filaggrin deficiency predisposes to atopy, atopy is also likely to impair the filaggrin-dependent skin barrier.

Regarding microbes, the normal skin defence is based on integrity of *stratum corneum* and on immune response by neutrophils and macrophages by production of substances which kill the microbes and by phagocytosis. Numerous antimicrobial peptides produced by keratinocytes and belonging to the classes of beta-defensins and cathelicidins are able to disrupt or penetrate the microbe membrane thus protecting the skin from infections (21). It has been demonstrated that in patients with AEDS there is a deficiency in the expression of beta-defensins and cathelicidins that may account for the susceptibility to skin infection, especially from *Staphilococcus aureus* (22). *S. Aureus* has a major role in AEDS, as indicated by the following features: 1) a very high density of colony-forming units *S. aureus* per cm^2 of inflamed atopic skin lesions (23); 2) the higher affinity for *S. aureus* of the atopic skin compared with nonatopic or psoriatic skin (24); 3) the reduction of *S. aureus* counts on atopic skin sites following effective topical treatment (25). In any form of AEDS, an additional pathophysiologic role is played by the cytokine IL-31 produced by keratinocytes, which exerts a potent pruritogenic effect (26). In fact, pruritus is associated with skin lesions caused by scratching or excessive washing and to consequent damage of keratinocytes and release of mediators, but also of autoantigens, and generation of autoantibodies (27). Moreover, autoreactivity phenomena also concur to pathogenesis of AEDS. In particular, manganese superoxide dismutase (MnSOD) of both human and foreign origin - especially from the long known *Malassezia spp* yeast (28) - may act as autoallergen. Specific IgE against human MnSOD correlating with the disease activity were detected in patients with AEDS, suggesting that human MnSOD with molecular mimicry with MnSOD from *Malassezia* may play a role, as showed by its capacity to induce in vitro T-cell reactivity and eczematous skin lesions, as an autoallergen in subjects with both atopic and nonatopic forms (29).

3. The allergy tests in diagnosis of AEDS

When food allergens are the cause of AEDS, the commonly used allergy tests, such as skin prick tests and in vitro measurement of specific IgE antibodies, have a role in the diagnostic work-up (30). Concerning food-specific IgE measurement, an useful application was suggested by Sampson and Ho, who identified in a group of 196 children and adolescents with AEDS the food-specific IgE levels predicting a positive result of a double-blind, placebo-controlled food challenge. Such levels, showing a positive predictive value higher than 95%, corresponded to 6 kU/L for egg, 32 kU/L for milk, 15 kU/L for peanut, and 20 kU/L for fish (31). The same author later confirmed the utility of specific IgE concentrations in predicting symptomatic allergy also for other foods such as wheat and soy (32). However, the advances in the knowledge of pathophysiology of AEDS, and particularly the understanding that in this disease the mechanisms of delayed hypersensitivity prevail, suggested the need of new diagnostic tools. The atopy patch test (APT) was recently defined as an important tool in diagnosis of AEDS, because it seems to have a greater significance than skin prick test or RAST, which simply detect the presence of specific IgE antibodies. Thus, allergy tests assessing only the immediate IgE-mediated phase of the allergic response can only partially detect the operating mechanisms. Instead, there is notable evidence supporting the capacity of the APT to reproduce the pathophysiologic events of AEDS.

In biopsy-based studies, a Th2 cytokine pattern was found 24 hours after APT, but a shift to a Th1 pattern, as occurs in chronic AEDS skin lesions, was noted after 48 hours (33, 34). A more frequent positivity to APT was reported in patients with allergen-specific lymphocyte proliferation and expression of activation markers on peripheral blood T-cells following *in vitro* stimulation with house dust mite, cat or grass pollen allergens, than in patients without lymphocyte proliferation (35). Application of the APT to skin of subjects with AEDS was followed by an influx of inflammatory dendritic epidermal cells (36). A significant increase of TEWL was reported in the site of the APT application, both after 48 and 72 hours, compared with the control skin site (37). By immunohistochemical analysis, the presence of IgE on Langerhans cells was demonstrated in positive APT reactions to *Dermatophagoides* in patients with mite-associated AEDS (38).

Clinically, patients with a diagnosis of intrinsic AEDS because of negative IgE tests actually had a positive APT for dust mites (39). This aspect is of particular interest, because AEDS patients with negative SPT and IgE measurement in serum should be defined as nonatopic unless APT is performed. A number of studies evaluated how common such patients are, with different observations. In one study the rate of positive APT in nonatopic patients was 23% (40), while in another study comparing AEDS patients with extrinsic and intrinsic forms, the rate of positive APT was 47.4% and 66.6%, respectively (41). In a European multicenter study, which included 314 patients with AEDS, the frequency of clear-cut positive APT reactions ranged from 39% with dust mites to 9% with celery. A notable observation from the study was that positive APT in face of all SPT and sIgE testing negative was found in 7% of the patients, whereas a positive APT without SPT or sIgE for the respective allergen was seen in 17% of the patients (42). This lead the authors to conclude that, as no gold standard for aeroallergen provocation in AEDS exists, the relevance of aeroallergens for AEDS may be evaluated by APT in addition to SPT and sIgE. Moreover, in children with respiratory symptoms an exclusive positivity to APT with dust mites was observed (43). On the other hand, it was reported that in 63 children with mite-induced asthma and rhinitis, all with positive SPT and sIgE in serum, 16 (25%) were positive to mite APT too, indicating that delayed hypersensitivity reactions were involved (44).

These observations lead us to investigate the possible factors underlying the positive result of APT in subjects with respiratory symptoms. In our first study, conducted on 297 children (45), we could demonstrate that in patients with asthma or rhinitis a positive APT to dust mite was strongly associated with the presence of current or past AEDS. Instead, most subjects with respiratory disease but a negative history for AEDS had a positive SPT. Multivariate analysis showed that there was a high probability of a positive APT result in patients with AEDS (odds ratio 17.4), in patients with AEDS and respiratory disease (odds ratio 21.9), and in patients with past AEDS and respiratory disease (odds ratio 22.8). These observations were confirmed in a study on a large population of 465 children aged 0.4 to 17.6 years. They were divided into four groups: group A, current AEDS (40 patients); group B, current AEDS with respiratory symptoms (156 patients); group C, past AEDS with respiratory symptoms (203 patients); and the control group, respiratory symptoms with no history of AEDS (66 patients). The APT was significantly more frequently positive in groups with current AEDS (groups A and B) or past AEDS (group C) than in the control group, while SPT and RAST were significantly more frequently positive in the control group (46). Such significant differences in response to APT in patients with diverse clinical expressions suggest that distinctive immunologic mechanisms lie beneath the different manifestations of hypersensitivity to dust mites. It seems conceivable that in subjects with a negative history for AEDS sensitization occurs by respiratory route and leads to the development of a Th2 pattern of response with ongoing production of specific IgE and consequent positive SPT and in vitro IgE tests. By contrast, in the case mite allergens enter through the skin, as it occurs in exposure to common indoor concentrations of the major allergen Der p 1 (47), such entering being facilitated by its proteolytic activity and in the presence of a filaggrin-dependent skin barrier dysfunction, a different chain of events is likely to take place. This is ultimately revealed by positive APT and negative SPT and *in vitro* IgE tests.

The recent observations on the diagnostic significance of APT in patients with different clinical expressions of the disease highlighted the importance of delayed hypersensitivity in AEDS. This brings into question the role of simple IgE sensitization in AEDS and also the appropriateness of the term atopic when applied to AEDS. In fact, current evidence shows that up to two thirds of patients with AEDS are not atopic, therefore even to continue using the term atopic dermatitis is to be considered problematic (48, 49). In fact, the definition of atopy as "a personal or familial tendency to produce IgE antibodies in response to low doses of allergens" (50) seems not to be appropriate for AEDS, as many patients show a positive result to APT but not to IgE tests. At the same time, the definition atopy patch test seems unfounded, because the test does not reveal atopy, i.e. a type I hypersensitivity, but a type IV hypersensitivity according to Gell and Coombs classification (51). A unifying solution should be the use, in both cases, of the term allergy, which is defined as "a hypersensitivity reaction initiated by immunologic mechanisms" (50) and includes all known mechanisms, as a replacement for atopy.

4. References

[1] Asher MI, Montefort S, Biorksten B, et al; ISAAC Phase Three Study Group Allergies. Worldwide time trends in the prevalence of asthma, rhinoconjunctivitis, and eczema in childood: ISAAC Phase One and Three repeat multicountry cross-sectional surveys. Lancet 2006; 368:733-743.

[2] Leung DY, Bieber T. Atopic dermatitis, Lancet 2003; 361:151-160.

[3] Mancini AJCS, Kaulback K. The socioeconomic impact of atopic dermatitis in the United States: a systematic review. Pediatr Dermatol 2008;25: 1-6.

[4] Boguniewicz M, Leung DYM. Atopic dermatitis. J Allergy Clin Immunol. 2006;117:S475-S480.

[5] Novak N, Bieber T, Leung DYM. Immune mechanisms leading to atopic dermatitis. J Allergy Clin Immunol 2003; 112:S128-S139.

[6] Giustizieri ML, Mascia F, Frezzolini A, et al. Keratinocytes from patients with atopic dermatitis and psoriasis show a distinct chemokine production profile in response to T-cell-derived cytokines. J Allergy Clin Immunol 2001;107:871-7.

[7] Sandilands A, Sutherland C, Irvine AD, McLean WH. Filaggrin in the frontline: role in skin barrier function and disease. J Cell Sci 2009;122:1285-4.

[8] Cookson W. The immunogenetics of asthma and eczema: a new focus on the epithelium. Nat Rev Immunol 2004;4:978-88.

[9] Palmer CN, Irvine AD, Terron-Kwiatkoski A, et al. Common loss-of-function variants of the epidermal barrier protein filaggrin are a major predisposing factor for atopic dermatitis. Nat Genet 2006;38:441-6.

[10] O'Regan GM, Sandilands A, McLean WHI, Irvine AD. Filaggrin in atopic dermatitis. J Allergy Clin Immunol 2008;122:689-93.

[11] Jungersted JM, Scheer M, Baurecht H, et al. Stratum corneum, skin barrier function and filaggrin mutations in patients with atopic eczema. Allergy 2010;65:911-8.

[12] Leung DYM. Our evolving understanding of the functional role of filaggrin in atopic dermatitis. J Allergy Clin Immunol 2009;124:494-5.

[13] Donnelly S, Dalton JP, Loukas A. Proteases in helminth- and allergen-induced inflammatory responses. Chem Immunol Allergy 2006;90:45-64.

[14] Novak N, Koch S, Allam JP, Bieber T. Dendritic cells: bridging innate and adaptive immunity in atopic dermatitis. J Allergy Clin Immunol 2010:125:50-9.

[15] Corrigan CJ, Jayaratmam A, Wang Y, et al. Early production of thymic stromal lymphopoietin precedes infiltration of dendritic cells expressing its receptor in allergen-induced late-phase cutaneous responses in atopic subjects. Allergy 2010;64:1014-22.

[16] Incorvaia C, Frati F, Verna N, et al. Allergy and the skin. Clin Exp Immunol 2008;153 (suppl 1):27-9.

[17] Spergel JM, Paller AS. Atopic dermatitis and the atopic march. J Allergy Clin Immunol 2003;112:S128-39.

[18] Palmer CN, Ismail T, Lee TH, et al. Filaggrin null mutations are associated with increased asthma severity in children and young adults. J Allergy Clin Immunol 2007;120:64-8.
[19] Illi S, von Mutius E, Lau S, et al. The natural course of atopic dermatitis from birth to age 7 years and the association with asthma. J Allergy Clin Immunol 2004;113:925-31.
[20] Howell MD, Kim BE, Gao P, et al. Cytokine modulation of atopic dermatitis filaggrin skin expression. J Allergy Clin Immunol 2009;124:S7-12.
[21] Nizet V, Ohtake T, Lauth X, et al. Innate antimicrobial peptide protects the skin from invasive bacterial infection. Nature 2001;414:454-7.
[22] Ong PY, Ohtake T, Brandt C, et al. Endogenous antimicrobial peptides and skin infections in atopic dermatitis. N Engl J Med 2002;347:1151-60.
[23] Cho SH, Strickland I, Tomkinson A, Fehringer AP, Gelfand EW, Leung FY. Preferential binding of Staphilococcus aureus to skin sites of Th2-mediated inflammation in a murine model. J Invest Dermatol 2001;116:658-63.
[24] Donnelly S, Dalton JP, Loukas A. Proteases in helminth- and allergen-induced inflammatory responses. Chem Immunol Allergy 2006;90:45-64.
[25] Nilsson EJ, Henning CG, Magnusson J. Topical corticosteroids and Staphilococcus aureus in atopic dermatitis. J Am Acad Dermatol 1992;27:29-34.
[26] Sonkoly E, Muller A. Lauerma AI, et al. IL-31: a new link between T cells and pruritus in atopic skin inflammation. J Allergy Clin Immunol 2006;117:411-7.
[27] Terui T. Analysis of the mechanisms for the development of allergic skin inflammation and the application for its treatment: overview of the pathophysiology of atopic dermatitis. J Pharmacol Sci 2009;110:232-6.
[28] Scheynius A, Johansson C, Buentke E, Zargari A, Linder MT. Atopic eczema/dermatitis syndrome and Malassezia. Int Arch Allergy Immunol 2002;127:161-9.
[29] Schmid-Grendelmeier P, Fluckiger S, Disch R, et al. IgE-mediated and T-cell mediated autoimmunity against manganese superoxide dismutase in atopic dermatitis. J Allergy Clin Immunol 2005;115:1068-75.
[30] Caubet JC, Eigenmann PA. Allergic triggers in atopic dermatitis. Immunol Allergy Clin North Am 2010;30:289-307.
[31] Sampson HA, Ho DG. Relationship between food-specific IgE concentrations and the risk of positive food challenge in children and adolescents. J Allergy Clin Immunol 1997;100:444-51.
[32] Sampson HA. Utility of food-specific IgE concentrations in predicting symptomatic food allergy. J Allergy Clin Immunol 2001;107:891-6.
[33] Sager N, Feldmann A, Schilling C, Kreitsch P, Neumann C. House dust mite-specific T cells in the skin of subjects with atopic dermatitis: frequency and lymphokine profile in the allergen patch test. J Allergy Clin Immunol 1992;89:801-10.
[34] van Reijsen FC, Bruijnzeel-Koomen CA, Kalthoff FS, et al. Skin-derived aeroallergen-specific T-cell clones of the Th2 phenotype in patients with atopic dermatitis. J Allergy Clin Immunol 1992;90:184-93.

[35] Wistokat-Wulfing A, Schmidt P, Darsow U, Ring J, Kapp A, Werfel T. Atopy patch test reactions are associated with T lymphocyte-mediated allergen-specific immune responses in atopic dermatitis. Clin Exp Allergy 1999;29:513-21.
[36] Kerschenlohr K, Decard S, Przybilla B, Wollenberg A. Atopy patch test reactions show a rapid influx of inflammatory dendritic epidermal cells (IDEC) in extrinsic and intrinsic atopic dermatitis patients. J Allergy Clin Immunol 2003;111:869-74.
[37] Gfesser M, Rakoski J, Ring J. The disturbance of epidermal barrier function in atopy patch test reactions in atopic eczema. Br J Dermatol 1996;135:560-5.
[38] Langeveld-Wildschut EG, Bruijnzel PL, Mudde GC, et al. Clinical and immunologic variables in skin of patients with atopic eczema and either positive or negative atopy patch test reactions. J Allergy Clin Immunol 2000;105:1008-16.
[39] Kerschenlohr K, Decard S, Darsow U, Ollert M, Wollnberg A. Clinical and immunologic reactivity to aeroallergens in "intrinsic" atopic dermatitis patients. J Allergy Clin Immunol 2003;111:195-7.
[40] Seidenari S, Giusti F, Pellacani G, Bertoni L. Frequency and intensity of responses to mite patch tests are lower in nonatopic subjects with respect to patients with atopic dermatitis. Allergy 2003;58:426-9.
[41] Ingordo V, D'Andria G, D'Andria C, Tortora A. Results of atopy patch tests with house dust mites in adults with "intrinsic" and "extrinsic" atopic dermatitis. J Eur Acad Dermatol Venereol 2002;16:450-4.
[42] Darsow U, Laifaoui J, Kerschenlohr K, et al. The prevalence of positive reactions in the atopy patch test with aeroallergens and food allergens in subjects with atopic eczema: a European multicenter study. Allergy 2004;59:1318-23.
[43] Fuiano N, Incorvaia C. Comparison of skin prick test and atopy patch test with dust mite extracts in patients with respiratory symptoms or atopic eczema dermatitis syndrome. Allergy 2003;58:828.
[44] Guler N, Kilerleri E, Tamay Z, Ones U. Atopy patch testing in children with asthma and rhinitis symptoms allergic to house dust mite. Pediatr Allergy Immunol 2005;17:346-50.
[45] Fuiano N, Incorvaia C, Prodam F, Procaccini DA, Bona G. Relationship between the atopy patch test and clinical expression of the disease in children with atopic eczema/dermatitis syndrome and respiratory symptoms. Ann Allergy Asthma Immunol 2008;101:174-8.
[46] Fuiano N, Fusilli S, Incorvaia C. House dust mite-related allergic diseases: role of the skin prick test, atopy patch test, and RAST in the diagnosis of different manifestations of allergy. Eur J Pediatr 2010;169:819-24.
[47] Huss-Marp J, Eberlein-Koenig B, Breuer K, et al. Influence of short-term exposure to airborne Der p 1 and volatile organic compounds on skin barrier function and dermal blood flow in patients with atopic eczema and healthy individuals. Clin Exp Allergy 2006;36:338-45.
[48] Flohr C, Johansson SG, Wahlgren CF, Williams H. How atopic is atopic dermatitis? J Allergy Clin Immunol 2004;114:150-8.
[49] Fuiano N, Incorvaia C. The atopy patch test: is it time to redefine its significance? Ann Allergy Asthma Immunol 2011;106:278-82.

[50] Johansson SGO, Hourihane JO, Bousquet J, et al. A revised nomenclature for allergy. An EAACI position statement from the EAACI nomenclature task force. Allergy 2001;56:813-24.
[51] Gell PGH, Coombs RRA, eds. Clinical Aspects of Immunology. 1st ed. Oxford, England: Blackwell 1963.

11

Advances in Assessing the Severity of Atopic Dermatitis

Zheng-Hong Di, Li Zhang, Ya-Ni Lv,
Li-Ping Zhao, Hong-Duo Chen and Xing-Hua Gao
Department of Dermatology, No.1 hospital of China Medical University
China

1. Introduction

Atopic dermatitis (AD) is a chronic, relapsing and pruritic inflammatory skin disorder. The prevalence of AD has been increasing significantly in recent decades, especially in developed nations. The pathogenesis of AD is still not completely understood. AD may be the results of interactions of abnormalities of immune system, genetics, environment and epidermal barrier defects. There is a wide spectrum of clinical manifestations in AD. Accordingly, there have been a number of methods and laboratory markers to assess the severity of AD. In spite of the facts that various severity assessing criteria and laboratory markers were reported or, more or less, applied, owing to the complexity of disease, race differences and environmental uncertainties, there is disagreement about the definitions and clinical application of these criteria or markers. Nevertheless, easy and quick assessing severity methods for AD are required to guide both the daily clinical and research studies. Here, we describe some recent advances in the assessment of the severity of AD.

1.1 Overview of the epidemiology of AD

AD is a chronic, inflammatory, itchy condition that usually begins in infancy but may continue into adult life; the disease is genetically predisposed, and its expression is modified by environmental factors. The prevalence of AD is unevenly distributed worldwide, varying between 0.73-23% (Levy et al., 2003).There is a tendency of increased prevalence of AD in recent years, especially in developed industrial nations. For example, the prevalence of AD at the ages of 12-15 almost doubled in the last 20 years of 20th century in Japanese, suggesting the strong impact of environmental factors in AD development(Sugiura et al., 1998).The incidence of an infant to develop AD is 25% in three months after birth, or 50% in two years after birth, given that the mother is an AD sufferer; The incidence of AD in the offspring reaches as high as 79%, if both the parents are atopic patients, suggesting the key role of genetic predisposition in the pathogenesis of AD(Bradley er al., 2000).Key clinical manifestations of AD include itchy, dry skin, inflammatory rashes and other atopic conditions. Though not fully clarified, the clinical phenotype characterizing AD is the product of interactions between susceptibility genes, the environment, defective skin barrier function, and immunologic responses. These complex interactions would induce biological and immunological responses at cellular or molecular levels, involving the skin, immune system or even the integument as a whole.

1.2 Diagnostic criteria of AD

During the past decades about 10 diagnostic criteria for AD have been set up(Brenninkmeijer et al., 2008),while the Hanifin and Rajka diagnostic criteria(in 1980) and Williams diagnostic criteria(in 1994) are the two most widely used methods in the world(Roguedas et al., 2004). The H-R criteria is such a detailed one (4 major and 23 minor criteria) that it is time consuming and not easy to operate, and thus mainly suitable for investigative studies and impractical for epidemiologic studies. What's more, some of the minor features described in the criteria, such as anterior neck folds and the Dennie-Morgan infra-orbital fold, has been challenged for their diagnostic significance in a study on Swiss AD (Mevorah et al., 1988). The concise Williams criteria (1 mandatory and 5 major criteria), are suitable for clinical and epidemiological studies. Williams criteria has been extensively validated(Brenninkmeijer et al., 2008). Due to its inherent nature of easy operation, this diagnostic criterion could be recommended in future international studies. In 1995, International Study of Asthma and Allergies in Childhood (ISAAC) set up ISAAC questionnaire for prevalence survey of childhood AD(Asher et al., 1995).Taken together, an ideal diagnostic criteria need to be well-validated ,easy to apply and suitable for interventional multicenter trials.

2. Assessment of the disease severity in AD

The methods of measuring disease severity of AD include the evaluation of lesion manifestations in combination with disease extent and intensity, subjective symptoms, quality of life (QOL), and the assessment of skin barrier function by bioengineering methods and laboratory parameters.

2.1 Assessment of clinical scoring systems

In the past, assessing the severity of AD, at levels of either overall or individual parameters, was mostly dependant on clinical scoring systems, such as the Scoring Atopic Dermatitis index (SCORAD)(European Task Force on Atopic Dermatitis, 1993), Atopic Dermatitis Area and Severity Index score(ADASIS) (Bahmer, 1992), Eczema Area and Severity Index (EASI) (Hanifin, 2001), are the most widespread used methods, to name a few(Charman &Williams, 2000).All of these tools, based on the entirely subjective score, have considerable inter-observer variability owing to the observers bias.

ADASIS was based on the lesion areas by point counting. On special body diagrams, the areas were color coded according to the severity of inflammation (green for mild, blue for moderate, and red for severe dermatitis).The result was evaluated by applying a transparent grid and fractionated lesion areas were weighted and multiplied by subjective pruritus intensity score. Haniffin et al suggested EASI index to assess the disease extent and percents of lesion area in four body regions (head and neck, lower limbs, upper limbs and trunk), borrowed from the psoriasis area and severity index (PASI) (Hanifin, 2001). The study by Rullo et al informed that EASI is more suitable for detection of subtle alterations of the severity of AD during drug effect studies, or follow-up of progression for research purposes (Rullo, 2008).

Charman and Williams evaluated 13 AD clinical scoring systems and confirmed that the simple and rapid SCORAD index was the most widely used one and its validity, reliability, sensitivity, and acceptability have been widely confirmed(Charman &Williams, 2000).The

SCORAD index includes objective symptoms (extent and intensity) and subjective criteria (daytime pruritus and sleep loss). The severity assessment of each items were evaluated at its average intensity. Due to that the subjective symptoms represented 20 % of total of inter-observer variation, European Task Force on Atopic Dermatitis recommended severity scale based only on the objective criteria of the SCORAD index to define mild, moderate, and severe AD (Kunz, 1997). It remains to be investigated that quite some laboratory parameters obtained from the lesion, serum, and other body fluids, have no significant correlation with SCORAD index. SCORAD index can not reflex the whole aspects of AD.

Most of the severity index has been applied for a given short-term therapeutic intervention, while they are insensitive in reflecting the overall disease activity to the chronic and fluctuating course of AD. Nottingham Eczema Severity Score (NESS) was introduced to be a clinical severity score method that documents AD severity over a long -term period of 12 months(Emerson et al., 2000; Hon et al., 2006).

For evaluating the life quality in AD, Quality of Life Index for Atopic Dermatitis (QoLIAD) is designed for adults with AD based on Quality of Life (QoL)and Children's Dermatology Life Quality Index (CDLQI) for children AD. These instruments could be used to evaluate the impact degree of AD and also measure the therapeutic effect (Whalley et al., 2004; Ben-Gashir et al., 2004).

Taken together, though well recognized and widely applied, the implementation of various scoring systems is complicated and subject to a variety of bias. Noninvasive, objective measurement has been developed and in use in recent year. The objective severity assessment of atopic dermatitis system (OSAAD) (Sugarman et al., 2003), which take advantage of instrumentations to measure water content (stratum corneum hydration, SCH), sebum content and trans-epidermal water loss (TEWL) of the skin, features the recent development of objective evaluation of AD.

OSAAD is a severity evaluation scale in AD including TEWL, SCH using a noninvasive bioengineering methods and estimation of affected body surface area (BSA). The method is suitable for both children and adults with AD compared with classical scoring system (Angelova-Fischer et al., 2005). The OSAAD score have several advantages over the clinical scoring methods. Measurement of TEWL and SCH is reproducible and reliable under given standard environment condition and instrument devices(Angelova-Fischer et al., 2005), able to evaluate quantitatively the severity scale of skin barrier impairment, sensitive to minor fluctuations in the course of AD development, and consequently applicable to assessment of treatment effects. The limitations of this technique are the inter- or intra- variability in AD patients, influenced by anatomic sites, environmental changes, etc. So the standardization of the conditions is very important in multicenter trials .There is no unified standard sites suitable for evaluation. Choi et al showed that antecubital fossa is the most favorable site for TEWL evaluation (Choi et al., 2003), while flexure surface is unsmooth. The '2 cm' site under the antecubital fossa resembles a flexure and is conveniently flat for measurements (Hon et al., 2008).

2.2 Evaluation of skin function and properties

The skin barrier is primarily in the outer 15μm of the epidermis, the stratum corneum (SC) (Landmann, 1988). Breakdown of skin barrier is the primary event in the development of AD, which may result in atopic march (Lipozencic & Wolf, 2007) . The evaluation of skin barrier and properties is based on several variances: such as TEWL, natural moisturizing factors (NMF), skin sebum content, skin pH and skin hydration (SH). The study

environment (controlled temperature and humidity level) of bioengineering research should be standardized.
From the skin surface, SH is relatively difficult to quantify objectively, instead, SCH level is measured .TEWL is a method to reflex SH, and also correlated well with objective SCORAD score (Gupta et al., 2008).There are two main systems which have been used to measure TEWL by comparing water flux rate following titrated water application: open chamber and closed chamber. The main drawback of open-chamber systems is the disturbance of air movements. The closed-chamber systems conquers this limitation by its closed-chamber, but a major problem with it is that it can not be used to perform continuous measurement, as there is a need of cleaning water vapor of the chamber after a site reading. Elkeeb et al introduced a new closed-chamber systems with a condenser to remove water vapor from chamber and enabling continuous measurement and confirmed significantly correlated with conventional closed and open-chamber systems(Elkeeb et al., 2010) .Later agreed standards of TEWL calibration method is needed to improve the comparability of TEWL measurement devices supplied by different manufacturers.
NMF is the most important factor for maintaining the skin proper moisture levels in SC. NMF largely comes from the acid degradation products of filaggrin, including pyrrolidone carboxylic acid (PCA) and urocanic acid (UCA), which also contribute to skin hydration acid mantle in outer SC (O'Regan et al., 2009) .While lowered expression of FLG in AD lesion was found universally (Howell et al., 2009), the loss-of-function mutations of FLG were observed in only less one-third of the general AD population (Marenholz et al., 2006; Palmer et al., 2006; Zhang et al., 2011; Ma et al., 2010). Reduced NMF levels were independently associated with FLG genotype and is a general feature of AD (Kezic et al., 2010).High-Performance Liquid Chromatograph (HPLC) is the common method used to evaluate NMF (Robinson et al., 2010a; Robinson et al., 2010b).
The skin surface sebum content, hydration and pH can be check by several commercialized instruments with respective probes on the surface of skin (Choi et al., 2003; Firooz et al., 2007; Man et al., 2009). They are easy to operate, but time consuming, difficult to use in infant AD patients. The temperature and humidity levels during their application also should be standardized.

2.3 Laboratory tests

Laboratory tests may also be applied for AD.

2.3.1 Skin tests (atopy patch test/ APT, skin prick test /SPT)

APT was traditionally used to assess sensitization to inhalant. Allergens/aeroallergen as a skin test, was used to diagnose AD (Ring et al., 1997).An eczematous reaction based on T cell-specific delayed-type allergic response to the allergens on the healthy skin of the patient's back or forearm is read after 48 and 72 hours. There is no golden standard for aeroallergen provocation of AD. Although the kinds of allergens are different in patients of different environment, race, and regions, the European APT model with standardization of allergen concentration and vehicle may be an useful diagnostic tool to AD patients. However, the clinical relevance of positive APT reactions depends on standardized provocation and avoidance testing verification (Lipozencic & Wolf, 2010).
Although the double-blind, placebo-controlled oral food challenges (DBPCFC) is the golden standard of diagnosis in food allergy(Sampson, 2003).The test is not always suitable to

interpret and operate, particularly in patients sensitive to several kinds of food or potential to anaphylactic Shock. Skin prick test (SPT) is designed for diagnosing food immediate hypersensitivity(Isolauri & Turjanmaa, 1996).The APT reflect delayed-phase allergic reactions, even with a late onset of symptoms (more than 2 hours after food ingestion). APT may provide further diagnostic information in addition to the SPT and serum IgE values used with standardized allergen concentration and vehicle (Niggemann et al., 2005). APT has higher sensitivity than SPT test for food allergy in young children with AD, and can be used to supplement the SPT in diagnosing food allergy in AD children(Stromberg, 2002) and those with late reactions were more easily to have positive APT tests to the relevant foods (Saarinen et al., 2001).The combination of APT, SPT and serum-specific IgE reduce the need for oral food challenges in children with AD (Roehr et al., 2001) and significantly enhance the accuracy in the diagnosis of food allergy when the total IgE is normal or SPT is negative(Boissieu&Dupont,2003). APT test may also help among children with AD to prevent unnecessary restrictive diets (Niggemann et al., 2000).While in a study of allergy to cow's milk and hen's egg in 3 year- old children, no hypersensitivity to cow's milk or hen's egg was predicted by APT alone. The real value of the APT in food allergy in children need to be further studied(Osterballe et al., 2004).

The sensitivity and specificity of the SPT of food allergen was 58% and 70%, while the sensitivity and specificity of the APT for late-phase clinical reactions of food allergen was 76% and 95% respectively (Niggemann et al., 2000). The negative predictive value is over 95%, while the positive predictive value is less than 40% of SPT (Sampson, 2003).So, a positive skin test cannot completely confirm a clinical food hypersensitivity, while a negative result can virtually rules out some kind of IgE-mediated food allergy. It should be noted that SPT may remain positive for many years after the loss of clinical food allergic reactivity. Patients should be re-challenged at intervals to determine whether their food allergy persists (egg, every 2-3 years; milk, soy, wheat, peanut, nuts, fish, and shellfish, every 1-2 years) (Sampson, 2001).

2.3.2 Biomarkers in serum or other body fluid

Seeking biomarkers in serum or other body fluid to reflect the severity of AD is an interesting topic. Though the fact that serum IgE level is elevated in more than half of AD has been well established, its correlation with disease severity is disputed, so was the interpretation for peripheral blood eosinophil count, which could be affected by many other factors except for hypersensitivity, such as parasite, drugs, hormone. There were reports that urine eosinophil protein X (Jenerowicz et al., 2006) and leukotriene E4 (Hon et al., 2004) may be used as biomarkers to reflect the severity of AD. Recently, Urinary aquaporin-2 was found to positively correlate with skin dryness of infant AD (Di et al., 2010). The clinical manifestations and distribution pattern of AD may vary at different age-related stages. AD is most prevalent in infants. An objective, easy and non-invasive test for evaluation of infant AD and corresponding management is much expected by both healthcare workers and parents.

2.3.2.1 Serum total IgE, specific IgE and IgE autoantibodies

IgE and specific IgE (ELISA or Radioallergosorbent test/RAST) can be used without the need of preparing lesion-free skin and waiting-up of antihistamines drug withdrawal, it is more practical than SPT for the screening of food allergies in most office settings due to its quick and easy- to operate merit. Serum IgE levels are increased in about 80% of adult AD

(C.A.Akdis et al., 2006). The remaining 20%-30% of patients exhibiting normal serum IgE levels and lack allergen-specific sensitization, are classified as intrinsic AD (IAD) (Novak &Bieber, 2003; Boguniewicz et al., 2006). 28% of AD serum contains IgE autoantibodies which target keratinocytes in AD patients (Altrichter et al., 2008).

For the total IgE and specific IgE, similar to skin tests, a negative result is fairly reliable in ruling out an IgE-mediated reaction. For a positive result, although the lesions significantly regress, there maybe no parallel decrease of serum IgE level. Further large-scale investigations of serum IgE levels between patients with extrinsic atopic dermatitis and intrinsic atopic dermatitis are needed (Ott et al., 2009).

2.3.2.2 Mast cell, eosinophil and its cellular contents

Mast cells play a very important role in the pathogenesis of AD. Tryptase and chymase are the major compound of mast cell granules. They have various effects on angiotensin, metalloproteases, lipoproteins, procollagen, neuropeptides and cytokines. The study by Badertscher et al confirmed that mast cell chymase is increased in chronic atopic dermatitis lesion (Badertscher et al., 2005), while there was no correlation of serum tryptase level with the severity of AD (Gerdes et al., 2009).

Eosinophils play an important role in inflammatory process of AD, the activated eosinophils release granule proteins including eosinophil cationic protein (ECP) and eosinophil derived neurotoxin/eosinophil protein X (EDN/EPX). ECP is released from activated eosinophils during the inflammation process. Serum ECP level increased in children with AD (Badertscher et al., 2005; Damps-Konstanska et al., 2005), but there was no correlation with the SCORAD index (Wu et al., 2011). While a study by Selnes et al suggest that there is no association between serum ECP and AD in an unselected population of children (Selnes &Dotterud,2005).Several investigative evidence indicate that serum EDN may reflect the disease severity in childhood phase AD(Taniuchi et al., 2001; Lee et al.,2009) and correlated with SCORAD index (K.Y.Lee et al.,2009).

2.3.2.3 T Lymphocytes and their subsets in peripheral blood

For a long time, two main types of effector CD4+ T cells, named as type 1 T helper (Th1) and type 2 Th (Th2) respectively, have been thought to be deeply involved in AD. Th2 cells produce IL-4, IL-5 and IL-13, Th1 cells produce interferon (IFN)-γ as the main cytokines. AD is an inflammatory skin disease characterized by the predominant infiltration of T cells, eosinophils, mast cell, dendric cell (DC) and macrophages in lesions. Disequilibrium between Th1/Th2 lymphocytes is an important feature of AD. Typically, AD has been considered the paradigm of a Th2-mediated disease, characterized by increase of Th2 and decrease of Th1 and their cytokines level in peripheral blood. Recently, research efforts have resulted in new subgroups of CD4+ T cells, such as IL-17-producing Th cells (Th17), the main cytokine they produce is IL-17A, and T-regulatory (Treg) (Agrawal et al., 2011; Souwer er al., 2010). There are two main groups of Treg cells identified. One is the natural Treg cells, characterized by CD4+CD25+ phenotype and develops under the control of the transcription factor FoxP3. The other is the adaptive Treg or T-regulatory type 1 (Tr1), characterized by the secretion of high levels of IL-10(M. Akdis et al., 2004; C.A.Akdis et al., 1998). It is suggested that the onset of allergic diseases are partly caused by insufficient development of allergen-specific Tregs. FoxP3+Treg could be found in the perivascular, dermis interstitial, and the dermoepidermal junction and the basal and suprabasal epidermal layers of AD (Caproni et al., 2007). But the study by Hayashida et al indicated that FoxP3+Treg subsets was similar to that of normal controls in peripheral blood of the acute phase AD and the decreased number of circulating Th17 cells is negatively correlated with CCL17, IgE and eosinophil levels in AD patients (Hayashida et al., 2011). IL-17 has been identified in acute AD lesions (Toda et al., 2003). The exact role of Treg and Th17 cell in AD is still unclear.

2.3.2.4 Cytokines and chemokine in the serum

A complex network of cytokines and chemokines are involved in atopic inflammation, at both the starting and maintainance stages of the inflammation. Scratching injury induce the production of proinflammatory cytokines (such as IL-1, TNF-α, GM-CSF), which in turn induce CCL27 and CCL17 development. Subsequently, CCL27 and CCL17 recruit skin-homing memory T cells into the skin. Within the skin, T cells are activated and release effector cytokines (eg, IL-4, IL-5, IL-13 in acute phase lesion, or IFN-r in the chronic lesion of AD).These effector cytokines will sustain and amplify the production of chemokines within atopic skin. In this complex procedure, many chemokines, (such as CCL1, CCL2, CCL11, CCL13, CCL18, CCL20, CCL21, and CCL26) interact with various immune effector cells through their receptors(D.Y.Leung et al., 2004; Homey et al., 2006). AD is a disease with the participation of whole body immune system, and that the immunologic abnormality is not limited to the skin. Generally, as is widely accepted that AD has been considered the paradigm of a Th2-mediated disease, characterized by increase Th2 and decrease Th1 and cytokines level, elevated serum IgE levels, eosinophilia in peripheral blood. Recent researched showed that the severity of AD has also been found to be associated with the levels of various other cytokines and chemokines in the lesion and serum, in addition to the conventional serum parameters, such as total serum IgE (tIgE), eosinophilic cationic protein (ECP), increased T helper type 2 (Th2)-skewed cytokine patterns(IL4,13) and decreased IFN-γ. Some of them in the serum of AD are correlated with disease severity, and thus may be new biomarkers to reflect AD disease severity. Clinical trials on interleukins and chemokines in the serum of patients with AD were summarized, in table1 and table 2.

Interleukin/IL

Many interleukins participate in AD and it is a consensus that increased IL4, 13 levels are seen in the serum of AD. Recently, many of other interleukins have been shown to play roles in the pathogenesis of AD, and increased serum levels have been detected (in table1). IL-10 is a powerful Th2 cytokines produced by LC in the lesion of AD and exerts its function through inhibition of the secretion of Th1 cytokines. While, the level of IL-10 in the serum may be not a significant marker (Shin et al., 2005). IL-22, a member of the IL-10 family and known to be preferentially produced by Th17 cells, is increased and has significant correlation with CCL17 levels in the serum of AD patients (Hayashida et al., 2011). On the contrary, IL-12 is prominently expressed in the chronic lesion of AD, it is a powerful inducer of Th0 to Th1 conversion and subsequent IFN-γ secretion from Th1.The level of IL-12 in the serum of AD is controversially reported. Piancatelli et al confirmed the serum IL-12 levels increased in paediatric AD (Piancatelli et al., 2008), while the study by Aral, M et al showed that there was no statistically significant difference between children AD and controls in respect of serum levels of IL-12(Aral et al., 2006). IL-16 is a natural ligand of CD4 molecules. Besides its chemotactic properties to CD4-expressing cells, IL-16 amplifies inflammatory processes and possesses immunoregulatory functions (Mathy et al., 2000; Nagy et al., 2011). IL-16 was found to be increased in the serum of AD, both in child and adult patients (Nagy et al., 2011; Belloni Fortina et al., 2006; Masuda et al., 2003).Also ,the level of IL-16 in the serum was significantly correlated with serum total IgE(Nagy et al., 2011), but not correlated with SCORAD index(Belloni Fortina et al., 2006) and eosinophils counting in peripheral blood(Nagy et al., 2011).The finding of Masuda K. et al confirmed IL-16 level in serum was significantly higher in patients with AD, and decreased significantly after topical treatment with corticosteroids or tacrolimus (Masuda et al., 2003). IL-18 is a pleiotropic cytokine that works both in Th1 and Th2 lymphocyte-mediated immunity. As a member of the IL-1 super family, IL-18 is a potent inducer of IFN-γ. IL-18 is involved in the pathogenesis of AD including Th1 and Th2 T lymphocyte-mediated immunity, including cytokine accumulation, and increase of IgE and histamine levels. Increased serum level of IL-18 and correlation with disease severity, eosinophil counts and serum sIL-2R levels was reported in several researches both in adult and children patients (Aral et al., 2006; Yoshizawa et al., 2002; Park &Youn, 2007; Sohn et al., 2004; Hon et al., 2004). IL-31 is a Th derived cytokine. Serum IL-31 was found over-expressed in both adults and paediatric AD and its serum level correlated positively with the disease severity (Raap et al., 2008; Ezzat et al., 2011).

Chemokines their receptors

Little is known about the very early events of atopic skin inflammation. The unceasing amplification inflammation cycle in AD lesions might start with pruritus and the injury induced by scratching, and skin barrier disruption, resulting in proinflammatory cytokine

Interle-ukins	Correlation with other clinical parameters	References	Expression in serum	Age of studied populations
IL-2	Inverse correlation with serum IgE	Yoshizawa et al., 2002	Increase	Adult (13–43years)
IL-12	Negative correlation with age and positive with SCORAD index	Piancatelli et al., 2008	Increase	Paediatric AD (1-184months)
	Positive correlation with SCORAD	Aral et al., 2006	No different with controls.	5–12 year old
	Positive correlation with IL-10	Yoshizawa et al., 2002	Increase	Adult (13–43years)
IL-16	Positive correlation with serum total IgE	Nagy et al., 2011	Increase	Mean :18.6 years; range: 7–49 years
	No correlation with SCORAD index	Belloni Fortina et al., 2006	Increase	Children
	Positive correlation with eosinophil count in peripheral blood and SCORAD	Masuda et al., 2003	Increase	Adult: aged 14 - 52 years, median 22
IL-18	Not done	Narbutt et al., 2009	Decrease under 10 years, no difference over 10 years	Mean age 11.4 years with moderate AD

Interle-ukins	Correlation with other clinical parameters	References	Expression in serum	Age of studied populations
	Positive correlation with SCORAD index	Park et al., 2007	Increase	15±10 years; range:2-41years
	Positive correlation with SCORAD index	Aral et al., 2006	Increase	5–12 year old
	Higher in sever AD than in mild AD	Sohn et al., 2004	Increase	Age range, 9 months to 11 years; mean, 4.28± 2.8 years
	Positive correlation with SCORAD index	Hon et al., 2004	Increase	Median age of 2.2 years (interquartile range 0.7-4.6 years)
	Positive correlation with eosinophil counts and serum soluble IL-2 receptor	Yoshizawa et al., 2002	Increase	Adult (13–43years)
IL-22	Positive correlation with CCL17	Hayashida et al., 2011	Increase	Adults (mean±SD age;27.2±6.1 years)
IL-31	Positive correlation with LSS, SSS and SCORAD index	Ezzat et al., 2011	Increase	Ages ranged between 1 and 10 years (mean ± SD: 5.75 ± 2.11 years)
	Positive correlation with SCORAD index both in extrinsic AD and intrinsic AD	Raap et al., 2008	Increase	Extrinsic AD (mean age, 37.8±14.1 years); Intrinsic AD (mean age, 31.8±11.2 years)

Table 1. Literatures about serum interleukins in AD

Chemo-kine	Correlation with other clinical parameters	References	Expressions in serum	Adult / childhood /infant phase
CXCL9	Not done	Narbutt et al., 2009	Decrease under 10 years old	Children (mean age 11.4 years with moderate AD
CXCL10/ IP-10	Not done	Narbutt et al., 2009	Decrease under 10 years old	Children (mean age 11.4 years with moderate AD
	Did not correlate with SCORAD index and its extend and intensity	T.F.Leung et al., 2003	No difference between mild and moderate AD	Median 2.1 years, range 0.6-4.2 years

Chemo-kine	Correlation with other clinical parameters	References	Expressions in serum	Adult / childhood /infant phase
CXCL12	Not done	Narbutt et al., 2009	Increase	Children
CCL2 /MCP-1	Did not correlate with SCORAD index and its extend and intensity	T.F.Leung et al., 2003	No difference between mild and moderate AD	Median 2.1 years, range 0.6-4.2 years
CCL11 /eotaxin /EOX	no significant relationship with TARC, MDC, IgE or SCORAD index	Jahnz-Rozyk et al., 2005	Increase	Age: Mean±SD of 24.7±10.7 years
	Positive correlate with SCORAD extent, but not SCORAD index.	T.F.Leung et al., 2003	Higher in moderate AD than in mild AD	Median 2.1 years, range 0.6-4.2 years
CCL17 /TARC	Positive correlation with soluble HLA-G. High umbilical cord serum levels were associated with infantile AD development	Miyahara et al., 2011	Umbilical cord serum levels from neonates destined to develop AD in infancy were higher than in those from neonates who showed no signs of AD during infancy; Serum levels were higher in mothers with AD than in those without AD.	Neonates and their mothers
	Not done	Narbutt et al., 2009	Decrease under 10 years old, increase over 10 years old	Children (mean age 11.4 years with moderate AD)
	Positive correlation with SCORAD index	Nakazato et al., 2008	Increase	Infants (mean age 4.5 months)
	Positive correlation with obj-SCORAD index, peripheral blood eosinophil counts and serum immunoglobulin E	Mostafa et al., 2008	Increase	Children (ages ranged between 2 and 10 years with a mean age of 5 ± 2.8 years)

Chemo-kine	Correlation with other clinical parameters	References	Expressions in serum	Adult / childhood /infant phase
	Positive correlation with SCORAD index	Hon et al., 2007	Increase	Aged younger than 18 years (mean ±SD: 10.7 ± 4.4 years)
	Positive correlation with serum CTACK and SCORAD index; decreased in accordance with ages	Song et al., 2006	Increase	Children (4.9±3.3 years, 2 months to 14 years)
	Positive correlation with SCORAD index	Jahnz-Rozyk et al., 2005	Increase	Age (Mean±SD of 24.7±10.7 years)
	Positive correlation with SCORAD extent and intensity components, Positive correlation with CCL22, but not SCORAD index	T.F.Leung et al., 2003	No different between mild and moderate AD	Median 2.1 years range 0.6-4.2 years
	Correlation with eosinophil number, SCORAD index, serum sE-selectin and weakly correlated with serum sIL-2 receptor	Kakinuma et al., 2001	Increase	Mean age ± SEM: 26.6 ± 8.9 years
CCL22 /MDC	Not done	Narbutt et al., 2009	Increase over 10 years old	Children (mean age 11.4 years with moderate AD
	Positive correlation with SCORAD index	Nakazato et al., 2008	Increase	Infants (mean age 4.5 months)
	Positive correlation with obj-SCORAD index, peripheral blood eosinophil counts and serum immunoglobulin E	Mostafa et al., 2008	Increase	Children (ages ranged between 2 and 10 years with a mean age of 5 ± 2.8 years)
	Positive correlation with SCORAD index	Jahnz-Rozyk et al., 2005	Increase	Age: Mean±SD of 24.7±10.7 years
	Positive correlation with SCORAD index and its extent and intensity components, Positive correlation with CCL17	T.F.Leung et al., 2003	Higher in moderate AD than in mild AD	Median 2.1 years range 0.6-4.2 years
	Positively related with SCORAD index, serum sE-selectin, sIL-2R, TARC and eosinophil numbers in peripheral blood	Kakinuma et al., 2002	Increase	Not described

Chemo-kine	Correlation with other clinical parameters	References	Expressions in serum	Adult / childhood /infant phase
CCL26 /eotaxin-3	Positive correlation with the serum CCL17 ,CCL22 levels, eosinophil numbers in peripheral blood and SCORAD index	Kagami et al., 2003	Increase	Adult (mean±SD: 28·7±7·1 years)
CCL27 /CTACK	Not done	Narbutt et al., 2009	Increase under 10 years old	Children (mean age 11.4 years with moderate AD
	Positive correlation with SCORAD index	Nakazato et al., 2008	Increase	Infants (mean age 4.5 months)
	Positive correlation with SCORAD index	Hon et al., 2007	Increase	Aged younger than 18 years (mean ±SD: 10.7 ± 4.4)
	Positive correlation with their serum TARC; SCORAD index; decreased in accordance with their ages	Song et al., 2006	Increase	Children: 4.9±3.3 years, 2 months to 14 years
	Positive correlated with SCORAD index	Hon et al., 2004	Increase	Children: median age of 5 (range: 1–11 years)
	Positive correlation with SCORAD index, sIL-2 receptor, sE-selectin,TARC, MDC in serum	Kakinuma et al., 2003	Increase	Adult(mean ± SEM age, 28.5 ± 6.8 years)
CCL28/ MEC	Positive correlation with LSS and SCORAD index, peripheral eosinophil counts, and serum LDH	Ezzat et al., 2009	Increase	Ages ranged between 8 and 120 months (mean ± SD: 47 ± 22 months)
	Not done	Kagami et al., 2005	Increase	Adults(mean±SD: 28.7± 6.7 years)
CX3CL1 /fracta-lkine	Positively associated with the scoring system proposed by Rajka and Langeland.	Echigo et al., 2004	Increase	Age: 24.7 ± 7.4 years

Table 2. Literatures about serum chemokines in AD. Abbreviations used in the table: CXCL10/IP-10, IFN-induced protein of 10 kd; CCL2/MCP-1, monocyte chemotactic protein 1; CCL11 /eotaxin (EOX); CCL17/TARC, thymus and activation-regulated chemokine; CCL22/MDC, macrophage-derived chemokine; CCL26/eotaxin-3; CCL27/CTACK, cutaneous T cell–attracting chemokine; CCL28/MEC, Mucosa-associated epithelial chemokine; CX3CL1/fractalkine; sE-selectin, serum soluble E-selectin; sIL-2R, soluble interleukin-2 receptor.

and chemokine production, directing the recruitment of pathogenic leukocytes to the skin (Steinhoff et al., 2006). There are many researches conformed that they are useful inflammatory markers for assessing severity of AD. Chemokines attract leukocytes transmigrate into the skin in AD by their gradients directing. Chemokine ligand-receptor interactions direct the multistep process of leukocyte migration. Chemokines can be classed into 4 subclasses according to the arrangement of N-terminal cysteine residues: CXC chemokines (CXCL); CC chemokines (CCL); C chemokines (XCL), and CX3C chemokine (CX3CL). To date, 45 human chemokine ligands and 10 CC chemokine, 7 CXC chemokine, 1 CX3C, and 1 XC receptors have been identified (Rossi & Zlotnik, 2000; Zlotnik &Yoshie, 2000; Balabanian et al., 2005). Many chemokines, including CCL1, CCL2, CCL3, CCL4, CCL5, CCL10, CCL11, CCL13, CCL17, CCL18, CCL20, CCL22, CCL26, CCL27, CCL28, CX3CL1, CXCL9, CXCL10, CXCL12, have been presumed to be involving in AD phenotype (Homey et al., 2006; Toda et al., 2003; Hayashida et al., 2011; Piancatelli et al., 2008; Jahnz-Rozyk et al., 2005; T.F.Leung et al., 2003; Miyahara et al., 2011; Hon et al., 2004,2007; Kagami et al., 2003,2005; Yoshizawa et al., 2002; Park&Youn, 2007; Kakinuma et al; 2003; Ezzat &Shaheen, 2009; Echigo et al., 2004) (in table2). These researches indicated that the imbalance in serum concentration of Th-1- and Th-2-derived chemokines may be one of the factors involved in pathogenesis of AD and biomarkers of AD disease severity.

CXCL9, CXCL10, and CXCL11 are Th-1-derived chemokines, while CCL11, CCL17, CCL22, CCL27 are Th-2-derived chemokines, leading to preferential influx of T1/Th2 lymphocytes to the lesion of AD respectively (Narbutt et al., 2009). CCL28 is recently identified to be selectively expressed by keratinocytes and its functional ligands are CCR3 and CCR10. CCL28 is similar to CCL27 in human, they shares 40% amino acid identity(Hieshima et al., 2003). CCL26, CCL11 through CCR3 contribute to eosinophils recruitment to the lesion of AD(Homey et al., 2006). CX3CL1 originates from the endothelial cell and its receptor is CX3CR1, which can direct several kinds of immunological effective cells (such as T cell, NK cell and monocytes and DC) (Echigo et al., 2004).

Research by Narbutt J et al indicated that the serum level of CXCL9 and CXCL10 was decreased in childhood AD (Narbutt et al., 2009). While there were many study indicating that CCL11, CCL17, CCL22, CCL27 level in the serum were increased in AD patients and correlated with disease severity (T.F.Leung et al., 2003; Mostafa et al., 2008; Nagy et al., 2011; Song et al., 2006; Sohn et al., 2004; Kakinuma et al., 2002,2008; Jahnz-Rozyk et al., 2005; Hijnen et al., 2004; Kakinuma et al., 2001). Among the Th2 chemokines, serum CCL27 correlated most significantly with the severity of AD (Nakazato et al., 2008).The research by Miyahara et al showed that increased level of CCL17 in umbilical cord serum of neonates destined to develop AD in infancy (Miyahara et al., 2011).But another research indicated that the serum level of CCL17 and IL-18 were decreased, and CXCL12 and CCL27 increased in kids younger than 10 years old. In childhood AD of over 10 years old, serum concentration of CXCL12, CCL17, CCL22 was higher (Toda et al., 2003).There are many research results confirmed that the increased CCL28 level in the serum of AD patients and correlated positively to the severity scores (Jahnz-Rozyk et al., 2005; T.F. Leung et al., 2003; Ezzat &Shaheen ,2009; Kagami et al., 2005; Ezzat et al., 2009), so CCL28 may be a useful parameter in the clinical diagnosis and prognosis after proper treatment. CCL26, as a chemokine attract eosinophils to the skin lesion is elevated in the serum and significantly correlated with the serum CCL17 and CCL22 levels, peripheral blood eosinophil numbers and SCORAD index (Kagami et al., 2003).

Taken together, interleukins and chemokines are important markers in AD. But the normal levels in infancy and age-specific analysis in atopic dermatitis of these markers have not been well determined, this should be taken into account when interpreting the results, especially in infant AD.

Tumor necrosis factor(TNF)

B cell-activating factor (BAFF) is a member of tumour necrosis factor superfamily. BAFF plays an important role in the survival and maturation of B lymphocyte cells. The level of serum BAFF in childhood AD patients increased and significantly correlated with total serum IgE level and total eosinophil count in peripheral blood(Jee et al., 2010).While , in another research, serum BAFF level was not elevated in patients with AD (Matsushita et al., 2008).

Neurotrophins and neuropeptides,Growth factors and hormones

The Neurotrophins (NT) family including Nerve growth factor (NGF), Brain-derived neurotrophic factor (BDNF), NT- 3,4,5, 6 and NT- 7 (Leibrock et al., 1989; Kolbeck et al., 1994). The biologic effects of NT family are not merely restricted to the central nervous system but also relevant to the nerve cells present in other organs including the skin. More and more studies have demonstrated that NTs play an important role in the pathogenesis of AD. Association of BDNF gene polymorphisms and the increased serum levels in AD patients was conformed. The level of BDNF in the serum was correlated with intrinsic type of AD severity (Ma et al.,2010; Raap et al., 2006).While the level of NGF in serum has no significant correlation with total IgE, or severity of disease assessed by SCORAD (Schulte-Herbruggen et al., 2007). Although serum levels of vasoactive intestinal peptide (VIP) are found to be increased in patients with AD, there was no correlation between serum VIP levels and disease severity, serum LDH levels, total serum IgE levels, and peripheral blood eosinophil counts in patients with AD (Umemoto er al., 2003). Also there was also no association between serum VIP concentration and itch intensity (C.H.Lee et al., 2006). A study showed TEWL, serum IgE and beta-endorphin were independent parameters for assessing itch intensity in AD (C.H.Lee et al., 2006).

Mast cell in the lesions is thought to play an important role in the pathogenesis of AD. Stem cell factor (SCF), and the interaction of SCF and its receptor, KIT (tyrosine kinase transmembrane receptor) are the key factors that induce mast cell growth, migration and differentiation. Serum levels of soluble SCF and soluble KIT were significantly elevated in AD patients, positively correlated with the disease severity, and decreased after effective treatment with topical corticosteroids (Kanbe et al., 2001).

Significantly higher expression of thymic stromal lymphopoietin (TSLP), an IL-7 - like cytokine, by lesional skin can induce DCs to express Th2 cell - polarizing signals in AD. DCs activated by TSLP can induce Th0 to differentiate into Th2 cells and play important roles in the maintenance and regulation of Th2 memory cells (Wang et al., 2006). While the serum TSLP level is inconsistent by different clinical study (E.B.Lee et al., 2010; Alysandratos et al., 2010; Nakamura et al., 2008).

The increasing level of serum antidiuretic hormone (ADH) in severe AD was confirmed , which was related with TEWL(Aoki, et al., 2005).

2.3.2.5 Enzymes

In the AD lesion, high lactate dehydrogenase(LDH) activity was found , especially in the epidermis. Also in the serum, the level of LDH and its isozyme (LDH4 and LDH5) is increased. After recovery of the patients, the serum LDH activity tended to decline. But there are no correlation between the LDH level and eosinocyte count in the peripheral blood or serum IgE level (Morishima et al., 2010).

Matrix metalloproteinases(MMPs) and their inhibitors, tissue inhibitors of metalloproteinases (TIMPs), are involved in inflammation mediated tissue destruction and remodeling. The maintenance of homeostasis of MMPs/TIMPs in the lesion is regulated by proinflammatory cytokines and growth factors (Woessner, 2001). In the study of Katoh N et al, they found that the level of TIMP-1 in the serum of AD patients was significantly increased, but reduced after treatments. The TIMP-1 level correlated with peripheral eosinophil counts, serum levels of IgE and LDH, eruption score, and eruption area. Moreover, the patients with chronic eruptions (lichenification and prurigo) had significantly higher TIMP-1 levels, while those with acute lesions were not correlated with TIMP-1 level in the serum. The authors gave a hypothesis that serum TIMP-1 level may be a useful marker to estimate the long-term disease activity of AD (Katoh et al., 2002).

Human tissue kallikreins, or kallikrein-related peptidases (KLKs), are the largest family of trypsin- or chymotrypsin-like serine proteases (SPs). At least eight KLKs are expressed in normal skin, of which KLK8, KLK5, KLK7 have been reported to be the most important KLKs involved in maintenance of the homeostasis of normal epidermis by cleaving corneodesmosomes. Moreover, KLK5 and KLK14 activate protease-activated receptor (PAR)-2, which is a signaling receptor in epidermal inflammation and a regulator of epidermal barrier function (Meyer-Hoffert, 2009). In the lesion of AD, the level of KLKs were increased (Voegeli et al., 2009). In the serum of AD, KLK8 was reported significantly elevated, while KLK5 and KLK11 were significantly decreased (Komatsu et al., 2007). The different expression between lesion and serum may be due to the diversity of the origins of KLKs from many tissues and organs.

Neopterin is biosynthesized from guanosine triphosphate and produced preferentially by monocytes and macrophages. Increased neopterin concentrations in serum or urine are connected with diseases linked with cellular immune reaction. Recently, serum neopterin levels was reported to increase and to be considered as a diagnostic marker of AD (Ciprandi et al., 2011).

2.3.2.6 Soluble immune receptors (SIRs)

The serum levels of SIRs ,such as sCD14, sCD23, sCD25 and sCD30 have been reported to be associated with AD (Ott et al., 2010; El Mongy et al., 2008; Di Lorenzo er al., 2003; Hon et al., 2005; Furue et al., 1999). CD30 released by CD30+ cells, a member of the TNF receptor superfamily, is a costimulatory molecule expressed on activated T and B cells. After cell activation, its extracellular domain generates soluble CD30 (sCD30) by enzymatic cleavage. Serum sCD30 is regarded as a indicator of Th2-type immune responses (El Mongy et al., 2008). Although there were several researches indicated that serum sCD30 levels were significantly higher and correlated positively with the severity of AD as assessed by SCORAD, age and duration of the disease (El Mongy et al., 2008; Di Lorenzo et al., 2003). Ott H et al indicated that the serum level of sCD23, sCD25 and sCD30 were highly aged dependent and can not be regarded as useful biomarkers for assessment of childhood AD (Ott et al., 2010).

2.3.2.7 Others in serum

Serum immunoglobulin free light chains (FLC) is classically associated with monoclonal gammopathies. An significantly increased level of FLC was observed in severe AD , while the association of FLC levels with age or total IgE levels was not confirmed (Kayserova et al., 2010).Vitamin D deficiency may be related to the severity of AD in the children patients. The level of serum in severe AD was significant lower than the mild AD (Peroni et al., 2010).

2.3.3 Biomarkers in urine

Leukotriene B4 (LTB4), LTC4, LTD4 and LTE4, the products of the oxidative metabolism of cell membrane arachidonic acid are secreted from eosinophils, mast cells and other inflammatory cells. As LTE4 is stable in urine, the urinal level of LTE4 may be a good marker for activation of mast cells and eosinophils in vivo. Urinary LTE4 increased in severe AD and correlated with severity of AD in children had been confirmed. Those having to sensitization to common allergens had higher LTE4 level than those without in the severe AD (Hon et al., 2004; Oymar &Aksnes, 2005).

EDN/EPX, one of the major proinflammatory mediators released by activated eosinophils, can induce severe tissue damage and maintenance and exacerbation of AD. A positive correlation between the SCORAD and serum ECP and urine EPX levels has been reported in children and adult patients (Breuer et al., 2001; Pucci et al., 2005; Pucci et al., 2000; Goto et al., 2007),also correlated with visual analog scales (VAS) scores for itching(Goto et al., 2007). While urinary EDN concentrations did not correlate with the number of eosinophils in the peripheral blood (Goto et al., 2007).

Urinary nitrate level significantly increased in AD patients. The severity and extent of AD significantly correlated with urinary nitrate and malondialdehyde level, but it did not correlate with urinary 8-hydroxydeoxyguanosine (8-OHdG) level (Nakai et al., 2009).

The increased TEWL in AD is attributable partly to impaired barrier function of the skin. Remarkable loss of body fluid would induce a series of systemic regulatory reactions. The functional antidiuretic hormone (ADH)-aquaporin (AQP)-2 axis is a major regulatory system to keep water balance. Increased serum ADH was detected in severe AD, a result possibly due to a dehydrated state caused by increased TEWL in these patients (Aoki, 2005). Recently, Urinary aquaporin-2 was found to be increased in infant AD patients, and positively correlate with skin dryness of infant AD, but its concentrations did not correlate with the number of eosinophils in the peripheral blood and the total IgE level in serum and disease severity (Di et al., 2010).

Increased neopterin levels in serum or urine are connected with diseases related with cellular immune reaction (Murr et al., 2002).In the association study by Horak E et al between neopterin in cord blood and urine in early childhood and the development of atopic dermatitisAD, they showed that family history of atopic disease was associated with lower urinary neopterin levels at age of 6 years (Horak er al., 2006).

Prostaglandin D2 (PGD2), the major cyclooxygenase product of mast cells, is a good marker for mast cell activation. In the lung, PGD2 converts to 9a, 11b-prostaglandin F2 (9a,11b-PGF2), which can be detected in the urine (O'Sullivan, 1999). The study of Oymar K and Aksnes L indicated that 9a, 11b-PGF2 level in the urine of severe childhood AD patients was increased and indicated that 9a, 11b-PGF2 may be a useful biomarker of mast cell activation in the urine (Oymar &Aksnes, 2004).

3. Conclusions

AD is a complex cutaneous disorder characterized by local and/or systemic immune reactions, and skin barrier dysfunction. Its clinical manifestations are affected by many factors, such as gene, environment, race, age etc. Further studies should be performed to findings of definitive biomarkers to assess the disease severity and evaluation of treatment effects. But the normal levels in infancy and age-specific analysis in AD of these markers have not been well determined, this should be taken into account when interpreting the results, especially in infant AD.

4. Abbreviations

Atopic dermatitis (AD);
Hanifin and Rajka diagnostic criteria (H-R criteria);
International Study of Asthma and Allergies in Childhood (ISAAC);
Quality of life (QoL);
Scoring Atopic Dermatitis index (SCORAD);
Dermatitis Area and Severity Index score (ADASIS);
Eczema Area and Severity Index (EASI);
Psoriasis area and severity index (PASI);
Nottingham Eczema Severity Score (NESS);
Children's Dermatology Life Quality Index (CDLQI);
Objective severity assessment of atopic dermatitis (OSAAD system);
Stratum corneum hydration (SCH);
Trans-epidermal water loss (TEWL);
Body surface area (BSA);
Stratum corneum (SC);
Natural moisturizing factors (NMF);
Pyrrolidone carboxylic acid (PCA);
Urocanic acid (UCA);
Atopy patch test (APT);
Skin prick test (SPT);
Eosinophil cationic protein (ECP);
Eosinophil derived neurotoxin/eosinophil protein X (EDN/EPX);
T-regulatory (Treg);
Interleukin (IL);
CCL2/MCP-1, monocyte chemotactic protein 1;
CCL11 /eotaxin (EOX);
CCL17 /TARC, thymus and activation-regulated chemokine;
CCL22 /MDC, macrophage-derived chemokine;
CCL26 /eotaxin-3;
CCL27/CTACK, cutaneous T cell-attracting chemokine;
CCL28/ MEC, Mucosa-associated epithelial chemokine;
CXCL10 /IP-10, IFN-induced protein of 10 kd;
CX3CL1 /fractalkine;
sE-selectin, serum soluble E-selectin ;
sIL-2R, soluble interleukin-2 receptor .
Tumor necrosis factor (TNF);
B cell-activating factor (BAFF);
Neurotrophins (NT);
Nerve growth factor (NGF);

Brain-derived neurotrophic factor (BDNF);
Vasoactive intestinal peptide (VIP);
Stem cell factor (SCF);
Tyrosine kinase transmembrane receptor (KIT);
Thymic stromal lymphopoietin (TSLP);
Dendric cell (DC);
Antidiuretic hormone (ADH);
Lactate dehydrogenase(LDH);
Matrix metalloproteinases(MMPs);
Tissue inhibitors of metalloproteinases (TIMPs);
Kallikreins (KLKs);
Soluble immune receptors (SIRs;)
Free light chains (FLC);
Leukotriene(LT);
Visual analog scales (VAS);
8-hydroxydeoxyguanosine (8-OHdG);
Aquaporin (AQP);
Prostaglandin D (PGD)

5. References

Agrawal, R.;Wisniewski, J.A. &Woodfolk, J.A. (2011). Curr Probl Dermatol. The role of regulatory T cells in atopic dermatitis, Vol.41, pp. 112-124,ISSN 1662-2944

Akdis, C.A.;Blesken, T.;Akdis, M. (1998). J Clin Invest. Role of interleukin 10 in specific immunotherapy, Vol.102, No.1, pp. 98-106,ISSN 0021-9738

Akdis, C.A.;Akdis, M.;Bieber, T. (2006). Allergy. Diagnosis and treatment of atopic dermatitis in children and adults: European Academy of Allergology and Clinical Immunology/American Academy of Allergy, Asthma and Immunology/ PRACTALL Consensus Report, Vol.61, No.8, pp. 969-987,ISSN 0105-4538

Akdis, M.;Verhagen, J.;Taylor, A. (2004). J Exp Med. Immune responses in healthy and allergic individuals are characterized by a fine balance between allergen-specific T regulatory 1 and T helper 2 cells, Vol.199, No.11, pp. 1567-1575,ISSN 0022-1007

Altrichter, S.;Kriehuber, E.;Moser, J. (2008). J Invest Dermatol. Serum IgE autoantibodies target keratinocytes in patients with atopic dermatitis, Vol.128, No.9, pp. 2232-2239, ISSN 1523-1747

Alysandratos, K.D.;Angelidou, A.;Vasiadi, M. (2010). Ann Allergy Asthma Immunol. Increased affected skin gene expression and serum levels of thymic stromal lymphopoietin in atopic dermatitis, Vol.105, No.5, pp. 403-404,ISSN 1534-4436

Angelova-Fischer, I.;Bauer, A.;Hipler, U.C. (2005). Br J Dermatol. The objective severity assessment of atopic dermatitis (OSAAD) score: validity, reliability and sensitivity in adult patients with atopic dermatitis, Vol.153, No.4, pp. 767-773, ISSN 0007-0963

Aoki, T. (2005). Br J Dermatol. Serum antidiuretic hormone is elevated in relation to the increase in average total body transepidermal water loss in severe atopic dermatitis, Vol.153, No.2, pp. 359-363, ISSN 0007-0963

Aral, M.;Arican, O.;Gul, M. (2006). Mediators Inflamm. The relationship between serum levels of total IgE, IL-18, IL-12, IFN-gamma and disease severity in children with atopic dermatitis, Vol.2006, No.4, pp. 73098, ISSN 0962-9351

Asher, M.I.;Keil, U.;Anderson, H.R. (1995). Eur Respir J. International Study of Asthma and Allergies in Childhood (ISAAC): rationale and methods, Vol.8, No.3, pp. 483-491, ISSN 0903-1936

Badertscher, K.;Bronnimann, M.;Karlen, S. (2005). Arch Dermatol Res. Mast cell chymase is increased in chronic atopic dermatitis but not in psoriasis, Vol.296, No.10, pp. 503-506, ISSN 0340-3696

Bahmer, F.A. (1992). Acta Derm Venereol Suppl (Stockh). ADASI score: atopic dermatitis area and severity index, Vol.176, pp. 32-33, ISSN 0365-8341

Balabanian, K.;Lagane, B.;Infantino, S. (2005). J Biol Chem. The chemokine SDF-1/CXCL12 binds to and signals through the orphan receptor RDC1 in T lymphocytes, Vol.280, No.42, pp. 35760-35766, ISSN 0021-9258

Belloni Fortina, A.;Tonin, E.;Pigozzi, B. (2006). Int J Immunopathol Pharmacol. IL-16 serum level in children with atopic dermatitis, Vol.19, No.4, pp. 841-845, ISSN 0394-6320

Ben-Gashir, M.A.; Seed, P.T. & Hay, R.J. (2004). Br J Dermatol. Quality of life and disease severity are correlated in children with atopic dermatitis, Vol.150, No.2, pp. 284-290, ISSN 0007-0963

Boguniewicz, M.; Schmid-Grendelmeier, P. & Leung, D.Y. (2006). J Allergy Clin Immunol. Atopic dermatitis, Vol.118, No.1, pp. 40-43, ISSN 0091-6749

Bradley, M.; Kockum, I.; Soderhall, C. (2000). Acta Derm Venereol. Characterization by phenotype of families with atopic dermatitis, Vol.80, No.2, pp. 106-110, ISSN 0001-5555

Brenninkmeijer, E.E.; Schram, M.E.; Leeflang, M.M. (2008). Br J Dermatol. Diagnostic criteria for atopic dermatitis: a systematic review, Vol.158, No.4, pp. 754-765, ISSN 0007-0963

Breuer, K.;Kapp, A. &Werfel, T. (2001). Allergy. Urine eosinophil protein X (EPX) is an in vitro parameter of inflammation in atopic dermatitis of the adult age, Vol.56, No.8, pp. 780-784, ISSN 0105-4538

Caproni, M.; Antiga, E.; Torchia, D. (2007). Allergy Asthma Proc. FoxP3-expressing T regulatory cells in atopic dermatitis lesions, Vol.28, No.5, pp. 525-528, ISSN 1088-5412

Charman, C. & Williams, H. (2000). Arch Dermatol. Outcome measures of disease severity in atopic eczema, Vol.136, No.6, pp. 763-769, ISSN 0003-987X

Choi, S.J.; Song, M.G.; Sung, W.T. (2003). J Korean Med Sci. Comparison of transepidermal water loss, capacitance and pH values in the skin between intrinsic and extrinsic atopic dermatitis patients, Vol.18, No.1, pp. 93-96, ISSN 1011-8934

Ciprandi, G.; De Amici, M.; Berardi, L. (2011). Clin Exp Dermatol. Serum neopterin levels in spontaneous urticaria and atopic dermatitis, Vol.36, No.1, pp. 85-87, ISSN 1365-2230

Consensus Report of the European Task Force on Atopic Dermatitis (1993). Dermatology. Severity scoring of atopic dermatitis: the SCORAD index., Vol.186, No.1, pp. 23-31,ISSN 1018-8665

Damps-Konstanska, I.; Gruchala-Niedoszytko, M.; Wilkowska, A. (2005). Pol Merkur Lekarski. [Serum eosinophil cationic protein (ECP) in patients with perennial rhinitis and atopic dermatitis, allergic to house dust mites], Vol.19, No.114, pp. 765-768, ISSN 1426-9686 de Boissieu, D. & Dupont, C. (2003). Eur Ann Allergy Clin Immunol. [Patch tests in the diagnosis of food allergies in the nursing infant], Vol.35, No.5, pp. 150-152, ISSN 1764-1489

Di Lorenzo, G.; Gangemi, S.; Merendino, R.A. (2003). Mediators Inflamm. Serum levels of soluble CD30 in adult patients affected by atopic dermatitis and its relation to age, duration of disease and Scoring Atopic Dermatitis index, Vol.12, No.2, pp. 123-125, ISSN 0962-9351

Di, Z.H.; Lv, Y.N.; Zhang, L. (2010). Br J Dermatol. Urinary aquaporin-2 is elevated in infant atopic dermatitis, Vol.163, No.5, pp. 1132-1134, ISSN 1365-2133

Echigo, T.; Hasegawa, M.; Shimada, Y. (2004). J Allergy Clin Immunol. Expression of fractalkine and its receptor, CX3CR1, in atopic dermatitis: possible contribution to skin inflammation, Vol.113, No.5, pp. 940-948, ISSN 0091-6749

El Mongy, S.; Metwaly, S.S.; Arafat, M.S. (2008). Egypt J Immunol. Serum levels of soluble CD30 in patients with atopic dermatitis: correlations with age, disease duration and severity, Vol.15, No.1, pp. 123-129, ISSN 1110-4902

Elkeeb, R.; Hui, X.; Chan, H. (2010). Skin Res Technol. Correlation of transepidermal water loss with skin barrier properties in vitro: comparison of three evaporimeters, Vol.16, No.1, pp. 9-15, ISSN 1600-0846

Emerson, R.M.; Charman, C.R. & Williams, H.C. (2000). Br J Dermatol. The Nottingham Eczema Severity Score: preliminary refinement of the Rajka and Langeland grading, Vol.142, No.2, pp. 288-297, ISSN 0007-0963

Ezzat, M.; Hasan, Z. & Shaheen, K. (2011). J Eur Acad Dermatol Venereol. Serum measurement of interleukin-31 (IL-31) in paediatric atopic dermatitis: elevated levels correlate with severity scoring, Vol.25, No.3, pp. 334-339, ISSN 1468-3083

Ezzat, M.H.; Sallam, M.A. & Shaheen, K.Y. (2009). Int J Dermatol. Serum mucosa-associated epithelial chemokine (MEC/CCL28) in atopic dermatitis: a specific marker for severity, Vol.48, No.8, pp. 822-829, ISSN 1365-4632

Ezzat, M.H. & Shaheen, K.Y. (2009). Indian J Dermatol. Serum mucosa-associated epithelial chemokine in atopic dermatitis: a specific marker for severity, Vol.54, No.3, pp. 229-236, ISSN 1998-3611

Firooz, A.; Gorouhi, F.; Davari, P. (2007). Clin Exp Dermatol. Comparison of hydration, sebum and pH values in clinically normal skin of patients with atopic dermatitis and healthy controls, Vol.32, No.3, pp. 321-322, ISSN 0307-6938

Furue, M.; Koga, T. & Yamashita, N. (1999). Br J Dermatol. Soluble E-selectin and eosinophil cationic protein are distinct serum markers that differentially represent clinical features of atopic dermatitis, Vol.140, No.1, pp. 67-72, ISSN 0007-0963

Gerdes, S.; Kurrat, W. & Mrowietz, U. (2009). Br J Dermatol. Serum mast cell tryptase is not a useful marker for disease severity in psoriasis or atopic dermatitis, Vol.160, No.4, pp. 736-740, ISSN 1365-2133

Goto, T.; Morioka, J.; Inamura, H. (2007). Allergol Int. Urinary eosinophil-derived neurotoxin concentrations in patients with atopic dermatitis: a useful clinical marker for disease activity, Vol.56, No.4, pp. 433-438, ISSN 1323-8930

Gupta, J.; Grube, E.; Ericksen, M.B. (2008). J Allergy Clin Immunol. Intrinsically defective skin barrier function in children with atopic dermatitis correlates with disease severity, Vol.121, No.3, pp. 725-730 e722, ISSN 1097-6825

Hanifin, J.M.; Thurston, M.; Omoto, M. (2001). Exp Dermatol. The eczema area and severity index (EASI): assessment of reliability in atopic dermatitis. EASI Evaluator Group, Vol.10, No.1, pp. 11-18, ISSN 0906-6705

Hayashida, S.; Uchi, H.; Moroi, Y. (2011). J Dermatol Sci. Decrease in circulating Th17 cells correlates with increased levels of CCL17, IgE and eosinophils in atopic dermatitis, Vol.61, No.3, pp. 180-186, ISSN 1873-569X

Hayashida, S.; Uchi, H.; Takeuchi, S. (2011). J Dermatol Sci. Significant correlation of serum IL-22 levels with CCL17 levels in atopic dermatitis, Vol.61, No.1, pp. 78-79, ISSN 1873-569X

Hieshima, K.; Ohtani, H.; Shibano, M. (2003). J Immunol. CCL28 has dual roles in mucosal immunity as a chemokine with broad-spectrum antimicrobial activity, Vol.170, No.3, pp. 1452-1461, ISSN 0022-1767

Hijnen, D.; De Bruin-Weller, M.; Oosting, B. (2004). J Allergy Clin Immunol. Serum thymus and activation-regulated chemokine (TARC) and cutaneous T cell- attracting chemokine (CTACK) levels in allergic diseases: TARC and CTACK are disease-specific markers for atopic dermatitis, Vol.113, No.2, pp. 334-340, ISSN 0091-6749

Homey, B.; Steinhoff, M.; Ruzicka, T. (2006). J Allergy Clin Immunol. Cytokines and chemokines orchestrate atopic skin inflammation, Vol.118, No.1, pp. 178-189, ISSN 0091-6749

Hon, K.L.; Leung, T.F.; Ma, K.C. (2004). Clin Exp Dermatol. Serum levels of cutaneous T-cell attracting chemokine (CTACK) as a laboratory marker of the severity of atopic dermatitis in children, Vol.29, No.3, pp. 293-296, ISSN 0307-6938

Hon, K.L.; Leung, T.F.; Ma, K.C. (2004). Clin Exp Dermatol. Urinary leukotriene E4 correlates with severity of atopic dermatitis in children, Vol.29, No.3, pp. 277-281, ISSN 0307-6938

Hon, K.L.; Leung, T.F.; Ma, K.C. (2004). Pediatr Dermatol. Serum concentration of IL-18 correlates with disease extent in young children with atopic dermatitis, Vol.21, No.6, pp. 619-622, ISSN 0736-8046

Hon, K.L.; Leung, T.F.; Ma, K.C. (2005). J Dermatolog Treat. Brief case series: montelukast, at doses recommended for asthma treatment, reduces disease severity and increases soluble CD14 in children with atopic dermatitis, Vol.16, No.1, pp. 15-18, ISSN 0954-6634

Hon, K.L.; Kam, W.Y.; Lam, M.C. (2006). Qual Life Res. CDLQI, SCORAD and NESS: are they correlated?, Vol.15, No.10, pp. 1551-1558, ISSN 0962-9343

Hon, K.L.; Lam, M.C.; Leung, T.F. (2007). Int J Dermatol. Are age-specific high serum IgE levels associated with worse symptomatology in children with atopic dermatitis?, Vol.46, No.12, pp. 1258-1262, ISSN 0011-9059

Hon, K.L.;Wong, K.Y.;Leung, T.F. (2008). Am J Clin Dermatol. Comparison of skin hydration evaluation sites and correlations among skin hydration, transepidermal water loss, SCORAD index, Nottingham Eczema Severity Score, and quality of life in patients with atopic dermatitis, Vol.9, No.1, pp. 45-50, ISSN 1175-0561

Horak, E.; Murr, C.; Streif, W. (2006). Pediatr Allergy Immunol. Association between neopterin in cord blood, urinary neopterin in early childhood and the development of atopic dermatitis, asthma and hay fever, Vol.17, No.1, pp. 11-16, ISSN 0905-6157

Howell, M.D.; Kim, B.E.; Gao, P. (2009). J Allergy Clin Immunol. Cytokine modulation of atopic dermatitis filaggrin skin expression, Vol.124, No.3 Suppl 2, pp. R7-R12, ISSN 1097-6825

Isolauri, E. & Turjanmaa, K. (1996). J Allergy Clin Immunol. Combined skin prick and patch testing enhances identification of food allergy in infants with atopic dermatitis, Vol.97, No.1 Pt 1, pp. 9-15, ISSN 0091-6749

Jahnz-Rozyk, K.; Targowski, T.; Paluchowska, E. (2005). Allergy. Serum thymus and activation-regulated chemokine, macrophage-derived chemokine and eotaxin as markers of severity of atopic dermatitis, Vol.60, No.5, pp. 685-688, ISSN 0105-4538

Jee, H.M.; Kim, K.W.; Hong, J.Y. (2010). Clin Exp Dermatol. Increased serum B cell-activating factor level in children with atopic dermatitis, Vol.35, No.6, pp. 593-598, ISSN 1365-2230

Jenerowicz, D.; Czarnecka-Operacz, M. & Silny, W. (2006). Acta Dermatovenerol Croat. Selected eosinophil proteins as markers of inflammation in atopic dermatitis patients, Vol.14, No.2, pp. 73-80, ISSN 1330-027X

Kagami, S.; Kakinuma, T.; Saeki, H. (2003). Clin Exp Immunol. Significant elevation of serum levels of eotaxin-3/CCL26, but not of eotaxin-2/CCL24, in patients with atopic dermatitis: serum eotaxin-3/CCL26 levels reflect the disease activity of atopic dermatitis, Vol.134, No.2, pp. 309-313, ISSN 0009-9104

Kagami, S.; Kakinuma, T.; Saeki, H. (2005). J Invest Dermatol. Increased serum CCL28 levels in patients with atopic dermatitis, psoriasis vulgaris and bullous pemphigoid, Vol.124, No.5, pp. 1088-1090, ISSN 0022-202X

Kakinuma, T.; Nakamura, K.; Wakugawa, M. (2001). J Allergy Clin Immunol. Thymus and activation-regulated chemokine in atopic dermatitis: Serum thymus and activation-regulated chemokine level is closely related with disease activity, Vol.107, No.3, pp. 535-541, ISSN 0091-6749

Kakinuma, T.; Nakamura, K.; Wakugawa, M. (2002). Clin Exp Immunol. Serum macrophage-derived chemokine (MDC) levels are closely related with the disease activity of atopic dermatitis, Vol.127, No.2, pp. 270-273, ISSN 0009-9104

Kakinuma, T.; Saeki, H.;Tsunemi, Y. (2003). J Allergy Clin Immunol. Increased serum cutaneous T cell-attracting chemokine (CCL27) levels in patients with atopic dermatitis and psoriasis vulgaris, Vol.111, No.3, pp. 592-597, ISSN 0091-6749

Kanbe, T.; Soma, Y.; Kawa, Y. (2001). Br J Dermatol. Serum levels of soluble stem cell factor and soluble KIT are elevated in patients with atopic dermatitis and correlate with the disease severity, Vol.144, No.6, pp. 1148-1153, ISSN 0007-0963

Katoh, N.; Hirano, S.; Suehiro, M. (2002). Clin Exp Immunol. Increased levels of serum tissue inhibitor of metalloproteinase-1 but not metalloproteinase-3 in atopic dermatitis, Vol.127, No.2, pp. 283-288, ISSN 0009-9104

Kayserova, J.; Capkova, S.; Skalicka, A. (2010). Scand J Immunol. Serum immunoglobulin free light chains in severe forms of atopic dermatitis, Vol.71, No.4, pp. 312-316, ISSN 1365-3083

Kezic, S.; O'Regan, G.M.; Yau, N. (2011). Allergy. Levels of filaggrin degradation products are influenced by both filaggrin genotype and atopic dermatitis severity, ISSN 1398-9995

Kolbeck, R.; Jungbluth, S. & Barde, Y.A. (1994). Eur J Biochem. Characterisation of neurotrophin dimers and monomers, Vol.225, No.3, pp. 995-1003, ISSN 0014-2956

Komatsu, N.; Saijoh, K.; Kuk, C. (2007). Exp Dermatol. Human tissue kallikrein expression in the stratum corneum and serum of atopic dermatitis patients, Vol.16, No.6, pp. 513-519, ISSN 0906-6705

Kunz, B.; Oranje, A.P.; Labreze, L. (1997). Dermatology. Clinical validation and guidelines for the SCORAD index: consensus report of the European Task Force on Atopic Dermatitis, Vol.195, No.1, pp. 10-19, ISSN 1018-8665

Landmann, L. (1988). Anat Embryol (Berl). The epidermal permeability barrier, Vol.178, No.1, pp. 1-13, ISSN 0340-2061

Lee, C.H.;Chuang, H.Y.;Shih, C.C. (2006). Br J Dermatol. Transepidermal water loss, serum IgE and beta-endorphin as important and independent biological markers for development of itch intensity in atopic dermatitis, Vol.154, No.6, pp. 1100-1107, ISSN 0007-0963

Lee, E.B.; Kim, K.W.; Hong, J.Y. (2010). Pediatr Allergy Immunol. Increased serum thymic stromal lymphopoietin in children with atopic dermatitis, Vol.21, No.2 Pt 2, pp. e457-460, ISSN 1399-3038

Lee, K.Y.; Cho, K.J.; Kim, Y.T. (2009). Ann Allergy Asthma Immunol. Serum eosinophil-derived neurotoxin in childhood atopic dermatitis: a useful marker of disease activity?, Vol.102, No.6, pp. 532-534, ISSN 1081-1206

Leibrock, J.; Lottspeich, F.; Hohn, A. (1989). Nature. Molecular cloning and expression of brain-derived neurotrophic factor, Vol.341, No.6238, pp. 149-152, ISSN 0028-0836

Leung, D.Y.; Boguniewicz, M.; Howell, M.D. (2004). J Clin Invest. New insights into atopic dermatitis, Vol.113, No.5, pp. 651-657, ISSN 0021-9738

Leung, T.F.; Ma, K.C.; Hon, K.L. (2003). Pediatr Allergy Immunol. Serum concentration of macrophage-derived chemokine may be a useful inflammatory marker for assessing severity of atopic dermatitis in infants and young children, Vol.14, No.4, pp. 296-301, ISSN 0905-6157

Levy, R.M.; Gelfand, J.M. & Yan, A.C. (2003). Clin Dermatol. The epidemiology of atopic dermatitis, Vol.21, No.2, pp. 109-115, ISSN 0738-081X

Lipozencic, J. & Wolf, R. (2007). Dermatol Clin. Atopic dermatitis: an update and review of the literature, Vol.25, No.4, pp. 605-612, x, ISSN 0733-8635

Lipozencic, J. & Wolf, R. (2010). Clin Dermatol. The diagnostic value of atopy patch testing and prick testing in atopic dermatitis: facts and controversies, Vol.28, No.1, pp. 38-44, ISSN 1879-1131

Ma, L.; Gao, X.H.; Zhao, L.P. (2009). J Eur Acad Dermatol Venereol. Brain-derived neurotrophic factor gene polymorphisms and serum levels in Chinese atopic dermatitis patients, Vol.23, No.11, pp. 1277-1281, ISSN 1468-3083

Ma, L.; Zhang, L.; Di, Z.H. (2010). Br J Dermatol. Association analysis of filaggrin gene mutations and atopic dermatitis in Northern China, Vol.162, No.1, pp. 225-227, ISSN 1365-2133

Man, M.Q.; Xin, S.J.; Song, S.P. (2009). Skin Pharmacol Physiol. Variation of skin surface pH, sebum content and stratum corneum hydration with age and gender in a large Chinese population, Vol.22, No.4, pp. 190-199, ISSN 1660-5535

Marenholz, I.; Nickel, R.; Ruschendorf, F. (2006). J Allergy Clin Immunol. Filaggrin loss-of-function mutations predispose to phenotypes involved in the atopic march, Vol.118, No.4, pp. 866-871, ISSN 0091-6749

Masuda, K.; Katoh, N.; Okuda, F. (2003). Acta Derm Venereol. Increased levels of serum interleukin-16 in adult type atopic dermatitis, Vol.83, No.4, pp. 249-253, ISSN 0001-5555

Mathy, N.L.; Scheuer, W.; Lanzendorfer, M. (2000). Immunology. Interleukin-16 stimulates the expression and production of pro-inflammatory cytokines by human monocytes, Vol.100, No.1, pp. 63-69, ISSN 0019-2805

Matsushita, T.; Fujimoto, M.; Echigo, T. (2008). Exp Dermatol. Elevated serum levels of APRIL, but not BAFF, in patients with atopic dermatitis, Vol.17, No.3, pp. 197-202, ISSN 1600-0625

Mevorah, B.; Frenk, E.; Wietlisbach, V. (1988). Dermatologica. Minor clinical features of atopic dermatitis. Evaluation of their diagnostic significance, Vol.177, No.6, pp. 360-364, ISSN 0011-9075

Meyer-Hoffert, U. (2009). Arch Immunol Ther Exp (Warsz). Reddish, scaly, and itchy: how proteases and their inhibitors contribute to inflammatory skin diseases, Vol.57, No.5, pp. 345-354, ISSN 1661-4917

Miyahara, H.; Okazaki, N.; Nagakura, T. (2011). Clin Exp Allergy. Elevated umbilical cord serum TARC/CCL17 levels predict the development of atopic dermatitis in infancy, Vol.41, No.2, pp. 186-191, ISSN 1365-2222

Morishima, Y.; Kawashima, H.; Takekuma, K. (2010). Pediatr Int. Changes in serum lactate dehydrogenase activity in children with atopic dermatitis, Vol.52, No.2, pp. 171-174, ISSN 1442-200X

Mostafa, G.A.; Tomoum, H.Y.; Salem, S.A. (2008). Pediatr Allergy Immunol. Serum concentrations of CCR4 ligands in relation to clinical severity of atopic dermatitis in Egyptian children, Vol.19, No.8, pp. 756-762, ISSN 1399-3038

Murr, C.; Widner, B.; Wirleitner, B. (2002). Curr Drug Metab. Neopterin as a marker for immune system activation, Vol.3, No.2, pp. 175-187, ISSN 1389-2002

Nagy, G.; Gaspar, K.; Irinyi, B. (2011). Int Arch Allergy Immunol. Association between Serum IL-16 Levels and the Degree of Sensitization in Patients with Atopic Dermatitis, Vol.156, No.1, pp. 69-74, ISSN 1423-0097

Nakai, K.; Yoneda, K.; Maeda, R. (2009). J Eur Acad Dermatol Venereol. Urinary biomarker of oxidative stress in patients with psoriasis vulgaris and atopic dermatitis, Vol.23, No.12, pp. 1405-1408, ISSN 1468-3083

Nakamura, K.; Tsuchida, T.; Tsunemi, Y. (2008). J Dermatol. Serum thymic stromal lymphopoietin levels are not elevated in patients with atopic dermatitis, Vol.35, No.8, pp. 546-547, ISSN 0385-2407

Nakazato, J.; Kishida, M.; Kuroiwa, R. (2008). Pediatr Allergy Immunol. Serum levels of Th2 chemokines, CCL17, CCL22, and CCL27, were the important markers of severity in infantile atopic dermatitis, Vol.19, No.7, pp. 605-613, ISSN 1399-3038

Narbutt, J.; Lesiak, A.; Sysa-Jedrzeiowska, A. (2009). Mediators Inflamm. The imbalance in serum concentration of Th-1- and Th-2-derived chemokines as one of the factors involved in pathogenesis of atopic dermatitis, Vol.2009, pp. 269541, ISSN 1466-1861

Niggemann, B.; Reibel, S. & Wahn, U. (2000). Allergy. The atopy patch test (APT)-- a useful tool for the diagnosis of food allergy in children with atopic dermatitis, Vol.55, No.3, pp. 281-285, ISSN 0105-4538

Niggemann, B.; Rolinck-Werninghaus, C.; Mehl, A. (2005). Allergy. Controlled oral food challenges in children--when indicated, when superfluous?, Vol.60, No.7, pp. 865-870, ISSN 0105-4538

Novak, N. & Bieber, T. (2003). J Allergy Clin Immunol. Allergic and nonallergic forms of atopic diseases, Vol.112, No.2, pp. 252-262, ISSN 0091-6749

O'Regan, G.M.; Sandilands, A.; McLean, W.H. (2009). J Allergy Clin Immunol. Filaggrin in atopic dermatitis, Vol.124, No.3 Suppl 2, pp. R2-6, ISSN 1097-6825

O'Sullivan, S. (1999). Acta Physiol Scand Suppl. On the role of PGD2 metabolites as markers of mast cell activation in asthma, Vol.644, pp. 1-74, ISSN 0302-2994

Osterballe, M.; Andersen, K.E. & Bindslev-Jensen, C. (2004). J Am Acad Dermatol. The diagnostic accuracy of the atopy patch test in diagnosing hypersensitivity to cow's milk and hen's egg in unselected children with and without atopic dermatitis, Vol.51, No.4, pp. 556-562, ISSN 1097-6787

Ott, H.; Stanzel, S.; Ocklenburg, C. (2009). Acta Derm Venereol. Total serum IgE as a parameter to differentiate between intrinsic and extrinsic atopic dermatitis in children, Vol.89, No.3, pp. 257-261, ISSN 0001-5555

Ott, H.; Wilke, J.; Baron, J.M. (2010). J Eur Acad Dermatol Venereol. Soluble immune receptor serum levels are associated with age, but not with clinical phenotype or disease severity in childhood atopic dermatitis, Vol.24, No.4, pp. 395-402, ISSN 1468-3083

Oymar, K. & Aksnes, L. (2004). Acta Derm Venereol. Urinary 9alpha,11beta-prostaglandin F(2) in children with atopic eczema/dermatitis syndrome: an indicator of mast cell activation?, Vol.84, No.5, pp. 359-362, ISSN 0001-5555

Oymar, K. & Aksnes, L. (2005). Allergy. Increased levels of urinary leukotriene E4 in children with severe atopic eczema/dermatitis syndrome, Vol.60, No.1, pp. 86-89, ISSN 0105-4538

Palmer, C.N.; Irvine, A.D.; Terron-Kwiatkowski, A. (2006). Nat Genet. Common loss-of-function variants of the epidermal barrier protein filaggrin are a major predisposing factor for atopic dermatitis, Vol.38, No.4, pp. 441-446, ISSN 1061-4036

Park do, S. & Youn, Y.H. (2007). Korean J Lab Med. [Clinical significance of serum interleukin-18 concentration in the patients with atopic dermatitis], Vol.27, No.2, pp. 128-132, ISSN 1598-6535

Peroni, D.G.; Piacentini, G.L.; Cametti, E. (2010). Br J Dermatol. Correlation between serum 25 (OH)-vitamin D levels and severity of atopic dermatitis in children, ISSN 1365-2133

Piancatelli, D.; Bellotta, L.; Del Beato, T. (2008). Int J Immunopathol Pharmacol. Total IL-12 levels are increased in paediatric atopic dermatitis: correlations with age and disease severity, Vol.21, No.2, pp. 359-365, ISSN 0394-6320

Pucci, N.; Lombardi, E.; Novembre, E. (2000). J Allergy Clin Immunol. Urinary eosinophil protein X and serum eosinophil cationic protein in infants and young children with atopic dermatitis: correlation with disease activity, Vol.105, No.2 Pt 1, pp. 353-357, ISSN 0091-6749

Pucci, N.; Novembre, E.; Cammarata, M.G. (2005). Allergy. Scoring atopic dermatitis in infants and young children: distinctive features of the SCORAD index, Vol.60, No.1, pp. 113-116, ISSN 0105-4538

Raap, U.; Werfel, T.; Goltz, C. (2006). Allergy. Circulating levels of brain-derived neurotrophic factor correlate with disease severity in the intrinsic type of atopic dermatitis, Vol.61, No.12, pp. 1416-1418, ISSN 0105-4538

Raap, U.; Wichmann, K.; Bruder, M. (2008). J Allergy Clin Immunol. Correlation of IL-31 serum levels with severity of atopic dermatitis, Vol.122, No.2, pp. 421-423, ISSN 1097-6825

Ring, J.; Darsow, U.; Gfesser, M. (1997). Int Arch Allergy Immunol. The 'atopy patch test' in evaluating the role of aeroallergens in atopic eczema, Vol.113, No.1-3, pp. 379-383, ISSN 1018-2438

Robinson, M.; Visscher, M.; Laruffa, A. (2010). J Cosmet Sci. Natural moisturizing factors (NMF) in the stratum corneum (SC). I. Effects of lipid extraction and soaking, Vol.61, No.1, pp. 13-22, ISSN 1525-7886

Robinson, M.; Visscher, M.; Laruffa, A. (2010). J Cosmet Sci. Natural moisturizing factors (NMF) in the stratum corneum (SC). II. Regeneration of NMF over time after soaking, Vol.61, No.1, pp. 23-29, ISSN 1525-7886

Roehr, C.C.; Reibel, S.; Ziegert, M. (2001). J Allergy Clin Immunol. Atopy patch tests, together with determination of specific IgE levels, reduce the need for oral food challenges in children with atopic dermatitis, Vol.107, No.3, pp. 548-553, ISSN 0091-6749

Roguedas, A.M.; Machet, L.; Fontes, V. (2004). Ann Dermatol Venereol. [Atopic dermatitis: which are the diagnostic criteria used in medical literature?], Vol.131, No.2, pp. 161-164, ISSN 0151-9638

Rossi, D. & Zlotnik, A. (2000). Annu Rev Immunol. The biology of chemokines and their receptors, Vol.18, pp. 217-242, ISSN 0732-0582

Rullo, V.E.; Segato, A.; Kirsh, A. (2008). Allergol Immunopathol (Madr). Severity scoring of atopic dermatitis: a comparison of two scoring systems, Vol.36, No.4, pp. 205-211, ISSN 0301-0546

Saarinen, K.M.; Suomalainen, H. & Savilahti, E. (2001). Clin Exp Allergy. Diagnostic value of skin-prick and patch tests and serum eosinophil cationic protein and cow's milk-specific IgE in infants with cow's milk allergy, Vol.31, No.3, pp. 423-429, ISSN 0954-7894

Sampson, H.A. (2001). J Allergy Clin Immunol. Utility of food-specific IgE concentrations in predicting symptomatic food allergy, Vol.107, No.5, pp. 891-896, ISSN 0091-6749

Sampson, H.A. (2003). Clin Dermatol. The evaluation and management of food allergy in atopic dermatitis, Vol.21, No.3, pp. 183-192, ISSN 0738-081X

Schulte-Herbruggen, O.; Folster-Holst, R.; von Elstermann, M. (2007). Int Arch Allergy Immunol. Clinical relevance of nerve growth factor serum levels in patients with atopic dermatitis and psoriasis, Vol.144, No.3, pp. 211-216, ISSN 1423-0097

Selnes, A. & Dotterud, L.K. (2005). J Eur Acad Dermatol Venereol. No association between serum eosinophil cationic protein and atopic dermatitis or allergic rhinitis in an unselected population of children, Vol.19, No.1, pp. 61-65, ISSN 0926-9959

Shin, H.D.; Park, B.L.; Kim, L.H. (2005). Allergy. Interleukin-10 haplotype associated with total serum IgE in atopic dermatitis patients, Vol.60, No.9, pp. 1146-1151, ISSN 0105-4538

Sohn, M.H.; Lee, K.E. & Kim, K.E. (2004). Allergy Asthma Proc. Interleukin-18 is associated with increased severity of atopic dermatitis in children, Vol.25, No.3, pp. 181-184, ISSN 1088-5412

Song, T.W.; Sohn, M.H.; Kim, E.S. (2006). Clin Exp Allergy. Increased serum thymus and activation-regulated chemokine and cutaneous T cell-attracting chemokine levels in children with atopic dermatitis, Vol.36, No.3, pp. 346-351, ISSN 0954-7894

Souwer, Y.; Szegedi, K.; Kapsenberg, M.L. (2010). Curr Opin Immunol. IL-17 and IL-22 in atopic allergic disease, Vol.22, No.6, pp. 821-826, ISSN 1879-0372

Steinhoff, M.; Bienenstock, J.; Schmelz, M. (2006). J Invest Dermatol. Neurophysiological, neuroimmunological, and neuroendocrine basis of pruritus, Vol.126, No.8, pp. 1705-1718, ISSN 0022-202X

Stromberg, L. (2002). Acta Paediatr. Diagnostic accuracy of the atopy patch test and the skin-prick test for the diagnosis of food allergy in young children with atopic eczema/dermatitis syndrome, Vol.91, No.10, pp. 1044-1049, ISSN 0803-5253

Sugarman, J.L.; Fluhr, J.W.; Fowler, A.J. (2003). Arch Dermatol. The objective severity assessment of atopic dermatitis score: an objective measure using permeability barrier function and stratum corneum hydration with computer-assisted estimates for extent of disease, Vol.139, No.11, pp. 1417-1422, ISSN 0003-987X

Sugiura, H.; Umemoto, N.; Deguchi, H. (1998). Acta Derm Venereol. Prevalence of childhood and adolescent atopic dermatitis in a Japanese population: comparison with the disease frequency examined 20 years ago, Vol.78, No.4, pp. 293-294, ISSN 0001-5555

Taniuchi, S.; Chihara, J.; Kojima, T. (2001). J Dermatol Sci. Serum eosinophil derived neurotoxin may reflect more strongly disease severity in childhood atopic dermatitis than eosinophil cationic protein, Vol.26, No.1, pp. 79-82, ISSN 0923-1811

Toda, M.; Leung, D.Y.; Molet, S. (2003). J Allergy Clin Immunol. Polarized in vivo expression of IL-11 and IL-17 between acute and chronic skin lesions, Vol.111, No.4, pp. 875-881, ISSN 0091-6749

Umemoto, N.; Kakurai, M.; Okazaki, H. (2003). J Dermatol Sci. Serum levels of vasoactive intestinal peptide are elevated in patients with atopic dermatitis, Vol.31, No.2, pp. 161-164, ISSN 0923-1811

Voegeli, R.; Rawlings, A.V.; Breternitz, M. (2009). Br J Dermatol. Increased stratum corneum serine protease activity in acute eczematous atopic skin, Vol.161, No.1, pp. 70-77, ISSN 1365-2133

Wang, Y.H.; Ito, T.;Homey, B. (2006). Immunity. Maintenance and polarization of human TH2 central memory T cells by thymic stromal lymphopoietin-activated dendritic cells, Vol.24, No.6, pp. 827-838, ISSN 1074-7613

Whalley, D.; McKenna, S.P.; Dewar, A.L. (2004). Br J Dermatol. A new instrument for assessing quality of life in atopic dermatitis: international development of the Quality of Life Index for Atopic Dermatitis (QoLIAD), Vol.150, No.2, pp. 274-283, ISSN 0007-0963

Woessner, J.F., Jr. (2001). J Clin Invest. That impish TIMP: the tissue inhibitor of metalloproteinases-3, Vol.108, No.6, pp. 799-800, ISSN 0021-9738

Wu, K.G.; Li, T.H.; Chen, C.J. (2011). Int J Immunopathol Pharmacol. Correlations of serum Interleukin-16, total IgE, eosinophil cationic protein and total eosinophil counts with disease activity in children with atopic dermatitis, Vol.24, No.1, pp. 15-23, ISSN 0394-6320

Yoshizawa, Y.; Nomaguchi, H.;Izaki, S. (2002). Clin Exp Dermatol. Serum cytokine levels in atopic dermatitis, Vol.27, No.3, pp. 225-229, ISSN 0307-6938

Zhang, H.; Guo, Y.; Wang, W. (2011). Allergy. Mutations in the filaggrin gene in Han Chinese patients with atopic dermatitis, Vol.66, No.3, pp. 420-427, ISSN 1398-9995

Zlotnik, A. & Yoshie, O. (2000). Immunity. Chemokines: a new classification system and their role in immunity, Vol.12, No.2, pp. 121-127, ISSN 1074-7613

12

Trigger Factors, Allergens and Allergy Testing in Atopic Dermatitis

Evmorfia Ladoyanni
Department of Dermatology, Dudley Group Hospitals, Corbett Hospital Vicarage Road, Stourbridge, West Midlands United Kingdom

1. Introduction

Atopic dermatitis (AD) is a chronic inflammatory skin disorder affecting between 10-20% of children and 1-3% of adults in the general population. It is associated with high morbidity and has major public health implications. AD is associated with hyper-reactivity of the skin to environmental trigger factors that are harmless in normal individuals. Major contributors to this hyperactivity are the many immune and inflammatory changes taking place in the skin and peripheral blood in AD individuals. AD can be classified into several subgroups, each with different immune and pathological features, suggesting a multifactorial disease and heterogeneity. Historically two types of AD have been identified. They include the "extrinsic or allergic" type of AD, which is characterized by Immunoglobulin E (IgE) mediated sensitization (immediate, type I hypersensitivity) and occurs in 70-80% of individuals. The "non-allergic or intrinsic" type of AD affects 20-30% of individuals and is defined by a more T-cell driven feature (delayed, type IV hypersensitivity), with low IgE levels and absent IgE sensitization. More recently a transition from the intrinsic to the extrinsic type has been reported in young children, and AD individuals can show a combination of above mentioned phenotypes or complete absence of the known features. The clinical diagnosis of AD does not cause major difficulties as there are fairly well defined criteria. Identifying the underlying pathophysiology for the affected individual can be more of a challenge, as there is no gold standard test available for AD and the AD individual might move from one pathophysiological "type" of AD to another. Clinically AD is divided into acute, subacute and chronic forms with correlated histopathological changes. The transition from one clinical form to another is fluent and can be very rapid. AD individuals frequently give a personal and or a family history of asthma and allergic rhinitis, the so called atopic triad. Exacerbation of one of the disorders in this triad can cause concomitant exacerbation of the other two suggesting some underlying common pathways and interdependence (Reitamo et al., 2008).

Predisposing factors for AD are multifactorial and involve genetic susceptibility, defects in skin barrier function, immune dysregulation, western life style and exposure to environmental trigger factors. The development of disease is an interplay of gene-gene and gene-environment interactions. The early age of onset and familial predisposition as well as the high concordance rate of AD in monozygotic (77%) and dizygotic (15%) twins suggest a genetically determined primary defect probably affecting the skin barrier thus playing a key role in the development of AD (Burns et al., 2004). The integrity of the skin barrier involves several components, including regulation of proteolysis of corneodesmosomes, the lipid lamellae and generation of natural moisturizing factor (MNF) from the breakdown products of the structural protein filaggrin. An imbalance of these components makes the epidermal barrier more susceptible to irritants, which in turn can lead to a disturbance of skin barrier function allowing penetration of microbes and allergens into the epidermis and dermis interdependence (Reitamo et al., 2008). In a recent meta-analysis filaggrin gene defects were shown to increase the risk of developing allergic sensitization, AD, and allergic rhinitis. The presence of filaggrin gene mutations correlated strongly with disease severity and treatment failure, and also increased the risk of asthma in AD patients (Van den Oord & Sheikh, 2009).

IgE is composed of two identical heavy and light chains, that form the constant Fc domain and the antigen-binding sites, through which the IgE molecule binds to its cell surface receptors. Raised serum IgE levels are most commonly seen in parasitic infections as a defensive response. IgE mediated hypersensitivity is largely regulated by T lymphocytes. AD is generally thought to be due to an imbalance between Th1 and Th2 cells, with a Th2 cell predominant immune profile in its active stage. Th2 cells produce interleukin (IL) -4, IL-5, IL-6 and IL-13, which induce IgE production and activation of eosinophils, producing the acute signs and symptoms of AD.

In general various cells contribute to the underlying pathomechanism of AD including Langerhans cells (LC), macrophages, T cells, B cells, keratinocytes, endothelial cells, eosinophils and mast cells. These cells communicate with each other in Th2 predominant cytokines as well as chemokines, prostanoids, proteases and reactive oxygen species products. High affinity IgE receptors play a crucial role in promoting this process.

A number of environmental factors can trigger and perpetuate the inflammatory skin cascade in AD including irritants, foods, aeroallergens, infection. All four classic Coombs' classification types of hypersensitivity (type I-IV) have been implicated in the pathophysiology of AD, including pseudo allergy. The hypersensitivity types can occur either alone or in combination in the AD individual. In the extrinsic type of AD high levels of specific IgE antibodies and raised total IgE levels in peripheral blood have been significantly associated with severity of dermatitis (Reitamo et al., 2008 & Burns et al., 2004).

2. Trigger factors, allergens and allergy testing in atopic dermatitis

The rate of increase in prevalence in AD in recent years is too rapid to be accounted for by changes in population genetics. Therefore environmental factors are the most likely modulating influences. The two principal aspects that have attracted attention are pollution and microbes. The identification of relevant pollutants that might contribute to the expression of atopic phenotype is still confused. Interaction with environmental microbes may be important in the causation of AD in a number of ways. Early-life exposure may condition maturation of the immune system so that apparent dysregulation associated with IgE production and allergy formation does not occur. Significant differences have been observed in the prevalence of allergies between urban and rural population within one country and observations confirm greater allergy sensitization in first-born and a lower frequency in children from large families. Evidence suggests that microbes entering via fecal-oral route have a greater protective effect against the development of atopic disease than those entering via the respiratory route (Burns et al., 2004).

AD has a Th2 cell predominant immune profile in its active stage. Th2 cells produce IL-4, IL-5, IL-6, IL-13, which induce IgE production and activation of eosinophils, producing the acute signs and symptoms of AD. Genetic factors, reduced bacterial stimulation in early infancy and a disruption in skin barrier and function are thought to contribute to the Th1-Th2 cell imbalance of skin in AD. Eczematous skin lesions evolve as a result of complex interactions between IgE bearing antigen presenting cells, T cell activation, mast cell degranulation, keratinocytes, eosinophils, and a combination of immediate and cellular immune response. A number of environmental factors have been reported to induce and perpetuate this inflammatory response of the skin including food and aeroallergens, microbes and irritants. All four classic types of hypersensitivity reactions have been implicated in the pathophysiology of AD including pseudo allergy. They can occur either alone or in combination in AD individuals (Reitamo et al., 2008 & Burns et al., 2004).

AD is a common chronic skin condition associated with high morbidity and major public health implications. As prevention of disease is not yet a real option, reducing morbidity is main aim of treatment. Identifying the underlying pathophysiology of the individual's AD is very crucial. To date no standard test is available to diagnose AD. Sensitization to various allergens is a major part of triggering and perpetuating the inflammatory skin response in AD. Various tests have been developed to investigate the underlying type(s) of hypersensitivity reaction(s) involved in AD patients. None of the available tests so far have proven sensitive and specific enough to identify reliably relevance between clinical disease and test result. Precise understanding of these tests including their limitations together with accurate correlation of patient symptoms and signs are required in order to differentiate between allergy, intolerances and hypersensitivities, and achieve an appropriate clinical diagnosis (Robinson & Smart, 2008).

Allergy tests commonly used in practice include measurement of total levels of IgE and allergen specific IgE levels in serum (radio-allergosorbent test/RAST), skin prick testing (SPT) and atopy patch testing (APT). A different positive predictive cut off point exists for each allergen tested respectively and similar test results do not imply a similar clinical reaction to each allergen (Robinson & Smart, 2008).

SPT is performed to detect the presence of allergen specific IgE to foods, aeroallergens, antibiotics and latex. A drop of a solution containing the allergen is applied to the skin and a lancet used to prick the skin. The allergen binds to IgE on mast cells causing degranulation and the release of histamine. This manifests as a weal and flare reaction, the diameter of which can be measured. SPT is easy to perform and results are immediately available. It can trigger off allergic reactions including anaphylaxis. Various medications including antihistamines, H2-antagonists, tricyclic antidepressants and neuroleptics can interfere with SPT and need to be withheld prior to testing. A positive SPT result indicates only sensitization and does not always equate to clinically relevant allergy. It must be interpreted in the context of clinical history, clinical signs and allergen exposure. The size of the weal does not necessarily correlate with severity of clinical reaction (Robinson & Smart, 2008 & Goodwin, 2008). The RAST detects free allergen specific IgE in serum. It is less sensitive and specific than SPT and is particularly useful where SPT is contraindicated. Testing is available for a wide range of food and environmental allergens. The RAST results are not affected by prior drug use and can be performed in patients with widespread skin disease. The RAST can be reported semi quantitatively as a score or as quantitative measurement by using the CAP RAST technology. The process involves an allergy-impregnated disc being incubated with patient's serum. Allergen specific IgE, if present binds to allergen. The disc is then incubated with radio-labeled anti IgE and radioactivity measured to give level of specific IgE present to particular allergen. Positive RAST results indicate the presence of IgE to an allergen or cross reacting allergen, and are difficult to interpret in the presence of high levels of total IgE (>1000kU/L). Results therefore must always be interpreted in the context of clinical history (Robinson & Smart, 2008 & Goodwin, 2008).

APT is epicutaneous application of inhalant and food allergens on unaffected skin of AD individuals eliciting a delayed, type IV hypersensitivity reaction. It was traditionally developed to investigate association between AD and allergy to aeroallergens and proved in that context to have a higher specificity when compared to SPT and RAST. More recently the APT has been used to supplement the SPT in the diagnosis of food allergy, in an attempt to identify delayed reactions to food products. Reproducibility of APT results raises unsolved issues and is to date poor for most food allergens and good for inhalant allergens. Variables that can strongly influence results are allergen concentration, skin site and devices used for allergen application as well as reading time and/or criteria for defining positive reactions. These variables seem to be specific for each allergen (Lipozencić & Wolf, 2010).

- Allergen concentration not standardized
- Different vehicles used
- Differences in skin sites and pre-treatment of skin
- Differences in reading time and duration of patch testing

Table 1. Factors affecting reproducibility of APT

Patch testing (PT) is an epicutaneous and the gold standard test in the diagnosis of contact allergic dermatitis (CAD). It is not a routine investigation for the diagnosis of AD, but ideal to rule out contact allergy (e.g. to topical medication) in the presence of AD. Recent evidence suggests that CAD is as common in AD individuals as in the general population and PT is recommended in AD patients with recalcitrant disease, hand eczema and in children (Fonacier & Aquino, 2010).

Oral food challenges are the "gold standard" for the diagnosis of food allergy. They can be open, single or double blinded, or placebo controlled. A range of vehicles can be used to disguise food (liquids or solid). Tolerance of a serving size of a food is generally considered evidence of lack of reactivity. In AD oral food challenges should be performed in a double-blind placebo-controlled manner (Robinson & Smart, 2008).

Negative RAST, SPT and APT results have a high negative predictive value and are fairly reliable methods of excluding allergy. Positive results however require careful consideration and correlation with clinical history and clinical presentation (Robinson & Smart, 2008 & Goodwin, 2008).

2.1 Aeroallergens

Clinical manifestations of allergy to aeroallergens involve allergic rhinitis, asthma and exacerbation of AD. Patients with atopic predisposition can express one or all of these clinical manifestations. Filaggrin gene defects have been shown to increase the risk of developing allergic sensitization, AD, and allergic rhinitis (Van den Oord & Sheikh, 2009). A variety of inhalants have been implicated in exacerbations of AD including house dust mite

(HDM), dust mites, HDM feces, animal dander (cat and dog), molds and pollens. Sensitization to aeroallergens appears to be more prevalent in older children and adults, leading to aggravation of AD after bronchial inhalation. Allergen specific T- cells have been identified in affected skin of AD to grass pollen, birch pollen and HDM supporting the concept of a T-cell mediated specific immune response to inhalant allergens with clinical implications. Sensitization to inhalant allergens is thought to occur via skin as well as respiratory route. Allergens penetrate the disturbed epidermal barrier fix on the specific IgE present on LCs and activate them. The activated LCs migrate to a lymph node and present the allergen to T cells, provoking an eczematous reaction. The appearance of eczematous skin lesions is due to cytotoxic T-cell activity and not to the aeroallergen specific IgE. Repeated epicutaneous allergen application has been shown to elicit eczematous lesions in AD individuals (Reitamo et al., 2008 & Goodwin, 2008).

Transcutaneous route
Mite allergen activates LCs via IgE fixation Documented presence of HDM on skin Induction of eczematous lesions following APT
Respiratory route
Flare up of AD following allergen inhalation Induction of new eczematous skin lesions upon allergen inhalation

Table 2. Routes of sensitization aeroallergens in AD

The respiratory route in the induction of new skin lesions may be relevant in a subset of patients with concomitant allergic asthma. Early studies reported that inhalation of house dust or pollen extract can provoke exacerbations of AD. Skin lesions have also been shown to develop in AD individuals after placebo-controlled bronchial provocation of HDM, cat allergen or tree pollen. Aggravation of eczema is more pronounced in AD individuals with concomitant allergic asthma than in patients suffering from AD alone. Two possible explanations have been offered for this phenomenon. Allergen exposed in airways enters the circulation and is transported to skin activating there the inflammatory cascade. Another possibility is allergen induced airway inflammation causes release of mediators from inflammatory cells in skin already primed for AD. Substantial clinical improvement has been reported to occur when sensitized AD individuals are exposed to environments lacking the allergens to which they react (Reitamo et al., 2008& Burns et al., 2004).

Mites belong to the most potent allergen sources and are considered a perennial allergen. Thirteen mite species have been identified in house dust so far, the two commonest mites in homes worldwide include *Dermatophagoides pteronyssimus* and *Dermatophagoides farinae*. Beds and overstuffed furniture are main foci for breeding dust mites. Airborne level of mite allergen during sleep in bedroom is tenfold higher than that found in living rooms of same house during daily activities. Mite allergens persist for months after death of mite. Exposure to high doses of mite allergen in early infancy has been associated with higher incidence of developing eczema. Efforts to create dust mite free environment yielded significant improvement in clinical symptoms although not complete remission. AD patients not sensitized or not exposed to mites benefited as much from exposure to mite free environment as those with mite sensitization and/or exposure.

- Evidence of aeroallergen specific T cells invading the skin
- Presence of aeroallergen specific IgE
- Exacerbation of AD following exposure to aeroallergen
- Exacerbation of AD following epicutaneous aeroallergen application
- New skin lesions induced by APT
- Clinical improvement in aeroallergen poor environment

Table 3. Factors implicating aeroallergens underlying pathomechanism of AD

Many AD patients are highly sensitized to aeroallergens and experience precipitation of AD upon epicutaneous or bronchial allergen exposure. RAST and SPT help to verify or exclude the presence of IgE mediated hypersensitivity, by measurement of allergen specific IgE in serum and evaluation of IgE bound on mast cells. Neither test procedure considers those AD patients characterized by cell-mediated sensitization. The APT was established as a provocation test for a subgroup of AD patients to study the induction of eczema by aeroallergens after 24-72 hours. It is similar to nasal or bronchial provocation test in allergic rhinitis and asthma. Allergen specific IgE is not obligatory for a positive APT reaction. APT has shown a higher specificity towards inhalants (69-92%) when compared to SPT (44-53%) and serum specific IgE (42-64%), suggesting a more appropriate screening role for SPT and RAST in this context. APT does not replace the classical methods of diagnosis of IgE-mediated allergy. APT are usually negative in individuals with respiratory allergy and healthy subjects pointing to AD specific triggering mechanisms required to produce APT positivity. Much effort has been undertaken to standardize APT procedures. The protocol of the European task Force on Atopic Dermatitis (ETFAD) provides a standardized APT technique (Ronchetti et al., 2008).

Despite above impressive data on APT as a diagnostic tool, final scientific proof for the relevance of aeroallergens as identified by positive APT, for clinical manifestation of AD is still missing. The question on how well APT can identify AD patients who would benefit from allergen avoidance remains to be answered.

- Suspicion of aeroallergen symptoms without proof of positive specific IgE or positive SPT
- Severe and/or persistent AD with unknown trigger factors
- Multiple IgE sensitizations without proven clinical relevance in patients with eczema

Table 4. ETFAD consensus on APT indications

In summary sensitization to inhalant allergens is a major contributing factor to the pathogenesis and perpetuation of AD. It is found more commonly in older children and later life of AD individuals and is demonstrated by presence of aeroallergen specific IgE and positive SPT to aeroallergens. Bronchial inhalation challenge, RAST, SPT, and APT to aeroallergens, are the main tests available for investigation. Using these tests in combination and in consideration of clinical history and signs is likely to yield a higher clinically relevant result. Negative results of above investigations are fairly reliable methods of excluding allergy.

2.2 Food allergens

The prevalence of AD and food allergies (FA) appears to have increased in recent years in many western countries. In this context it is important to define the terms. FA and food hypersensitivity (FH) indicate an adverse clinical reaction to food due to interaction of food proteins with one or more immune mechanisms. Food intolerance (FI) is the result of non-immunological reactions to foods and food additives (Reitamo et al., 2008).

• Food allergy due to IgE mediated mechanism (Coombs' classification, type I)
• Food allergy involving other immunological mechanisms (type IV)
• Non-allergic food intolerance (pharmacological, metabolic, or toxic reaction to food)
• Food aversion (often non-specific symptoms, unconfirmed by blinded food challenge)

Table 5. Types of adverse reactions to foods

FA has the greatest incidence in infancy and early childhood. Around 8% of children are thought to develop adverse reactions to food, most of them within the first year of life. The prevalence of FA varies between regions and is influenced by culture and genetic factors. The spectrum of food allergens has remained relatively unchanged despite the rise of FA incidence. Seven food items account for 90% of FA in children. These include cow's milk, egg, peanuts, soybeans, wheat, fish, and tree nuts. By three years of age the majority of children will have developed tolerance to these food items with the exception of peanuts/ tree nuts and seafood. In adults, IgE mediated FA is rare. The main food allergens in adults are peanuts, tree nuts, fish and shellfish (Kim, 2008).

Infants and children	Adults
Cow's milk Egg Peanut Tree nuts Soy Wheat Fish	Peanut Tree nuts Fish Shellfish

Table 6. Major food allergens in children and adults

In general high-protein food allergens are considered to be more allergenic. Most food allergens are water-soluble glycoproteins that are particularly resistant to food processing, cooking and digestion.

Food Item	Protein
Cow's milk	*Caseins* α_1-casein α_2-casein β-casein κ-casein γ-casein *Whey proteins* β-lactoglobulin α-lactalbumin Bovine serum albumin (BSA)
Egg white	Ovomucoid Ovalbumin Ovotransferrin/conalbumin Lysozyme
Peanut	Vicillin Conglutin Glycinin
Soy bean	Gly m 1 Trypsin inhibitor

Table 7. Common food allergens

FA in infancy is thought to be due to a failure of the gastrointestinal tract (GIT) to develop oral tolerance (OT). No down regulation occurs of GIT immune system in its responsiveness towards ingested soluble food antigens. Factors predisposing to impaired OT include increased antigen uptake, decreased production of secretory IgA, and an imbalance towards Th2 response. Other factors include dose and frequency of antigen exposure, biological characteristics of antigens as well as early intestinal inflammation affecting gut permeability and mucosal antigen uptake. IgE sensitization can occur as early as during fetal period and maternally ingested antigens can be excreted in the breast milk. An additional mode of sensitization to food allergens in AD individuals may involve the impaired skin barrier function, so that sensitization to food allergens may occur even though the food in question has not yet been integrated into the diet (Reitamo et al., 2008 & Kim, 2008).

Immunologically triggered FA can clinically present as immediate (oral allergy syndrome, urticaria, angioedema, bronchospasm and anaphylaxis), intermediate (predominantly GIT symptoms), and late-onset reactions (AD flares, development of cough and wheeze).

• Specific food antigen can be identified • Timing of symptoms closely related to food intake • Symptoms can involve more than one organ (oral itching and/or swelling, nausea, vomiting, abdominal pain, diarrhea, asthma, rhinitis, urticaria, angioedema, anaphylaxis) • Positive personal or family history of other atopic disorders

Table 8. Factors suggesting classic IgE mediated food allergy

FA is the earliest manifestation of atopy affecting both breast- and formula-fed infants. Early sensitization to food allergens is typically transient. It affects AD individuals mainly in the first 2 to 3 years but particularly in the first 12 months of life and is often followed by inhalant sensitization as demonstrated by presence of aeroallergen specific IgE and positive SPT to aeroallergens. These may in turn contribute to ongoing eczema later in life (older children and adults). Multiple studies have established that approximately 35% of children with moderate to severe AD have FA. Double-blind placebo-controlled food challenge (DBPCFC) is the gold standard for diagnosis of FA. Children with AD, that were assessed for FA by DBPCFC showed reactions in 40% of challenges. Of the positive challenges skin symptoms occurred in 84% of AD subjects, 56% showed either skin, GIT or respiratory symptoms and only 30% developed isolated skin reactions. Children with positive DBPCFC were younger than those without. Generally, the younger the patient and the more severe the AD, the more likely FA is to be a causative factor (Reitamo et al., 2008 & Kim, 2008). In adults with AD IgE-mediated FA plays only a minor role (1-3%). In this group birch pollen related food allergens have been shown to be a major predisposing factor. In recent years pseudo allergens have been reported to exacerbate symptoms in adults with AD, although it is still controversial if these observations always reflect a true pseudo allergic underlying pathomechanism. Pseudo allergic reactions are more known in the clinical context of urticaria and angioedema. To date no reliable laboratory or skin tests are available to diagnose pseudo allergy, so that for the identification of possible pseudo allergen trigger factors elimination diet and oral challenge are the norm (Reese et al., 2009).

Approximately 85% of AD individuals have specific IgE to food- and aeroallergens, making diagnosis of FA based on laboratory testing alone inadvisable. The importance of a careful history cannot be overemphasized. The history combined with diagnostic tests, should point toward a few possible offending foods or groups of food products. Food allergen specific IgE is a useful tool in the assessment of FA. A different positive predictive cut off point exists for each allergen tested and similar test results do not imply a similar clinical reaction to different allergen. Higher levels of specific IgE indicate increased likelihood of allergic reaction with exposure. Levels though cannot predict the severity of allergic reaction. In general positive RAST results only indicate the presence of IgE to an allergen or cross-reacting allergen and may not correlate with true clinical reactions. Patients with AD can have very high levels of non-specific IgE, which can be detected and give rise to false positive results (Robinson & Smart, 2008 & Goodwin, 2008 & Kim, 2008).

SPT in the diagnosis of FA in infancy is thought to be unreliable. It can provide rapid results with high sensitivity, and has a high negative predictive value (>95%), with a negative skin test essentially excluding IgE- mediated FA. In contrast the positive predictive value is

<50%; suggesting that an isolated positive SPT cannot be predictive for FA. A cut off weal diameter of 6-8mm has been demonstrated to be associated with a positive oral food challenge (predictive value >95%). In this context SPT can reduce the need for oral food challenges by 23% when compared to RAST testing. SPT with fresh fruits and vegetables is a better predictor of clinical relevant reaction in comparison to the use of commercial extracts for SPT (Robinson & Smart, 2008 & Goodwin, 2008 & Kim, 2008).

FA in children with AD is thought to be an IgE- and T-cell mediated phenomenon, making the use of the APT a useful diagnostic tool. Clinical studies have demonstrated the APT to be particularly useful in predicting late-phase clinical reactions. However different studies have published contradicting results regarding sensitivity of unstandardized food APT and further clinical studies are required for standardization and patient group selection for food APT. APT cannot replace oral food challenges. Finally APT in conjunction with positive RAST and positive SPT to food allergens has been shown to reliably predict positive food challenges (Robinson & Smart, 2008 & Goodwin, 2008 & Kim, 2008 & Ronchetti et al., 2008).

In summary, a proper dietary and clinical history combined with available testing are more likely to yield a clinical relevant result. Involvement of a dietitian is paramount in AD patients complaining of FA in order to avoid malnutrition in the long run.

2.3 Microbial allergens

Interaction with environmental microbes may be important in the causation of AD in a number of ways. Early-life exposure may condition maturation of the immune system so that apparent dysregulation associated with IgE production and allergy formation does not occur. The possible role of microbes in the early maturation of the immune system may be the major factor that could explain the differences between western and developing world regarding the incidence of atopy and allergic diseases. Microbes entering via fecal-oral route have been shown to have a greater protective effect against development of allergic diseases than those entering via respiratory route. Early exposure to Hepatitis A virus, *Helicobacter pylori* or *Toxoplasma gondii* has been associated with a reduced risk for atopy by 60%. The burden of exposure of microbial endotoxins in early infancy is thought to play a major role in driving the immune system towards protective responses and away from nuisance responses that are associated with allergy (Burns et al., 2004). A number of observations suggest the relevance of skin flora in clinical manifestation of AD. In individuals with atopic phenotype, eczema may be induced or exacerbated by staphylococcal toxins or by the presence of *Malassezia* yeasts on the skin.

Staphylococcus aureus is found on the skin of 90% of chronic AD individuals, but only on 5% of healthy subjects. When present on healthy normal skin *S. aureus* is usually low in number and mainly confined to intertriginous areas and nasal nares. The presence of *S. aureus* on atopic skin depends on the skin lesion. *S. aureus* has been isolated in 55-75% of clinically unaffected AD skin, 85-91% of chronic lichenified lesions and 80-100% of acute exsudative eczematous lesions. The density of *S. aureus* on acutely inflamed AD skin can be 1000-fold higher than on uninvolved skin in AD individuals suggesting a good correlation between the degree of bacterial colonization and clinical disease severity

The ability of *S. aureus* to cause human disease is dependent on production of cell surface adhesions, antiphagocytic factors and secreted exotoxins, whose function appear to be both securing nutrient for microbes and delaying function of immune system. Among the factors secreted by *S. aureus* is the large family of superantigen exotoxins.

The factors influencing colonization and infection of *S. aureus* in AD skin are not yet well understood and likely to be multifactorial. Defective skin barrier function, reduced content of skin lipids, loss of certain innate antibacterial activities via changes of antibacterial peptides on skin, and a more alkaline pH of skin surface are all thought to play a role in this context. Antimicrobial peptides such as β-defensins and cathelicidins are critical elements of the skin's innate immunity. These peptides eliminate not only *S. aureus*, but also fungal, viral and other bacterial pathogens. The decreased antimicrobial peptide levels in AD skin are not caused by intrinsic defect in keratinocyte production but rather to inhibition mediated by the Th2 cytokine milieu in the AD microenvironment (Schlievert et al., 2008).
Scratching disturbs the epidermal barrier and releases pro-inflammatory cytokines that up regulate the extracellular matrix molecules to act as adhesins to *S. aureus*. Cracks in the skin expose underlying extracellular matrix molecules to *S. aureus* attachment (Reitamo et al., 2008).

- Disturbed skin barrier and function
- Reduced content of skin lipids
- pH of skin surface more alkaline
- Increased adherence of *S. aureus* to skin due to raised fibronectin and fibrinogen (so called adhesins)
- Reduced keratinocyte production of β-defensins and LL-37 (antimicrobial peptides)

Table 9. Factors influencing colonization and infection with *S. aureus* in AD

Staphylococcal super antigens include staphylococcal enterotoxins, classically the common cause of food poisoning and non menstrual toxic shock syndrome (TSS), and TSS toxin1 (TSST-1), the cause of both menstrual and non menstrual TSS. Staphylococcal enterotoxin serotypes A-E (SEA-SEE) and SEG-SEQ are well documented in the literature. Super antigens are defined by their ability to stimulate cytokine release from both T cells and macrophages. They bind directly without antigen processing to constitutively expressed HLD-DR molecules on professional antigen-presenting cells precipitating marked T cell stimulation (Macias et al., 2011).
Most AD individuals show raised specific IgE levels in serum against staphylococcal superantigens and rarely make IgE against constituents of *S. aureus* cell wall. They also demonstrate super antigen specific IgE on their skin. Basophils from patients with superantigen specific IgE release histamine on exposure to relevant superantigen, but not when exposed to super antigens they are not sensitized to. A correlation between presence of superantigen specific IgE and clinical AD severity has been identified and colonization with superantigen producing *S. aureus* is greatest with IgE to staphylococcal superantigen. Skin homing peripheral T cells have also been shown to respond to superantigen and contribute to eosinophilia and IgE production in AD. Epicutaneous application of SEB to unaffected AD skin is followed by exacerbation of eczema suggesting that superantigens can precipitate and sustain the dermal inflammatory cascade in AD individuals. Combined treatment of AD with antibiotics and corticosteroids is more effective than corticosteroid treatment alone suggesting that *S. aureus* secrets products that can induce steroid resistance (Schlievert et al., 2008). In a recent study *S. aureus* strains isolated from steroid resistant AD showed an ability to

produce larger numbers of superantigen types per organism. There was also dysregulated production of super antigens and production of unusual superantigen combinations. Reduction of *S. aureus* on AD skin controls the skin inflammation which predisposes to *S. aureus* colonization and/or infection. Discrepancies in antibiotic sensitivity pattern have been documented among *S. aureus* strains colonizing different sites of AD skin (affected and unaffected) and also in AD individuals with prior antibiotic therapy. Repeat microbial susceptibility testing on different body sites is therefore recommended (Kedzierska et al., 2008).

• Efficacy of topical antiseptic treatment • Efficacy of topical antibiotic therapy • Efficacy of application of gammaglobulins • Efficacy of oral antibiotic and antifungal therapy

Table 10. Relevance of skin flora for AD

In recent years there is an increasing body of evidence suggesting that yeasts particularly of the genera of *Malassezia* and *Candida* can be relevant for AD pathogenesis. Many studies have demonstrated colonization of AD skin with *Malassezia* yeasts with subsequent deterioration of clinical disease (Darabi et al., 2009). *Malassezia* yeasts are members of the normal human skin flora, and often associated with different dermatological disease. The concentration of yeasts on skin does not have to be raised in AD individuals, suggesting that skin barrier dysfunction and typical changes in skin inflammatory response in AD play a major role. Great variation in density and presence of *Malassezia* yeasts in different sites of AD skin has been documented with the highest concentrations affecting the scalp and upper trunk and the lowest on hands. Sensitization to *Malassezia* yeasts have been exclusively demonstrated in AD individuals, via SPT with *Malassezia* extracts and the presence of *Malassezia* specific IgE antibodies. The density of the yeasts reduces with progressing age, although the yeast cells are larger in adults than in children. *Malassezia* specific IgE in serum has been identified in 20-100% of AD subjects depending on trial. Prevalence was highest in adults with head and neck AD (HNAD) and lowest in children with AD. A strong correlation between *Malassezia* specific IgE levels and severity of HNAD has been found, with *Malassezia* specific IgE being a good marker for HNAD (Darabi et al., 2009). Positive SPT to *Malassezia* extracts have been reported in 13.5-79% of AD individuals, compared to small minority in individuals with other *Malassezia* induced skin conditions. This suggests an exclusive presence of *Malassezia* sensitization in AD subjects. *Malassezia* antigens have been used to APT in some trials and positive results were observed in AD patients suggesting a possible role of *Malassezia* yeasts in eliciting and perpetuating eczema in already sensitized AD individuals (Reitamo et al., 2008 & Darabi et al., 2009). *Malassezia* extracts are not yet part of the standardized APT panel provided by ETFAD. No consistent correlation has been shown between HNAD and positive APT. In many trials oral antifungal therapy has been shown to improve clinical manifestations of AD, particularly in the context of HNAD, exacerbations during adolescence and young childhood, severe AD recalcitrant to conventional therapy, and presence of other atopic diseases. It is not clear yet if this is due to the anti-inflammatory effects of antifungals or due to their antifungal properties. Despite the available positive data on *Malassezia* species and AD there is not convincing proof for the importance of this yeast in AD pathogenesis. *Malassezia* sensitization has been reported in both types of AD, extrinsic and intrinsic, and skin barrier dysfunction in AD enabling easier access and therefore cross reactivity between human and fungal manganese superoxide dismutase might be another explanation for the sensitization to *Malassezia* yeasts seen in AD.

Colonization with *Candida albicans* has been found in higher numbers on involved and uninvolved skin of AD individuals than on normal subjects. More importantly colonization of the gastrointestinal tract with *Candida* yeasts was identified in 70% of AD patients compared to 54% of healthy volunteers. 22-94% of AD individuals have shown positive SPT to *C. albicans* and positive correlation existed between the number of positive SPTs and clinical disease severity. *C. albicans* specific IgE has been reported in 25-88% of AD patients and cross reactivity to *Malassezia* has been described. Interestingly PT with *C. albicans* extracts have shown fewer positive results than the healthy controls. In summary the evidence on *C. albicans* is too small to allow any conclusions about its role in AD pathogenesis (Reitamo et al., 2008).

2.4 Autoallergens

IgE autoreactivity has been implicated in the immune pathogenesis and in particular perpetuation of AD. Striking similarities between environmental allergens and human proteins have been identified on molecular analysis of allergens, and IgE-reactive autoantigens against human proteins have been cloned from human epithelial copy DNA expression libraries. Autoantigens have been detected in IgE-mediated immune complexes in serum of AD individuals and release of autoallergens following tissue (skin barrier) damage has been reported. More importantly reduced levels of IgE autoallergen levels have been noted following successful treatment of AD. It is possible that following initiation of the AD immune and inflammatory cascade in skin and peripheral blood by environmental allergens, these mechanisms are then partially perpetuated by autoallergens. More studies are required in the future to allow any sensible conclusion (Reitamo et al., 2008).

2.5 Contact allergens

It is clear that AD individuals are at greater risk in developing irritant contact dermatitis than non-atopic subjects, as contact allergens are likely to penetrate the defective skin barrier more easily. In this context hand eczema has been reported to occur in higher frequency in AD patients. AD individuals, who are particularly employed in occupations involving wetwork are prone to develop an intractable hand dermatitis in their occupational setting leading to considerable occupational disability. Urticaria is frequently encountered in AD individuals, and an allergic basis is found more often in atopic subjects than in the normal population. Contact urticaria of hands may lead to exacerbation of clinical disease in AD particularly in food handlers and slaughterhouse workers (food allergens) as well as health care workers (latex protein sensitivity) (Burns et al., 2004).

There has been dispute about whether atopic individuals are at greater risk to developing contact allergic reactions. CAD has a reported prevalence of as high as 28% in certain European countries, and similarity in clinical symptoms between AD and CAD makes correct diagnosis of CAD a challenge and can easily lead to misdiagnosis. A recent PT study found that a family history of AD (85%), female sex (74%), and age 11-16 (63%) were predisposing risk factors to contact allergen sensitization. Another study evaluating contact sensitization in a series of atopic pediatric patients, that were patch tested, identified 43% positive reactions without commenting on clinical relevance of these reactions (Fonacier & Aquino, 2010 & Jacob S et al., 2008). AD individuals can develop sensitivity to a variety of contact allergens such as topical medicaments including emollients and corticosteroids as well as fragrances, particularly in the presence of recalcitrant periorbital dermatitis. A positive past medical history of AD (44% in patients with periorbital dermatitis) has been found to be a predisposing factor for periorbital dermatitis when compared with all patch-tested individuals (29% with peri-orbital dermatitis). Statistically significantly more patients with AD were found in the group of patients with than without periorbital dermatoses. The periorbital region is a prime location for AD and in consequence a defective skin barrier alleviates sensitization to contact allergens as well as aeroallergens.

Hand eczema and compositae allergy may be more common in AD, whereas allergies to topical corticosteroids and antiseptic solutions are only positive in a small subset of AD patients (15%) (Fonacier & Aquino, 2010).

Oat sensitization and its clinical manifestations in the form of digestive, respiratory and cutaneous symptoms (including CAD) has been identified in 15-20% of AD children, compared to none in the normal population. It is likely to be due to repeated applications of oat proteins through topical emollients and hygiene products on a predisposed impaired epidermal skin barrier of AD individuals. Oat can also be added to the list of food products (e.g. peanut, ovalbumin, almond) responsible for FA triggered by a possible percutaneous sensitization. Avoiding application of topical containing oat protein products in AD infants is paramount in reducing sensitization to oat (Boussault P et al., 2007).

- New-onset dermatitis
- Progression or deterioration of existing dermatitis (AD/Psoriasis)
- Recalcitrant dermatitis by standard therapies
- Clinical presentation of dyshidrosis

Table 11. Factors that make a diagnosis of CAD likely

A lower frequency of positive quinoline allergy has been documented in AD individuals, whereas contact allergy to neomycin among atopic subjects is usually found to be equivalent or slightly raised in comparison to non-AD individuals. AD subjects appear to have increased efficiency in orally tolerising haptens but are inefficient in orally tolerising proteins. The reduced contact allergy to quinoline in AD patients might be explained by a higher exposure of haptens in the gut and skin at a young age producing "hapten"-tolerance (McFadden & White, 2008).

History for CAD should always include the patient's personal hygiene environment, medical and medicament history as well as home and care giver environment. PT should be performed in all AD patients where CAD is considered and particularly in children with AD. However because of irritancy interpretation of PT may be difficult in AD individuals and the severity of AD might have an impact on the results obtained through PT. PT should always include the emollients used.

In summary more and more studies suggest, that CAD might occur as common in AD individuals and particularly in children with AD as in the general population.

Consideration of CAD is recommended in each case of recurrent and recalcitrant clinical disease, and PT should be considered and offered to AD patients in those circumstances. However the relevance between a positive PT reaction and clinical severity of AD remains to be answered.

3. Conclusion

AD is a common chronic skin condition associated with high morbidity and major public health implications. As prevention of disease is not yet a real option, reducing morbidity is main aim of treatment. Identifying the underlying pathomechanism of the individual's AD is very crucial. High levels of specific IgE antibodies and or total IgE levels in serum are significantly associated with severity of dermatitis in individuals with the extrinsic type of AD. Raised specific IgE antibodies can be detected in the peripheral blood for most trigger factors and allergens. Food and aeroallergens, microbes including *S. aureus* and *Malassezia* yeasts, contact allergens and autoallergens have been identified to trigger AD and perpetuate so the underlying immune and inflammatory cascade of AD.

To date no standard test is available to diagnose AD. Sensitization to various allergens is a major part of triggering and perpetuating the inflammatory skin response in AD. Various tests have been developed to investigate the underlying type(s) of hypersensitivity reaction involved in AD patients. None of the available tests so far have proven sensitive and specific enough to identify reliably relevance between clinical reaction and test result. Allergy tests commonly used in practice include measurement of total levels of IgE and allergen specific IgE levels in serum (RAST), SPT, APT, PT and DBPCFC.

Precise understanding of these tests including their limitations together with accurate correlation of patient history, symptoms and signs are required in order to differentiate between allergy, intolerances and hypersensitivities, and achieve an appropriate clinical diagnosis. Results must always be interpreted in the context of clinical history.

In a recent meta-analysis filaggrin gene defects have shown to increase the risk of developing allergic sensitization, AD, and allergic rhinitis. The presence of filaggrin gene mutations correlated strongly with disease severity and treatment failure, and also increased the risk of asthma in AD patients. Gene testing for filaggrin gene mutations might be an additional way to identify atopic individuals in future. Restoring skin barrier function in filaggrin deficient individuals early in life may help prevent the development of sensitization and halt the development and progression of allergic disease.

4. References

Boussault P et al. (2007). *Oat sensitization in children with atopic dermatitis: prevalence risks and associated factors* Allergy 2007: 62: 1251–1256

Burns T, Brethnach S, Cox N, Griffiths C (2004). *Rook's Textbook of Dermatology,* (7th ed. Chapter 18). Blackwell Publishing. ISBN 0-632-06429-3

Czarnobilska Ket al (2010). *A half of school children with "ISAAC eczema" are ill with allergic contact dermatitis.* J Eur Acad Dermatol Venereol; 4.

Darabi K et al. (2009). *The role of Malassezia in atopic dermatitis affecting the head and neck of adults.* J Am Acad Dermatol;60(1):125-36

Fonacier LS, Aquino MR (2010). *The role of contact allergy in atopic dermatitis.* Immunol Allergy Clin North Am;30(3):337-50

Goodwin H (2008). *Eczema and allergy: how useful is allergy testing?* Paediatr Nurs; 20(10): 25-30

Jacob S et al.(2008) *Patch testing: Another steroid-sparing agent to consider in children.* Paed Dermatol;25 (1):81-87

Kedzierska A et al. (2008). *Susceptibility testing and resistance phenotype detection in Staphylococcus aureus strains isolated from patients with atopic dermatitis, with apparent and recurrent skin colonization.* Br J Dermatol;159(6):1290-9

Kim JS (2008). *Paediatric atopic dermatitis: The importance of food allergens.* Semin Cutan Med Surg;27(2):156-60

Lipozencić J, Wolf R (2010). *The diagnostic value of atopy patch testing and skin prick testing in atopic dermatitis:facts and controversies.* Clin Dermatol;28(1):38-44

Macias ES et al (2011) *Superantigens in dermatology,* J Am Acad Dermatol;64(3):455-72

McFadden JP, White JM (2008). *Reduced frequency of atopic dermatitis quinoline-allergic patients: the "hapten-atopy hypothesis".* Contact Dermatitis.;58(5):291-5

Most tables in the text have been taken from Reitamo S, Luger TA, Steinhoff M (2008). Textbook of Atopic Dermatitis, (Chapters 3-5 and 7-9) Informa healthcare, ISBN 978-1-84184-246-2

Reese I et al (2009). *Diagnostic approach for suspected peudoallergic reaction to food ingredients.* J Dtsch Dermatol Ges;7(1):70-7

Reitamo S, Luger TA, Steinhoff M (2008). *Textbook of Atopic Dermatitis,* (Chapters 3-5 and 7-9) Informa healthcare, ISBN 978-1-84184-246-2

Robinson M, Smart J (2008). *Allergy testing in children,* Aust Fam Physician.;37(4):210-3

Ronchetti R et al. (2008). *Reproducibility of atopy patch tests with food and inhalant allergens.* J Biol Regul Homeost Agents;22(1):27-33

Schlievert PM et al. (2008). *Superantigen Profile of Staphylococcus aureus Isolates from Patients with Steroid-Resistant AtopicDermatitis.* Clin Infect Dis;15;46(10):1562-7

Van den Oord RA, Sheikh A (2009). *Filaggrin gene defects and risk of developing allergic sensitisation and allergic disorders: systematic review and meta-analysis.* Brit Med J;339:b2433

13

Physical and Chemical Factors that Improve Epidermal Permeability Barrier Homeostasis

Mitsuhiro Denda
Shiseido Research Center
Japan

1. Introduction

For terrestrial creatures, the water-impermeable barrier function of the skin is essential to maintain life in the face of environmental dryness. Stratum corneum, which plays a crucial role in the barrier function, is composed of two components, i.e., protein-rich nonviable cells and intercellular lipid domains. When the barrier function is damaged by a surfactant, organic solvent or tape stripping, a series of homeostatic systems operates to restore the barrier function to its original level. At the first stage of the barrier repair process, exocytosis of lipid-containing granules, lamellar bodies, is accelerated and the internal lipid is secreted into the intercellular domain between the stratum granulosum and stratum corneum, forming a water-impermeable membrane.

The barrier function is strongly associated with skin pathology. Abnormality of the barrier function is observed in a variety of skin diseases, such as atopic dermatitis. Although the barrier function of healthy skin can recover automatically after damage, the recovery is delayed by emotional stress or by aging. Moreover, under low environmental humidity, barrier damage induces epidermal hyperplasia and inflammation.

On the other hand, acceleration of the barrier recovery prevents epidermal hyperplasia induced by barrier disruption in a dry environment. Thus, methods to improve the barrier function are very important for clinical dermatology. In the last two decades, various chemical and physical factors that accelerate the barrier recovery process have been reported. In this chapter, I will describe those findings and discuss some new biological aspects of epidermal barrier function.

2. Physical factors that influence barrier function

2.1 Temperature

2.1.1 Exposure to high temperature for one hour

Since the end of the last century, a series of thermo-activated receptors, called the transient receptor potential protein (TRP) superfamily, has been found in the peripheral nervous system and cloned. Julius and his co-workers found TRPV1 (VR1) as a polymodal detector of pain-producing heat (>43°C) or chemicals, such as capsaicin and protons, in primary afferent neurons (Caterina et al. 1997). We showed that TRPV1 is also expressed in human epidermal keratinocytes (Denda et al. 2001), and demonstrated its functional activity in human cultured keratinocytes (Inoue et al. 2002). Subsequently, TRPV3 (Peier 2002a) and

TRPV4 (Chung et al. 2003), both of which are activated by high temperature (around 30°C), were also found to be expressed in keratinocytes.

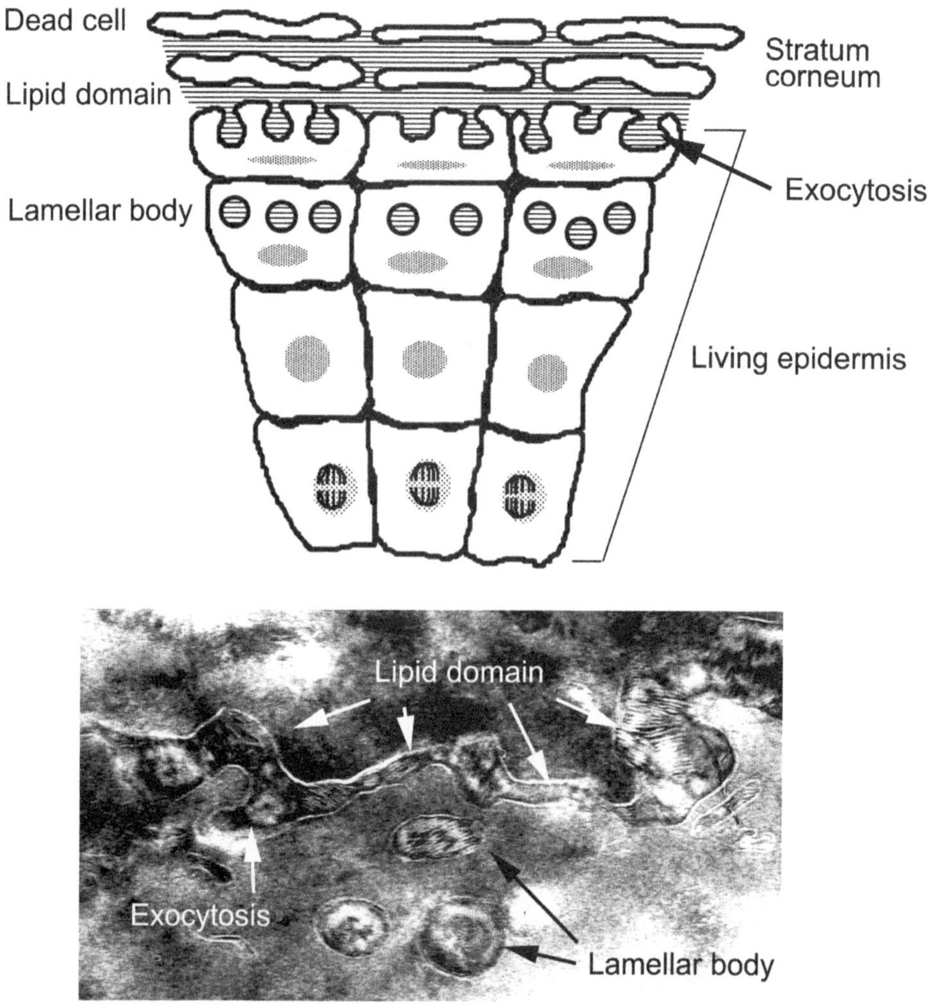

Fig. 1. Schematic diagram of skin (top) and photomicrograph illustrating the skin structures (bottom).

We have shown that changes of calcium dynamics are associated with epidermal permeability barrier homeostasis [Denda 2003a]. TRPs are cation-permeable channels. Thus, we hypothesized that activation of TRPs might influence barrier homeostasis. To evaluate the influence of these receptors on barrier homeostasis, we incubated hairless mouse skin and human skin at various temperatures immediately after tape stripping

(Denda 2007). At temperatures from 36°C to 40°C, barrier recovery was accelerated in both species compared with the area kept at 34°C. At 34°C or 42°C, barrier recovery at occluded sites was delayed compared with un-occluded sites. Topical application of 4α-phorbol 12,13-didecanone, an activator of TRPV4, accelerated barrier recovery, while ruthenium red, a blocker of TRPV4, delayed it. Capsaicin, an activator of TRPV1, delayed barrier recovery, while capsazepin, an antagonist of TRPV1, blocked this delay. 2-Aminoethoxydiphenyl borate and camphor, TRPV3 activators, did not affect the barrier recovery rate. Since TRPV4 is activated at about 35°C and above, while TRPV1 is activated at about 42°C and above, these results suggest that TRPV1 and TRPV4 both influence skin permeability barrier homeostasis.

2.1.2 Exposure to low temperature for one minute

Previous studies have identified cold-sensitive proteins, TRPA1 and TRPM8, that are activated by low temperature (<22°C) in peripheral nerve cells [Story 2003][Peier 2002b]. Recently, TRPA1 was also found in epidermal cells, in which it is activated by lower temperature (<17°C) [Atoyan 2009]. We demonstrated that exposure of cultured human keratinocytes to low temperature induced elevation of intracellular calcium [Tsutsumi 2010]. When the temperature of the medium was reduced to 17~22°C, elevation of intracellular calcium was observed. The extent of elevation was greater in non-differentiated cells than in differentiated cells. Application of Ruthenium Red (a non-selective TRP blocker) and HC030031 (a specific antagonist of TRPA1) reduced the elevation. These results suggest that functional cold-sensitive calcium channels, TRPA1and/or TRPM8, are present in human epidermal keratinocytes. Thus, we hypothesized that modulation of TRPA1 and/or TRPM8 might influence epidermal permeability barrier homeostasis.

To test this idea, we first examined the effects of topical application of agonists of TRPA1 and brief cold exposure on the barrier recovery rate after barrier disruption [Denda 2010a]. Topical application of a TRPA1 agonist, allyl isothiocyanate or cinnamaldehyde, accelerated the barrier recovery after tape stripping. The effect of both agonists was blocked by HC030031, an antagonist of TRPA1. Brief exposure (1 minute) to cold (10-15°C) also accelerated barrier recovery and this acceleration was also blocked by HC030031. Electron-microscopic studies indicated that brief cold exposure accelerated lamellar body secretion between stratum corneum and stratum granulosum, while pre-treatment with HC030031 inhibited the secretion. These results support the hypothesis that TRPA1 is associated with epidermal permeability barrier homeostasis.

We next examined the effect of topical application of TRPM8 modulators on epidermal permeability barrier homeostasis [Denda 2010b]. Immunohistochemical study and RT-PCR confirmed the expression of TRPM8 or TRPM8-like protein in epidermal keratinocytes. Topical application of TRPM8 agonists, menthol and WS 12, accelerated barrier recovery after tape stripping. The effect of WS12 was blocked by a non-selective TRP antagonist, Ruthenium Red, and a TRPM8-specific antagonist, BTCT. Topical application of WS12 also reduced epidermal proliferation associated with barrier disruption under low humidity, and this effect was blocked by BTCT. Our results indicate that TRPM8 or a closely related protein in epidermal keratinocytes plays a role in epidermal permeability barrier homeostasis and epidermal proliferation after barrier insult.

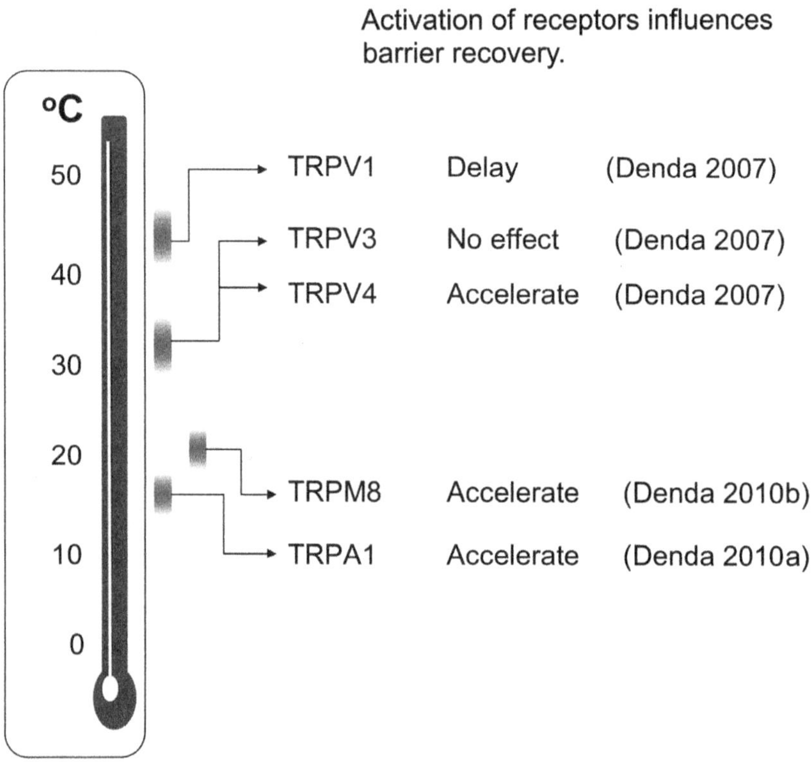

Fig. 2. Temperature ranges within which various TRP receptors are activated, and effect of their activation on epidermal permeability barrier homeostasis.

2.2 Visible light

The effects of ultraviolet or infrared radiation on skin are well known, but only a few reports describe the effect of visible radiation. We have shown that visible radiation influences the epidermal barrier recovery rate after barrier disruption (Denda & Fuziwara 2008). The effects of visible radiation on epidermal permeability barrier recovery were evaluated by using light-emitting diodes as light sources. The flank skin of hairless mice was tape-stripped, and immediately exposed to blue (430-510 nm), green (490-560 nm), red (550-670 nm) or white (400-670 nm) light (20 W each) for 1 hour, followed by measurement of transepidermal water loss. Control mice were kept in a dark box during the experiments. During the irradiation, the skin surface temperature was kept constant at 37°C in all mice. Irradiation with red light significantly accelerated barrier recovery, while irradiation with blue light delayed it, compared with the control. White or green light did not affect the barrier recovery rate. We next carried out a study using hairless mouse skin organ culture. The permeability barrier was disrupted by means of acetone treatment, then each section was incubated afloat on the medium (37°C) and irradiated with blue, red or white light (20 w) for one hour. Immediately after the end of irradiation, we evaluated the barrier function. Again, red light accelerated barrier recovery, while blue light delayed it. An electron-microscopic study suggested that red light accelerated lamellar body secretion, while blue light blocked it. These results indicate that visible radiation affects skin barrier homeostasis. That is, epidermal keratinocytes might have a sensory system for visible radiation.

Rhodopsin is a well-known photosensitive protein found in rod cells of the retina and detects light/dark contrast. Cone opsins are also photosensitive receptors in the cone cells of the retina and detect color. We have reported immunochemical studies using anti-rhodopsin and anti-opsin antibodies on human skin (Tsutsumi 2009). Both mouse retina and human epidermis showed clear immunoreactivity with each antibody. Interestingly, immunoreactivity against longer-wavelength opsin antibody was observed in the basal layer of the epidermis, while immunoreactivity against rhodopsin and shorter-wavelength opsin was observed in the upper layer. PCR analysis confirmed the expression of rhodopsin-like and opsin-like genes in human retina and skin. These results suggest that a series of proteins, which play a crucial role in visual perception, are also expressed in human epidermis.

In retina, transducin and phosphodiesterase 6 play key roles in signal transmission. Thus, we hypothesized that these proteins might exist in epidermal keratinocytes and be associated with barrier homeostasis (Goto 2011). Immunohistochemical study and reverse transcription-PCR assays confirmed the expression of both transducin and phosphodiesterase 6 in epidermal keratinocytes. Topical application of 3-isobutyl-1-methylxanthine, a non-specific phosphodiesterase inhibitor, blocked the acceleration of barrier recovery by red light. Topical application of zaprinast, a specific inhibitor of phosphodiesterases 5 and 6, also blocked the acceleration, while T0156, a specific inhibitor of phosphodiesterase 5, had no effect. Red-light exposure reduced the epidermal hyperplasia induced by barrier disruption under low humidity, and the effect was blocked by pretreatment with zaprinast. Our results indicate phosphodiesterase 6 is involved in the recovery-accelerating effect of red light on the disrupted epidermal permeability barrier. Also, epidermal keratinocytes have a similar energy conversion system to that of the retina.

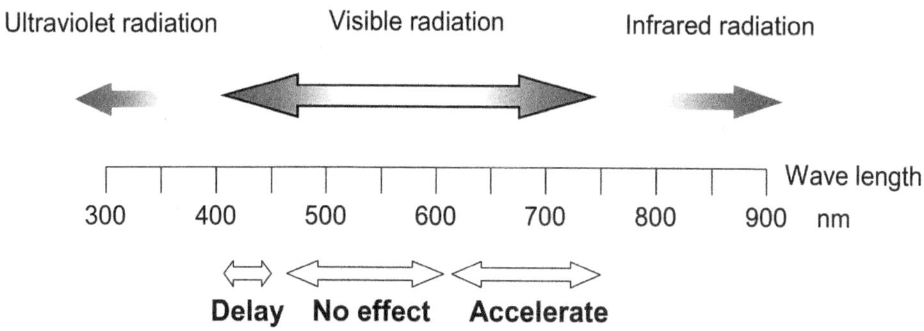

Fig. 3. Effects of visible radiation on epidermal permeability barrier homeostasis.

2.3 Sound

The frequency range of audible acoustic sound for adult humans is approximately 20-16000 Hz (Heffner 2004). However, Oohashi and his coworkers demonstrated that ultrasound at a frequency above 20000 Hz (20 kHz) influences human brain electrical activity and systemic hormonal levels (Oohashi 2000)(Oohashi 2006)(Kawai 2001)(Yagi 2003). Interestingly, these effects did not involve the ear (Oohashi 2006). On the other hand, recent work has demonstrated that a slight, inaudible puff of air on the skin influences auditory perception (Gick & Derrick 2009). These results suggest that an unknown system that is responsive to ultrasound exists at the human body surface. Based on these findings, we considered that audible or inaudible sound frequencies might influence epidermal barrier homeostasis.

First, we evaluated the effects of 5, 10, 20 and 30 kHz sound on intact skin of hairless mice (Denda & Nakatani 2010). We disrupted the permeability barrier by tape stripping and immediately exposed the skin to sound for one hour. The speaker cone lightly touched one side of the flank, and we attached a silent speaker cone to the other flank as a control. Application of sound at a frequency of 10, 20 or 30 kHz accelerated barrier recovery, while 5 kHz sound had no effect. The effects on barrier recovery were observed 23 hours after cessation of the sound application.

To determine whether the effect was induced by sound or skin vibration, we next placed the speaker 1 or 3 cm away from the skin surface. In this case, too, significant acceleration of the barrier recovery by sound was observed. The sound pressure levels were 0 cm: 83 dB, 1 cm: 78 dB, 3 cm: 70 dB.

We also evaluated the effect of different sound pressures on the barrier recovery rate. The sound source was placed 1 cm away from the skin surface, and the frequency was 20 kHz. The barrier recovery rate increased with increasing sound pressure. An electron-microscopic study indicated that exposure to sound at a frequency of 20 kHz accelerated lamellar body secretion between stratum corneum (SC) and stratum granulosum (SG). These results indicate that epidermis might have an unknown system for sensing sound.

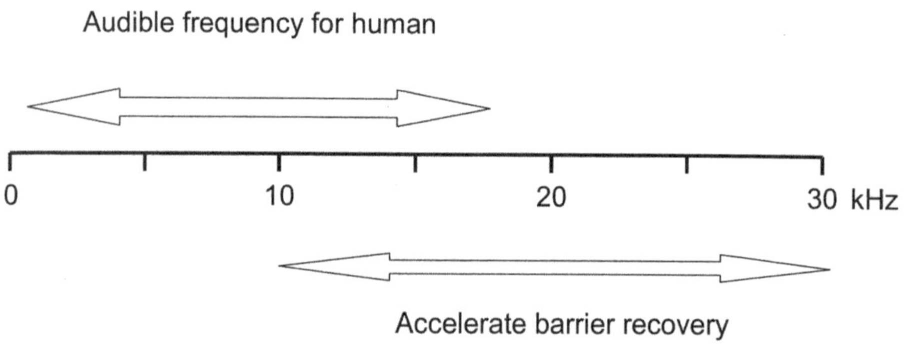

Fig. 4. Effects of sound on epidermal permeability barrier homeostasis

2.4 Electrical potential

It has been demonstrated that cultured human keratinocytes migrate to the negative pole in direct current electrical fields (Nishimura 1996). This result suggested that keratinocytes might have a sensory system for the external electrical field. Thus, we hypothesized that external electrical potential would influence epidermal barrier homeostasis. We applied negative and positive direct electric potential (0.5 V) to hairless mouse flank skin immediately after barrier disruption for one hour, and then we evaluated barrier recovery by the measurement of transepidermal water loss. At the area of applied negative potential, the barrier recovery rate was significantly accelerated, while the recovery was delayed at the area of positive applied potential (Denda & Kumazawa 2002).

We subsequently found that several interfacial electrical conditions also affect barrier homeostasis. For example, topical application of barium sulfate or aqueous solution of ionic polymers formed an electrical double layer on the skin surface and affected the barrier recovery rate (Fuziwara 2004)(Denda 2005). Moreover, just placing metals on the skin surface after barrier disruption accelerated the barrier recovery, presumably because free electrons were supplied from metal to the skin surface (Denda & Kumazawa 2010). When chemically different materials are in contact, electro-chemical phenomena, such as formation of an electrical double layer, are induced. We previously demonstrated that a voltage-gated calcium channel is expressed at the upper layer of the epidermis (Denda 2006). Thus, when the skin touches other materials, physiological phenomena might be induced.

3. Chemical factors that influence barrier function

3.1 Ions

Lipid metabolism is regulated by a series of enzymes in the epidermis (Feingold & Elias 2000) and each of them has optimal conditions of pH (Mauro 1998), concentrations of other ions (Denda 1999), etc. for activity. For example, the pH value of the healthy stratum corneum is kept acidic because the lipid-processing enzymes have an acidic optimal pH. Mauro et al. demonstrated that topical application of a basic buffer after barrier disruption delayed the repair process because the basic condition perturbed lipid processing (Mauro 1998).

It has also been shown that topical application of calcium or potassium reduced barrier repair [Lee 1992], while magnesium and a mixture of calcium and magnesium salts accelerated the repair process [Denda 1999]. Topical application of an aqueous solution containing 10 mM magnesium chloride, magnesium sulfate, and magnesium lactate accelerated barrier repair. Application of magnesium bis(dihydrogen phosphate) or magnesium chloride in PBS solution did not affect the barrier recovery rate. Application of 10 mM calcium chloride aqueous solution delayed barrier repair, but a mixture of calcium chloride and magnesium chloride accelerated it when the calcium-to-magnesium molar ratio was lower than 1. Application of the mixture also improved the condition of dry, scaly skin induced by SDS treatment. These results suggest that ions are important in barrier homeostasis.

3.2 Hexose

Hexose is known to influence the stability of phospholipid bilayers. Therefore, the effects of topical application of all 12 stereoisomers of dextro-hexose on the epidermal barrier recovery rate after barrier disruption were evaluated (Denda 2011). Immediately after tape stripping, a 0.1 M aqueous solution of each hexose was applied on hairless mouse skin. Among the 8 dextro-aldohexoses, topical application of altose, idose, mannose and talose accelerated barrier recovery, while allose, galactose, glucose and gulose had no effect. Among the 4 dextro-ketohexoses, psicose, fructose, sorbose and tagatose all accelerated barrier recovery. Because the effects of hexoses on the barrier recovery rate appeared within one hour, the mechanism is unlikely to be genomic. Instead, these hexoses may influence phase transition of the lipid bilayers of lamellar bodies and cell membrane, a crucial step in epidermal permeability barrier homeostasis.

3.3 Physiological lipids

Lipids play a crucial role in the water-impermeable barrier function of the skin. Damaged barrier function can be restored by topical application of a water-impermeable substance such as petrolatum (Man 1995). In this case, the petrolatum stays in the stratum corneum and forms a water-impermeable membrane. However, Man et al. demonstrated that a topically applied mixture of stratum corneum lipids, i.e., ceramide, cholesterol and free fatty acids, was incorporated in the nucleated layer of epidermis and accelerated repair of the barrier function after damage (Man 1996). They were the first to report a method to accelerate the barrier recovery by regulating endogenous factors in the epidermis. Interestingly, when they applied ceramide, cholesterol, or free fatty acid alone, or a mixture of two of these, the barrier recovery was delayed. Only when they applied a mixture of all three lipids at a specific relative ratio was the barrier recovery accelerated (Man 1996). These results suggest that a balance of the three lipids is crucial for skin barrier homeostasis.

Physical factors	Accelerate barrier recovery	Delay barrier recovery
Temperature (Denda 2007)	36~40°C (1 hour)	>42°C
(Denda 2010a,b)	10~15°C (1 min)	
Visible light (Denda 2008)	Red (550~670 nm)	Blue (430~510 nm)
Electrical potential (Denda&Kumazawa 2002)	Negative	Positive
Sound (Denda&Nakatani 2010)	10~30 kHz	
Chemical factors		
Ionic polymers (Denda 2005)	sodium salt anionic	cationic
Barium sulphate (Fuziwara 2004)	ζ negative	ζ positive
Metal (Denda& Kumazawa 2010)	Pt, Au, Ag, In, Zr, Sm	
Ions (Lee 1991) (Denda 1999)	magnesium	calcium, potassium
Hexose (Denda 2011)	most hexoses	
Physiological lipids balanced mixture (Man 1996)	balanced mixture	unbalanced mixture

Table 1. Summary of the effects of physical, chemical and biological factors on skin permeability barrier recovery.

In the case of aging, different treatment might be necessary because of the different metabolism of aged skin. Ghadially et al. demonstrated that skin barrier function in elderly subjects was destroyed more easily than that in young individuals (Ghadially 1995). Moreover, the barrier recovery rate after barrier disruption was significantly slower for the elderly subjects than for younger ones. The same tendency was observed in both humans and hairless mice. They also suggested that synthesis of cholesterol is reduced more than that of other lipids, i.e., ceramide and fatty acids, in aged mice. The delay of barrier recovery with aging was improved by topical application of cholesterol (Ghadially 1996) or mevalonic acid (Haratake 2000), presumably because the delay of the aged skin was caused by a decrease of cholesterol synthesis.

4. Biochemical factors that influence barrier function

4.1 Endocrine factors

Sex hormones are strongly associated with epidermal permeability barrier homeostasis (Hanley 1996). Moreover, when the balance of these hormones alters at menopause or during the menstrual cycle, skin sensitivity or barrier function is changed. These results suggest that the relative composition of hormones influences barrier function and skin sensitivity. We recently studied the effects of topical application of sex hormones on the permeability barrier recovery rate of hairless mice after tape stripping (Tsutusmi and Denda 2007). Application of androgens, testosterone and androsterone, delayed barrier recovery. The delay was blocked by application of beta-estradiol. Application of progesterone also delayed barrier recovery. However, the delay was enhanced by the application of beta-estradiol. These results suggest that the alteration of the sex hormone balance at menopause or during the estradiol cycle might be the cause of skin problems at the corresponding period of time.

4.2 Neurotransmitters

Epidermal keratinocytes express a series of receptors, which were originally found in the central nervous system as neurotransmitter receptors. These receptors can be categorized two groups: ionotropic receptors and G-protein-coupled receptors.

Among the former group, receptors that act as calcium ion or chloride ion permeable channels plays crucial roles in epidermal permeability barrier homeostasis. Topical application of calcium channel agonists delays barrier recovery, while antagonists accelerate barrier repair (Denda et al. 2002a) (Denda 2003) (Fuziwara 2003). Topical application of chloride ion channel agonists accelerates barrier recovery (Denda 2003) (Denda 2002b).

The G-protein coupled receptors influence intracellular cAMP level, which plays a crucial role in epidermal barrier homeostasis (Denda 2003b). Increase of intracellular cAMP in epidermal keratinocytes by topical application of forskolin delays barrier recovery, while cAMP antagonist treatment accelerates barrier recovery. Activation of dopamine 2-like receptors (Fuziwara 2005), melatonin receptors, and serotonin receptor (type 5-HT1) decreases intracellular cAMP and consequently accelerates barrier recovery, while activation of adrenergic β2 receptors increases the intracellular cAMP and delays barrier repair (Denda 2003b). Barrier disruption induces an increase of intracellular cAMP. Thus, topical application of agonists of receptors that reduce the intracellular cAMP level accelerates barrier repair. (Denda 2004, Denda 2005)

Histamine receptors are related to skin barrier function [Ashida and Denda 2001]. Three different types of histamine receptors, H1, H2, H3, and H4 have been reported. First, topical application of histamine H1 and H2 receptor antagonists accelerated barrier repair. Histamine itself, H2 receptor agonist, and histamine releaser delayed barrier repair. Histamine H3 receptor antagonist and agonist did not affect the barrier recovery rate. Topical application of H1 and H2 receptor antagonists prevented the epidermal hyperplasia induced by barrier disruption under low humidity. The mechanism of the interactions between the histamine receptors and the barrier repair process have not been elucidated yet

Nitric oxide (NO) is also involved in barrier homeostasis. We first demonstrated that neuronal nitric oxide synthase knockout (nNOS-/-) mice showed a faster barrier recovery rate than did wild-type mice. nNOS is expressed in epidermal keratinocytes [Ormerod 1998]. Thus, NO generated by keratinocytes might delay barrier repair. To examine this possibility, we next evaluated the effects of NO donor and NOS inhibitor on the barrier recovery rate. Topical application of a NO donor, S-nitroso-N-acetyl-D,L-penicillamine delayed barrier recovery. The application of a nNOS inhibitor accelerated barrier recovery, while the application of a inducible nitric oxide synthase (iNOS) inhibitor did not affect it. Moreover, topical application of a guanylyl cyclase inhibitor accelerated barrier recovery. We observed the release of NO from a skin organ culture after barrier disruption. Thus, regulation of nNOS in epidermal keratinocytes might be useful approach to improve barrier homeostasis (Ikeyama 2007).

Ionotropic receptors	Accelerate Barrier Recovery	Delay Barrier Recovery
P2X receptor (Denda 2002a)	Antagonist	Agonist
NMDA receptor (Fuziwara 2003)	Antagonist	Agonist
Cholinergic receptor (Denda 2003)	Antagonist	Agonist
GABA(A) receptor (Denda 2002b)	Agonist	-
Glycine receptor (Denda 2003)	Agonist	-
G-Protein coupled receptors		
Adrenergic β2 receptor (Denda 2003b)	Antagonist	Agonist
Dopamine 2-like receptor (Fuziwara 2005)	Agonist	Antagonist
Serotonin receptor (Denda 2005)	Agonist	-
Melatonin receptor (Denda 2005)	Agonist	-

No effect, or experiment has not been done.

Table 2. Effects of agonists and antagonists of neurotransmitter receptors on skin permeability barrier recovery.

Ryanodine receptors (RyR) play an important role as calcium channels in the regulation of intracellular calcium levels in the nervous system and muscles. We investigated the expression of RyR in human epidermis. (Denda 2011) Immunohistochemical studies and RT-PCR indicated the expression of RyR type 1, 2, and 3 proteins in epidermal keratinocytes. The expression level of each RyR subtype was higher in differentiating keratinocytes than in proliferative cells. We also demonstrated the functional expression of RyR by means of calcium imaging. In cultured human keratinocytes, application of the RyR agonist 4-chloro-*m*-cresol (CMC) induced elevation of the intracellular calcium concentration and co-application of the RyR antagonist 1,1′-diheptyl-4,4′-bipyridinium dibromide (DHBP) blocked the elevation. Application of CMC accelerated keratinocyte differentiation *in vitro*. On the other hand, topical application of CMC after tape-stripping of hairless mouse skin delayed barrier recovery, while application of an RyR antagonist, dantrolene or DHBP, accelerated the barrier recovery. These results suggest that RyR expressed in epidermal keratinocytes is associated with both differentiation of keratinocytes and epidermal barrier homeostasis (Denda S 2011).

4.3 Protease inhibitors

Topical application of specific protease inhibitors accelerates barrier recovery after barrier disruption (Denda 1997). Topical application of 4-(aminomethyl)cyclohexane carboxylic acid (tranexamic acid), a well known anti-plasmin reagent, also accelerates barrier recovery. In contrast, inactive analogs of tranexamic acid do not influence barrier recovery. Application of several trypsin-like serine protease inhibitors, e.g., leupeptin, TLCK and PMSF, accelerates barrier recovery, while other protease inhibitors, e.g., EDTA, pepstatin, N-ethylmaleimide, chymostatin, and TPCK, have no effect on barrier recovery. Although the mechanism was not clarified, it was shown that protease activated receptor type 2 is associated with barrier homeostasis (Hachem 2006).

4.4 Nuclear hormone receptor activators

Feingold and his co-workers demonstrated an important influence of nuclear hormone receptors on epidermal differentiation and stratum corneum barrier formation. Activation of PPARα by farnesol stimulated the differentiation of epidermal keratinocytes (Feingold 1999)(Hanley 2000). Cornified envelope formation and involucrin and transglutaminase protein and mRNA levels were also increased by the activation of PPARα (Feingold 2000). Interestingly, the inflammatory response was also inhibited (Sheu 2002). Topical application of PPARα activators accelerated barrier recovery after tape stripping or acetone treatment and prevented the epidermal hyperplasia induced by repeated barrier disruption (Feingold 1999). Regulation of nuclear hormone receptors might therefore be a possible approach for improvement of the cutaneous barrier.

5. Psychological factors that influence barrier function

As described above, psychological stress impairs barrier homeostasis. To study the effects of stress on barrier homeostasis, we used three models of stress, i.e., immobilization, a crowded environment and a change of living place [Denda 1998][Denda 2000]. In each case, the barrier recovery rate was delayed after barrier disruption. The plasma corticosterone level was increased by each stress, and it was reduced by application of a sedative drug [Denda 2000]. The delay of barrier repair induced by psychological stress was also prevented by application of a sedative drug or glucocorticoid receptor antagonist [Denda 2000]. These results suggest that psychological stress stimulates increased production of glucocorticoids, which adversely affect skin barrier homeostasis. The effect of psychological stress on skin barrier homeostasis in humans has also been examined [Garg 2001]. Reduction of psychological stress might accelerate the skin barrier repair process. Several studies have demonstrated that certain odorants can reduce stress, acting like a sedative drug [Tsuchiya 1992]. These odorants prevented the delay in skin barrier recovery induced by psychological stress in both mice and humans [Denda 2000a][Denda 2000b]. These results suggest the feasibility of a new skin care strategy based on inhalation of specific odorants.

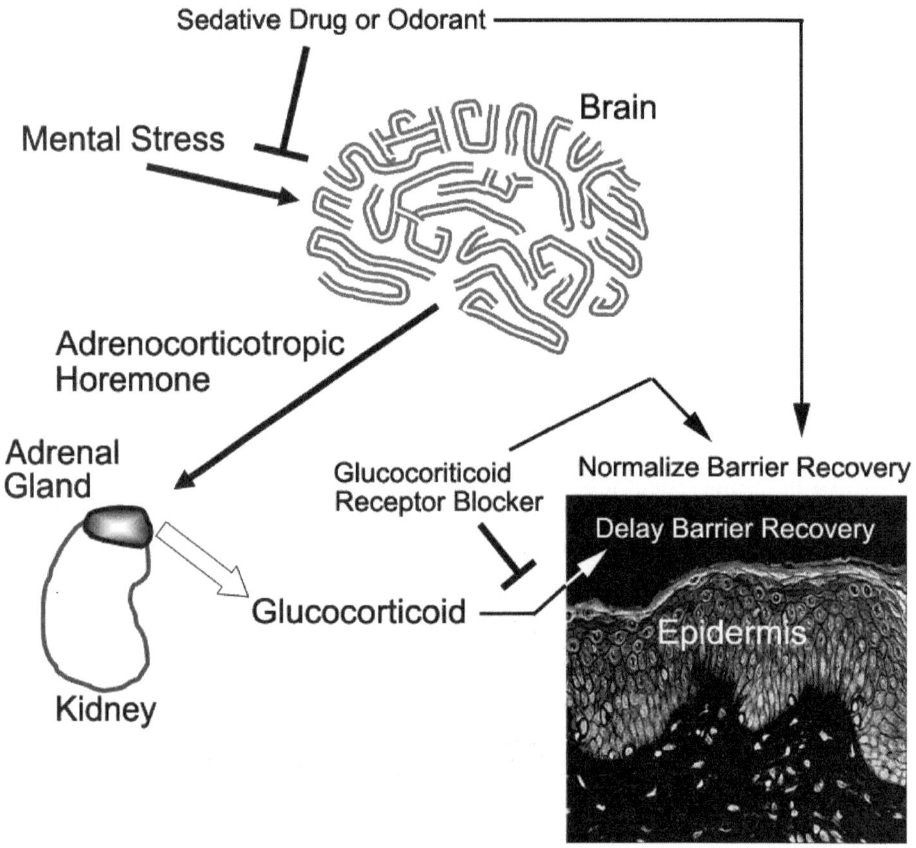

Fig. 5. Schematic illustration of the effect of mental stress on the endocrine system and on skin barrier function.

6. Conclusion

Epidermal barrier dysfunction is observed in a variety of skin diseases, such as atopic dermatitis, psoriasis, and contact dermatitis, and barrier disruption induces an inflammatory response that might aggravate dermatitis (Grice 1980). On the other hand, acceleration of barrier recovery was shown to improve epidermal hyperplasia (Denda 1997)(Fuziwara 2004). Since a wide range of physical or chemical factors, as described here, influence barrier homeostasis, control or modulation of these factors is expected to open up new possibilities for the treatment of human skin diseases involving barrier abnormality.

7. References

Ashida Y. and Denda M. (2001) Histamine H1 and H2 receptor antagonists accelerate skin barrier repair and prevent epidermal hyperplasia induced by barrier disruption in a dry environment. J Invest Dermatol 11 ,261-265, 2001

Atoyan R., Shander D., Botchkarvera NV. (2009) Non-neural expression of transient receptor potential type A1 (TRPA1) in human skin. J Invest Dermatol 129:2312-2315

Caterina MJ, Schumacher MA, Tominaga M, et al. (1997) The capsaicin receptor: a heat-activated ion channel in the pain pathway. Nature; 389:816-24.

Chung MK, Lee H, Caterina MJ. (2003) Warm temperatures activate TRPV4 in mouse 308 keratinocytes. J Biol Chem. 278:32037-46.

Denda M. (2011) Effects of topical application of aqueous solutions of hexoses on epidermal permeability barrier recovery rate after barrier disruption. Exp Dermatol in press

Denda, M. (2005) New methodology to improve epidermal barrier homeostasis. in: *Skin Moisturizer, 2nd Edition: Chemistry and Function,* (Loden M and Maibach H ed)pp155-160 CRC Press, 2005

Denda, M. Fuziwara, K. Inoue, et al. (2001) Immunoreactivity of VR1 on epidermal keratinocyte of human skin. Biochem Biophys Res Commun 2001; 285:1250-1252

Denda M and Nakatani M. (2010) Acceleration of permeability barrier recovery by exposure of skin to 10-30 kilohertz sound. Br J Dermatol 162: 503-507

Denda M and Kumazawa N. (2010) Effects of metals on skin permeability barrier recovery. Exp Dermatol 19:e124-e127

Denda M., Fuziwara S., Hibino T. (2006) Expression of voltage-gated calcium channel subunit aC1 in epidermal keratinocytes and effects of agonist and antagonists of the channel on skin barrier homeostasis. Exp Dermatol 15:455-460

Denda M, Tsutsumi M, Denda S. (2010a) Topical application of TRPM8 agonists accelerates skin permeability barrier recovery and reduces epidermal proliferation induced by barrier insult: The role of cold-sensitive TRP receptors in epidermal permeability barrier homeostasis. Exp Dermatol 19:791-795

Denda M., Tsutsumi M., Goto M., Ikeyama K., Denda S. (2010b) Topical application of TRPA1 agonists and brief cold exposure accelerate skin permeability barrier recovery. J Invest Dermatol 130:1942-1945

Denda M., Kumazawa N., (2002) Negative electric potential induces epidermal lamellar body secretion and accelerates skin barrier recovery after barrier disruption. J Invest Dermatol 118:65-72 (2002)

Denda, M. and Fuziwara, S. (2008) Visible radiation affects epidermal permeability barrier recovery: Selective effects of red and blue light. J Invest Dermatol 128, 1335-1336

Denda M., Fuziwara S., Inoue K. (2003a) Influx of calcium and chloride ions into epidermal keratinocytes regulates exocytosis of epidermal lamellar bodies and skin permeability barrier homeostasis. J Invest Dermatol 121: 362-367,

Denda, M., Fuziwara, S., Inoue, K. Association of cyclic AMP with permeability barrier homeostasis. (2004) J Invest Dermatol 122, 140-146

Denda, M., Fuziwara, S., Inoue, K. (2003b) Beta-2-adrenergic receptor antagonist accelerates skin barrier recovery and reduces epidermal hyperplasia induced by barrier disruption. J Invest Dermatol 121, 142-148, 2003

Denda, M., Inoue, K., Fuziwara, S., Denda, S. (2002a) P2X purinergic receptor antagonist accelerates skin barrier repair and prevents epidermal hyperplasia induced by skin barrier disruption. J Invest Dermatol 119, 1034-1040

Denda, M., Inoue, K., Inomata, S., Denda, S. (2002b) GABA (A) receptor agonists accelerate cutaneous barrier recovery and prevent epidermal hyperplasia induced by barrier disruption. J Invest Dermatol 119, 1041-1047

Denda, M., Katagiri, C., Maruyama, N. (1999) Some magnesium salts and a mixture of magnesium and calcium salts accelerate skin barrier recovery. Arch Dermatol Res 291, 560-563, 1999

Denda, M., Kitamura, K., Elias, P.M., Feingold, K.R., (1997) Trans-4-(aminomethyl) cyclohexane carboxylic acid (t-AMCHA), an anti-fibrinolytic agent, accelerates barrier recovery and prevents the epidermal hyperplasia induced by epidermal injury in hairless mice and humans. J. Invest Dermatol 109, 84-90

Denda M., Nakanishi K., Kumazawa N. (2005) Topical application of ionic polymers affects skin permeability barrier homeostasis. Skin Pharmacology and Physiology 18:36-41,2005

Denda, M., Sokabe, T., Tominaga, T., Tominaga, M. (2007) Effects of skin surface temperature on epidermal permeability barrier homeostasis. J Invest Dermatol 127, 654-659.

Denda, M., Tshuchiya, T., Hosoi, J., (1998) Immobilization-induced and crowded environment-induced stress delay barrier recovery in murine skin. Br. J. Dermatol. 138, 780-785

Denda, M., Tsuchiya, T., Elias, P.M., Feingold, K.R., (2000) Stress alters cutaneous permeability barrier homeostasis. Am J Physiol 278, R367-R372 (2000)

Denda, M. and Tsuchiya, T., (2001) Barrier recovery rate varies time-dependently in human skin. Br. J. Dermatol 142, 881-884

Denda, M., Tsuchiya, T., Shoji, K., Tanida, M. (2000) Odorant inhalation affects skin barrier homeostasis in mice and humans. Br J Dermatology 142, 1007-1010

Denda, M., Tanida, M., Shoji, K., Tsuchiya, T. (2000) Inhalation of a sedative odorant prevents the delay of cutaneous barrier repair induced by psychological stress. The Autonomic Nervous System 37, 419-424,2000

Denda S., Kumamoto S., Takei K., Tsutsimi M., Aoki H., Denda M., Ryanodine receptors are expressed in epidermal Keratinocytes and assosiated with Keratinocyte differentiation and epidermal permeability barrier homeostasis. J. Invest Dermatol 2011 in press.

Feingold KR. (1999) Role of nuclear hormone receptors in regulating epidermal diffrentiation. Program and Preprints of Annual Scientific Seminar, Society of Cosmetic Chemists.(1999) 30-31

Feingold KR, (2000) Farnesol stimulates differentiation in epidermal keratinocytes via PPARalpha. J Biol Chem. 275: 11484-91.

Feingold, K.R., Elias, P.M. (2000) The environmental interface: regulation of permeability barrier homeostasis. In *Dry Skin and Moisturizers. Chemistry and Function.* (Loden M and Maibach HI ed) pp45-58 CRC Press, Boca Raton, USA (2000)

Friel DD. TRP: its role in phototransduction and store-operated Ca^{2+} entry. Cell.1996; 85:617-9.

Fuziwara, S., Inoue, K., Denda, M. (2003) NMDA-type glutamate receptor is associated with cutaneous barrier homeostasis. J Invest Dermatol 120, 1023-1029, 2003

Fuziwara S., Ogawa K., Aso D., Yoshizawa D., Takata S., Denda M. (2004) Barium sulfate with a negative z potential accelerates skin permeable barrier recovery and prevents epidermal hyperplasia indueced by barrier disruption. Br J Dermarol 151:557-564

Fuziwara S., Suzuki A., Inoue K., Denda M., (2005) Dopamine D2-like receptor agonists accelerate barrier repair and inhibit the epidermal hyperplasia induced by barrier disruption. J invest Dermatol 125: 783-789

Garg, A., Chren, M.M., Sands, L.P., Matsui, M.S., Marenus, K.D., Feingold, K.R., Elias, P.M. (2001) Psychological stress perturbs epidermal permeability barrier homeostasis: implications for the pathogenesis of stress-associated skin disorders. Arch Dermatol. 137, 53-59

Ghadially R, Brown BE., Sequeira-Martin SM., Feingold KR, Elias PM, (1995) The aged epidermal permeability barrier. Structural, functional, and lipid biochemical abnormalities in humans and asenescent murine model. J Clin Invest 95: 2281-2290

Ghadially R, Brown BE, Hanley K, Reed JT, Feingold KR, Elias PM, (1996) Decreased epidermal lipid synthesis accounts for altered barrier function in aged mice. J Invest Dermatol 106: 1064-1069

Gick B, Derrick D. (2009) Aero-tactile integration in speech perception. Nature. 462: 502-4.

Goto M, Ikeyama K, Tsutsumi M, Denda S, Denda M. (2011) Phosphodiesterase inhibitors block the acceleration of skin permeability barrier repair by red light. Exp Dermatol 20:568-57

Grice KA. (1980) Transepidermal water loss in pathologic skin. In: Jarrett A (ed) The Physiology and Pathophysiology of the Skin. Academic Press, London, UK; 2147-55

Hachem JP, Houben E, Crumrine D, Man MQ, Schurer N, Roelandt T, Choi EH, Uchida Y, Brown BE, Feingold KR, Elias PM. (2006) Serine protease signaling of epidermal permeability barrier homeostasis. J Invest Dermatol.126:2074-86.

Hanley K.M. Rassner U., Jiang Y., Vansomphone D., Crumurine D., Komuves L., Elias P.M., Feingold K.R., Williams M.L. (1996) Hormonal basis for the gender difference in epidermal barrier formation in the fetal rat. Acceleration by estrogen and delay by testosterone. J Clin Invest 97:2576-2584

Hanley K, Kömüves LG, Ng DC, Schoonjans K, He SS, Lau P, Bikle DD, Williams ML, Elias PM, Auwerx J, Feingold KR. (2000) Farnesol stimulates differentiation in epidermal keratinocytes via PPARalpha. J Biol Chem. 275:11484-91

Haratake A, Ikenaga K, Katoh N, Uchiwa H, Hirano S, Yasuho H, (2000) Topical mevalonic acid stimulates de novo cholesterol synthesis and epidermal permeability barrier homeostasis in aged mice. J Invest Dermatol 114:247-252

Heffner RS. (2004) Primate hearing from a mammalian perspective. Anat Rec A Discov Mol Cell Evol Biol 281:1111-1122.

Ikeyama, K., Fuziwara, S., Denda, M. (2007) Topical application of neuronal nitric oxide synthase inhibitor accelerates cutaneous barrier recovery and prevents epidermal hyperplasia induced by barrier disruption. J Invest Dermatol 127, 1713-1719, 2007

Inoue K, Koizumi S, Fuziwara S, et al. (2002) Functional vanilloid receptors in cultured normal human keratinocytes. Biochem Biophys Res Commun 291:124-129

Kawai N, Honda M, Nakamura S, et al. (2001) Catecholamines and opioid peptides increase in plasma in humans during possession trances. Neuroreport 12:3419-23.

Lee, S.H., Elias, P.M., Proksch, E., Menon, G.K., Man, M.Q., Feingold, K.R., (1992) Calcium and potassium are important regulators of barrier homeostasis in murine epidermis. J. Clin. Invest. 89, 530-538

Man MQ, Brown BE, Wu-Pong S, Feingold KR, Elias PM. (1995) Exogenous nonphysiologic vs physiologic lipids. Arch Dermatol 131:809-816

Man MQ, Feingold KR, Thornfeld CR, Elias PM. (1996) Optimization of physiologic lipid mixtures for barrier repair. J Invest Dermatol 106:1096-1101, 1996

Mauro T, Grayson S, Gao WN, Man MQ, Kriehuber E, Behne M, Feingold KR, Elias PM. (1998) Barrier recovery is impeded at neutral pH, independent of ionic effects: implications for extracellular lipid processing. Arch Dermatol Res 290: 215-222,

Nishimura KY, Isseroff RR, Nuccitelli R. (1996) Human keratinocytes migrate to the negative pole in direct current electric fields comparable to those measured in mammalian wounds. J Cell Sci. 109:199-207.

Oohashi T, Kawai N, Nishina E, et al. (2006) The role of biological system other than auditory air-conduction in the emergence of the hypersonic effect. Brain Res. 1073-1074:339-47.

Oohashi T, Nishina E, Honda M, et al. (2000) Inaudible high-frequency sounds affect brain activity: hypersonic effect. J Neurophysiol. 83:3548-58.

Ormerod, A.D., Weller, R., Copeland, P., Benjamin, N., Ralston, S.H., Grabowski, P. (1998) Deletion of nitric oxide syntases in psoriasis. Arch Dermatol Res 290, 3-8

Peier AM, Moqrich A, Hergarden AC, et al. (2002b) A trp channel that senses cold stimuli and menthol. Cell.108:705-15.

Peier AM, Reeve AJ, Andersson DA, Moqrich A, Earley TJ, Hergarden AC, Story GM, Colley S, Hogenesch JB, McIntyre P, Bevan S, Patapoutian A (2002a) A heat-sensitive TRP channel expressed in keratinocytes. Science. 2002;296:2046-9.

Sheu MY, Fowler AJ, Kao J, Schmuth M, Schoonjans K, Auwerx J, Fluhr JM, Man MQ, Elias PM, Feingold KR, (2002) Topical peroxisome proliferator activated receptor-alpha activators reduce inflammation in irritant and allergic contact dermatitis models. J Invest Dermatol. Jan;118(2002):94-101.

Story GM, Peier AM, Reeve AJ, et al. (2003) ANKTM1, a TRP-like channel expressed in nociceptive neurons, is activated by cold temperatures. Cell.112 :819-29.

Tsuchiya T., Tanida M., Uenoyama S. (1992) Effects of olfactory stimulation with jasmin and its component chemicals on t the duration of pentobarbital-induced sleep in mice. Life Sci, 50(15),1097-1102, 1992

Tsutsumi M., Denda S., Ikeyama K., Goto M., Denda M. (2010) Exposure to low temperature induces elevation of intracellular calcium in cultured human keratinocytes. J Invest Dermatol 130: 1945-1948

Tsutsumi M., Ikeyama K., Denda S., Nakanishi J, Fuziwara S., Aoki H., Denda M. (2009) Expressions of rod and cone photoreceptor-like proteins in human epidermis. Exp Dermatol 18:567-570

Tsutsumi, M. and Denda, M. (2007) Paradoxical effects of beta-estradiol on epidermal permeability barrier homeostasis. Br J Dermatol 157, 776-779

Yagi R, Nishina E, Honda M, et al. (2003) Modulatory effect of inaudible high-frequency sounds on human acoustic perception. Neurosci Lett 351:191-5.

14

Clinical Management of Atopic Dermatitis

Soheyla Mahdavian, Patty Ghazvini, Luis Pagan,
Angela Singh and Todd Woodard
Florida A&M University College of Pharmacy and Pharmaceutical Sciences
USA

1. Introduction

Atopic Dermatitis (AD) is a common inflammatory, pruritic skin disorder. It is a chronic disease with often relapse. Several factors including genetic predisposition, allergies to specific foods, irritant chemicals, and aeroallergens are thought to be the cause of AD. Diagnosis is difficult, and often occurs after ruling out other disorders with a clinical presentation resembling atopic dermatitis.

2. Definition

Atopic Dermatitis is a chronic relapsing inflammatory condition of the skin that occurs most frequently in childhood and may spontaneously resolve or continue throughout a person's life span leading to lifelong sensitivity to irritants and allergens (Habif, 2008). It occurs as a result of several interrelated factors including genetic, immunologic and environmental issues, which ultimately cause a disruption in the epidermal barrier function leading to the development of dry, pruritic skin. The itching can be severe lasting throughout the day and worsening at night, which can lead to sleep disruptions and dramatically reduce the patients' quality of life (Bieber, 2008). Episodes of AD can be triggered by events such as psychological stress, exposure to irritants and allergens or as a result of seasonal or climate changes (Habif, 2008). Additionally, patients with AD are at an increased risk of developing infections especially due to *Staphylococcus Aureus* and Herpes Simplex Virus, asthma and allergic rhinitis (Bieber, 2008).

3. Epidemiology

Over the past several decades' industrialized nations have seen a dramatic rise in the incidence of AD (Ghazvini, et al. 2010). This disease occurs primarily in childhood affecting 15-30% of children and 2-10% of adults. It most frequently begins in early childhood with 45% of cases occurring within the first six months of life and 85% of cases diagnosed within the first five years (Bieber, 2008).

4. Pathophysiology

The pathophysiological mechanism of AD is multifactorial involving genetic, structural and immunological elements. The hallmark characteristic of AD is epidermal barrier dysfunction.

In normal individuals there are three factors that contribute to intact epidermal barrier function; structural proteins, lipids and proteases. Alterations in these components contribute to epidermal barrier dysfunction in AD patients. Additionally, genetic dysfunctions can be classified into two distinct groups; mutations occurring in genes encoding for epithelial structures and mutations occurring in genes encoding for elements of the immune system (Bieber, 2008). Lastly, immunological dysfunction appears to play a critical role in the pathogenesis of AD and involves alterations in T-cells, B-cells, eosinophils and IgE production.

4.1 Structural factors

There are several factors that lead to epidermal barrier dysfunction including changes in the stratum corneum, decreases in lipid levels and loss of function of a crucial protein called filaggrin. This is compounded by alterations in the expression of enzymes, such as peptidases within the epidermal layer leading to further breakdown of this protective barrier. Ultimately, the disruption of the epidermal barrier facilitates the penetration of environmental allergens and promotes allergic skin inflammation (Bieber 2008; Caubet & Eigenmann 2010).

4.2 Genetic factors

Researchers have identified several candidate genes that contribute to both the structural and immunological dysfunctions seen in AD. There is a genetically determined dominance of Th_2 cells, which produce cytokines including Interleukin-4 (IL-4), Interleukin-5 (IL-5) and Interleukin-13 (IL-13). These cytokines play a role in the synthesis of IgE, which is upregulated in 85% of patients with AD. Additionally, there is a loss of function mutation in the gene encoding for the protein filaggrin, which is a crucial protein in cutaneous barrier function (Bieber 2008; Caubet & Eigenmann, 2010).

4.3 Immunological factors

The immunological factors that contribute to AD are multifactorial and complex. As stated previously, disruptions in the epidermal barrier facilitate the penetration of allergens. These allergens are presented to the Langerhans Cells (LCs) located within the epidermal layer, which migrate to the lymphoid organs where they present the allergen to the Th_2 cells. (Callard & Harper 2007) Additionally, activated dendritic cells serve to stimulate memory Th_2 cells and migrate to the lymph nodes where they further increase the systemic pool of Th_2 cells by stimulating naïve T-cells. This increase in circulating T-cells results in the development of skin lesions through the production of inflammatory cytokines IL-4, IL-13, IL-5 and IL-12. Further promotion of the inflammatory response is modulated by Th_2 cells through the upregulation of adhesion molecules on endothelial cells and increases in high affinity receptors for IgE on LCs and other antigen presenting cells. Lastly, eosinophils appear to play a role through secretion of cytolytic proteins resulting in further damage to the epithelial cells (Caubet & Eigenmann 2010).

Other immunological factors that contribute to the pathogenesis of the disease include a down regulation of toll-like receptors (TLRs) within the epidermal cells. These TLRs serve to bind bacterial, fungal and viral structures leading to the activation of epithelial cells to produce antimicrobial peptides. These receptors are down regulated in the presence of IL-4, IL-13 and IL-10 in patients with AD The result is patients are at an increased risk of developing skin infections and are often colonized with *Staphylococcus Aureus* (Bieber, 2008).

5. Clinical presentation

The clinical appearance of AD varies with disease severity. At all stages, patients have dry skin. Intensely pruritic, erythematous papules associated with exudates are seen in the acute phase of AD in infants. In the infantile stage (0-2 years old), the distribution of the rash is normally located on the face, chin, cheeks, scalp, trunk and extensor surfaces, but not on the nose or the diaper area (Deshazo, 2009). As the disease becomes more chronic, there is associated lichenification and the distribution of the rash is mostly seen on the wrists, ankles and neck in the childhood stage (2 years old-puberty) (Deshazo, 2009; Lipozencic, 2010). Approximately, 40% of childhood AD persists into adulthood (Bettrani, 2007). The distribution of rash in adults is similar to the childhood form mostly noticeable on the upper arms, back, wrists, dorsa of hands, fingers, feet and toes (Deshazo, 2009). The presence of pustules within areas of dermatitis suggests a secondary infection. Lesions with a less distinct distribution should prompt a search for an alternative diagnosis.

6. Diagnosis

The diagnosis of atopic dermatitis is based on a constellation of clinical signs and symptoms, physical examination and history. Laboratory tests are unnecessary and skin biopsy has been found to be little value, but they can exclude other diagnosis in adults. Although the majority of AD patients have elevated total serum IgE, up to 30% of these patients have normal total serum IgE and show no allergic sensitization to food or aeroallergens (Schmid-Grendelmeier, et al. 2005). However, monitoring of IgE remains a nonspecific finding of AD.

Normally, diagnosis is confirmed by chronicity of symptoms, pruritis, and age-specific morphology and distribution of symptoms (Ong P, et al. 2008). However, well-defined criteria are important in the diagnosis of AD and diagnostic criteria developed by Hanifin and Rajka are widely accepted (see Table 1). The American Academy of Dermatology has also developed diagnostic criteria for AD (Leung & Hong, 2007). Please see Table 2.

There are many exacerbating factors that are triggers, which can expedite the progress of inflammation. These triggers are found in food allergens, bacteria, viruses, stress and opportunistic pathogens. One of the major triggers is the microorganism *Staphylococcus Aureus* due to the fact that is organism secretes a toxin which can stimulate action of T cells (Ghazvini, et al. 2010). Among viruses, herpes simplex virus has been identified as one of the possible triggers of AD (Ghazvini, et al. 2010). Diagnostic testing is mainly utilized to determine specific allergens that may be causing the condition. These tests include:

- Allergy or skin prick test - a positive prick test indicates the presence of IgE antibodies specific for a certain antigen. However, the positive predictive value is only 50%, which means a patient who has a positive test should undergo confirmatory testing through food challenges (Ghazvini, et al. 2010).
- Atopy patch test- an atopy patch test (APT) is currently used to evaluate allergen without comparison with another accurate and reliable method, because no gold standard exists for aeroallergen provocation in AD. The APT is presumed to reflect delayed-phase clinical reactions. The patch test is performed by applying a patch consisting of large test chambers containing allergens. The patch is applied to the back for 48-72 hours on areas that are affected by AD or have not been treated with topical creams or ointments (Akdis, et al. 2006; Lipozencic, 2010).

- Food challenge - This is the most accurate test to diagnose allergy to food; skin reactions are expected to present up to 24 hours after testing. There are three patterns of skin reactions which can be observed with this test:
    - Immediate type reactions such as urticaria, erythema and angioedema may occur without worsening the AD symptoms and they may occur within a few minutes after food intake (Ong P, et al. 2008).
    - Pruritis may be noted after ingestion of food, which makes the patient scratch and may trigger AD.
    - Late reactions may occur as 6 to 8 hours after food ingestion (Ong P, et al. 2008).
- Serum IgE measurement - Even though a larger number of AD patients have elevated serum IgE levels, approximately 30% have normal levels and do not present with allergic sensitization to allergens (Ong P, et al. 2008).
- Skin biopsy - This is not necessary for diagnosis, however it may be essential for excluding other differentials of AD (see Table 3).

Major Features	Minor Features
Pruritis	Xerosis
Typical morphology and distribution	Cutaneous infections
Flexural lichenification of linearity in adults	Early age of onset
Chronic or relapsing dermatitis	Ichthyosis, palmar hyperlinearity and keratosis pilaris
Facial or extensor involvement in infants and children	Nonspecific dermatitis of the hands or feet
Personal or family history of atopy (asthma, atopic dermatitits, contact urticaria)	Raised serum immunoglobulin (Ig) E levels
	Nipple eczema
	Pityriasis alba
	White dermatographism and delayed blanch response
	Anterior subcapsular cataracts
	Perifollicular accentuation
	Course influenced by environmental/emotional factors
	Facial erythema or pallor
	Dennie-Morgan infraorbital folds, orbital darkening

**At least 3 major and minor features must be present for a diagnosis of atopic dermatitis.

Table 1. Hanifin-Rajka Diagnostic Criteria for Atopic Dermatitis (Ghazvini, et al. 2010)

Essential Features (must be present)	Pruritis Eczema (with typical morphology for age) Chronic or relapsing history
Important Features (seen in most cases; add support to diagnosis)	Early age at onset Personal or family history of atopy or IgE reactivity Xerosis Cutaneous infections Nonspecific dermatitis of the hands or feet Elevated serum IgE levels Positive skin test for immediate-type allergy
Associated Features (nonspecific; help suggest diagnosis)	Atypical vascular response (facial pallor, white dermatographism) Keratosis pillaris, hyperlinearity of palms Pityriasis alba Nipple eczema Ocular or periorbital changes, including anterior subcapsular cataracts, Dennie-Morgan infraorbital folds, orbital darkening Perioral or periauricular lesions Perifollicular accentuation, lichenification or prurigo lesions

Table 2. Diagnostic Criteria for Atopic Dermatitis by the American Academy of Dermatology (Ong P, et al. 2008)

Other dermatosis - Contact dermatitis - Irritant dermatitis - Nummular dermatitis - Seborrheic dermatitis - Psoriasis ichthyosis	Immunodeficiency syndromes - Wiskott-Aldrich syndrome - Severe combined immunodeficiency syndrome with Omen's - Immune dysregulation, polyendocrinopathy, enteropathy, X-linked - Graft vs host disease - Dermatitis herpetiformis
Infections - Dermatophytosis - Scabies	Metabolic and nutritional deficiencies - Phenylketonuria - Zinc deficiency - Niacin deficiency - Pyridoxine deficiency
Malignancies - T cell lymphoma/mycosis fungoides - Letterer-Siwe disease	

Table 3. Differential Diagnosis in Atopic Dermatitis (Deshazo, 2009)7. Treatment

7. Treatment

7.1 Nonphamacological interventions

7.1.1 Dietary restrictions

Hen's egg, milk, wheat, soy, peanuts, nuts, and fish are responsible for 90% of the food allergy in patients with atopic dermatitis (Sircherer & Sampson, 1999). Avoiding these foods, and other foods suspected to cause flares may be helpful in reducing disease exacerbation, especially in children. Several studies identified the effects of dietary restriction in children with atopic dermatitis. One of these trials, conducted by Sloper and associates evaluated 78 children with atopic dermatitis. Patients were on a diet, which excluded cow's milk, eggs, and foods known to trigger exacerbations. At the end of the trial, 64 patients experienced an improvement in their atopic dermatitis symptoms (Sloper, et al. 1991). Few studies in this meta-analysis used validated diagnostic criteria, which could have given skewed results. Because there are no precise findings in these studies, foods containing milk, eggs, or other known causes of disease flares should be avoided in patients with atopic dermatitis.

7.1.2 Aeroallergen reduction

Like with food allergens, different aeroallergens such as dust mites, pollen, mold, and animal dander can cause AD exacerbation. This exacerbation can be triggered either by inhalation or direct contact. Fungus and cockroaches have also been suspected (Michel, et al. 2009; Simon-Nobbe, et al. 2008). There have been conflicting studies that show avoidance of aeroallergens, particularly dust mites, reduce disease symptoms. A double-blind, placebo controlled study using dust mite reducing measures in the home proved to improve the symptoms of atopic dermatitis (Tan, et al. 1996). By contrast, there are also trials that show the reduction in aeroallergens have no affect on symptoms of atopic dermatitis (Koopman, et al. 2001; Oosting, et al. 2002). Although the data varies, there is no harm in taking dust mite reducing measures. Aeroallergen reduction techniques that can be used include: using dust mite-proof encasings on pillows, mattresses, and box springs, washing bedding in hot water weekly, removal of bedroom carpet, and decreasing indoor humidity levels with air conditioning (Arlian & Platts-Mills, 2001).

7.1.3 Detergent and chemical avoidance

Because there is a higher chance of skin irritation in patients with atopic dermatitis, it is important to avoid those products or chemicals that can cause disease exacerbation (Nassif, et al. 1994). Certain soaps, fabric softeners, perfumes, cosmetics, and lotions contain alcohol and other ingredients that can be irritating to the skin of those patients with AD. These products can induce the itch-scratch cycle and worsen symptoms. It is suggested that laundry detergents containing enzymes can also worsen symptoms. A blinded crossover trial of 25 adults looked at the affect on atopic dermatitis symptoms with enzyme-enriched detergent, and a control detergent, which contained no enzymes. Although no diagnostic criteria were described in the trial, the SCORAD index was used to evaluate the patients' severity of symptoms. There was no statistical difference in symptomatic relief between the two groups of patients (Andersen, et al. 1998). However, enzyme-enriched products should be avoided in patients with known hypersensitivity to enzyme proteins.

7.1.4 Phototherapy

The use of natural sunlight for the treatment of atopic dermatitis has been shown to be beneficial, but sunburn should be avoided. If sunlight occurs in the presence of high humidity, or heat which triggers sweating, aggravation of symptoms can occur. Ultraviolet (UV) light (UVB, narrowband UVB, and high-intensity UVA) therapy can be useful in adjunct with other treatments options for patients. Topical glucocorticoid therapy, high-dose UVA1 phototherapy, and UVA-UVB phototherapy were compared in patients with atopic dermatitis. This was a randomized, multi-center trial that found significant differences in favor of high-dose UVA1 and fluocortolone therapy were observed ($p < 0.0001$), as compared with UVA-UVB therapy. At day 10, high-dose UVA1R was superior to fluocortolone ($p < 0.002$) therapy. (Krutmann, et al. 1998). There are also several small trials that look at specific wavelengths of and equipment for UV therapy. Chemophototherapy, psoralen with UVA (PUVA), has also been shown to be effective, but should be limited to those patients with widespread AD. Comparison studies with PUVA are limited. Short-term adverse events of UV phototherapy are mild and include: erythema, pruritis, and pigmentation. Potential long-term adverse effects include: premature skin aging, and cutaneous malignancies (Leung, et al. 2004). UV phototherapy is proven to be an effective method of therapy, because of this it is usually used as a second or third line of treatment.

7.1.5 Psychological approaches

Patients with atopic dermatitis are shown to have significant issues with anxiety, anger, and emotional stress (Bender 2002). They usually respond to embarrassment, frustration, anxiety, or other upsetting events with increased pruritis and scratching (Kodama, et al. 1999). Although emotional factors do not cause atopic dermatitis, studies show that psychological techniques, such as stress reduction approaches, behavior modifications, and group counseling sessions may reduce the exacerbation of atopic dermatitis, particularly those prone to habitual scratching (Melin, et al. 1986).

7.2 Pharmacological therapies

7.2.1 Nonprescription therapies

7.2.1.1 Antihistamines

Oral antihistamines are usually recommended for pruritis. However, a recent study of 16 trials showed no little evidence associated with the relief of pruritis with sedating or non-sedating antihistamines (Klein & Clark, 1999). These observations, however, do not exclude the possibility that individual patients may benefit from antihistamines. Because pruritis can be worse at night, oral histamines have been beneficial at bedtime for their sedative properties in patients experiencing symptoms, and can be used as a short-term adjuvant to topical therapy (Kristal & Klein, 2000). The first generation antihistamines, hydroxyzine, diphenhydramine, and cyproheptadine all have sedative effects, but it is shown hydroxyzine to be more effective than the latter (Denman, 1986; Leung, et al. 1998). Newer generation antihistamines ceterizine, loratadine, and fexofenadine may not be beneficial since they lack the sedating properties of the first generation antihistamines. Topical antihistamines should be avoided to the risk of irritating the skin further (Shelley, et al.

1996). Common side effects of antihistamines include: sedation, dry mouth, constipation, blurred vision, and dizziness.

7.2.1.2 Coal tar preparations

Coal tar has been used to treat skin disorders for centuries. Although the exact pharmacologic effects are unknown, it is thought coal tar has antibacterial, antifungal, antipruritic, and keratoplastic effects (Andrew & Moses, 1999; Grupper, 1971; Lavker, et al. 1981). There is a theoretical risk that coal tar being a carcinogen based on observational studies of workers who use tar components in their occupation, however there have been no increase in cancer with clinical use (Callen, et al. 2007). Coal tar preparations have many disadvantages. Their odor, dark staining color, and side effects make them less desirable to patients. Coal tar comes in a variety of formulations, including creams, gels, shampoos, lotions and soaps. Newer formulations make the preparations more tolerable than older versions (Niordson & Stahl, 1985). It is suggested that coal tar be applied at night to avoid the odor and staining of daytime clothing. Adverse effects associated with coal tar preparations include burning, stinging, folliculitis, and photosensitization (Kristal & Klein, 2000).

7.2.1.3 Emollients

Xerosis contributes to microfissures and cracks which can introduce microbes and allergens under the skin. This usually becomes exacerbated in the cold, dry winder months. Because AD is characterized by a decrease in skin barrier function, moisturizing and skin protection play an important role in the disease. Emollients have long been used for this. Although emollients have not been found to improve atopic dermatitis directly, they are a vital source of skin hydration and protection for these patients. The moisturizing aids are available in the forms of lotions, creams, and ointments, and are usually used in conjunction with corticosteroids. Formulations that contain certain dyes, alcohols, or fragrances can exacerbate atopic dermatitis and should be avoided. Because lotions are less viscous than the other formulations, they contain more water, which can cause an evaporative effect causing further skin drying. Ointments may interfere with appropriate sweat removal and result in sweat retention dermatitis. Emollients are better at maintaining skin hydration when applied after the patient soaks in a lukewarm bath.

7.2.2 Prescription therapies

7.2.2.1 Topical preparations

7.2.2.1.1 Topical corticosteroids

Topical corticosteroids have been a standard for treatment of atopic dermatitis and other skin disorders for years. Clinicians who are not familiar with topical corticosteroids can be challenged when providing care, due to the various strengths and formulations in which these medications are available. The decision to use a more or less potent corticosteroids depends on the severity of the dermatitis, location of the lesions, and the type of skin involved. Based on their vasoconstrictor assays, there are six potentcies of topical corticosteroids that are available though prescription, please refer to Table 4. Potency of topical corticosteroids depends on the concentration of the medication, but also the delivery vehicle. For example, betamethasone valerate ointment is considered more potent than a foam or cream containing the same medication. In general, the lowest potency that will control symptoms should be used. Low potency corticosteroids are recommended for the

Group 1: Super-High Potency	Vehicle
Betamethasone dipropionate augmented 0.05%	Gel, lotion, ointment
Clobetasol propionate 0.05%	Cream, gel, foam, ointment, solution
Fluocinonide 0.1%	Cream
Halobetasol propionate 0.05%	Cream, ointment
Group 2: High Potency	Vehicle
Amcinonide 0.1%	Ointment
Betamethasone dipropionate 0.05% augmented	Cream
Betamethasone dipropionate 0.05%	Ointment
Desoximetasone 0.25%	Cream, gel, ointment
Desoximetasone 0.05%	Gel
Diflorasone diacetate 0.05%	Ointment
Fluocinonide 0.05%	Cream, gel, ointment, solution
Halcinonide 0.1%	Cream, ointment
Mometasone furoate 0.1%	Ointment
Triamcinolone acetonide 0.5%	Ointment
Group 3: Medium-High Potency	Vehicle
Amcinonide 0.1%	Cream, lotion
Betamethasone dipropionate 0.05%	Cream
Betamethasone valerate 0.1%	Ointment
Desoximetasone 0.05%	Cream
Diflorasone diacetate 0.05%	Cream
Fluocinonide emollient 0.05%	Cream
Fluticasone propionate 0.005%	Ointment
Triamcinolone acetonide 0.1%	Ointment
Triamcinolone acetonide 0.5%	Cream
Group 4: Medium Potency	Vehicle
Betamethasone valerate 0.12%	Foam
Fluocinolone acetonide 0.025%	Ointment
Hydrocortisone valerate 0.2%	Ointment
Mometasone furoate 0.1%	Cream, lotion
Triamcinolone acetonide 0.1%	Cream
Group 5: Medium-Low Potency	Vehicle
Betamethasone dipropionate 0.05%	Lotion
Betamethasone valerate 0.1%	Cream
Desonide 0.05%	Ointment
Fluocinolone acetonide 0.025%	Cream
Flurandrenolide 0.05%	Lotion
Fluticasone propionate 0.05%	Cream
Group 6: Low Potency	Vehicle
Alclometasone Desonate 0.05%	Cream, ointment
Fluocinolone acetonide 0.01%	Oil, cream,
Desonide 0.01%, 0.05%	Cream, gel, foam, lotion

Table 4. Topical Steroids Preparations

face, eyelids, genitalia, and sensitive areas, as well as on young children and infants (Leung & Barber, 2003). More potent corticosteroids are used on other areas of the body in adults and children over 12 years of age.

The dosing application of topical corticosteroids is important in the management of the disease, but there are limited trials on the optimal dose. Potent topical corticosteroids should be used for the shortest duration of time and an emollient used in combination during flare-ups to prevent steroid-related side effects (Akdis, et al. 2006). Corticosteroids should be applied once to twice a day; frequent use does not improve efficacy and increases the risk of side effects (Bleehen, et al 1995; Leung & Barber, 2003). The risk of adverse reactions depends on the drug potency, skin integrity, and length of treatment (Fleischer, 1999). It is the clinician's responsibility to balance the need for a potent corticosteroid with the potential for adverse reactions. Adverse effects of topical corticosteroids can be local or systemic. The latter, which occurs rarely, include adrenal suppression, Cushing's syndrome, cataracts, and glaucoma (Correale, et al. 1999; Ruiz-Maldonado, et al. 1982; Stoppoloni, et al. 1983). Local adverse reactions include skin atrophy, contact dermatitis related to the vehicle, depigmentation, rosacea, steroid acne, and folliculitis (Correale, et al. 1999; Fleischer, 1999; Raimer, 2000). Treatment with topical corticosteroids can also reduce the colonization of S. Aureas, which may trigger exacerbations (Lipozencic & Wolf, 2007).

7.2.2.1.2 Topical calcineurin inhibitors

Pimecrolimus and tacrolimus are topical immunosuppresants that selectively inhibit the activation of T cells by inhibiting calcineurin, an enzyme required for the transcription of certain genes that code for specific inflammatory cytokines (Bornhovd, et al. 2002; Grassberger, et al. 2009). These are not recommended as first-line therapy or for mild atopic dermatitis. Pimecrolimus cream 1% and Tacrolimus ointment 0.03% are recommended for second-line therapy for mild to moderate AD in non-immunocompromised patients over two years old who have not been successful with other topical treatments.

Short-term (up to four years) treatment with Tacrolimus has been shown safe and effective in children older than two years of age. In a 12-week randomized, vehicle-controlled, double blind, multicenter study of 351 children, 2 to 15 years of age, with moderate to severe atopic dermatitis, tacrolimus ointment (0.03% and 0.1% concentrations) was safe and significantly more efficacious than the vehicle (Paller, et al. 2001). Studies also show that the calcineurin inhibitors are more effective that topical cortical steroids. In a multicenter, randomized, double-blind, parallel-group comparison of tacrolimus ointment 0.03% and 0.1% with hydrocortisone acetate ointment 1% involved 560 children 2 to 15 years of age (Reitamo, et al. 2002). Both concentrations of tacrolimus were significantly more effective than hydrocortisone acetate.

Pimecrolimus has also shown similar results to tacrolimus. Two identically designed, multicenter, randomized, controlled trials compared pimecrolimus cream 1% with vehicle in 403 children 2 to 17 years of age. Both groups received treatment twice daily for 6 weeks. Results showed significant alleviation of symptoms and signs with pimecrolimus compared with the vehicle (Van Leent, et al. 1998.)

Adverse effects of these two agents are similar. The most common adverse reactions are mild to moderate transient burning, stinging, itching, and erythema at the application site, which tends to resolve after the first few days of treatment (Bekersky, et al. 2001; Kang, et al. 2001; Paller, et al. 2001; Reitamo, et al. 2002; Soter, et al. 2001). They are, however, contraindicated in pregnant or breast feeding women. These agents have been studied for short term use (two years for pimecrolimus and 4 years for tacrolimus) and have been shown to have favorable outcomes, but have been advised that they be used in accordance to their guidelines due to the potential cancer risk. Long term studies for these drugs are still needed.

7.2.2.2 Systemic immunosuppressants

There are those individuals in which topical steroid use does not result in complete remission. As result, systemic immunosuppressant along with novel therapeutic options are warranted for severe refractory cases to provide increase in therapeutic options with effective remission rates and limited adverse effects. These subsets of patients should be referred to a specialist (i.e., dermatologist or allergist) for further evaluation. Severe atopic dermatitis may be described as the presence of widespread skin lesions or physically and/or emotionally disabling disease that significantly compromises a patient's quality of life. The following will describe available systemic therapies for atopic dermatitis.

7.2.2.2.1 Corticosteroids

Systemic corticosteroids are not recommended for chronic or maintenance treatment of atopic dermatitis due to many common side effects associated with their use and possible rebound flaring upon discontinuation (Akdis et al, 2006). Typical side effects include; osteoporosis, cataracts, growth suppression, and poor wound healing. A short course of systemic corticosteroids with taper is recommended to abort an acute flare-up. Recommended dosing with prednisone is 40 to 60 mg daily for three to four days followed by 20 to 30 mg daily for three to four days can be beneficial.

7.2.2.2.2 Cyclosporine

Cyclosporine has proven beneficial in attenuating exacerbations in adults and children with severe atopic dermatitis. It also may be used for intermittent chronic not just short-term therapy. Cyclosporine is classified as a calcineurin inhibitor, which blocks T cell activation. A dose of 5mg/kg/day divided every 12 hours has been evaluated. Monitoring of trough levels, renal, and hepatic function is essential. A taper by 1mg/kg/day every one to three months is recommended. (Sowden et al, 1991; Brazelli et al, 2002). Common side effects associated with cyclosporine include increased risk of infection, malignancy, nephrotoxicity, hypertension, and seizures.

7.2.2.2.3 Interferons

Interferon-gamma (IFN-gamma) works by suppressing T helper cell activity along with other immunomodulatory effects (Schmitt 2007). Interferon-gamma (IFN-gamma) has shown varying results in the treatment of severe atopic dermatitis although a couple of trials have shown a reduction in symptoms and body surface involvement (Hanifin et al 1993). Side effects that may occur include granulocytopenia, fever/chills, myalgias, headache, and inject site pain.

Several biological therapies have been studied for severe atopic dermatitis and only a few have shown benefit in small subset of patients. Further studies are necessary before any of these medications can be routinely recommended. Some of the biological therapies that have been evaluated are Omalizumab, Rituximab, Infliximab, Etanercept, Alefacept, and Mepolizumab (Graves et al 2007).

7.2.2.2.4 Antimetabolites, azathiaprine, and methotrexate

Antimetabolites azathioprine and methotrexate have shown usefulness in severe atopic dermatitis. Azathioprine is an antagonist of purine metabolism that inhibits T cell proliferation. Methotrexate is a folic acid antagonist that inhibits reactions and promotes release of adenosine. It also inhibits lymphocyte proliferation. Adverse effects associated with azathioprine and methotrexate are myelosupression, hepatotoxicity, gastrointestinal disturbances, and increased risk of infection. Monitoring of hematologic and liver function tests is mandatory (Hon et al 2009; Weatherhead et al 2007).

7.3 Emerging therapies

As discussed, atopic dermatitis is an important skin disorder that leads to significant costs and morbidity to patients, families, and society. Effective therapeutic agents are limited in number, and all have side effects that impede successful long-term use. Consequently, there is a high medical need for better therapies. Bimosiamose, nanocrystalline silver cream, phosphodiesterase-4 inhibitors, and IL-4/IL-3 receptor blockers are considered here.

7.3.1 Bimosiamose

Bimosiamose is a selectin antagonist that blocks the initial slowing of leukocyte traffic, preventing leukocytes from migrating into the tissue, and may alter cell activation and cell-cell signalling pathways. Currently Bimosiamose is in Phase II clinical testing for asthma, psoriasis, and atopic dermatitis (Revotar Biopharmaceuticals 2011).

7.3.2 Nanocrystalline silver cream

Nanocrystalline Silver Cream completed preliminary studies evaluating its use in atopic dermatitis. Silver has proven for decades to be an effective antimicrobial agent. It has been the active ingredient for the treatment of burns and other wounds. It has also demonstrated anti-inflammatory activity in animal studies. Human studies are currently in Phase II trials evaluating nanocrystalline silver cream applied twice daily using placebo, 0.5% or 1% cream (ClinicalTrials.gov 2005).

7.3.3 Phosphodiesterase-4 Inhibitors

Phosphodiesterases play a key role in degrading cAMP, which is an important process in virtually all the cell types involved in the pathophysiology of allergic and inflammatory diseases including asthma and chronic obstructive pulmonary disease (COPD), but also skin diseases such as psoriasis and atopic dermatitis. PDE-4 is the major and most abundant in almost all inflammatory and immune cells. PDE-4 suppresses several pro-inflammatory mechanisms like cytokine generation and secretion, IgE production, proliferation, and histamine generation just to name a few. Topical and systemic therapies are being studied. One general problem is the group associated side effect profile with nausea, emesis, and enhanced gastric acid production being the most critical commonly occurring with systemic therapies. Some examples are topical Atizoram and orally Arofylline. The newly FDA approved Roflumilast (Darilesp®) for severe COPD is being investigated for its utility in atopic dermatitis (Baumer et al 2007).

7.3.4 Interleukin receptor blockers

Elevated IgE responses and eosinophilia is observed in many patients with atopic dermatitis. This is thought to reflect the increased expression of Th2 cytokines, in particular IL-4, IL-5, and IL-13. Cutaneous infiltration of activated T-cells and their release of cytokines are thought to be key events in the development of atopic dermatitis. There are three ways of inhibition of IL-4; synthesis inhibitors, binding site inhibitors, and inhibiting intracellular signal transduction. Suplatast tosylate is an example of a synthesis inhibitor developed in Japan and may prove useful for steroid resistant asthma, but data about possible effects in atopic dermatitis are lacking. There are several compounds being studied as therapeutic agents inhibiting the binding site and signal transduction (Hennekes & Asadullah 2002).

8. Complications

If AD is not appropriately treated there can be several complications that can arise. It is shown that patients with atopic dermatitis are more susceptible to microorganisms, particularly S. aureus. Untreated lesions can result in bacterial infections, and acute inflammatory responses of the skin. Patients with atopic dermatitis can also present with eyelid dermatitis, nipple dermatitis, and cheilitis of the lips. Eyelid dermatitis and chronic blepharitis can result in visual impairment from corneal scarring. Other ocular complications include atopic keratoconjunctivitis, vernal conjunctivitis, and keratoconus (Leung, et al. 2003). Management of AD is important in the prevention of other conditions.

9. Role of a clinician

Patient education, in addition to treatment, is a factor that can drastically help improve the health of any patient. The healthcare practitioner plays a very important role in a patients' improvement of atopic dermatitis. They can assist a patient in determining what the causative agent is, and provide counselling on how to avoid that particular agent. A physician's knowledge on appropriate diagnosis and the available treatment options is very important in ensuring optimal care. As the drug experts, pharmacists are also responsible for the care of the patient. By providing practical advice concerning the appropriate use of drug products, such as topical corticosteroids and calcineurin inhibitors, compliance can be optimized and adverse effects minimized. In addition, the pharmacist can diminish the stress and anxiety often experienced by patients and caregivers, particularly parents of infants and children with atopic dermatitis. In addition, a pharmacist can advise undiagnosed or untreated patients' on when it is necessary to receive treatment from a physician.

10. Conclusion

Atopic dermatitis is a condition that has no cure, but the main goal of treatment is to reduce disease flares and improve the patients' quality of life. Avoidance of triggering factors, optimal skin care, and pharmacotherapy can produce control of exacerbations in patients. Although there is no cure, there are many safe and effective treatment options available. Corticosteroids remains the standard for therapy, but those unresponsive to corticosteroids have other options including systemic and topical immunomodulators, and non-prescription agents.

11. References

Akdis C., Bieber T., Akdis M., et al. Diagnosis and treatment of atopic dermatitis in children and adults: European Academy of Allerogology PRACTALL Consensus Report. *J*

Allergy Clin Immunol 2006:118:152-169. Andersen P, Bindslev-Jensen C, Mosbech H, et al. Skin Symptoms in Patients with Atopic Dermatitis Using Enzyme-containing Detergents. A Placebo-controlled Study. *Acta Derm Venereol.* 1998; 78: 60–62

Andrew N, Moses K. Tar revisited. Int J Dermatol 1985; 24: 216–8.

Arlian L, Platts-Mills T. The biology of dust mites and the remediation of mite allergens in allergic disease. *J Allergy Clin Immunol.* 2001;107(Suppl):S406–S413.

Baumer W, Hoppmann J, Rundfeldt C, et al. Highly selective phosphodiesterase 4 inhibitors for the treatment of allergic skin diseases and psoriasis. *Inflamm Allergy Drug Targets.* 2007 Mar;6(1):17-26.

Bekersky I, Fitzsimmons W, Tanase A, et al. Nonclinical and early clinical development of tacrolimus ointment for the treatment of atopic dermatitis. *J Am Acad Dermatol.* 2001;44:S17-S27.

Bender B. Psychological dysfunction associated with atopic dermatitis. *Immunol Allergy Clin North Am.* 2002; 22:43–53.

Bettrani V. The clinical spectrum of atopic dermatitis. *J Allergy Clin Immunol* 2007;104 (Suppl 2):S87-S98.

Bieber, T. 2008. Mechanisms of Disease Atopic Dermatitis. *New England Journal of Medicine,* 358,14, 1483-1494.

Bleehen SS, Chu AC, Hamann I, et al. Fluticasone propionate 0.05% cream in the treatment of atopic eczema: a multicentre study comparing once-daily treatment andonce-daily vehicle cream application versus twice-daily treatment. Br J Dermatol. 1995;133(4):592-597.

Bornhovd E, Burgdorf W, Wollenberg A: Immunomodulatory macrolactams for topical treatment of infl ammatory skin diseases. *Curr Opin Investig Drugs* 2002; 3: 708–712.

Brazzelli V, Prestinari F, Chiesa M, et al. Sequential treatment of severe atopic dermatitis with cyclosporin A and low-dose narrow-band UVB phototherapy. *Dermatol* 2002; 204:252.

Callard R, Harper J. The Skin Barrier, Atopic Dermatitis and Allergy: A Role for Langerhans Cells? *Trends Immunol.* 2007. Jul;28(7):294-8.

Callen J, Chamlin, S, Eichenfield, L, et al. A systematic review of the safety of topical therapies for atopic dermatitis. *Br J Dermatol.* 2007;156: 203–221.

Clinical Trials. Preliminary Study of Safety and Efficacy of Nanocrystalline Silver Cream in Atopic Dermatitis (Eczema). Accessed 5/11/11. Available from: www.clinicaltrials.gov

Correale C, Walker C, Murphy L, et al. Atopic dermatitis: a review of diagnosis and treatment. *Am Fam Physician.* 1999;60:1191-1198.

Caubet, J, Eigenmann, P. 2010. Allergic Triggers in Atopic Dermatitis. *Immunology Allergy Clinics North America,* 30, 289-307.

Denman S. A review of pruritus. *J Am Acad Dermatol.* 1986;14:375-392.

Deshazo R. Atopic dermatitis. *Am J Med* 2009;122-121-125.

Fleischer A Jr. Treatment of atopic dermatitis: role of tacrolimus ointment as a topical noncorticosteroid therapy. *J Allergy Clin Immunol.* 1999;104:S126-S130.

Ghazvini, P, Pagan L, Rutledge T, Goodman, S. 2010. *Journal of Pharmacy Practice,* 23,2, 110-116.

Grassberger M, Baumruker T, Enz A, et al. A novel anti-infl ammatory drug, SDZ ASM 981, for the treatment of skin diseases: in vitro pharmacology. *Br J Dermatol* 1999; 141: 264–273.

Graves J, Nunley K, Heffernan M. Off-label uses of biologics in dermatology: rituximab, omalizumab, infliximab, etanercept, adalimumab, efalizumab, and alefacept (part 2 of 2). *J Am Acad Dermatol* 2007; 56:e55.

Grupper C. The chemistry, pharmacology and use of tar in treatment of psoriasis. In: Farber EM, Cox AJ, eds. Psoriasis: Proceeding of International Symposium. Stanford: Stanford University, 1971: 347–56.

Habif, T. 2008. *Clinical Dermatology*. Mosby, 978-0-7234-3541-9. Britain.

Hanifin J, Schneider L, Leung D, et al. Recombinant interferon gamma therapy for atopic dermatitis. *J Am Acad Dermatol* 1993; 28:189.

Hennekes H and Asadullah K. Strategies for Targeting IL-4 as a Novel Therapeutic Approach for theTreatment of Atopic Dermatitis. *Curr. Med. Chem. – Anti-Inflammatory & Anti-Allergy Agents*, 2002, 1, 41-53

Hon K, Ching G, Leung T, et al. Efficacy and tolerability at 3 and 6 months following use of azathioprine for recalcitrant atopic dermatitis in children and young adults. *J Dermatol Treat* 2009; 20:141.

Kang S, Lucky A, Pariser D, et al. Long-term safety and efficacy of tacrolimus ointment for the treatment of atopic dermatitis in children. *J Am Acad Dermatol.* 2001;44:S58-S64.

Klein P, Clark R. An evidence-based review of the efficacy of antihistamines in relieving pruritus in atopic dermatitis. *Arch Dermatol.* 1999;135:1522–1525. (Ia)

Kodama A, Horikawa T, Suzuki T, et al. Effect of stress on atopic dermatitis: investigation in patients after the great hanshin earthquake. *J Allergy Clin Immunol.* 1999;104:173–176.

Koopman L, van Strien R, Kerkhof M, et al. Placebo-controlled trial of house dust mite-impermeable mattress covers: effect on symptoms in early childhood. *Am J Respir Crit Care Med* 2002;166(3):307–13.

Kristal L, Klein P. Atopic dermatitis in infants and children. *Pediatr Clin North Am.* 2000;47: 877-895.

Lavker R, Grove F, Kligman A. The atrophogenic effect of crude coal tar on human epidermis. *Br J Dermatol* 1981; 105: 77–81.

Leung A, Hon K. Atopic Dermatitis. *Adv Pediatr* 2007;54:241-273.

Leung A, Barber K. Managing Childhood Atopic Dermatitis. *Adv Dermatol.* 2003; 20: 129-137.

Leung A, Wong B, Chan P, et al. Pruritus in children. *J R Soc Health.* 1998;118:280-286.

Leung D, Eichenfield LF, Boguniewicz M. Atopic dermatitis (atopic eczema). In: Freeberg IM, Eisen AZ, et al., eds. Dermatology in General Medicine, 6th ed. New York: McGraw-Hill, 2003:1464–1480.

Leung D, Nicklas R, Li J. et al. Disease management of atopic dermatitis: an updated practice parameter. Joint Task Force on Practice Parameters. *Ann Allergy Asthma Immunol.* 2004 Sep;93(3 Suppl 2):S1-21.

Lipozencic J. The diagnostic value of atopy patch testing and prick testing in atopic dermatitis. *Clin Dermatol* 2010:28:38-44.

Lipozencic J, Wolf R. Atopic Dermatitis: an Update and Review of the Literature. *Dermatol Clin* 2007; 25: 605–612

Melin L, Frederiksen T, Noren P, et al. Behavioural treatment of scratching in patients with atopic dermatitis. *Br J Dermatol.* 1986;115:467–474.

Michel S, Yawalkar N, Schnyder B, et al. Eczematous skin reaction to atopy patch testing with cockroach in patients with atopic dermatitis. *J Investig Allergol Clin Immunol* 2009;19(3):173–9.

Nassif A, Chan S, Storrs FJ, et al. Abnormal skin irritancy in atopic dermatitis and in atopy without dermatitis. *Arch Dermatol.* 1994;130:1402–1407.

Niordson A, Stahl D. Treatment of psoriasis with Clinitar cream: a controlled clinical trial. *Br J Clin Pract.* 1985;39: 67–68, 72.

Ong P, Boguniewicz M. Atopic Dermatitis. *Primary Care: Clinics in Office Practice* 2008;134:1348-1359.

Oosting A, de Bruin-Weller M, Terreehorst I, et al. Effect of mattress encasings on atopic dermatitis outcome measures in a double-blind, placebo-controlled study: the Dutch mite avoidance study. *J Allergy Clin Immunol* 2002;110(3):500–6.

Paller A, Eichenfield L, Leung D, et al. A 12 week study of tacrolimus ointment for the treatment of atopic dermatitis in pediatric patients. *J Am Acad Dermatol.* 2001;44:S47-S57.

Raimer S. Managing pediatric atopic dermatitis. *Clin Pediatr.* 2000;39:1-14.

Reitamo S, Van Leent E, Ho V, et al. Efficacy and safety of tacrolimus ointment compared with that of hydrocortisone acetate ointment in children with atopic dermatitis. *J Allergy Clin Immunol.* 2002;109:539-546.

Ruiz-Maldonado R, Zapata G, Tamayo L, et al. Cushing's syndrome after topical application of corticosteroids. *Am J Dis Child.* 1982;136:274-275.

Shelley W, Shelley E, Talanin N. Self-potentiating allergic contact dermatitis caused by doxepin hydrochloride cream. *J Am Acad Dermatol.* 1996;34:143–144.

Sicherer S, Sampson H. Food hypersensitivity and atopic dermatitis: pathophysiology, epidemiology, diagnosis, and management. *J Allergy Clin Immunol* 1999;104(3 Pt 2):S114–22.

Simon-Nobbe B, Denk U, Poll V, et al. The spectrum of fungal allergy. *Int Arch Allergy Immunol* 2008;145(1):58–86.

Sloper K, Wadsworth J, Brostoff J. Children with atopic eczema. I: Clinical response to food elimination and subsequent double-blind food challenge. *Q J Med.* 1991;80(292):677-693.

Schmid-Grendelmeier P, Simon D, Simon H, et al. Epidemiology, clinical features and immunology of atopic dermatitis. *Allergy* 2005;56:845-851.

Schmitt J, Schäkel K, Schmitt N, Meurer M. Systemic treatment of severe atopic eczema: a systematic review. *Acta Derm Venereol* 2007; 87:100

Soter N, Fleischer A Jr, Webster G, et al. Tacrolimus ointment for the treatment of atopic dermatitism in adult patients, part II: safety. *J Am Acad Dermatol.* 2001;44(suppl):S39-S46.

Sowden J, Berth-Jones J, Ross J, et al. Double-blind, controlled, crossover study of cyclosporin in adults with severe refractory atopic dermatitis. *Lancet* 1991; 338:137.

Stoppoloni G, Prisco F, Santinelli R, et al. Potential hazards of topical steroid therapy. *Am J Dis Child* 1983;137:1130-1131.

Tan B, Weald D, Strickland I, et al. Double-blind controlled trial of effect of housedust-mite allergen avoidance on atopic dermatitis. *Lancet* 1996;347(8993):15–8.

Van Leent F, Gräber M, Thurston M, et al. Effectiveness of the ascomycin macrolactam SDZ ASM 981 in the topical treatment of atopic dermatitis. *Arch Dermatol.* 1998;134:805-809.

Weatherhead S, Wahie S, Reynolds N, et al. An open-label, dose-ranging study of methotrexate for moderate-to- severe adult atopic eczema. *Br J Dermatol* 2007; 156:346.

15

Food Allergy in Atopic Dermatitis

Geunwoong Noh[1] and Jae Ho Lee[1,2]
[1]*Subdivision of Allergy and Clinical Immunology*
Department of Paediatrics, Chungnam National University Hospital, Daejoen
[2]*Department of Paediatrics, Chungnam National University*
College of Medicine, Daejeon
Korea

1. Introduction

Atopic dermatitis (AD) is a form of allergic skin inflammation characterized by late eczematous skin lesions [1]. These skin lesions occur through non-Immunoglobulin E (non-IgE)-mediated immune responses, and therefore, AD can be regarded as a non-IgE-mediated allergic inflammatory skin disease [2]. Many causes, including inhalant allergens, food allergens, and other factors, have been implicated in AD [1]. In addition to information about the causes, knowledge of the immunologic nature of AD is extremely important in order to understand AD. Without an understanding of the immunologic nature of AD, the cause of food allergy in patients with AD may be wrongly identified. Because of this confusion in establishing the cause of a food allergy in AD, the role of food allergy in AD remains poorly understood [2]. However, with the recent advance in the diagnosis and treatment of food allergy, it is necessary inevitably to distinguish between IgE- and non-IgE-mediated food allergies that co-exist with AD in order to better understand and control AD [2].

It is well-known that food allergy is an important cause of atopic dermatitis [3]. Although food allergies can be either IgE- or non-IgE-mediated, due to a lack of diagnostic modalities such as laboratory tests to diagnose non-IgE-mediated food allergy [4], it is difficult to clarify the nature of the food allergy, leading to confusion about role of food allergy in AD. Tests that determine IgE levels cannot predict the likelihood of an eczematous reaction because eczematous reactions are the result of non-IgE-mediated food allergies [2].

Until recently, discrimination of IgE-mediated and non-IgE-mediated food allergies was not considered necessary for diagnosis or treatment. Therapeutic modalities, including tolerance induction for food allergy (TIFA), have been developed for patients with food allergy [5,6]. However, the principles for diagnosing and treating IgE-mediated or non-IgE-mediated food allergies are quite different [7]. Presently, a differential diagnosis is absolutely necessary for relevant, proper, and successful treatment of IgE-mediated and non-IgE-mediated food allergies, independently. Clinical approaches to treat food allergy in AD patients, including laboratory tests and diagnosis, should consider the conceptual differences between IgE-mediated and non-IgE-mediated food allergies.

In the past, avoidance has been suggested as the main principle for treating food allergies [8]. More recently, however, the clinical and laboratory characteristics of IgE-mediated and non-IgE-mediated food allergy in atopic dermatitis have been well-characterized, and the relevant treatment techniques, including tolerance induction for food allergy (TIFA), have been markedly advanced and well-established [7]. In this chapter, updates on the diagnosis and relevant treatments for food allergy in AD are described

2. Atopic dermatitis

2.1 Definition

Atopic dermatitis (AD) is a chronic, relapsing inflammatory skin disease [1] that is characterized by non-IgE-mediated allergic skin inflammation, in which allergen-specific Th2 cells play a major role in the pathogenesis of the inflammation [2]. The appearance of atopic dermatitis is characterized by late eczematous reactions, which result from an allergen-specific Th2 immune response.

2.2 Immunopathogenesis of AD with food allergy

The immunologic phases of food allergy in AD include a sensitization phase and an effector phase (Fig. 1) [2]. During the sensitization phase, the tolerance of a subject to a specific allergen is determined. Response to that allergen, either allergic or tolerant, occurs in the effector phase.

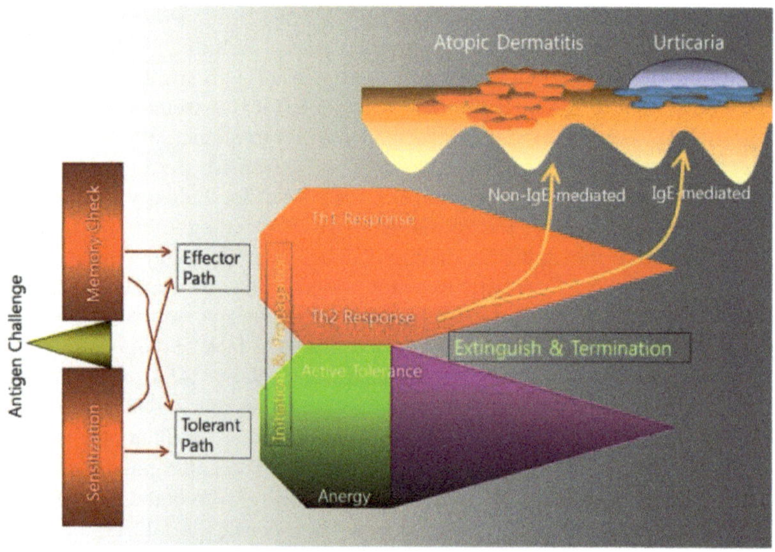

Fig. 1. Scheme of immunopathogenesis of food allergy in atopic dermatitis. When allergen is challenged, the immune system check the memory. In the neosensitization, immunologic memory of allergy is induced in the Th2 polarized status, or tolerized in normal status. In the immunologic process, IgE-mediated allergy or non-IgE-mediated allergy is formed when food allergen is to be memorized to react as allergic reactions. If food allergen is re-challenged, atopic dermatitis is appeared by non-IgE-mediated food allergy or IgE-mediated allergy including urticaria to anaphylactic shock occured. If allergen is memorized being tolerant, there is no reaction even by any further challenge by allergen. IgE-mediated food allergy and non-IgE-mediated allergy is apparently different in the immunopathogenesis as well as clinical manifestations.

Humans are continually challenged by foreign particles, including pathogens and foods. Protection from these foreign substances is mediated by effective immune responses (effectors). Protection from immune responses directed against food occurs by an immune tolerance response (tolerance). Allergy is one type of effector immune response that is the consequence of allergic sensitization. Allergic sensitization occurs from a Th1/Th2 imbalance [9]. There are 2 classes of allergic effector mechanisms: IgE-mediated and non-IgE-mediated allergic reactions. An IgE-mediated allergic response occurs if allergen-specific IgE is activated after exposure to the specific allergen. IgE-mediated immune reactions include urticaria, asthma, and rhinitis.

IgE has been positioned at the center of focus in allergy and allergic disease research. However, a major characteristic of AD is its non-IgE-mediated response.

3. Clinical characteristics of food allergy in AD

3.1 Clinical features of AD

The clinical phenotype of AD varies with age and course of the disease [10]. The eczematous lesions may present as acute (oozing, crusted, or eroded vesicles or papules on erythematous plaques), subacute (thick and excoriated plaques), or chronic (lichenified, slightly pigmented, or excoriated plaques) forms. Furthermore, xerosis and a lowered threshold for itching are usual hallmarks of AD. Pruritus attacks can occur throughout the day and worsen at the night, causing insomnia, exhaustion, and a substantial impairment in quality of life. To date, the symptoms and signs of AD have been listed horizontally. However, the primary clinical manifestations of AD include eczematous skin lesions and itching caused by allergen-specific Th2 immune responses. Some clinical manifestations of AD, including papule, plaque, and xerosis, are descriptions of skin manifestations; some manifestations, including excoriation, are related to the primary AD symptoms and signs; and some manifestations, including viral infection and impetigo, insomnia, and exhaustion, are secondary to the primary symptoms and signs.

3.2 Clinical features of food allergy in AD

The clinical manifestations of IgE-mediated food allergy (IFA) are uniform in AD and in the absence of AD; they include dermatologic manifestations, such as immediate urticaria and rashes, as well as other cardiovascular and respiratory symptoms and signs [2].

The clinical manifestations of non-IgE-mediated food allergy (NFA) are not uniform. Although IFA has been described as a central immunopathogenesis of atopic dermatitis, the symptoms and signs of IFA do not correspond to those of atopic dermatitis. Rather, the symptoms and signs of NFA are those of atopic dermatitis itself.

Food allergies have clinical manifestations on the skin as well as gastrointestinal and respiratory systems. Cutaneous reactions have been categorised as non-eczematous versus eczematous and early versus late [11]. Non-eczematous reactions tend to occur immediately after exposure to the food, usually immediately or within less than 1 hour. The typical reactions include pruritus, urticaria, angioedema, and diffuse morbilliform erythema. These reactions do not cause immediate exacerbations of AD, and they are commonly associated with gastrointestinal or respiratory symptoms. Acute urticaria and angioedema are among the most common symptoms, and acute contact urticaria or allergy can also occur. One-half of the reactions after the ingestion of milk are not mediated by specific IgE antibodies to milk protein and are lost by the age of 3 years. Eczematous reactions has been regarded as occurring less frequently. They usually manifest as a late event, generally defined as occurring 2 to 6 hours or more after exposure to the food. As has already been shown, eczematous reactions can develop infrequently as an early event or in combination with non-eczematous reactions.

The symptoms and signs of NFA are not uniform; they vary according to subjects and foods [2]. In addition, in one subject, various symptoms and signs often develop according to the food ingested. The onset time of symptoms and signs of NFA ranges from 2 hours to several days, up to even a week, after intake [12]. Because it is very difficult to predict the onset time of NFA symptoms, physicians should observe patients long enough to cover the maximum onset time following challenge or intake during daily life. The clinical manifestations of NFA show patterns of their own with respect to onset time, the severity of clinical manifestations, and type of allergy.

It should be kept in mind that AD patients, as well as other food allergy patients, may be allergic to multiple food allergens [13]. These patients may also have multiple types of food allergy, such as IFA and NFA, together. However, when this is the case, patients will not necessarily have both IFA and NFA simultaneously to the same food. The diagnosis, management, and treatment of food allergy in AD should be approached keeping in mind that subjects may have food allergies to multiple foods and that they may exhibit multiple types of food allergies including both IFA and NFA.

3.3 Types of foods that cause atopic dermatitis

Based on OFC outcomes, the most common food allergens in the United States, accounting for the vast majority of food allergies in patients, are known as cow's milk, hen's eggs, peanuts, soy, wheat, tree nuts, and shellfish [14]. Although some children prove to be truly allergic to meats, fruits, vegetables, or other grains, the vast majority have negative OFCs for these foods.

As confirmed in several studies, cow's milk, hen's eggs, wheat, soy, and peanuts are responsible for approximately 75% of food-associated AD [15,16] in IFA, whereas for NFA, meats as well as cow's milk, hen's eggs, soy and wheat were the major causes of AD [13].

In Western country, Hen's eggs and cow's milk are significantly more likely to result in IFA and are associated with elevated food-specific IgE [11]. Soy and wheat are more likely to cause late eczematous flares, but reactions to cow's milk were also observed. Although some of these reactions are observed in the context of elevated food-specific IgE, some also occur in the absence of food-specific IgE.

The same food can provoke IFA and NFA. In recent studies, foods were mapped according to the kinds of food allergy (IFA or NFA) and severity [7]. Such mapping is necessary for the proper management of food allergy in atopic dermatitis.

3.4 Mixed-type allergy: The simultaneous presence of two different types of food allergy, IFA and NFA, in AD

Because IFA and NFA are present together in atopic dermatitis, the characteristics of AD that result from each of these two types of food allergy should be clarified [7]. It is generally understood that IFA, rather than NFA, plays a central role in the immunopathogenesis of AD until recently [12]. Immediate reactions in IFA often lead to increased scratching and, eventually, secondary exacerbation of eczematous lesions [11], whereas direct exacerbation of AD with development of new eczematous outbreaks tends to occur as a late reaction and infrequently as an early reaction. However, in its clinical and immunopathogenic aspects, NFA is similar to AD. With the advent of successful treatments for food allergy, IFA is less so. In this chapter, AD are described, especially in the viewpoint of non-IgE-mediated food allergy.

3.5 Multiple food allergies in AD

Multiple sensitisation to foods in IFA

Multiple sensitisation with foods has not been generally considered a possible cause of AD; this is another point that can easily confuse clinicians and patients. The prevalence of data describing multiple food allergies in published studies provides an estimate of multiple food allergy prevalence [7, 13]. In a study of food allergies in a highly atopic group of children, all of whom had atopic dermatitis and 50% of whom had concurrent asthma or allergic rhinitis, 57% reacted to two or three foods during double-blind, placebo-controlled food challenges [17]. Most children in this subset had positive skin prick tests (SPTs) to several foods, although only approximately one third of positive tests correlated with positive food challenge [13]. However, few children reacted to more than three foods [18]. Five foods (eggs, peanuts, milk, wheat, and soy) accounted for approximately 60% of the positive clinical responses in this study [19].

More than 500 random serum samples were evaluated for specific IgE against six common food allergens (milk, eggs, wheat, soy, peanuts, and cod) [17]. They addressed that having evidence of IgE-mediated sensitisation to a food does not necessarily imply a true food allergy. This study found that 27% of children were sensitised to more than one of the six foods. The main limitation of this retrospective study was that information regarding clinical reactivity to foods was not available; therefore, it is not known how many of these patients were truly allergic to more than one food.

A recent study examining the prevalence of multiple food allergies found that most (>70%) food-allergic children were allergic to or were avoiding multiple foods [17]. On average, each child was avoiding three or four foods or food groups. These children were generally very atopic, with 56% showing atopic dermatitis, 47% having allergic rhinitis, and 38% having asthma. Thus, highly atopic children may be at greater risk for allergies to multiple foods.

Sensitisation to multiple foods in AD

Although food allergies are not the only cause of AD, in many cases AD is caused by multiple food allergies. Over 50% of AD patients also exhibited NFA to a mean of 2.8 food items [18]. Moreover, IFA co-exists simultaneously with AD and NFA [7]. Interestingly, in most cases, patients with isolated IFA did not have AD. From these results, it seems clear that NFA is the major type of food allergy in AD, although IFA is the aggravating cause of AD.

4. Diagnosis of food allergy in AD

The diagnosis of food allergy should be made following the discrimination of IgE- and non-IgE-mediated allergies. Diagnostic protocols for IFA have been proposed by various researchers, institutes and academic societies; however, the concept of dosage quantitation, along with the measurement of clinical severity changes on the basis of discrimination of IgE- and non-IgE-mediated food allergy, has clearly become the most important point in successful immunotherapy [7]. Because both the diagnostic and the therapeutic protocols for IgE- and non-IgE-mediated food allergies differ greatly, the major points in these protocols should be revised.

The two most important points regarding diagnosis of food allergy in atopic dermatitis are as follows: 1) distinction should be made between IFA and NFA and 2) the treatment dosage must be calibrated and the clinical severity assessed for the purposes of therapy and follow-up [7].

4.1 Allergy history

A detailed clinical history is the key first step in the diagnosis of potential food allergy, followed by skin testing and immunoassay testing when indicated by the history [14]. Ultimately, however, in cases of non-anaphylactic reactions and especially non-IgE-mediated food allergies, OFCs may be required for an accurate diagnosis.

Parents often consider their child's AD as an "allergic" manifestation of a presumed food allergy [11]. Although the influence of the media and popular culture may play a role, parents also receive differing opinions from primary care providers and dermatologists [11]. Greater than 90% of parents and 60% of primary care providers may suspect food allergy as the cause of AD, resulting in referrals to allergists and extensive testing.

Food allergies should be suspected from the patient's history of experiences of allergy provocation, especially in case of IgE-mediated food allergy [7]. However, apart from major immediate anaphylactic reactions, patient history has proven to be an unreliable way to diagnose food allergies [3]. A poor correlation between food allergy and medical history, with only 25%-48% sensitivity overall and a 72%-97% specificity for IFA, has been reported. Moreover, in NFA it is more difficult for patients and parents to recognise the relationship between the ingested food and allergy provocation because of the difficult clinical characteristics as well as delayed reactions of this condition, and a history of NFA is inconsistent with the final diagnosis of NFA [18]. The additional possibility of exercise-induced food allergy should be considered and excluded by history.

4.2 Laboratory approaches to food allergy in AD

Blood eosinophil numbers

Increases in blood eosinophil counts due to NFA provocation by OFC have been demonstrated and blood eosinophilia is useful simply as a clue in the diagnosis of allergy [20]. The level of blood eosinophils has clinical significance as a predictor of the efficacy of IFN-γ therapy in atopic dermatitis [21].

Total IgE

Although not all patients with AD have elevated IgE, as many as 40% to 80% [11] have been found to have high food-specific IgE levels. Total IgE does not seem to be associated with current allergic disease activity.

ECP

Eosinophil cationic protein (ECP) is produced by activated eosinophils [22]. Food additives were shown to elevate blood ECP in atopic dermatitis [23]. Interestingly, ECP is elevated without the elevation of blood eosinophil numbers in AD patients and even in normal subjects in recent studies conducted [24]. In this report, food additives were shown to provoke xerosis (dry skin) and resultant pruritus consistent with AD. Among patients suspected to have AD, over 30% showed pseudoallergies to food additives [25]. The signs and symptoms caused by food additives can interfere with the interpretation of OFC and with the therapeutic process. ECP is specifically elevated in patients who ingest artificial chemical food additives [24] and elevated ECP has been used as a marker of pseudoallergic reactions due to food additives, particularly when blood eosinophil numbers are normal.

Skin prick test and specific IgEs in IFA

IFA is approached initially by tests for allergen-specific IgE. The skin prick test (SPT) has a high negative predictive value (approximately 95%) and is most informative when it is negative; the positive predictive value ranges between 30% and 50% [3]. Therefore, SPT is useful for excluding IFA, but a positive result may only be suggestive of IFA. Laboratory testing for food-specific IgEs also has a high negative predictive value, estimated to be 75%, but its positive predictive value is low, ranging from 20% to 60%. Recently, the diagnostic levels of food-specific IgEs have been determined. The presence of specific IgEs at or above these levels offers a positive predictive value of approximately 95% for IFA. Although skin prick tests and serum IgE measurements can confirm sensitisation, neither of these tests can on its own prove clinical allergy to a specific food with reliability or consistency. Moreover, IgE-based laboratory tests will only predict IFA; IgE-based tests are not useful for the diagnosis of NFA in AD [18].

In spite of the extremely high specific IgE and strong SPT usually associated with HDM, HDM rarely induces anaphylactic reactions following exposure. In contrast, food-induced IgE-mediated allergies, including systemic urticaria and anaphylactic allergic reactions, can occur when a patient has high specific IgE levels or strong skin reactivity for a food allergen.

Interpretation of polysensitisation from the results by the SPT or allergen-specific IgE

Polysensitisation to multiple allergens as the result of allergen-specific IgE and skin prick tests, especially to multiple food allergens, may be embarrassing to the physician. Sensitisation of the skin caused by the skin prick test and the presence of specific IgE do not indicate the presence of allergy [2].

In cases of skin sensitisation, patients often show similar reactions (itching, rash, or urticaria) to contact with allergen in the skin prick test. Therefore, patients should avoid allergens which are positive by the skin prick test. Sensitisation to specific allergens by allergen-specific IgE does not always provoke allergy. Based on the level of allergen-specific IgE, IgE-mediated allergy can be predicted, especially for food allergens. Therefore, physicians should just consider IgE-mediated food allergy if patients have high food-specific IgE.

Allergy patch test

The immunopathogenesis of eczematous allergic reactions to food that occurs in non-IgE-mediated food allergy is similar to that of allergic contact dermatitis in that it is T lymphocyte-mediated and associated with food-specific T lymphocytes [3]. For these reasons, atopic patch testing (APT) has been used to investigate food-induced eczema.

Laboratory follow-up

Blood eosinophils provide information on current disease activity of the non-IgE-mediated type [20]. For the evaluation of disease progress and continuing disease activity and for the effective management of non-IgE-mediated allergy including NFA, blood eosinophil levels are tested repeatedly on a regular schedule.

Serum ECP should also be followed to determine changes in the disease activity of non-IgE-mediated allergy and the effectiveness of an elimination diet for food additives in atopic dermatitis.

The interpretation of the results of allergen-specific tests, such as the skin prick test and allergen-specific IgE, is often complicated because the number of positive SPT responses, the spectrum of IgE sensitisation and even the results for the same allergen often change in the same individual over time [26]. This variability may be related to the number of allergens tested and the age at which the measurements are performed. The most common food allergens determined with the SPT are soy, cow's milk, peanuts, carrot, hen's eggs whites, wheat, and corn [27].

However, changes in reactivity to allergens must be considered to be a natural phenomenon that is affected by the natural outgrowing of food allergy and the gradual acquisition of allergy to inhaled allergens, including house dust mites and pollen [2]. The change in the number of allergens to which a patient responds over time and the change in response to one allergen over time provides the physician with information on the progress of the disease. If the number of sensitised allergens decreases, the allergy itself may be regarded to be decreasing systemically. In addition, if the strength of SPT or the level of food-specific IgE is decreasing, the patient may be outgrowing the allergy.

4.3 Oral food challenge

The gold standard to confirm or disprove food allergy is the OFC, particularly double-blinded, placebo-controlled OFCs [8]. In the case of NFA, OFCs are safe, whereas in IFA, OFCs are time-consuming and carry the potential for severe reactions. They should be performed by experienced health-care professionals who have access to emergency equipment. Despite the mentioned caveats, OFCs are especially useful because observation for 24 hours or more after food exposure allows the assessment of both early and late reactions to the food and thus can detect both IgE- and non-IgE-mediated processes.

4.3.1 Prerequisites for oral food challenge in atopic dermatitis

Evaluation of clinical severity scores

For the diagnosis of food allergy, a clinical severity scoring system is necessary. This scoring differs between IFA and NFA. The diagnosis of IFA is straight forward because of the apparent clinical manifestation following a challenge. There are several scoring systems for IFA described by Clark [28] and Noh [6]. The diagnosis of NFA is difficult due to its clinical characteristics, which are almost the same as those of atopic dermatitis, and the SCORAD index and clinical severity scoring systems for AD can be used for NFA [29]. Clinical severity scoring should be done at the initial evaluation, at every visit, and before and after every procedure.

1. Diet record

A dietary diary should be kept during diagnosis and treatment [2]. In the process of management of food allergies in AD, daily diet diaries should be used to record complete basic recipes for each meal. For the supervision of dietary management, all food should be recorded, including elimination diets, open OFCs, and tolerance induction. This is especially important for breast-feeding infants. In such cases, the diet of the mother should be recorded along with the diet of the infant, including the times of ingestion and the time of the appearance of new AD lesions or aggravation of old AD lesions.

2. Elimination diet

An elimination diet should precede an oral food challenge. Without complete elimination of the causes of the allergy provocation, it is difficult to interpret the results of an oral food challenge [2].

For IFA, the causative foods are typically easily recognised by parents and patients; it is therefore easy to eliminate and challenge with foods. However, it is very difficult to recognise the triggers for the diagnosis to be made in NFA. The accumulated statistics for NFA in atopic dermatitis are absolutely necessary [2]. Moreover, in cases of NFA associated with atopic dermatitis, the causative agents are more complicated and may include HDM [30]; thus, all possible allergens must be eliminated for a proper oral food challenge. Fortunately, the proper control of the causative allergens, including food and inhaled allergens, can be evaluated based on stable improvement during an elimination diet. An initial elimination diet is important as an indicator of the proper control of allergy provocation [2].

Once patients show improvement through an initial elimination diet, oral food challenges are conducted. Foods that were not addressed in the initial elimination diet should also be considered. IFN-γ therapy can be considered when patients do not improve following the initial elimination diet [2] because IFN-γ therapy itself does not affect allergy provocation during the next OFC [20].

3. Basic general management

Without basic care and the control of allergens other than foods, the precise diagnosis of food allergies may be confusing. This type of management includes the following: 1) Skin care using non-steroid drugs and emollients including moisturizer and aroma oil, 2) House dust mite and other inhaled allergen care (dander, pollen, fungi and others); patients should be tested for allergy provocation by inhaled or environmental allergens, 3) Other factors (infection control, others), 4) Discontinue all medications that affect allergy provocation (steroids, antihistamines, other immunosuppressants, drugs with unknown effects (herbal medications), etc [2].

4.3.2 Elimination diets as a first step in the diagnosis of food allergies

1. Elimination diet and elementary diet

Diet control for the elimination of food allergy can be assessed using an elimination diet and an elementary diet. An elimination diet is a restriction of the possibly causative foods, whereas an elementary diet permits several safe foods. Both approaches require clinical data from studies [18, 19, 21]; such data are very important because if the clinical statistics are not proper, dietary restriction does not result in clinical improvement. The proper OFC then cannot be advanced further.

For an effective elementary diet, the absolutely safe foods in atopic dermatitis should be addressed. An effective elimination diet is a higher modality because it requires the accumulation of clinical data for statistics regarding the causative foods for atopic dermatitis. Noh and Lee focused on these points, and an effective elimination diet is now available for atopic dermatitis [12, 13, 18, 19, 21].

More than 50% of AD patients have NFA . Without the control of allergy provocation, AD cannot be effectively controlled [21]. As a first step in the diagnosis of food allergy, dietary restrictions should be initiated. If a patient shows improvement on an elimination diet, a food allergy to the restricted foods should be strongly suspected. An optimal elimination diet can be achieved by providing a list of the foods to be restricted, which in turn can be determined by clinical statistics.

2. Breast-fed infants

In the case of breast-fed infants, maternal elimination diets are recommended. Once a maternal elimination diet is implemented, improvements are often observed in the infant [31]. If eczema improves during the elimination diet, the clinical relevance of the eliminated foods should be confirmed with standardised, physician-supervised oral food challenges to the mother.

4.3.3 Oral food challenge

Through OFC, the suspected foods should be listed with the classification of type of allergy, and a relevant elimination diet that eliminates only suspected foods should result in an improvement of AD symptoms [2]. The order for the OFC should prioritise NFA before IFA. Additionally, the importance of certain foods should be considered according to the patient's wishes. An OFC for NFA should generally precede an OFC for IFA. Each OFC is conducted according to the relevant protocols.

1. Principle of oral food challenge in AD (Goldmann's triad): intake, elimination diet and challenge test

The diagnosis of food allergy follows the standard principle of Goldmann's triad [19]. When patients show symptoms and signs after the ingestion of suspected causative foods, an elimination diet is initiated. If the patient shows improvement with this diet, the eliminated food is strongly suspected as the cause of AD. If the patient again shows the clinical manifestation with subsequent food challenge, the challenged food is confirmed as the cause of AD.

2. Proper elimination of foods as an absolute condition for OFC

An elimination diet is the first effective way to confirm a food allergy in AD. However, a proper elimination diet is necessary [2]. Unless such a diet is performed, it is likely that elimination will be ineffective. A proper elimination diet is essential and should not be omitted.

4.3.4 Types of OFC

There are various types of OFC that may be clinically indicated, including open, single-blind, double-blind, and placebo-controlled trials. The choice of the type of OFC is based on a clinical assessment of the potential for bias in the interpretation of the results) [32]. Open OFC is the unmasked, unblinded administration of a food in its natural form. Open OFC is recommended for IFA because IFA is associated with a clear clinical manifestation. Moreover, in NFA, open OFC is effective in the clinical setting and can be performed on an out-patient basis. Open OFC is a cost-efficient procedure that saves substantial time and resources. It is thus considered to be a reasonable first choice for evaluating an adverse reaction to a food when the need for an OFC has been established.

Blinding and masking by mixing the challenge food with a masking vehicle or placing the food in vehicles, including opaque capsules or powders, reduces bias [32]. In the single-blind OFC, the observer but not the patient knows the food being tested. In the double-blind

OFC, the challenge material is provided by a third party, such as a dietitian, and the patient, the patient's family, and the observer are unaware of when the test food is administered. Bias is thus minimised. Placebo-controlled challenges may be administered in either a single-blind or double-blind fashion.

4.3.5 Indications for an OFC

Indications for an OFC in AD are listed below [2, 20, 32]; 1) Identify foods causing AD for the initial diagnosis of a food allergy and for monitoring resolution of the food allergy, 2) Discriminate between IFA and NFA, 3) Calibrate the provoking dose and determine the clinical severity of the reaction for therapeutic purposes in IFA and in order to monitor progress in IFA treatment, 4) Expand the diet in persons who have multiple dietary restrictions because of subjective complaints, such as headaches or hyperactive behaviour, 5) Assess the status of tolerance to cross-reactive foods, 6) Assess the effect of food processing on food tolerability, e.g., fruits and vegetables that may be tolerated in cooked form in the pollen-food allergy syndrome.

4.3.6 OFC procedures for IFA and NFA

The basic concept of OFC is the same for IFA and NFA. However, due to the different clinical characteristics of the two types of allergy, the OFC protocols for each differ significantly in principle and in dosage protocol [7]. OFC is conducted with relevant protocols for IFA or NFA. An OFC for IFA is relatively easy and simple, with higher risk, whereas an OFC for NFA is intricate and all aspects of this OFC should be carefully considered.

- IFN-γ in OFC

IFN-γ does not inhibit allergy provocation [19]; however, it does improve the pre-existing symptoms and signs of atopic dermatitis, including eczematous skin lesions and pruritus [19, 21]. The clinical characteristics of AD are of the non-IgE-mediated type, and the onset and duration of symptoms and signs are relatively longer [7]. It is difficult to handle or proceed to the next challenge when the patient shows a severe NFA reaction during the challenge. The use of steroids or antihistamines for symptomatic treatment can inhibit the allergic reaction caused by OFC or hide the symptoms of allergy provocation during an OFC.

4.3.7 Clinical characteristics of OFC

1. IFA and NFA

Rapid onset and apparent clinical manifestations are typical of IFA [7]. During proceeding with the OFC for food allergy, the onset time following challenge, the duration of symptoms and signs, and the various clinical manifestations should be considered. Although the diagnosis of NFA is made based on the change of clinical severity scores, expertise is necessary in the OFC for NFA because the same food may provoke variable clinical manifestations with an unexpected onset time during the challenge.

2. Characteristics of OFC

The characteristics of food allergy are well described by Noh and Lee [7]. The clinical characteristics of food allergy to the same food may differ among patients and may differ in the same patient according to the type of food. Some foods, such as shrimp and mackerel, tend to provoke IgE-mediated food allergy, whereas other foods, such as milk, eggs, soybeans and wheat, tend to provoke both IgE- and non-IgE-mediated food allergies. Other foods, such as meats, tend to predominantly provoke non-IgE-mediated food allergy. According to the characteristics of the region, the kinds of foods that cause food allergy also differ. Patients who live near the sea tend to have allergies to seafood, whereas patients who live in land tend to have less frequent allergies to seafood. Allergy to rice is less frequent in Oriental countries than in Western countries, whereas wheat allergy is more frequent in Oriental countries than in Western countries.

The statistics on food allergy are very important in clinical practice. Basically, the foods that should be restricted in the initial elimination diet for the control of food allergy in atopic dermatitis have been identified based on the statistics on food allergy [12, 13, 18, 19, 21]. The necessary statistics should be based on challenge tests conducted at least with open OFC and not on laboratory results because IgE-based tests cannot predict the presence of food allergy, particularly for non-IgE-mediated food allergy in atopic dermatitis.

Interestingly, meat (beef, chicken, pork) has not been recognised as an important cause of food allergy in atopic dermatitis because meats induce predominantly non-IgE-mediated food allergies [12, 13, 18, 19, 33]. From the statistics, fewer than 5% of patients have allergies to chicken and pork simultaneously. Therefore, if a patient shows an allergy to either chicken or pork, the physician can predict the possibility that the other may not provoke allergy in the patient. Approximately 10% of patients have allergies to both milk and eggs; thus, if a patient is allergic to either milk or eggs, the possibility that the patient has allergy to the other is less than 10%. Similar data are available for soybeans and wheat. The use of statistics is thus very helpful in managing food allergies related to atopic dermatitis.

Patients sometimes think that they may be allergic to beef if they are allergic to milk because milk comes from cows. However, this is not the case. Milk and beef have no statistical relationship as causes for food allergy in atopic dermatitis [12, 13, 18, 19, 33]. The same is the case for chicken and eggs. Physicians and dietitians should consider these points in the management of food allergy in atopic dermatitis.

4.4 Diagnosis of food allergy in infants

4.4.1 Breast-feeding infants and children

If an infant develops severe eczema while it is exclusively breast-fed, it is essential to consider a food allergy provoked by proteins in the breast milk. All food proteins can pass from the maternal diet into breast milk [31]. If an allergy due to exposure to a protein via maternal milk is diagnosed, it is necessary to modify the diet of the mother with professional dietetic support and supervision. Previously, in cases where multiple foods were implicated or there were concerns about maternal nutrition, it was appropriate to suggest the substitution of an appropriate milk formula. However, with the advent of tolerance induction, TIFA for allergenic foods is also available.

For the diagnosis of food allergy in the breast-feeding infant, OFC is performed through the mother [2]. Improvement of the baby following an elimination diet in the mother should occur before proceeding with an OFC. The mother ingests the challenge food and the baby consumes the breast milk. The baby is then evaluated following the same processes. The important point is that the baby should consume breast milk within a specified time (1-2 hours) after the mother ingests the challenge food. If the baby does not improve with the mother's elimination diet, IFN-γ therapy can be administered to the baby to elicit clinical improvement.

Because of its nutritional purpose, this process is designed to identify completely safe foods rather than allergenic foods [2]. According to the OFC protocol for breast-fed babies, it is very important to list the foods that can be ingested by the mother that are completely safe for the baby. The primary purpose of the diagnosis of food allergy is to provide safe recipes for the infant and the mother. Subsequently, the test results will be applied to the infant during the phase of solid food introduction. Safe foods will be introduced with priority. An OFC is conducted on the mother using normal protocols; the sole difference is that the food is given to the mother and reactions are observed in the infant.

4.4.2 Formula-feeding infants

In formula-feeding babies, the OFC is simpler than in breast-feeding infants [2]. The primary purpose of treatment is to set up safe formula feeding with casein hydrolysate, soy formula or other foods. To rule out milk allergy, challenge with casein hydrolysate will be performed for the diagnosis of allergy, especially to casein. If the infant improves with casein hydrolysate, he or she is allergic to casein and casein hydrolysate formula is be used until weaning.

If the baby does not improve on casein hydrolysate formula, it is subsequently challenged with amino acid-based formula. If the baby improves, the baby is allergic to components other than casein in milk or together with allergic to casein. The baby can then be fed the amino acid-based formula or be tested on soy formula. If the baby cannot tolerate the amino acid-based formula and has an allergy to casein hydrolysate, or if the parents wish to feed the baby soy formula, a soy formula challenge can be performed. If the baby improves with the soy formula, the baby is allergic to milk and can be fed with soy formula until weaning.

TIFA for any formula is indicated when the baby does not improve with either soy formula or casein hydrolysate or when the baby does not tolerate amino acid-based formula [2]. Parents can select the kinds of foods (milk or soy) to be tolerised. After tolerance induction for formula, the baby is fed the tolerised formula until weaning.

4.4.3 Mixed-feeding baby (breast-feeding with formula feeding)

An initial elimination diet for the mother is conducted with simultaneous feeding of a safe formula, as described above [2]. After initially setting the baby up with safe formula feeding and diet restriction of the mother, an OFC of the mother for the diagnosis of food allergy in the infant should be performed as described above.

4.4.4 Solid food introduction for baby (approximately 5-12 months)

The primary purpose of diagnosis is to set up a safe recipe for the infant to prevent nutritional deficiencies due to elimination diets or food allergies [2]. Transiently, an elimination diet should be conducted in the mother and all solid foods should be stopped in the infant (elimination diet of infant and mother). Due to nutritional considerations, elimination for the infant and the mother should not be conducted for more than 3 days. If the baby does not improve, IFN-γ therapy for the baby is indicated during subsequent OFCs of the baby. If the baby improves following an elimination diet of the mother and baby with or without IFN-γ, sequential introduction of solid foods may be performed according to the weaning schedule. However, the sequence of foods can be changed according to the circumstances of the infant and the mother. The mother and infant should be simultaneously fed with the same challenge foods. In case of formula feeding infants, stop all solid foods to the infant (elimination diet in the infant) and simultaneously set up a safe formula feeding during the elimination diet in the infant, as described above. Sequential introduction of solid foods should be performed according to the weaning schedule. Nutritional care for the infant is essential.

5. Immunotherapy for food allergy in AD

Presently, there are 3 therapeutic approaches for food allergies. In all cases, the allergen should be avoided until proper treatment is administered [9]. In infants and young children, the allergenic food(s) should be excluded from the diet until the allergy is outgrown unless exclusion results in nutritional deficiency or the allergen cannot be avoided; in such cases, active treatment, such as tolerance induction for food allergy (TIFA), is performed [2]. If exclusion cannot be practiced, patients may experience discomfort caused by non-IgE-mediated food allergy and atopic dermatitis or reactions as serious as anaphylaxis from repetitive ingestion of the allergenic food(s). However, with the recent advent of TIFA treatment, management of atopic dermatitis has improved remarkably [7].
Clinical tolerance can develop over time; this process is also called "outgrowing" the allergy. Allergies to milk and eggs are common food allergies that are outgrown: 80% of children with milk and egg allergies show tolerance by the age of 3 to 5 years [8]. In contrast, only about 20% of young children develop tolerance to peanuts, and less than 10% outgrow an allergy to tree nuts. However, the persistence of food allergy is variable and depends on the specific food allergen.

5.1 Specific Immunotherapy for food allergy

Allergen-specific therapies have been investigated to achieve desensitization and/or tolerance to an allergen [34]. Desensitization is defined as a change in the threshold dose of ingested food allergen necessary to cause allergic symptoms. Tolerance is the induction of long-term immunologic changes associated with the ability to ingest a food without showing symptoms and without ongoing therapy. In a recent pilot study [35], subcutaneous immunotherapy (SCIT) was well tolerated in children with milk allergy. Despite its efficacy in treating food allergy as well as allergic rhinoconjunctivitis and venom hypersensitivity, this traditional approach to allergen immunotherapy is impractical and unsafe for the treatment of food allergies because of an unacceptably high rate of anaphylactic reactions in IgE-mediated food allergy [34]. Sublingual immunotherapy (SLIT) has a broad efficacy for the treatment of inhalant allergies. SLIT has been used to treat hazelnut allergy and a life-threatening kiwi allergy. Currently, trials are in progress to evaluate the efficacy of SLIT in treating other food allergies. Traditional Chinese Medicine represents an innovative approach with the potential to treat food allergies although this approach is not allergen-specific. Food Allergy Herbal Formula (FAHF-2) is reported to promote tolerance and protection from anaphylaxis in mouse models. Further, human clinical trials are just beginning and hold promise for future clinical efficacy. Omalizumab is a recombinant, humanized, monoclonal anti-IgE antibody that was demonstrated to significantly increase the threshold peanut protein dose necessary for allergic response in oral food challenge, thereby providing potential protection from accidental peanut ingestion. Clinical trials are in progress to evaluate both anti-IgE monotherapy for food allergy and the use of omalizumab as an adjunct to oral immunotherapy. While this therapy is suitable for IgE-mediated food allergy, it is not applicable for treatment of non-IgE-mediated food allergy. Protection from peanut allergic response has also been demonstrated in a report where rectal immunization with mutated peanut protein allergens protected mice from anaphylaxis, Peptide immunotherapy has also been investigated using the immunodominant epitopes of ovalbumin.

5.2 Oral immunotherapy for food allergy: Tolerance induction for food allergies (TIFA) or specific oral tolerance induction (SOTI)

Oral immunotherapy appears to be effective in inducing desensitization in most patients, as well as oral tolerance in a subset of patients with food allergy [34]. Oral immunotherapy was officially introduced in 1996 in "Monographs in Allergy" [36, 37]. Noh & Lee reported the first successful use of oral immunotherapy for food allergy [38]. They used IFN-γ as the adjuvant for oral immunotherapy for food allergy and named this therapy "specific oral tolerance induction (SOTI)" in 2003. SOTI was attempted for IgE-mediated food allergy in humans by several investigators [5, 34, 39-43]. The complete SOTI protocol for IgE-mediated food allergy was accomplished by also using IFN-γ in 2009 by Noh & Lee [6].

Several terms are used to describe oral immunotherapy for food allergy. These terms are based on an escalating dosage of orally ingested foods or food protein to induce immune tolerance for allergenic food(s). Tolerance induction for food allergy (TIFA) was first coined by Noh & Lee in 2003 [38]. Specific oral tolerance induction (SOTI) is currently the more precise term to describe oral tolerance induction for specific allergens in food allergy, and this term, SOTI, was also used first by Noh in 2003 in a report on milk-specific oral tolerance induction for non-IgE-mediated food allergy in atopic dermatitis. Tolerance induction for food allergy (TIFA) is a similar term that has a broader immunologic meaning: to induce immune tolerance for allergenic foods by any method.

5.3 IFN-γ in food allergy and AD

IFN-γ was introduced for the correction of Th1/Th2 imbalance, which is the basic immunologic mechanism in allergies, including food allergy [21]. As expected, desensitization for house dust mites was successful when IFN-γ was used, but was ineffective without IFN-γ [30]. Moreover, IFN-γ seemed to show tolerogenic effects in addition to its corrective effects in Th1/Th2 imbalance [7]. Especially, IFN-γ was absolutely necessary for TIFA for non-IgE-mediated food allergy. Other than SOTI, effective treatment methods for non-IgE-mediated food allergy by using IFN-γ have not been established. Without IFN-γ, tolerance is not induced in non-IgE-mediated food allergy.

5.4 Indication for SOTI

Tolerance induction for food allergy is indicated when (1) nutritional deficiency is expected, (2) the patient is inevitably unable to avoid the allergen (e.g., wheat allergy in a baker), (3) an infant displays allergy to all available formulae, and (4) the patients or parents want an improved quality of life [2].

6. Prevention of food allergy

6.1 Breastfeeding for the prevention of food allergy

Breast milk is the gold standard for protective nutrients fed to newborn infants, and present clinical evidence supports the strong protective effect of breast milk against age-related infectious gastroenteritis [44]. An important function of early breastfeeding is its anti-inflammatory effect on the immature, excessive inflammatory response in newborns.

Several components of breast milk, including transforming growth factor (TGF)-beta, interleukin (IL)-10, erythropoietin, and lactoferrin, can reduce the inflammatory response to stimuli in the newborn intestine. Although, historically, there has been widespread support for the concept that breast-feeding is protective against atopic disease in general, breastfeeding could facilitate food allergies in certain cases by allowing transfer of the allergens from the mother's diet through breast milk. Exclusive breastfeeding for 4 months should be recommended to prevent atopic disease; however, there is no evidence to support the protective effect of exclusive breastfeeding beyond this period. Mixed feeding should be encouraged until 6 months of age.

6.2 Delayed introduction to solid foods to prevent the development of food allergy

An additional question regarding food allergy and AD is whether delaying the introduction of solid foods to infants at a high risk for AD can delay or prevent the development of AD. The most recent clinical report states that exclusive breast feeding for 4 to 6 months for infants who are at a high risk for AD (i.e., positive family history) can help prevent or delay AD; furthermore, cow's milk should not be introduced until 2 years of age in order to prevent allergy [11]. No convincing evidence exists to delay the introduction of any solid food beyond 4 to 6 months of age. In contrast, dairy products are recommended to be introduced at 12 months; hen's egg at 24 months; and peanuts, tree nuts, fish, and seafood at 36 months.

Attempts to avert the development of food allergy through primary prevention strategies such as early restriction of dietary allergens and modified timing of complementary solid food introduction to infants have proven to be frustrating and possibly counter-productive. Early dietary restriction of peanuts is recommended to avoid sensitization [34]. However, early consumption of food proteins and subsequent oral tolerance induction in infants and children may be a key element in preventing the development of food allergies. In another study, neither the diversity nor the timing of introduction of complementary foods had any association with development of eczema. The most recent recommendations for high-risk infants do not endorse restriction of maternal diet during pregnancy and lactation or restriction of allergenic foods in infants after 4-6 months of age.

Elimination of highly allergic foods is plausible to prevent the development of food allergy [34]. Concerning the timing of solid food introduction, a delay does not seem to prevent the development of food allergy, but it may enhance sensitization to some foods. Introducing solid food at 4-6 months might result in the lowest allergy risk and the recommended duration of exclusive breast feeding and age of introduction of solids were confirmed to be 6 months [46]. Exclusive breastfeeding for at least 4 months for infants at a high risk of developing atopic disease but no current convincing evidence that delaying solid food introduction, including fish, eggs, and foods containing peanut protein, beyond 4–6 months of age had a significant protective effect on the development of atopic disease [47]. In contrast, early introduction of peanuts during infancy, rather than avoidance, was reported to prevent the development of peanut allergy [48]. Their data might be a good example of oral immune tolerance in a human model.

In contrast, some reports have suggested that delaying the introduction of hyperallergenic solid foods during weaning is not effective in preventing the development of food allergy. A new concept about the timing of weaning and the introduction of solid foods was suggested

[49]. Avoidance of highly allergenic foods beyond 4-6 months might not be effective in preventing the development of food allergy in most children, and the effect of specific early introduction of allergenic foods was being investigated. Significantly, delaying the introduction of solid foods until 4 to 6 months of age in infants at a high risk for atopic disease appears to reduce the incidence of AD [11].

6.3 Elimination of hyperallergenic foods from the diet of prenatal or breastfeeding mothers

Opinions about a mother's diet during breast feeding differ. Whether a mother should follow an elimination diet for hyperallergenic foods to prevent food allergy remains a matter of debate [2]. From prenatal development studies, however, there is no evidence to support the assumption that an elimination diet can prevent food allergy because the mother's immune system protects the fetus from foods ingested by the mother.

6.4 Correction of Th1/Th2 imbalance

The development of food allergy is related to Th2-deviant immune status in the sensitization phase of AD [9]. Although IFN-γ has tolerogenic effects on pre-existing food allergy, the development or prevention of a food allergy is primarily associated with sensitization. IFN-γ plays a role in preventing food allergy by correcting the Th1/Th2 imbalance [21].

6.5 Prevention of allergy provocation

The diagnosis of food allergy and subsequent elimination diet of all possible allergenic foods is important to prevent further sensitization from repetitive allergy provocation. Repetitive allergy provocation and the resultant further Th2-polarization make patients more likely to develop additional allergies [2]. Sensitization to more food allergens, as well as aeroallergens, can occur with repeated allergy flares. It follows that allergy provocation by known allergens should be avoided to prevent further sensitization. For this reason, AD should be evaluated for repetitive allergy provocation and not simply the severity of AD. Furthermore, patients with mild AD should be treated early to prevent repeated allergic responses.

6.6 IL-10 for the prevention of food sensitization

Helminths induce generation of IL-10 in the gut and prevent sensitization to foods in mice [50]. Promotion of an IL-10-rich environment in the gut was investigated for its role in preventing or even treating food allergies. The prevention of food allergies by administering either an IL-10-secreting *Lactococcus lactis* [51] or an avirulant *Salmonella typhimurium* strain that promotes IL-10 secretion in the gut [52] was demonstrated. In this study, transiently expanded IL-10-secreting T cell populations played an important role in keeping the allergen-specific effector T cell responses in check. From these results, it was possible to explain how skin exposure to high doses of allergens led to a decreased immune response with subsequent allergen exposures [53].

6.7 Skin hydration

Physical injury leads to a Th2-deviant status in the local skin and resultant allergic status (Fig. 2) [54]. These changes result in sensitization to simultaneously exposed allergens as described above. Dryness is one of the main causes of itching. For all aspects of AD symptoms, skin hydration is very important to prevent further sensitization through the skin.

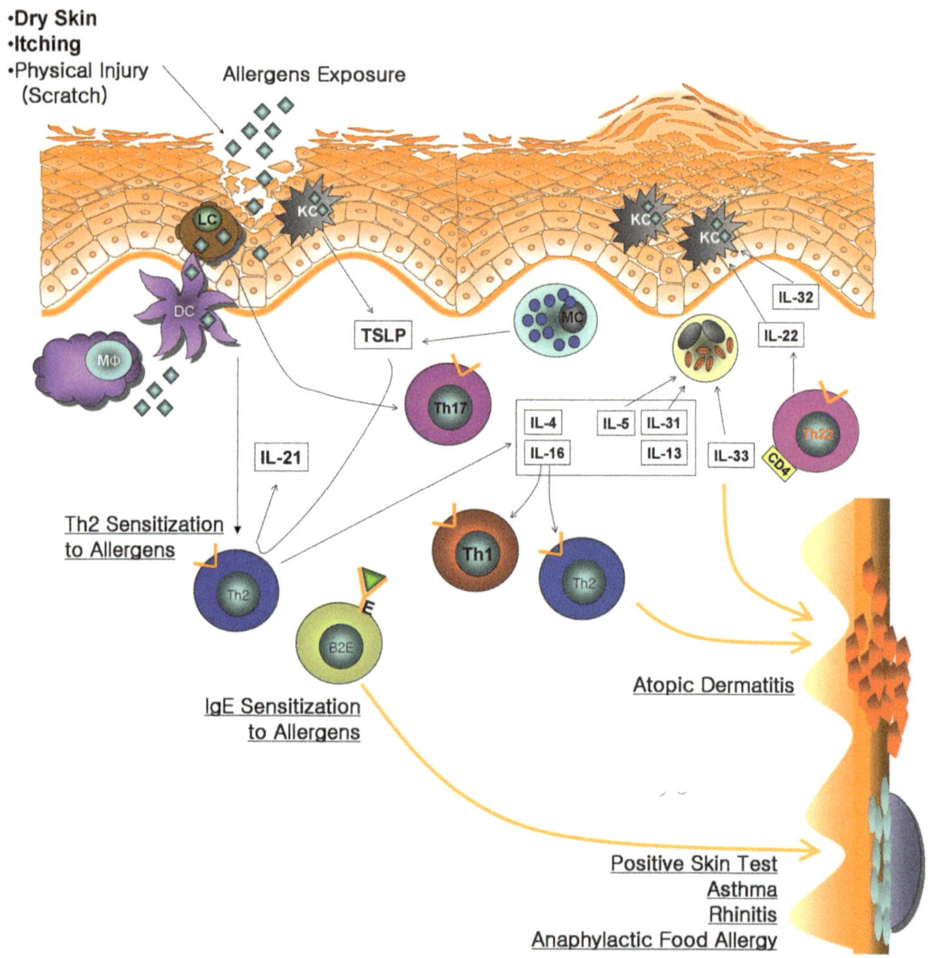

Fig. 2. Immunopathogenesis of sensitization through skin. Physical injury induced the release of thymus stromal lymphopoietin (TSLP) in the skin and subsequently IL-21 is released from Th2 cell by TSLP. By the multiple actions of IL-21, the skin is Th2-polarized. In this process, also many Th2-related cytokines are involved including IL-4, IL-5, IL-13, IL-16, IL-31, IL-32. Any allergens exposed simultaneously in this status, are sensitized in skin. If skin is sensitized by IgE-mediated allergy, skin prick test to sensitized allergens becomes positive, while if skin is sensitized by non-IgE-mediated allergy, allergy patch test may become positive with the development of atopic dermatitis.

6.8 Restriction of food additives

Food additives play a role in food allergy and AD by acting as pseudoallergens [25]. Ingestion of food additives leads to dryness and itching [24]. Physical injury by scratching due to dryness and itching results in sensitization to additional allergens [54]. This cycle of dryness and injury caused by scratching contributes to repeated allergic responses (Fig. 2). In order to prevent sensitization to multiple allergens, use of food additives should be restricted.

7. Acknowledgement

First of all, I dedicate this manuscript to Yeahee Yoo, for her excellent support in finishing this work. Also, this work was supported by the grant of the Korean Ministry of Education, Science and Technology (The Regional Core Research Program/Chungbuk BIT Research-Oriented University Consortium).

8. Abbreviations

IFA, IgE-mediated food allergy; NFA, non-IgE-mediated food allergy; TIFA, tolerance induction for food allergy; SOTI, specific oral tolerance induction

Keywords

Food allergy, IgE-mediated food allergy, Non-IgE-mediated food allergy, Tolerance, Oral tolerance induction, IFN-γ

9. References

[1] Bieber T. Atopic dermatitis. New England Journal of Medicine 2008;358:1483-1494.

[2] Noh G, Lee JH, Lee SS. Food allergy and atopic dermatitis. In Handbook of Diet, Nutrition and the Skin. Preedy VR (Ed). Wageningen, Netherlands: Wageningen Academic Publishers 2011 in press.

[3] Suh, K.Y., 2010. Food Allergy and Atopic Dermatitis: Separating Fact from Fiction. Seminars in Cutaneous Medicine and Surgery 29, 72-78.

[4] Jyonouchi, H., 2008. Non-IgE mediated food allergy, Inflammation and Allergy Drug Targets 3, 173-180.

[5] Longo G, Barbi E, Berti I, et al. Specific oral tolerance induction in children with very severe cow's milk-induced reactions. J Allergy Clin Immunol 121:343-347, 2008.

[6] Noh G, Lee SS. A pilot study of IFN-γ-induced specific oral tolerance induction for IgE-mediated anaphylactic food allergy. Journal of Interferon and Cytokine Research 2009; 29:667-676.

[7] Lee JH, Noh G, Noh J, Lee S, Choi WS, Kim HS, Lee K, Choi S, Jin H, Cho S, Lee S. Clinical characteristics of oral tolerance induction of IgE-mediated and non-IgE-mediated food allergy using interferon gamma. Allergy and Asthma Proceedings , 2010;31:e39-e47.

[8] Kim JS. Food Allergy: Diagnosis, Treatment, Prognosis, and Prevention. Pediatric Annals 2008;37:546-551.

[9] Lancour M. Acute infections in atopic dermatitis. A clue for a pathogenic role of a Th1/Th2 imbalance. Dermatol 1994;188: 255-7.

[10] Ricci G, Patrizi A, Giannetti A, Dondi A, Bendandi B. Masi M. Does improvement management of atopic dermatitis influence the appearance of respiratory allergic diseases? A follow-up study. Clinical and Molecular Allergy 2010;8: 8-19.

[11] Suh KY. Food Allergy and Atopic Dermatitis: Separating Fact from Fiction. Semin Cutan Med Surg 2010;29:72-78.
[12] Noh G, Ahn HS, Cho NY, Lee S, Oh JW. The clinical significance of food specific IgE/IgG4 in food specific atopic dermatitis. Pediatric Allergy and Immunology 2007;18:63-70.
[13] Lee SS, Noh G, Lee KY. Clinical application of histamine prick test for food challenge in atopic dermatitis. Journal of Korean Medical Science 2001;16:276-282.
[14] Fleischer DM, Bock A, Spears GC, Wilson CG, Miyazawa NK, Gleason MC, Gyorkos EA, Murphy JR, Atkins D, Leung DYM. Oral Food Challenges in Children with a Diagnosis of Food Allergy. J Pediatr 2011 158:578-583.e1.
[15] Burks, A.W., Mallory, S.B., Williams, L.W. and Shirrell, M.A., 1988. Atopic dermatitis: Clinical relevance of food hypersensitivity reactions. The Journal of Pediatrics 113, 447-451.
[16] Burks, A.W., James, J.M., Hiegel, A., Wilson, G., Wheeler, J.G., Jones, S.M. and Zuerlein, N., 1998. Atopic dermatitis and food hypersensitivity reactions. The Journal of Pediatrics 132, 132-136.
[17] Wang J. Management of the Patient with Multiple Food Allergies. Curr Allergy Asthma Rep (2010) 10:271–277
[18] Noh G, Ji EJ, Park JN, Kim KH, Do MH, Lee EK, Lee SS. The importance of food open challenge test in atopic dermatitis: The comparison of allergy history, skin-prick test, and specific IgE detection. Nutritional Science, 1999;2:119-124.
[19] Lee SS, Lee KY, Noh G. The necessity of diet therapy for successful interferon-γ therapy in atopic dermatitis. Yonsei Medical Journal 2001;42:161-171.
[20] Noh G, Jin H, Lee J, Noh J, Lee WM, Lee SS. Eosinophilia as a predictor of food allergy in atopic Dermatitis Allergy and Asthma Proceedings 2010;31:e18-e24.
[21] Noh GW, Lee KY. Blood eosinophils and serum IgE as predictors for prognosis of interferon gamma therapy in atopic dermatitis. Allergy 1998: 53: 1202-1207.
[22] Dahl R, Venge P. Blood eosinophil leucocyte and eosinophil cationic protein. In vivo study of the influence of beta-2-adrenergic drugs and steroid medication. Scand J Respir Dis. 1978;59:319-22.
[23] Worm M, Ehlers I, Sterry W, Zuberbier T. Clinical relevance of food additives in adult patients with atopic dermatitis. Clinical and Experimental Allergy 2000;30:407-414.
[24] Lee JM, Jin HY, Noh G, Lee SS. Effect of processed foods on serum levels of eosinophil cationic protein among children with atopic dermatitis. Nutr Res Pract. 2011;5:224-229
[25] Vieluf D, Wieben A. Ring J. Oral provocation tests with food additives in atopic eczema. International Achieves of Allergy and immunology 1999;118:232-233.
[26] Flohr C, Johansson SGO, Wahlgren CF, Williams H. How atopic is atopic dermatitis? J Allergy Clin Immunol 2004;113:150-8.
[27] Rokaitė R, Labanauskas L, Vaidelienė L. Role of the skin patch test in diagnosing food allergy in children with atopic dermatitis. Medicina (Kaunas) 2004;40:1081-7.
[28] Clark AT, Ewan PW. Food Allergy in childhood. Arch Dis Child 2003:88;79-81.
[29] Sprikkelman AB, Tupker RA, Burgerhof H, et al. Severity scoring of atopic dermatitis: a comparison of three scoring systems. Allergy 1997;52:944-949.

[30] Noh G, Lee KY. Pilot study of IFN-g-induced specific hyposensitization for house dust mites in atopic dermatitis: IFN-g-induced immune deviation as a new therapeutic concept for atopic dermatitis. Cytokine 2000;2:472-6.
[31] Rance F. Food allergy in children suffering from atopic eczema. Pediatric Allergy and Immunology 2008;19:279-284.
[32] Nowak-Wegrzyn A, Assa'ad AH, Bahna SL, Bock SA, Sicherer SH, Teuber SS. Work Group report: Oral food challenge testing. Journal Allergy and Clinical Immunology 2009;123:s365-s383.
[33] Kim, T.E., Park, S.W., Noh, G. and Lee, S., 2002. Comparison of skin prick test results between crude allergen extracts from foods and commercial allergen extracts in atopic dermatitis by double-blind placebo-controlled food challenge for milk, egg, and soybean. Yonsei Medical Journal 43, 613-620.
[34] Scurlock AM, Jones SM. An update on immunotherapy for food allergy. Cur Opin Allergy Clin Immunol 2010, 10:587-93.
[35] Dupont C, Kalach N, Soulaines P, et al. Cow's milk epicutaneous immunotherapy in children: a pilot trial of safety, acceptability, and impact on allergic reactivity. J Allergy Clin Immunol 2010; 125:1165-1167.
[36] Bahna SL. Oral desensitization with cow's milk in IgEmediated cow's milk allergy. Contra! Monogr Allergy 1996; 32:233-5.
[37] Wuthrich B. Oral desensitization with cow's milk in cow's milk allergy. Pro! Monogr Allergy 1996;32:236-40.
[38] Noh, G. and Lee, S.S., 2003. Effects of IFN-γ on milk-specific oral tolerance induction for milk allergy in atopic dermatitis: Food specific oral tolerance induction using IFN-γ as adjuvant. In Clinical Immunology and Allergy in Medicine. Marone G (Ed). Naples, Italy: JGC Editions, 475-496.
[39] Skripak JM, Nash SD, Rowley H et al. A randomized, double-blind, placebo-controlled study of milk oral immunotherapy for cow's milk allergy. J Allergy Clin Immunol 2008;122:1154-60.
[40] Martorell A, Felix R, Cerda JC, Martorell CA. Oral rush desensitization to cow's milk. Following of desensitized patients during three years. Allergolo Immunopathol (Madr) 2007;35:174-6.
[41] Staden U, Blumchen K, Blankenstein N et al. Rush oral immunotherapy in children with persistent cow's milk allergy. J Allergy Clin Immunol 2008;122:418-9.
[42] Niggemann B, Staden U, Rolinck-Werninghaus C, Beyer K. Specific oral tolerance induction in food allergy. Allergy 2006;61:808-11.
[43] Staden U, Rolinck-Werninghaus C, Brewe F, Wahn U, Niggemann B, Beyer K. Specific oral tolerance induction in food allergy in children: efficacy and clinical patterns of reaction. Allergy 2007;62:1261-9.
[44] Walker A. Breast milk as the gold standard for protective nutrients. J Pediatr. 201b;156:S3-7.
[45] Du Toit G, Katz Y, Sasieni P, et al. Early consumption of peanuts in infancy is associated with a low prevalence of peanut allergy. J Allergy Clin Immunol 2008; 122:984-991.
[46] Anderson J, Malley K, Snell R. Is 6 months still the best for exclusive breastfeeding and introduction of solids? A literature review with consideration to the risk of the development of allergies. Breastfeed Rev 2009;17:23-31.

[47] Greer F, Sicherer S, Burks W. Effects of early nutritional interventions on the development of atopic disease in infants and children: The role of maternal dietary restriction, breastfeeding, timing of introduction of complementary foods, and hydrolyzed formulas. Pediatrics 2008;121: 183-91.

[48] Du Toit G, Katz Y, Sasieni P et al. Early consumption of peanuts in infancy is associated with a low prevalence of peanut allergy. J Allergy Clin Immunol 2008;122:984-91.

[49] Kazuyuki Kurihara. Immunotherapy for Food Allergy. Allergology International. 2010;59:9-14

[50] Bashir ME, Andersen P, Fuss IJ, Shi HN, Nagler-Anderson C. An enteric helminth infection protects against an allergic response to dietary antigen. J Immunol 2002; 169: 3284-92.

[51] Frossard CP, Steidler L, Eigenmann PA. Oral administration of an IL-10-secreting Lactococcus lactis strain prevents food-induced IgE sensitization. J Allergy Clin Immunol 2007; 119: 952-9.

[52] Eigenmann PA, Asigbetse KE, Frossard CP. Avirulant Salmonella typhimurium strains prevent food allergy in mice. Clin Exp Immunol 2008; 151: 546-53.

[53] Fujio K, Okamura T, Yamamoto K. The Family of IL-10-Secreting CD4(+) T Cells. Adv Immunol 2010; 105: 99-130.

[54] Ogawa T, Gunawan H, Ikeda S, Okumura K, Ogawa H. Cytokine milieu modulates release of thymic stromal lymphopoietin from human keratinocytes stimulated with double-stranded RNA. J Allergy Clin Immunol 2009; 123: 179-86.

Part 4

New Treatments

16

Suplatast Tosilate for Prophylaxis of Pediatric Atopy

S. Yoshihara, M. Ono, Y. Yamada, H. Fukuda, T. Abe and O. Arisaka
Department of Pediatrics, Dokkyo University School of Medicine, Tochigi Japan

1. Introduction

The onset of asthma may be related to Th2 cytokine dominance at the time when food allergies occur several months after birth. This study investigated the effectiveness of early intervention with a Th2 cytokine inhibitor (suplatast tosilate) for prevention of asthma in infants with food allergies and atopic dermatitis. Suplatast tosilate dry syrup (6 mg/kg daily) or a histamine H1-blocker (ketotifen fumarate dry syrup: 0.06 mg/kg daily) was administered randomly to 53 infants with atopic dermatitis caused by food allergies. The primary endpoints were the incidence of asthma and the time to the onset of wheezing. The peripheral blood Th1/Th2 ratio, total IgE level, and eosinophil count were measured before and after treatment. After 24 months of treatment, the prevalence of asthma was significantly lower in the suplatast group (20.8%) than in the ketotifen group (65.6%, $p < 0.01$). Additionally, the time from the start of treatment to the initial episode of wheezing for infants who developed asthma was significantly longer in the suplatast group than the ketotifen group ($p < 0.01$). Furthermore, the eosinophil count was significantly decreased by suplatast treatment ($p < 0.05$), and there was a significant difference between the suplatast and ketotifen groups with respect to both the eosinophil count ($p < 0.01$) and the Th1/Th2 ratio ($p < 0.05$). The results of the present pilot study suggest that suplatast tosilate is useful for the primary prevention of wheezing and asthma in children.

2. Atopic dermatitis is associated with asthma

Asthma frequently develops by the age of 3 yr (1) and recent research has demonstrated that its onset is tending to occur at a younger age (2). Various hypotheses have been suggested with respect to the etiology of asthma. According to the Tucson cohort study performed in the United States, there is a low probability of atopic asthma developing in infants with recurrent wheezing up to the age of 3 yr, and they are considered to be a separate population from the infants in whom recurrent wheezing persists until later childhood (3). In the former group, viral infection is the direct cause of wheezing, while the latter group have an atopic constitution and their asthma may persist during the school years and even into adulthood. Thus, this latter group may be a population for which early intervention is important. It is known that chronic asthma is more likely to develop in patients who are positive in tests for food or house dust allergens (4, 5). The rate of progression to adult asthma is also high among individuals who test positive for food allergens, such as those in eggs or milk, during early infancy (6), while another study has shown that the strongest risk factor for life- threatening asthma is the presence of food allergy (7). Atopic dermatitis was reported to be associated with asthma that has a later onset (8), while inhibition of the occurrence of asthma has been reported in dermatitis patients treated with H1-blocker therapy (9, 10).

2.1 Th2 cytokine inhibitor: Suplatast tosilate

We have tested the preventive effect of treatment with a Th2 inhibitor, suplatast tosilate. In previous in vitro and in vivo studies, suplatast tosilate has been shown to inhibit the production of IgE antibodies, reduce tissue eosinophil infiltration, and block the production of IL-4 and IL-5 (11–13). More recently, it was shown to prevent goblet cell hyperplasia by blocking IL-13 production (14). According to a study performed in a mouse model of food allergy, suplatast tosilate decreases IL-4 and IL-6 production in the small intestine, and also ameliorates small bowel necrosis (15). In adults with asthma, suplatast tosilate shows comparable anti-inflammatory activity to inhaled steroids (16), as well as improving lung function, asthma symptoms, and airway hyperresponsiveness (16, 17). In patients receiving high-dose inhaled steroids, addition of suplatast tosilate allows the steroid dose to be reduced (18). Furthermore, evaluation by bronchial biopsy has shown that this drug decreases the number of eosinophils and EG2-positive cells in the airway mucosa, as well as inhibiting goblet cell hyperplasia (17, 19). Infants with a family history of atopy and infants in whom atopic disease occurs soon after birth have been reported to show a shift of the Th1-Th2 cytokine balance towards Th2 dominance (20, 21). Accordingly, the Th1-Th2 balance during the early postnatal period is believed to be a key factor in determining whether or not allergy develops.

2.2 Aim and method of this study

The present study was designed to investigate early intervention in atopic dermatitis patients with food allergies, a population considered to be at high risk for the development of asthma. Suplatast tosilate was chosen for early intervention therapy in the present study based on the hypothesis that selective inhibition of Th2 cytokines would improve the Th1-Th2 balance in the high-risk group for asthma (children with Th2 cytokine dominance). Comparison was made with a histamine H1-blocker, ketotifen fumarate, as the control drug.

2.2.1 Subject

We studied 60 consecutive infants who presented to our department with symptoms of atopic dermatitis caused by food allergies that had persisted for at least 2 month. All of the infants had a family history (at least one parent) of atopic disease, such as bronchial asthma, allergic rhinitis, or atopic dermatitis. The diagnosis of atopic dermatitis was based on the criteria of the Japanese Dermatological Association (22), and all of the infants had predisposing factors for atopic disease (a family history of atopy, a history of allergic disease, or a predisposition to IgE production). They primarily developed pruritic eczema that showed repeated episodes of exacerbation and remission. Only infants with chronic dermatitis that had persisted for 2 months or more were diagnosed as having atopic dermatitis. Food allergies were diagnosed from the history using the following criteria: (i) a history of skin disease influenced by food, and (ii) a raised serum level of specific IgE for cow's milk or egg white (CAP RAST class ‡2). Children were excluded who had a history suggesting the prior existence of asthma, such as wheeze and chronic cough unrelated to respiratory tract infection. Infants who had used oral sodium cromoglycate or other antiallergy drugs within the previous 4 wk (agents that could potentially affect the outcome of this study) were also excluded, but those using topical steroids rated as medium strength or weak to control atopic dermatitis were permitted to enter the study.

2.2.2 Study design

Thirty children were randomly assigned to oral treatment with suplatast tosilate dry syrup (IPD dry syrup 5%, Taiho Pharmaceutical Co. Ltd, Tokyo Japan) at a dose of 3 mg/kg twice daily (the total daily dose was 6 mg/kg) and 30 were assigned to receive ketotifen fumarate dry syrup at dose of 0.03 mg/kg twice daily (the total daily dose was 0.06 mg/kg). Both these drugs were administered for at least 2 yr, and could be continued for up to 4 yr at the request of the parents. After the start of the study, subjects were reviewed at the outpatient department once monthly until completion of the study. Blood was collected at the start and after 6 months of treatment for measurement of the total IgE level; the specific IgE levels for egg white, cow's milk, Der P, and house dust mite; the eosinophil count; and the Th1/Th2 ratio. The primary endpoints of this study were the incidence of asthma and the time to the initial episode of wheezing among the patients in whom asthma occurred. Wheezing was confirmed by the authors via auscultation, and the date of the initial of wheezing, as well as subsequent episodes of wheezing and persistent cough excluding those caused by infection, was recorded in each infant. Asthma was defined as the occurrence of three or more episodes of wheezing associated with expiratory dyspnea, and the day of onset of asthma was defined as the day when the initial episode of wheezing occurred in each patient with asthma. The secondary endpoints of this study were the percentage of patients admitted to hospital because of asthma and changes of the peripheral blood eosinophil count, IgE level, and Th1/Th2 ratio. For the treatment of atopic dermatitis and food allergies, the use of concomitant drugs other than medium-strength to weak topical steroids was not allowed during the study period. After the onset of asthma, antiasthma medications, mainly anti-inflammatory drugs, could be prescribed.

2.2.3 Measurement of the Th1/Th2 ratio

The Th1/Th2 ratio was measured by flow cytometry using a FACScan (23). In brief, CD4-positive cells (helper T cells) were isolated. Then Th2 cytokine-positive cells were detected and counted after staining with an anti-IL-4 antibody, while Th1 cytokine - positive cells were identified with an anti-IFN-c antibody, after which the Th1/Th2 ratio was calculated.

2.2.4 Measurement of serum total IgE and specific IgE

Serum total IgE was measured using a fluoroenzyme immunoassay (FEIA) (CAP RIST FEIA, Pharmacia, Uppsala, Sweden). The levels of specific IgE for house dust mite, Der P, egg white, and cow's milk were measured using FEIA (CAP RAST FEIA, Pharmacia).

2.2.5 Ethics

This study was approved by the Regional Ethics Committee for Human Research at Dokkyo University School of Medicine Hospital. The parents of all patients participating in this study gave oral and written informed consent.

2.2.6 Statistical analysis

The initial wheezing episodes were plotted by the Kaplan–Meier method, and p-values were calculated with the log-rank test. Pearson's chisquared test was used to analyze the incidence of asthma. The Th1/Th2 ratio, total IgE level, and eosinophil count were compared between before and after treatment using the paired t-test. It was employed to determine the significance of differences between the two treatments. Results were expressed as the mean ± s.e., and p-values of <0.05 were considered to indicate statistical significance.

2.3 Result of this study

A total of seven infants were excluded from the study: three infants were excluded because their parents did not allow their children to receive suplatast tosilate, while four infants were excluded because they stopped attending the hospital for various reasons. As a result, there were 29 infants in the ketotifen group and 24 in the suplatast group. The clinical profile of each group is shown in the Table 1.

	Ketotifen group (n = 29)	Suplatast group (n = 24)	p-value
Sex	Males 22, female 7	Males 18, female 6	0.942
Age (days)	370.9±78.7	365.5±80.5	0.728
Age at onset (days)	145.1±34.5	134.4±19.7	0.633
No. of days from onset to drug treatment (days)	225.8±69.4	231.0±77.7	0.837
Total IgE (IU/ml)	509.2±209.6	745.7±207.0	0.24
Egg IgE (Class)	2.50±0.26	3.36±0.31	0.0188
Milk IgE (Class)	2.09±1.87	3.69±0.37	0.0273
House dust mite IgE (Class)	1.25±0.49	1.56±0.59	0.814
Der P IgE (Class)	1.31±0.48	1.73±0.64	0.752

Table 1. Clinical profile

There were no significant differences between the two groups with respect to the sex ratio, age, time of onset of atopic dermatitis, number of days from onset to drug treatment. The mean age at the start of treatment was 365.5 ± 80.5 days in the 24 infants who received suplatast tosilate and 370.9 ± 78.7 days in the 29 who received ketotifen fumarate.

There were no differences between the suplatast group and the ketotifen group with respect to the total IgE level or the levels of specific IgE for house dust mite or Der P before treatment. However, the specific IgE levels for egg white and milk were significantly higher in the suplatast group.

The incidence of asthma was significantly lower in the suplatast group than the ketotifen group, with asthma occurring in five out of 24 patients from the former group (20.8%) vs. 19 out of 29 patients from the latter group (65.6%, $p < 0.01$). Additionally, the time from the start of drug treatment to the onset of wheezing among patients in whom asthma occurred was significantly longer in the suplatast group than the ketotifen group ($p < 0.01$, Fig. 1). The percentage of infants who were admitted to hospital for the treatment of asthma was significantly lower ($p < 0.05$) in the suplatast group (one out of 24 patients, or 4.2%) than in the ketotifen group (seven out of 29 patients, or 24.1%).

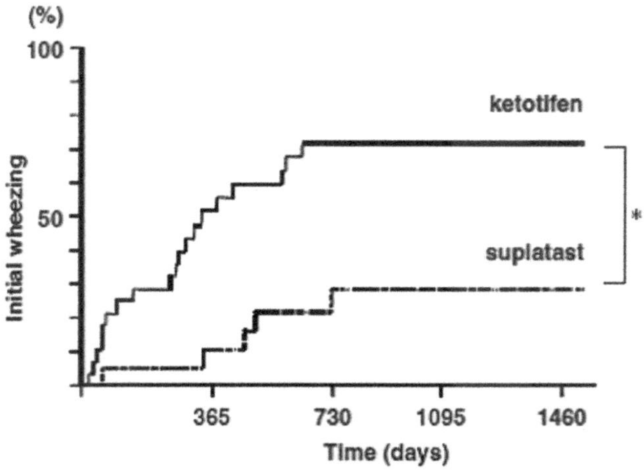

Fig. 1. Onset of wheezing during treatment with a Th2 cytokine inhibitor (suplatast tosilate) or a histamine H1-blocker (ketotifen fumarate).

The eosinophil count decreased significantly from 1.212 ± 174 to 679 ± 111/lL ($p < 0.05$) after 219 ± 42 days of suplatast treatment (n = 21), while no significant change was observed after 280 ± 44 days of ketotifen treatment (n = 19). The change after treatment was significantly larger ($p < 0.01$) in the suplatast group (-532.4 ± 120.0) compared with the ketotifen group (-2.1 ± 126.0) (Fig. 2). Although there was no significant change of the Th1/Th2 ratio after treatment in either the suplatast group (from 4.88 ± 1.07 to 6.76 ± 1.58%, n = 16) or the ketotifen group (from 10.00 ± 8.52 to 6.44 ± 1.88% n = 10), there was a significant difference of the ratio between the two groups ($p < 0.05$) (Fig. 3). However, there was no significant difference between the groups with respect to changes of the total IgE level (data not shown).

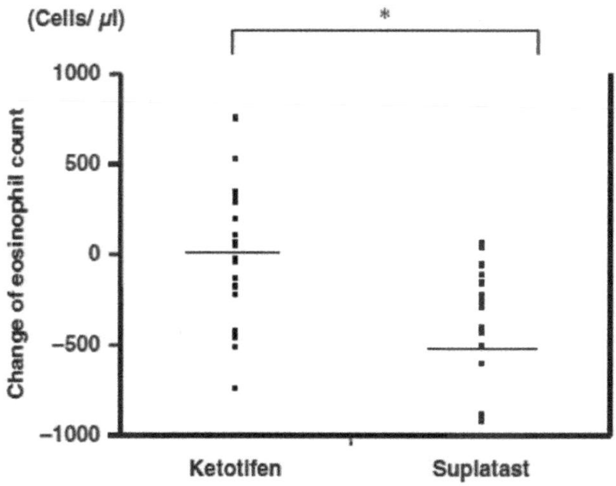

Fig. 2. Eosinophil count before and after treatment with suplatast tosilate (-532.4 ± 120.0) or ketotifen fumarate (-2.1 ± 126.0); *$p < 0.01$ by the t-test.

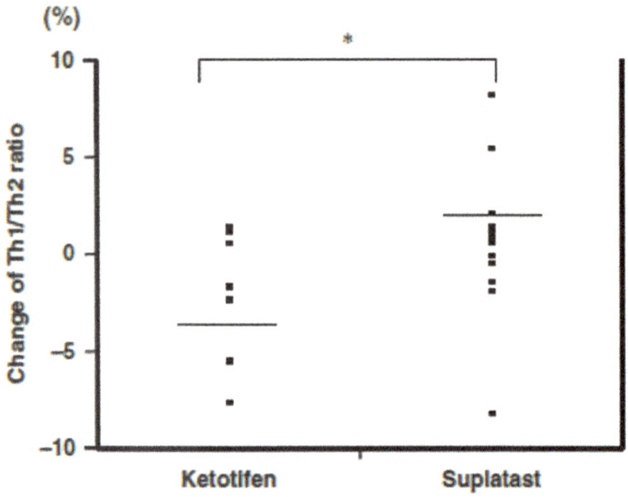

Fig. 3. Th1/Th2 ratio before and after treatment with suplatast tosilate (1.88 ± 1.57) or ketotifen fumarate (-3.56 ± 1.99); *$p < 0.05$ by the t-test.

No adverse events and no laboratory abnormalities were observed in the suplatast group. Two episodes of sedation occurred in the ketotifen group, but these were transient and did not result in the discontinuation of therapy.

2.4 Effectiveness of early intervention with a Th2 cytokine inhibitor

Children with a family history of allergic disease are likely to have a predisposition to atopy and the processes leading to the development of such diseases may commence in utero. After birth, continuous exposure to certain food antigens may sequentially trigger allergic reactions that manifest as food allergies, atopic dermatitis, asthma, and allergic rhinitis. Such reactions are involved in the progression of allergic disease (24, 25). Treatment designed to suppress the exacerbation of allergic airway inflammation may potentially have an important role in the prophylaxis and management of these diseases.

We compared the inhibitory effect of suplatast tosilate and the H1-blocker ketotifen fumarate on the onset of asthma in patients with atopic dermatitis who were positive for egg-white or milk allergens. When ketotifen was previously tested in 121 infants with atopic dermatitis who were treated for a 1-yr period, it reduced the occurrence of asthma compared with placebo, and the subgroup of children with a high IgE level showed a significant benefit (9). After 24 months of treatment in the present study, however, asthma developed in 65.6% of the patients receiving ketotifen vs. only 20.8% of those treated with suplatast. To assess the prevention of progression to severe asthma, we analyzed the number of patients who required hospital treatment for their asthma. Seven out of 29 infants from the ketotifen group and only one out of 24 infants from the suplatast group were admitted to hospital for the treatment of asthma, with the percentage being significantly lower in the suplatast group. This finding suggests the possibility that suplatast can prevent progression of mild asthma to severe asthma.

To examine the systemic effects of suplatast (a Th2 cytokine inhibitor) vs. those of ketorifen (an antihistamine), the Th1/Th2 ratio, total IgE level, and eosinophil count were measured before and after treatment. As a result, the Th1/Th2 ratio was found to be significantly higher after treatment in the suplatast group than in the ketotifen group, but neither drug decreased the serum IgE level. Based on the previous report that 3 or 6 months of treatment with suplatast tosilate decreased the serum levels of IgE and IL-4 in adults with perennial allergic rhinitis (26), we assessed the changes of parameters over a 6-month period in this study. The failure of suplatast tosilate to suppress IgE production may have been related to the low age of the subjects in the suplatast group (mean age at the start of treatment with suplatast: 365.5 days), because there is a gradual increase of tolerance to food allergens such as egg white and cow's milk, while sensitization to inhaled allergens like Der P and house dust mite shows a rapid increase at this age and infants with an atopic tendency show increased IgE synthesis at this age (27). Accordingly, we were not able to assess the efficacy of suplatast from the total IgE level. The Early Treatment of the Atopic Child (ETAC) study investigated the use of cetirizine, an H1-blocker like ketotifen for preventing the onset of asthma and found no significant overall benefit compared with the placebo, although asthma was prevented in patients sensitized to house dust mite or grass pollen (10). Our patients had high antibody titers for food allergens, but their mean baseline CAP RAST scores were 2 or less for both house dust mite and Der P. This suggests that suplatast was more effective than H1-blockers for patients who were not strongly sensitized to inhaled allergens. As we did not initially plan to assess changes of specific IgE levels in the present study, these parameters were only measured in a few patients after the start of treatment. Therefore, drawing firm conclusions is impossible, but we plan to investigate further whether suplatast has a similar effect to that of immunotherapy, which prevents the development of new allergies (e.g., suppresses reactions to inhaled allergens) (28). In the present study, we directed our attention to the Th1/Th2 ratio. At birth, the production of INF-c is very low and infants are in a state where the immune response is Th2 dominant. If IFN-c production increases during the 6 months after birth, the immune response will become Th1 dominant and the production of IL-4 will be inhibited, preventing the acquisition of an atopic predisposition. In an environment that does not cause induction of IFN-c, however, its level gradually increases with maturity, but IL-4 also continues to be produced until an atopic predisposition is acquired (29). Our preliminary study showed that persons with a strong atopic predisposition, who developed food allergies followed by atopic dermatitis, asthma, and allergic rhinitis, actually had a higher Th1/Th2 ratio than healthy subjects and had a Th1-Th2 balance skewed toward Th2 dominance (unpublished observation). Such findings suggest that there is a tendency for Th2 dominance in infancy and that an increase of inflammation due to eosinophils, etc. may lead to the eventual onset of asthma. Suplatast has been shown to inhibit the activity of eosinophils by in vitro and in vivo studies, including research performed using peripheral blood, sputum, and bronchial tissue specimens obtained by biopsy (12–14, 16, 17). In the present study, suplatast significantly decreased the peripheral blood eosinophil count compared with ketotifen. There have been several reports of a relationship between the onset of asthma and eosinophils. For example, Bromchoalveolar lavage fluid (BALF) levels of Eosimophilic Catiomic Protein (ECP) are higher in patients with childhood asthma than in those with infantile wheeze (30), and persons who subsequently develop asthma have more Eosimophil Granulocyte-2 (EG2)- positive cells in the epithelium or lamina propria on bronchial biopsy than those who do not (31).

It appears that inhibition of the onset of asthma may be attributable to two factors, which are a decrease of the eosinophil count and a shift of the Th1/Th2 ratio toward Th1 dominance. The results of our study provide some corroboration for the hypothesis that inhibition of eosinophilic inflammation and improvement of the Th1/Th2 balance can contribute to preventing the onset of asthma.

The present investigation was only a pilot study, but it is still clinically significant that more than half of our patients with atopic dermatitis and food allergies developed asthma before age three during treatment with ketotifen, while only 20% of the suplatast group did so. Among the criteria in the asthma predictive index (API) (32), which is based on the Tucson Children's Respiratory Study, as well as the major and minor criteria in the modified asthma predictive index (mAPI) (33) based on the PEAK trial, a parental history of asthma, physician-diagnosed atopic dermatitis, and allergic sensitization to milk, egg, or peanuts correspond to the criteria used in the present study. These other studies have suggested that early intervention with suplatast can prevent progression to chronic asthma if patients meeting the criteria that suggest an increased likelihood of progression to chronic asthma in the future are treated before they develop wheezing. Both the API and the mAPI include the criterion of an eosinophil count ‡4%. Most of the patients in the present study met this criterion and showed a significant decrease of eosinophils after treatment with suplatast. Therefore, early intervention with suplatast may prevent progression to chronic asthma even in patients with a high eosinophil count, who have an increased risk of developing chronic asthma. The finding that a lower percentage of patients in the suplatast group needed hospital admission for asthma also serves as evidence that this drug may prevent progression to chronic asthma.

3. Conclusion

There have only been a few reports about early intervention for patients with a high risk of developing asthma. Iikura et al. reported a research of early intervention (34). To evaluate the prophylactic effect of ketotifen against the onset of asthma they selected 121 infants with atopic dermatitis. A placebo syrup group and an active syrup group were followed for 1 year, with bimonthly evaluations. During the 1 year study, asthma was observed in eight children of the ketotifen group (13.1%) and in 25 children of the placebo group (41.6%) (P less than .001). As a result, they concluded that Ketotifen is effective for early intervention in children with atopic dermatitis.

Suplatast tosilate is an oral agent that has been available in Japan for 12 yr since 1995. It is highly safe, and there have been no reports of serious adverse reactions to this drug (35). The manufacturer of Suplatast, (Taiho Pharmaceutical Co., Ltd., Tokyo, Japan) summarized the adverse events that were detected among 154 children under 3 yr old in a study of actual use. According to this report, adverse reactions were only noted in two patients. This shows that Suplatast is also safe for patients under 3 yr old and thus is thus suitable for long-term administration to high risk patients in order to prevent the onset of asthma. It is one of the few drugs available that act as a non-specific regulator of the immune system. Then, it showed that the allergic predisposition is improved in suppressing the symptom. Therefore it can be said that suplatast tosilate is an antiallergic fundamentally curative drug. In the future, we hope to collect more cases and explore whether this drug can change the natural history of asthma.

4. References

[1] Martinez FD, Wright AL, Taussig LM, Holberg CJ, Halonen M, Morgan WJ. Asthma and wheezing in the first six years of life. N Engl J Med 1995: 332: 133–8.

[2] Sly RM. Changing prevalence of allergic rhinitis and asthma. Ann Allergy Asthma Immunol 1999: 82: 233–48.

[3] Taussig LM, Wright AL, Holberg CJ, Halonen M, Morgan WJ, Martinez FD. Tucson Children's Respiratory Study.1980 to present. J Allergy Clin Immunol 2003: 111: 661–75.

[4] Kulig M, Bergmann R, Tacke U, Wahn U, Guggenmoos-Holzmann I. Long-lasting sensitization to food during the first two years precedes allergic airway disease. The MAS Study Group, Germany. Pediatr Allergy Immunol 1998: 9: 61–7.

[5] Sporik R, Holgate ST, Platts-Mills TA, Cogswell JJ. Exposure to house-dust mite allergen (Der p I) and the development of asthma in childhood. A prospective study. N Engl J Med 1990: 323: 502–7.

[6] Rhodes HL, Sporik R, Thomas P, Holgate ST, Cogswell JJ. Early life risk factors for adult asthma: a birth cohort study of subjects at risk. J Allergy Clin Immunol 2001: 108: 720–5.

[7] Roberts G, Patel N, Levi-Schaffer F, Habibi P, Lack G. Food allergy as a risk factor for life-threatening asthma in childhood: a case-controlled study. J Allergy Clin Immunol 2003: 112: 168–74.

[8] Bergmann RL, Edenharter G, Bergmann KE, et al. Atopic dermatitis in early infancy predicts allergic airway disease at 5 years. Clin Exp Allergy 1998: 28: 965–70.

[9] Iikura Y, Naspitz CK, Mikawa H, et al. Prevention of asthma by ketotifen in infants with atopic dermatitis. Ann Allergy 1992: 68: 233–6.

[10] Warner JO, ETAC Study Group. Early treatment of the atopic child. A double-blinded, randomized, placebo-controlled trial of cetirizine in preventing the onset of asthma in children with atopic dermatitis: 18 months-treatment and 18 months-posttreatment follow-up. J Allergy Clin Immunol 2001: 108: 929–37

[11] Yanagihara Y, Kiniwa M, Ikizawa K, Shida T, Matsuura N, Koda A. Suppression of IgE production by IPD-1151T (suplatast tosilate), a new dimethylsulfonium agent: (2) regulation of human IgE response. Jpn J Pharmacol 1993: 61: 31–9.

[12] Iijima H, Tamura G, Hsiue TR, Liu Y, Taniguchi H, Shirato K. Suplatast tosilate inhibits late response and airway inflammation in sensitized guinea pigs. Am J Respir Crit Care Med 1999: 160: 331–5.

[13] Zhao GD, Yokoyama A, Kohno N, Sakai K, Hamada H, Hiwada K. Effect of suplatast tosilate (IPD-1151T) on a mouse model of asthma: inhibition of eosinophilic inflammation and bronchial hyperresponsiveness. Int Arch Allergy Immunol 2000: 121: 116–21.

[14] Shim JJ, Dabbagh K, Takeyama K, et al. Suplatast tosilate inhibits goblet-cell metaplasia of airway epithelium in sensitized mice. J Allergy Clin Immunol 2000: 105: 739–45.

[15] Ueno K, Samson K, Chen H, et al. Food allergy and liver/intestines. Effect of suplatast tosilate and chinese traditional medicines. Allergy Clin Immunol Int 2004: 1: 310–6.

[16] Tamaoki J, Takeyama K, Aoshiba K, Nakata J, Nishimura K, Nagai A. A Th2 cytokine inhibitor for airway inflammation in mild asthma. J Allergy Clin Immunol 2003: 111: 197–8.

[17] Sano Y, Suzuki N, Yamada H, et al. Effects of suplatast tosilate on allergic eosinophilic airway inflammation in patients with mild asthma. J Allergy Clin Immunol 2003: 111: 958–66.

[18] Tamaoki J, Kondo M, Sakai N, et al. Effect of suplatast tosilate, a Th2 cytokine inhibitor, on steroiddependent asthma: a double-blind randomized study. Lancet 2000: 356: 273–8.

[19] Hoshino M, Fujita Y, Saji J, Inoue T, Nakagawa T, Miyazawa T. Effect of suplatast tosilate on goblet cell metaplasia in patient with asthma. Allergy 2005: 60: 1394–400.

[20] Warner JA, Jones CA, Jones AC, Warner JO. Prenatal origins of allergic disease. J Allergy Clin Immunol 2000: 2 (Pt2): S493–8.

[21] Prescott SL, Macaubas C, Smallacombe T, Holt BJ, Sly PD, Holt PG. Development of allergen-specific T-cell memory in atopic and normal children. Lancet 1999: 353: 196–200.

[22] Yamamoto S, Kohmo Y. Guidelines For The Management of Atopic Dermatitis. Japan: Kyowakikaku, 2006.

[23] Kohsaka T, Miyazaki T, Noma Y, et al. Examination for detection of intracellular cytokines by flow cytometry. J Med Pharm Sci 1997: 38: 875–82.

[24] Rhodes HL, Thomas P, Sporik R, Holgate ST, Cogswell JJ. A birth cohort study of subjects at risk of atopy: twenty-two-year follow-up of wheeze and atopic status. Am J Respir Crit Care Med 2002: 165: 176–80.

[25] Ohshima Y, Yamada A, Hiraoka M, et al. Early sensitization to house dust mite is a major risk factor for subsequent development of bronchial asthma in Japanese infants with atopic dermatitis: result of a 4-year followup study. Ann Allergy Asthma Immunol 2002: 89: 265–70.

[26] Washio Y, Ohashi Y, Tanaka A, et al. Suplatast tosilate affects the initial increase in specific IgE and Interleukin-4 during immunotherapy for perennial allergic rhinitis. Acta Otolaryngol 1998: 538: 126–32.

[27] Laan MP, Baert MR, Bijl AM, et al. Markers for early sensitization and inflammation in relation to clinical manifestations of atopic disease up to 2 years of age in 133 high-risk children. Clin Exp Allergy 2000: 30: 944–53.

[28] Des Roches A, Paradis L, Menardo JL, Bouges S, Daures JP, Bousquet J. Immunotherapy with a standardized dermatophagoides pteronyssinus extract. VI specific immunotherapy prevents the onset of new sensitizations in children. J Allergy Clin Immunol 1997: 99: 450–3.

[29] Sigrus N, Bjarnason R, Sigurbergsson F, Kjellman B. Respiratory syncytical virus bronchiolitis in infancy is an important risk factor for asthma and allergy at age 7. Am J Respir Crit Care Med 2000: 161: 1501–7.

[30] Marguet C, Dean TP, Basuyau JP, Warner JO. Eosinophil cationic protein and interleukin-8 levels in bronchial lavage fluid from children with asthma and infantile wheeze. Pediatr Allergy Immunol 2001: 12: 27–33.

[31] Pohunek P, Warner JO, Turzikova J, Kudrmann J, Roche WR. Markers of eosinophilic inflammation and tissue re-modelling in children before clinically diagnosed bronchial asthma. Pediatr Allergy Immunol 2005: 16: 43–51.

[32] Castro- Rodriguez JA, Holberg CJ, Wright AL, Martinez FD. A clinical index to define risk of asthma in young children with recurrent wheezing. Am J Respir Crit Care Med 2000: 162: 1403–6.

[33] Guilbert TW, Morgan WJ, Zeiger RS, et al. Atopic characteristics of children with recurrent wheezing at high risk for the development of childhood asthma. J Allergy Clin Immunol 2004: 114: 1282–7.

[34] Iikura Y, Naspitz CK, Mikawa H, Talaricoficho S, Baba M, Sole D, Nishima S. Prevention of asthma by ketotifen in infants with atopic dermatitis. Ann Allergy. 1992: Mar: 68(3): 233-6.

[35] Sano Y, Yamada H. Progress in suplatast tosilate reserch. Clin Exp Allergy 2007: 37: 970–2.

17

Thinking Atopic Dermatitis Treatment Differently: Specific Immunotherapy as an Option

Massimo Milani
ALK Abellò Medical Department,
Lainate, Milan
Italy

1. Introduction

Atopic Dermatitis (AD) is a common inflammatory itching skin disease[1]. This skin disorder affects a large number of children and adults[2]. Epidemiological studies show that up to 25% of children and up to 3% of adult are affected worldwide[3]. Several studies in addition suggest an increasing prevalence of AD. The clinical picture of AD is dominated by chronic eczematous skin lesions in typical localizations[4]. In infants and small children, the rash is often present on the skin around the knees and elbows and the cheeks[5]. In teenagers and adults, the rash is often present in the creases of the wrists, elbows, knees or ankles, and on the face or neck. Symptoms commonly could vary from person to person. The most common symptoms are dry, itchy skin and rashes on the face, inside the elbows and behind the knees, and on the hands and feet[6]. Itching is the most relevant and common symptom of atopic dermatitis. Scratching and rubbing in response to itching irritates the skin, increases inflammation, and actually increases itchiness. Itching is a particular problem during sleep when conscious control of scratching is lost. The appearance of the skin that is affected by atopic dermatitis depends on the amount of scratching and the presence of secondary skin infections. The skin may be red and scaly, be thick and leathery, contain small raised bumps, or leak fluid and become crusty and infected. These features can also be found in people who do not have atopic dermatitis or who have other types of skin disorders. Atopic dermatitis may also affect the skin around the eyes, the eyelids, and the eyebrows and lashes. Scratching and rubbing the eye area can cause the skin to redden and swell. Some people with atopic dermatitis develop an extra fold of skin under their eyes. Patchy loss of eyebrows and eyelashes may also result from scratching or rubbing. In addition clinically unaffected skin in AD is not normal. It is frequently dry and has a greater irritant skin response than normal healthy skin[7]. Microscopic studies reveal a sparse perivascular T-cell infiltrate in unaffected AD skin that is not seen in normal healthy skin[8].

There is a marked infiltration of CD41 activated memory T cells in acute AD[9]. Antigen-presenting cells (eg, Langerhans cells inflammatory dendritic epidermal cells and macrophages) in lesional and, to a lesser extent, in nonlesional skin bear IgE molecules[10].

Mast cell degranulation can be observed. Macrophages dominate the dermal mononuclear cell infiltrate. Eosinophils also contribute to the inflammatory response, and T cells remain present, although in smaller numbers than seen in acute AD[11]. Chronic AD skin lesions undergo tissue remodeling caused by chronic inflammation. These skin lesions are associated with thickened plaques with increased skin markings (lichenification), increased collagen deposition in the dermis, and dry fibrotic papules[12]. AD is characterized by dry skin, even involving nonlesional skin and increased transepidermal water loss[13]. In particular, ceramides serve as the major water-retaining molecules in the extracellular space of the cornified envelope, and the barrier function of these complex structures is provided by a matrix of structural proteins, which are bound to ceramides[14]. A reduced content of ceramides has been reported in the cornified envelope of both lesional and nonlesional skin in patients with AD. Changes in stratum corneum pH levels have been found in patients with AD and might impair lipid metabolism in the skin. Overexpression of stratum corneum chymotryptic enzyme is also likely to contribute to the breakdown of the AD epidermal barrier[15].

Atopic dermatitis is very common: it affects males and females and accounts for 10 to 20 percent of all visits to dermatologists[16]. Although atopic dermatitis may occur at any age, it most often begins in infancy and childhood. Scientists estimate that 65 percent of patients develop symptoms in the first year of life, and 90 percent develop symptoms before the age of 5[17]. The cause of atopic dermatitis is not known, but the disease seems to result from a combination of genetic and environmental factors[18]. Children are more likely to develop this disorder if one or both parents have had it or have had other allergic conditions like asthma or allergic rhinitis[19]. While some people outgrow skin symptoms, approximately three-fourths of children with atopic dermatitis go on to develop hay fever or asthma[20]. Environmental factors can bring on symptoms of atopic dermatitis at any time in individuals who have inherited the atopic disease trait[21].

2. Atopic dermatitis and immune system: AD as an allergic disease

Atopic dermatitis is associated with malfunction of the body's immune system: the system that recognizes and helps fight bacteria and viruses that invade the body[22]. Scientists have found that people with atopic dermatitis have a low level of Interferon gamma (INF-γ) a cytokine (a protein) that is essential to the healthy function of the body's immune system and a high level of other cytokines such as IL-4 and IL-5 and IL-13 that lead to allergic reactions. The immune system can become misguided and create inflammation in the skin even in the absence of a major infection[23]. This can be viewed as a form of autoimmunity, where a body reacts against its own tissues. AD is also an important component of the atopic diathesis. AD frequently is associated with allergic respiratory disease and often is the first manifestation of allergic disease[24]. Patients suffering from AD will develop allergic rhinitis and asthma. The onset of AD generally occurs during the first 6 months of life. In adults with AD only 17% had onset after adolescence[25]. AD may arise from disregulation of IgE and T cell mediated hypersensitivity reactions[26]. Atopy is significantly associated with manifestation and severity of AD, especially in children. Exposure to aeroallergen (mites and pollen) has been shown to increase the risk factors for AD and AD severity[27]. Children with AD are at a high risk of allergic asthma and allergic rhinitis. Furthermore, aeroallergens are a trigger for exacerbations in adult AD. In about 80% of adult patients with

AD, the disease is associated with increased serum IgE levels, sensitization against aeroallergens and concomitant allergic rhinitis and asthma. Patients with AD can have very high serum IgE levels, often more than 10,000 IU/mL. It is important to note that specific IgE against allergens, whether measured in vivo by using SPTs or by using in vitro assays, does not equate to clinical disease or define clinical relevance in a given patient. In general, properly done SPTs to food allergens have a high negative predictive value, but the positive predictive value is only slightly higher than 50% for all patients. The inflammatory process in the skin initiates with the allergen uptake by epidermal dendritic cells which share in their surface the IgE-receptor. These cells, after the contact with the allergens, start the homing process of T cells. This process plays a central role for the inflammatory damage of skin[28]. Up to 80% of patients suffering from AD are sensitised against different aero and food allergens. This sensitisation is reflected by an increased total and allergen-specific IgE and/or by a positive Skin prick test[29].

2.1 AD as an allergic disease: The role of allergens sensitization

Sensitization to inhalant allergens is often seen in patients with AD[30]. Allergens can exacerbate AD either by means of inhalation, direct contact with the skin, or ingestion. Sensitization can be detected by means of SPTs (if the skin is free from eczema) or by measurement of specific IgE antibodies. In addition, Atopy Patch Test can be used to assess the response in the skin. Most important allergens include dust mite, animal dander, and pollen confirmed by clinical trials and avoidance measures[31]. The role of dust mite allergen exposure is supported by patch tests, avoidance studies, and the very high titers of IgE antibodies to mite proteins in a large proportion of adults, as well as children older than 7 years with AD. The positive effect of house dust mite avoidance with special encasings has been shown in various studies[32]. Allergen avoidance however has limited efficacy in HMD allergic patients.

2.2 Traditional therapeutic approach of AD

Basic therapy of AD should comprise optimal skin care, addressing the skin barrier defect with the regular use of moisturizing and emollient topical products and skin hydration[33]. An additional relevant therapeutic approach is the identification and the avoidance of both specific and nonspecific trigger factors. Non specific irritants include clothing made from occluding or irritating synthetic or wool material. A key feature of AD is severe dryness of the skin caused by a dysfunction of the skin barrier with increased transepidermal water loss. This is typically accompanied by intense itch and inflammation. The regular use of emollients is important for addressing this problem, and together with skin hydration, it represents the mainstay of the general management of AD[34]. Emollients should be applied continuously, even if no actual inflammatory skin lesions are obvious. Corticosteroid creams and ointments have been used for many years to treat atopic dermatitis and other autoimmune diseases affecting the skin[35]. Sometimes over-the-counter preparations are used, but in many cases the doctor will prescribe a stronger corticosteroid cream or ointment. The side effects of uncontrolled topical steroid use, particularly on delicate skin areas, are well documented, and therefore topical steroid preparations should be applied no more than twice daily as short-term therapy for acute eczematous lesions[36]. Only mild to moderately potent preparations should be used on genital, facial, or intertriginous skin areas. New medications known as *immuno modulators* have been developed that help control inflammation and reduce immune system reactions when applied to the skin. Examples of these medications are tacrolimus ointment and pimecrolimus cream[37]. They can be used in patients older than 2 years of age and have few side effects (burning or itching the first few days of application). They not only reduce flares, but also maintain skin texture and reduce the need for long-term use of corticosteroids. However corticosteroids and immunomodulators are not eziologic treatments of AD. These approaches in fact are mostly limited to control symptoms and suppress inflammatory reactions but they are not causal treatments of this skin condition.

2.3 Thinking AD treatment approach differently: The specific allergen immunotherapy as an option

Several anecdotal and case reports suggest clinical benefit from allergen-specific desensitization (specific immunotherapy [SIT]) in AD[38]. SIT is effective in the management of allergic asthma, allergic rhinitis/conjunctivitis, and stinging insect hypersensitivity[39]. There is some evidence it might be effective in the treatment of atopic dermatitis in patients with aeroallergen sensitivity. At least 12 placebo controlled trials have been conducted to evaluate the efficacy of SIT in AD patients[40]. A total of 9 trials (75%) reported significant positive effect of SIT in comparison with placebo. More recently, one double-blind controlled trial in children with dust mite allergy and AD failed to show efficacy of SIT compared with placebo after 8 months of therapy[41]. However, treatment for an additional 6 months resulted in clinical improvement, suggesting that prolonged desensitization might be more effective than placebo. A more recent multicenter, randomized, blinded, dose-response trial with house dust mite SIT in 89 adults with chronic AD sensitized to dust mite showed that the SCORAD score decreased in the 3 dose groups in a dose-dependent manner and was significantly lower in the 2 high-dose groups compared with the low-dose group after 1 year of SIT[42]. The use of topical corticosteroids was also significantly reduced with higher doses, suggesting that SIT might be useful for patients with AD sensitized to house dust mite. This study demonstrated that adult atopic patients with severe form of AD could benefit from SIT. Children with AD with or without respiratory allergies or asthma have also been treated with allergen-specific oral desensitization (SLIT), with 69% of the group without respiratory allergies-asthma versus 74% of the group with respiratory allergies-asthma showing complete resolution of their skin disease after 24 months of therapy. To date, specific immunotherapy (SIT) is not an established therapeutic approach for the treatment of AD even if the recent Immunotherapy Practice Parameter states that AD could be a clinical indication for SIT. Some controlled trials have failed to show clinical efficacy of SIT in the treatment of AD. However, SIT with house dust mite (HDM) subcutaneous preparation has been recently shown, in a randomized double-blind trial, to improve eczema in patients with AD.

2.4 Clinical efficacy of sublingual immunotherapy in AD

In comparison with subcutaneous SIT, sublingual immunotherapy (SLIT) is considered a more convenient and safer approach for the treatment of some forms of allergies. So far, there is few and conflicting data regarding the efficacy and safety of Specific Sublingual Immunotherapy (SLIT) in patients with AD. In a randomised double blind trial a total of

56 children with AD were treated with SLIT HDM allergen extracts or the corresponding placebo for 18 months. Significant improvement of SCORAD (Scoring Atopic Dermatitis) in the active group was observed as soon as 9 months of treatment. Lower use of rescue medication in the active group was observed after 18 months[43]. We have conducted a multicenter trial evaluating the efficacy of SLIT in 96 AD patients showing that this therapeutic option is efficacious and safe[44]. More in details, 96 subjects (58 women and 38 men; between 18 and 60 years of age) with AD and IgE-proved HDM sensitivity (Class >2) were enrolled in the trial after their informed consent. Exclusion criteria were severe asthma and treatment with systemic or high potent topical corticosteroids or immunosuppressant agents. Patients were treated with SLIT for at least 12 months. SCORAD was evaluated at baseline and after 12 months of treatment. Results: baseline SCORAD value (mean±SD) was 43.3±13.7 (range: 18-84). After 1 year of SLIT, SCORAD value was reduced to 23.7±13.3 (range: 0-65; p=0.0001; unpaired T-Test vs baseline). This was a 46% reduction in SCORAD in comparison with baseline time. A significant improvement, defined as a SCORAD reduction of >30%, was observed in 57 out of 96 patients (59.2%). In 6 patients (5.9%) the SCORAD value did not change at the end of the observation period. In 33 patients (34.9%) the SCORAD reduction after SLIT was ≤30% in comparison with baseline (Figure 1). Specific-IgE serum levels were significantly

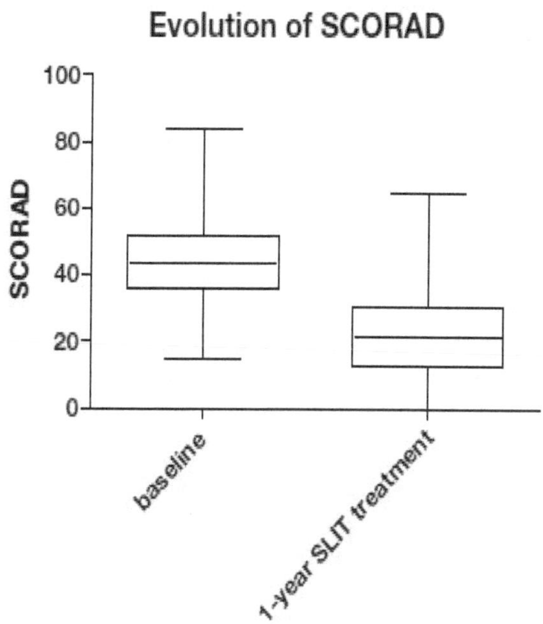

Fig. 1. Evolution of SCORAD index at baseline and after1 year of SLIT treatment (n = 96); (p = 0.0001 paired t-test)

(p=0.001) reduced after SLIT (Figure 2). No severe adverse events were observed during the trial. In this trial the SLIT with HDM extracts in patients with mild-moderate AD was effective in reducing the SCORAD after 1 year of SLIT treatment. In addition, the treatment was very well tolerated. Treatment with SLIT, furthermore, has allowed a gradual and relevant reduction of concomitant therapies with corticosteroids and immunosuppressants. SLIT can modulate the immuno-system in patients with AD and HDM sensitivity. In conclusion the data available from different trials suggest that SIT (both SCIT and SLIT) could be a relevant therapeutic option in the management of AD.

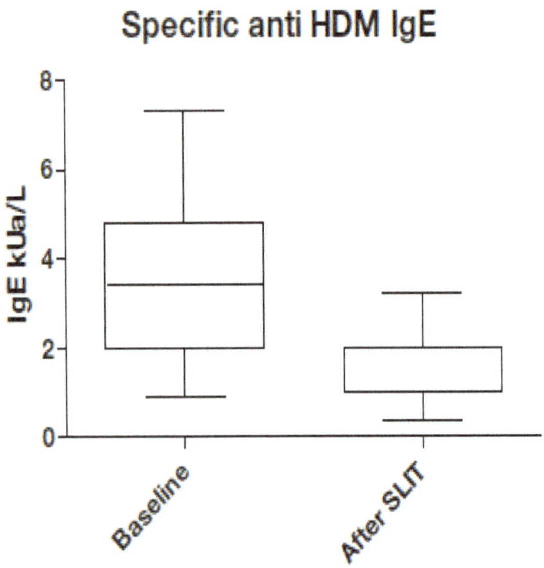

Fig. 2. Modification of specific anti HDM IgE serum levels at baseline and after1 year of SLIT treatment (n = 96); p = 0.0001 paired t-test.

3. Conclusion

Atopic Dermatitis (AD) is a common inflammatory itching skin disease affectings a large number of children and adults. Symptoms commonly could vary from person to person. The most common symptoms are dry, itchy skin and rashes on the face, inside the elbows and behind the knees, and on the hands and feet. Itching is the most relevant and common symptom of atopic dermatitis. Scratching and rubbing in response to itching irritates the skin, increases inflammation, and actually increases itchiness. The cause of atopic dermatitis is not known, but the disease seems to result from a combination of genetic and environmental factors. Children are more likely to develop this disorder if one or both parents have had it or have had other allergic conditions like asthma or allergic rhinitis. While some people outgrow skin symptoms, approximately three-fourths of children with atopic dermatitis go on to develop hay fever or asthma. AD frequently is associated with allergic respiratory disease and often is the first manifestation of allergic disease. Patients suffering from AD will develop allergic rhinitis and asthma. The inflammatory process in the skin of patients with AD initiates with the allergen uptake by epidermal dendritic cells which share in their surface the IgE-receptor. These cells, after the contact with the allergens, start the homing process of T cells. This process plays a central role for the inflammatory damage of skin. Up to 80% of patients suffering from AD are sensitised against different aero and food allergens. This sensitisation is reflected by an increased total and allergen-specific IgE and/or by a positive Skin prick test. So far not causative treatments are available for the treatment of AD. Topical corticosteroids and calcineurin inhibitors could ameliorate the clinical manifestation of AD. AD is frequently the first clinical manifestation of atopic disease in infancy. Basic therapy of AD comprises optimal skin care, emollient creams, topical corticosteroids and/or topical calcineurin inhibitors. Despite a strong rationale, hyposensitization with specific immunotherapy is not an established strategic treatment of AD. However, a recent study has shown that SCIT with HDM allergen extracts in adults AD patients with positive skin test toward HDM allergens is effective in reducing the SCORAD index and reducing, in the mean time, the need for topical corticosteroids. A wide clinical use of SCIT is, however, limited by the inconvenience and safety profile of this route of administration. A sublingual route has emerged as an effective alternative to subcutaneous immunotherapy. A recent trial, performed in children with AD, has shown that SLIT with HDM extracts could be effective in mild and moderate disease. SIT could be an effective and causal treatment of atopic dermatitis in patients with aeroallergen sensitivity. SLIT can modulate the immuno-system in patients with AD and HDM sensitivity. Several clinical trials (both controlled or uncontrolled) have shown that SIT is able to reduce the SCORAD and to reduce the use of symptomatic topical products. In conclusion the data available from different trials suggest that SIT (both SCIT and SLIT) could be a relevant therapeutic option in the management of AD.

4. Acknowledgment

ALK-Abello supported this study by providing immunotherapy extract. MM is ALK Abellò employee.

5. References

[1] Adkis C, Akdis M, Bieber T. Diagnosis and treatment of atopic dermatitis in children and adults: European Academy of Allergology and Clinical Immunonology / American Academy of Allergy, Asthma and Immunology / PRACTALL consensus report. *J Allergy Clin Immunol* 2006;118:152-69

[2] Williams HC, Strachan DP. The natural history of childhood eczema: observation from British 1958 birth cohort study. *Br J Dermatol* 1998;139:834-9

[3] Illi S, von Mutius E. The natural course of atopic dermatitis from birth to age 7 years and the association with asthma. *J Allergy Clin Immunol* 2004;113:925-31

[4] Hanafin J, Raijka G. Diagnostic features of atopic dermatitis. *Acta Derm Venereol Suppl* 1980;92:44-7

[5] Anon. Severity scoring of atopic dermatitis: the SCORAD index. Consensus report of European Task Force on Atopic Dermatitis. *Dermatology* 1993;186:23-31

[6] Seidenari S, Giusti G. Objective assessment of the skin of children affected by atopic dermatitis: a study of pH, capacitance and TEWL in eczematous and clinically uninvolved skin. Acta Derm Venereol 1996;75:429–33.

[7] Boguniewicz M, Leung DYM. Atopic dermatitis. *J Allergy Clin Immunol* 2006; 117(suppl):S475-80.

[8] Leung DYM, Bhan AK, Schneeberger EE, Geha RS. Characterization of the mononuclear cell infiltrate in atopic dermatitis using monoclonal antibodies. *J Allergy Clin Immunol* 1983;71:47–56

[9] Leung DY, Boguniewicz M, Howell MD, Nomura I, Hamid QA. New insights into atopic dermatitis. *J Clin Invest* 2004;113:651–7.

[10] Novak N, Kraft S, Bieber T. IgE receptors. *Curr Opin Immunol* 2001;13:721–6.

[11] Novak N, Valenta R, Bohle B, et al. Fcepsilon RI engagement of Langerhans cell-like dendritic cells and inflammatory dendritic epidermal cell-like dendritic cells induces chemotactic signals and different T-cell phenotypes in vitro. *J Allergy Clin Immunol* 2004;113:949–57.

[12] Leung DY, Bieber T. Atopic dermatitis. *Lancet* 2003;361:151-60.

[13] Proksch E, Folster-Holst R, Jensen JM. Skin barrier function, epidermal proliferation and differentiation in eczema. *J Dermatol Sci* 2006;43:159-69.

[14] Hudson TJ. Skin barrier function and allergic risk. *Nat Genet* 2006;38:399-400.

[15] Cork MJ, Robinson DA, Vasilopoulos Y, et al. New perspectives on epidermal barrier dysfunction in atopic dermatitis: gene-environment interactions. *J Allergy Clin Immunol* 2006;118:3-21

[16] Williams H, Flohr C. How epidemiology has challenged 3 prevailing concepts about atopic dermatitis. J Allergy Clin Immunol 2006;118:209-13.

[17] Anonymous. Worldwide variation in prevalence of symptoms of asthma, allergic rhinoconjunctivitis, and atopic eczema: ISAAC. The International Study of Asthma and Allergies in Childhood (ISAAC) Steering Committee. *Lancet* 1998;351:1225–32.

[18] Hoffjan S, Epplen JT. The genetics of atopic dermatitis: recent findings and future options. *J Mol Med* 2005;83:682–92.

[19] Bradley M, Soderhall C, Luthman H, Wahlgren CF, Kockum I, Nordenskjold M. Susceptibility loci for atopic dermatitis on chromosomes 3, 13, 15, 17 and 18 in a Swedish population. HumMol Genet 2002;11:1539–48.

[20] Williams HC, Strachan DP. The natural history of childhood eczema: observations from the British 1958 birth cohort study. *Br J Dermatol* 1998;139:834–9.

[21] Gustafsson D, Sjoberg O, Foucard T. Development of allergies and asthma in infants and young children with atopic dermatitis—a prospective follow-up to 7 years of age. *Allergy* 2000;55:240–5.

[22] Novak N, Bieber T, Leung DY. Immune mechanisms leading to atopic dermatitis. *J Allergy Clin Immunol* 2003;112(suppl):S128–39.

[23] Strachan DP. Hay fever, hygiene, and household size. *BMJ* 1989;299:1259-60.

[24] Purvis DJ, Thompson JM, Clark PM, Robinson E, Black PN, Wild CJ et al. Risk factors for atopic dermatitis in New Zealand children at 3.5 years of age. *Br J Dermatol* 2005;152:742–9.

[25] Ozkaya E. Adult-onset atopic dermatitis. *J Am Acad Dermatol* 2005;52:579–82.

[26] Novak N, Kruse S, Potreck J, Weidinger S, Fimmers R, Bieber T. Single nucleotide polymorphisms of the IL18 gene are associated with atopic eczema. *J Allergy Clin Immunol* 2005;115:828–33.

[27] Adinoff AD. Atopic dermatitis and aeroallergen contact sensitivity. *J Allergy Clin Immunol* 1988;81:736-42

[28] Novak N, Valenta R, Bohle B, Laffer S, Haberstok J, Kraft S et al. Fcepsilon RI engagement of Langerhans cell-like dendritic cells and inflammatory dendritic epidermal cell-like dendritic cells induces chemotactic signals and different T-cell phenotypes in vitro. *J Allergy Clin Immunol* 2004;113:949–57.

[29] Scalabrin DM, Bavbek S, Perzanowski MS,.Use of specific IgE in assessing the relevance of fungal and dust mite allergens to atopic dermatitis: a comparison with asthmatic and non asthmatic control subjects. *J Allergy Clin Immunol* 1999;104: 1273-9.

[30] Maintz L, Novak N. Getting more and more complex: the pathophysiology of atopic eczema. Eur J Dermatol 2007; 17:267–283.

[31] Werfel T, Kapp A. Environmental and other major provocation factors in atopic dermatitis. *Allergy* 1998;53:731-9.

[32] Tan BB, Weald D, Strickland I, et al. Double-blind controlled trial of effect of house dust mite allergen avoidance on atopic dermatitis. *Lancet* 1996;347:15–8.

[33] Subramanyan K. Role of mild cleansing in the management of patient skin. *Dermatol Ther* 2004;17:26–34.

[34] Loden M. Role of topical emollients and moisturizers in the treatment of dry skin barrier disorders. *Am J Clin Dermatol* 2003;4:771–88

[35] McHenry PM, Williams HC, Bingham EA. Management of atopic eczema: Joint Workshop of the British Association of Dermatologists and the Research Unit of the Royal College of Physicians of London. BMJ 1995;310:843–7.

[36] Korting HC, Kerscher MJ, Schafer- Korting M. Topical glucocorticoids with improved benefit/risk ratio: do they exist? *J Am Acad Dermatol* 1992;27:87–92.

[37] Wahn U, Bos JD, Goodfield M, Caputo R, Papp K, Manjra A et al. Efficacy and safety of pimecrolimus cream in the longterm management of atopic dermatitis in children. *Pediatrics* 2002;110:e2.

[38] Mastrandrea F. The potential role of allergen-specific sublingual immunotherapy in atopic dermatitis. *Am J Clin Dermatol* 2004;5:281–94.

[39] Bousquet J. Sublingual immunotherapy: validated. *Allergy* 2006;61:5-6

[40] Novak N, Simon Atopic dermatitis - from new pathophysiologic insights to individualized therapy. *Allergy*. 2011 Mar 3. doi: 10.1111/j.1398-9995.2011.02571.x

[41] Bussmann C, Bockenhoff A, Henke H, et al. Does allergen-specific immunotherapy represent a therapeutic option for patients with atopic dermatitis? *J Allergy Clin Immunol* 2006; 118:1292–1298

[42] Werfel T, Breuer K, Rueff F, Przybilla B, Worm M, Grewe M et al. Usefulness of specific immunotherapy in patients with atopic dermatitis and allergic sensitization to house dust mites: a multicentre, randomized, dose-response study. *Allergy* 2006;61:202–5.

[43] Pajno G, Caminiti L. Sublingual immunotherapy in mitesensitized children with atopic dermatitis: a randomized double blind, placebo-controlled study. *J Allergy Clin Immunol* 2007 120(1):164-70.

[44] Cadario G, Galluccio AG, Pezza M, Appino A, Milani M, Pecora S, Mastrandrea F Sublingual immunotherapy efficacy in patients with atopic dermatitis and house dust mites sensitivity: a prospective pilot study. *Curr Med Res Opin.* 2007 Oct;23(10):2503-6.

18

Occlusive Therapy in Atopic Dermatitis

Misha M. Heller[1], Eric S. Lee[2], Faranak Kamangar[3], Wilson Liao[4] and John Y. M. Koo[4]
[1]*University of Southern California, Keck School of Medicine, Los Angeles, California*
[2]*University of Nebraska Medical Center, College of Medicine, Omaha, Nebraska*
[3]*University of California Davis, School of Medicine, Sacramento, California*
[4]*University of California San Francisco, Department of Dermatology San Francisco, California*
USA

1. Introduction

The treatment of atopic dermatitis (AD) can be challenging for dermatologists and other healthcare professionals. Conventional treatments consisting of emollients and topical corticosteroids are often insufficient for severe and/or refractory AD. Other therapies include systemic corticosteroids, photochemotherapy using psoralen and ultraviolet-A light, and cyclosporine. However, all of these approaches have potentially serious side effects and relative contraindications, especially in children. Over the past two decades, occlusive therapy has been advocated as a safe and effective treatment modality for individuals with acute erythrodermic AD and those with severe and/or refractory AD. (Nicol 1987; Goodyear et al. 1991; Bridgman 1995; Devillers and Oranje 2005)

Occlusive therapy usually involves the application of emollients, antiseptics, or topical corticosteroids under either wet wrap dressings (WWD) or dry wrap dressings (DWD). This consists of moistened open-weave cotton tubular bandages (eg. Tubifast®, Tubigauz®) in WWD occlusion, versus dry gauze, plastic wraps, or hydrocolloid dressings (eg. Duoderm®) in DWD occlusion. (Nicol 1987; Goodyear et al. 1991; Bridgman 1995)

More recently, however, occlusion alone using a hydrogel patch has been utilized. The theory is that a major component in the pathophysiology of AD is barrier dysfunction. In fact, many current therapies target this barrier defect (i.e., pseudoceramide moisturizers and skin barrier emulsions). As such, an ideal repair mechanism would completely eliminate microbe and allergen penetration and transepidermal water loss in AD, both of which lead to xerosis, hypersensitivity, pruritus, and inflammation. The hydrogel patch, therefore, offers an innovative approach to *complete* barrier repair. (Park et al. 2011)

Regardless of the treatment approach, occlusive therapy offers many advantageous such as a cooling effect on inflamed skin, increased penetration of topical agents, enhanced skin hydration, and a barrier to external antigens and trauma (i.e. scratching). Reported disadvantages include the cumbersome and time-consuming nature of the application process, risk of allergic reaction to the occlusive material itself, and possible increased risk of infectious complications such as folliculitis, furunculosis, or cellulitis. An additional concern is that occlusion may cause skin maceration if used incorrectly, or can paradoxically promote skin dryness if too little topicals are applied. (Nicol 1987; Goodyear et al. 1991; Bridgman 1995; Krakowski et al. 2008)

Occlusion alone of both normal and lesional eczematous skin can result in increased density of cutaneous microbial flora. (Aly et al. 1978; Rajka et al. 1981) Moreover, there is a positive association between *Staphylococcus aureus* (*S. aureus*) colonization and disease severity. (Williams 2000) These findings suggest that occlusion, by increasing the density of *S. aureus*, might push already colonized eczematous skin into the realm of clinical infection. In addition, innate production of cutaneous anti-microbial peptides, such as sphingosine and β-defensin, is depressed in patients with AD such that eczematous skin possesses decreased natural resistance to bacterial invasion (Arikawa et al. 2002; Ong et al. 2002) Thus, evidence of clinically apparent skin infection may be a contraindication to occlusive therapy, as it may exacerbate the infection. (Aly et al. 1978) However, the possibility that *S. aureus* colonization may complicate occlusive therapy has not been adequately addressed to date.

Another concern is that the use of topical corticosteroids under occlusion may relate to an increased potential for absorption and greater incidences of possible adverse effects. Most attention has been focused on the risk of skin atrophy and striae, hypothalamic-pituitary-adrenal (HPA) axis suppression, as well as growth impairment in children.

Ultimately, this chapter aims to examine current evidence on the safety and efficacy of occlusive therapy in the treatment of AD.

2. Methods

Studies on the use of occlusive therapy for the treatment of atopic dermatitis were identified in PubMed and Embase Medline databases from January 1966 to April 2011, using the key terms "occlusion," "occlusive dressings", "occlusive therapy," "wet wrap," "wet dressings," "dry wrap," "dry dressings," "atopic dermatitis," "dermatitis," and "eczema." Key terms were also searched in combination. Reference lists of relevant publications were manually searched for additional relevant studies. The search was limited to original studies and review articles published in English or with English abstracts, in humans. Studies of small size and those that did not use a controlled or randomized study design were included due to the dearth of published literature on this topic. Publications meeting these criteria were then reviewed for study design, population, disease severity or type, study size, efficacy, and safety. The topical agent used, dilution, and type and period of occlusive therapy were also noted, when such information was made available in the publication. In addition, response to therapy was seen as improvement in disease severity or symptoms from baseline, improvement in SCORing Atopic Dermatitis (SCORAD), and/or improvement in Eczema Area and Severity Index (EASI) score, depending on what information was provided. Of note, SCORAD is composite score of eczema severity based on the surface area involved, intensity of symptoms, and subjective symptoms such as sleep disturbance and pruritus. EASI is a 12-point scoring system of disease severity assessing erythema, induration, lichenification, pruritus, and excoriation. Finally, conclusions were drawn from the results of these studies bearing in mind standard clinical practice.

3. Studies on occlusive therapy

There are a total of 19 studies evaluating the use of occlusive therapy in AD (Table 1). Fourteen studies used WWD, 5 of which were randomized controlled trials. All WWD

Study Design	Disease Severity	Size (n)	Population (age)	Type of Occlusion	Treatment Regimen	
					Topical agents*	Frequency & Duration
Goodyear et al.,1991 (Prospective)	Acute erythrodermic eczema	30	Children (9 months – 16 years), inpatient	WWD	HCT 1% or 25% dilution betamethasone cream	Twice daily, x 2-5 days
Mallon et al., 1994 (Prospective)	Chronic severe eczema	21	Children, outpatient with nursing visits	WWD	HCT 0.5% or 10% dilution betamethasone 0.1% cream	Daily, x < 5 days
Abeck et al., 1999 (Prospective)	Acute exacerbated eczema	6	Adults, children	WWD	Chlorhexidine, emollients	Frequency not reported, x 3 days
Wolkerstorfer et al. 2000 (Prospective, left-right comparison study)	Severe AD	31	Children (5 months – 13 years), inpatient	WWD	10-50% dilution fluticasone propionate 0.05% cream	Daily, re-wet every 2 hours, x 1 week
Tang, 2000 (Prospective)	Flare of facial eczema	10	Children (4 - 15 years)	WWD	10% dilution mometasone furoate 0.1% cream or ointment	Daily for 2-3 hours, x "few days"
Pei et al., 2001 (RCT)	Moderate-to-severe AD	40	Children (1 - 15 years)	WWD	10% dilution of mometasone furoate 0.1% ointment or 10% dilution of fluticasone propionate 0.005% ointment	Topical applied once daily, x 4 weeks open application (control group), versus topical applied once daily, x 2 weeks open application and then 2 weeks using WWD (study group)
Schnopp et al., 2002 (RCT, left-right comparison study)	Exacerbated AD	20	Children (2 - 17 years), inpatients	WWD	Mometasone furoate 0.1%, or its vehicle	Twice daily, x 5 days
Devillers et al., 2002 (Retrospective, left-right comparison study)	Refractory AD	26	Adults (6 months – 10 years), children (18 – 61 years), inpatient	WWD	5% (on face), 10% and 25% (on body, adults), 5% and 10% (on body, children) dilution fluticasone propionate 0.05% cream	Daily, re-wet every 2-3 hours, x 1 week
McGowan et al., 2003 (Prospective)	Atopic eczema	8	Children (3 - 8years)	WWD	10% or 25% dilution beclomethasone dipropionate	Daily, x 2-18 weeks (median = 12 weeks)
Beattie and Lewis-Jones, 2004 (RCT)	Moderate AD (requiring HCT 1% or less potent)	19	Children (4 months - 3 years)	WWD	HCT 1%	Topical applied twice daily, x 2 weeks open application (control group), versus topical applied daily, with WWD applied twice daily for the 1st week and then daily for the 2nd week (study group)

Study Design	Disease Severity	Size (n)	Population (age)	Type of Occlusion	Treatment Regimen	
					Topical agents*	Frequency & Duration
Foelster-Holst et al., 2006 (RCT, left-right comparison study)	Severe AD	24	Adults (18-63 years), children (6-16 years)	WWD	Prednicarbat alone or prednicarbat under WWT	Not reported, x 48-72 hours
Hindley et al., 2006 (RCT)	Moderate-to-severe AD	50	Children (4-27 months)	WWD	HCT 1%	Topical applied twice daily, x 4 weeks (control group), versus topical applied daily with WWD for 24-hours for the 1st week and then topical applied twice daily with WWD for 12- or 24- hours for 3 more weeks (study group)
Lee et al. (Prospective)	Severe AD	10	Adults (22 years)	WWD	0.9% saline solution	Daily (8 hours), x 7-14 days
Hon et al., 2007 (Prospective)	Moderate-to-severe AD	6	Children (3 - 15 years)	WWD	Mometasone furoate 0.1%	Overnight, x 3 days
Rajka et al., 1981 (Prospective)	Active AD	10	Adults, outpatient	DWD	None	Not reported, x 24 hours
Geraldez et al., 1989 (RCT)	Lichen simplex chronicus	60	Not reported	DWD	Diflucortolone valerate 0.3% ointment	Twice daily occlusion nightly, x 2 weeks
Volden et al., 1992 (Prospective)	Chronic, therapy-resistant AD	48	Adults	DWD	Clobetasol propionate lotion	Weekly, x 8-18 days
Gauger et al., 2003 (Prospective)	Generalized or localized AD	15	Adults, children (24.6 years), outpatient	DWD	Silver-coated textile	Daily, x1 week
Park et al, 2011 (Prospective)	Generalized or localized AD	15	Adults, outpatient	Hydrogel patch	Triamcinolone 0.1% cream	Hydrogel patch applied daily for 6-8 hours on one lesion, versus topical applied twice daily on another lesion, x 6 weeks

*Dilution and concentration noted when provided in the article

Table 1. Studies on Occlusive Therapy (HCT = Hydrocortisone, RCT = randomized control trial)

occlusion studies demonstrated efficacy in severe or acute, moderate and chronic AD. Among the 4 studies examining DWD, only one used a randomized controlled design. All, except one, DWD studies demonstrated improvements in AD. There is also one study that used an impermeable hydrogel patch consisting of about 50% water content. The hydrogel patch alone demonstrated improvements in AD, comparable to that of corticosteroid use alone. Increased cutaneous bacterial counts or clinical infections were reported in 4 out of the 15 studies using WWD and all 4 studies using DWD.

3.1 Wet wrap dressings

The following is a detailed description of the 14 studies evaluating the efficacy of WWD in the treatment of AD (Table 2). Occlusive therapy was first introduced by Goodyear et al. in 1991. Goodyear et al. (1991) evaluated the inpatient use of WWD occlusion for acute erythrodermic eczema. This WWD technique involved the application of open-weave cotton tubular dressings (Tubegauz®) impregnanted with hydrocortisone 1% cream (if child <2 years of age) or 10% dilution of bemethasone valerate (if child > 2 years of age) twice daily. All 30 children responded well to WWD occlusion, with no relapses noted at 2 weeks follow-up. Interestingly, an attempt at long-term home therapy using WWD, following the inpatient therapy, in 5 patients was unsuccessful due to reports of inconvenience, increased bacterial infections, and prolonged HPA axis suppression. (Goodyear 1991)

Mallon et al. (1994) studied the use of WWD in chronic severe eczema in 21 children. Eczema was managed using topical steroid creams (i.e. hydrocortisone 0.5% or 10% dilution betamethosone 0.1% cream) and emollients under WWD daily for less than 5 days. All patients responded well to WWD therapy. The treatment was also well-tolerated. Majority of parents (20/21) reported decreased use topical steroid per week following the introduction of WWD therapy. (Mallon et al. 1994)

Abeck et al. (1999) treated 6 patients (3 children and 3 adults) with acute exacerbated atopic eczema with basic emollients in combination with chlorhexidine-soaked dressings for 3 days. The study observed improvements in disease severity based on SCORAD score. Patients also reported decreased itch and sleep loss following WWD therapy. In addition, there was a reduction of *S. aureus* counts that paralleled skin improvement. (Abeck et al. 1999)

In a study of 31 children with severe refractory AD, Wolkerstorfer et al. (2000) investigated the efficacy of various cortiocosteroid dilutions under WWD occlusion. Participants were divided into 3 treatment groups. The first group consisted of 18 children, who were treated with 50% dilution of fluticasone propionate 0.05% (FP) cream under WWD for 2 weeks. In the second group, 5 children with symmetrically localized AD were treated with different dilutions (10%, 25% and 50%) of FP cream on the left and the right side of the body under WWD for one week and then 10% dilution of FP cream under WWD the following week. In the third group, 8 children were treated with 0% (i.e. only emollient), 5%, 10%, or 25% dilutions of FP cream applied to the entire body under WWD. After just one week of therapy, significant improvement in disease severity was observed, without noticeable differences between 5%, 10%, or 25% dilutions of FP cream under WWD. Less improvement was observed in the second week of therapy. In terms of skin infections, mild-to-moderate folliculitis was reported in a large proportion of the children, with 33% (6/18) children in the first group, 40% (2/5) children in the second group, and 63% (5/8) children in the third group. There was also one case of furunculosis in the third group. Interestingly, generalized folliculitis was noted in both of the children treated with only emollient during the first week. These findings suggests that although WWD occlusion may foster bacterial growth,

Study Design	Results		Adverse Events		
	Response to therapy	Additional Information	Infection	Skin Atrophy	Systemic
Goodyear et al., 1991 (Prospective)	All 90-100% clearance	Home maintenance WWD therapy was unsuccesful	N/A	N/A	Transient low morning cortisol levels
Mallon et al., 1994 (Prospective)	"All responded well"	20/21 parents reported using less topical steroids	None	N/A	N/A
Abeck et al., 1999 (Prospective)	Improved SCORAD	Decreased itch and sleep loss	Decreased *S. aureus* counts	N/A	N/A
Wolkerstorfer et al., 2000 (Prospective, left-right comparison study)	Improved SCORAD, most improvement observed in the 1st week of therapy	No difference between dilutions; dose-response (80%) and adrenal suppression with absolute amount (1.6 g/day)	Folliculitis reported in 6/18 (33%) children in 1st group, 2/5 (40%) children in 2nd group, 5/8 (63%) children in 3rd group. Furunculosis reported in 1/8 (13%) children in 3rd group.	None	HPA axis suppression related to the absolute amount of applied corticosteroid
Tang, 2000 (Prospective)	"Good response"		None	None	N/A
Pei et al., 2001 (RCT)	Improved subjective and clinical scores	No difference between topical agents, one child unable to tolerate WWD	N/A	N/A	N/A
Schnopp et al., 2002 (RCT, left-right comparison study)	Improved SCORAD	Topical corticosteriods are superior to steroid-free emollients under WWT	Decreased *S. aureus* counts in steroid group, no clinical infections in steroid or vehicle groups	N/A	N/A
Devillers et al., 2002 (Retrospective, left-right comparison study)	Improved SCORAD	No difference in improvement between dilutions applied to each side of the body	Long-term home treatment: 9 reported cases of infectious complications, including folliculitis, secondary impetigo, *Pseudomonas aeruginosa* infection, and cellulitius, and conjunctivitis	1 adult (also taking inhaled steroids) with striae	2 children and 1 adult had transient low morning cortisol, and 1 adult (also taking inhaled steroids) developed prolonged HPA suppression
McGowan et al., 2003 (Prospective)	N/A	No change in lower leg length (short-term bone growth) and urinary-DPD (bone turnover marker)	N/A	N/A	N/A

Study Design	Results		Adverse Events		
	Response to therapy	Additional Information	Infection	Skin Atrophy	Systemic
Beattie and Lewis-Jones, 2004 (RCT)	No difference in improvement between treatment groups	Greater HRQoL and sleep improvement in non-WWD control group	Folliculitis reported in 2/10 (20%) children (1 child withdrawn)	N/A	N/A
Foelster-Holst et al., 2006 (RCT, left-right comparison study)	Improved SCORAD in both treatment groups	Significantly better SCORAD improvement in the WWT group	None	None	None
Hindley et al., 2006 (RCT)	Improved SCORAD in both treatment groups	No significant difference observed in SCORAD improvement between two treatment groups	5/23 (22%) children in the WWD group received antibiotics for infective exacerbations of eczema	N/A	N/A
Lee et al. (Prospective)	Improved SCORAD	Epidermal water content increased, transepidermal water loss decreased, increased release of lamellar bodies and restoration of intercellular lipid lamellar structure observed	N/A	N/A	N/A
Hon et al., 2007 (Prospective)	Improved SCORAD	Scratching reduced by 20-60% as assessed by nocturnal wrist motion monitor, improved QoL	N/A	N/A	N/A

Table 2. Outcomes of Studies on Wet Wrap Dressing Occlusion (DPD = deoxypyridinoline, HPA = hypothalamic-pituitary-adrenal, HRQoL = Health Related Quality of Life)

the addition of topical corticosteroids to the treatment regimen appeared to provide some protective benefits. (Wolkerstorfer et al. 2000)

Tang (2000) treated 10 children experiencing a flare of facial eczema with WWD occlusion. Children were initiated on an intermittent treatment regimen involving 10% dilution of mometasone furoate 0.1% cream or ointment under WWD applied for 2-3 hours once daily for a few consecutive days. All parents reported good treatment response. No cutaneous side effects were observed from topical corticosteroid use. (Tang 2000)

Pei et al. (2001) performed a randomized control trial of 40 children with moderate-to-severe AD. Prior to starting the study, all patient were instructed to apply 0.005% flucinolone acetonide cream twice daily for 2 weeks to standardize treatment medications. Patient were then randomized to receive 10% dilution of 0.1% mometasone furoate ointment or 10% dilution of 0.005% fluticasone propionate ointment. These topical agents were applied once a day for 2 weeks without WWD. After this 2-week period of open application, patients were further randomized to receive the same topical agent for 2 more weeks without WWD, or for 2 more weeks under WWD. Only 30 patients (75%) entered into this second phase of the study since their disease severity had failed to improve by more than 50% after the initial 2 weeks of open topical application. In other words, only patients whose disease was refractory to a 2-week period of conventional open therapy continued in the study. Ultimately, there were a total of 27 patients who completed the study. One child receiving fluticasone propionate ointment dropped out of the study because the patient was unable to tolerate WWD. The study found that significantly greater improvements in disease severity and extent in patients using WWD, as compared to controls. These results suggest that WWD may be an effective second-line therapy in children whose disease is refractory to conventional open topical corticosteroids. (Pei et al. 2001)

Schnopp et al. (2002) examined the effect of WWD in a randomized control study of 20 inpatients with exacerbated AD. Children received either a topical corticosteroid preparation (mometasone furoate 0.1%) or a steroid-free preparation (its vehicle) under WWD, applied twice daily for 5 days to the tested area in a left-right study. Disease severity at day 3 and day 5 continuously improved in both groups; however, the mometasone furoate-treated group showed significantly greater irmprovements. *Staphylococcus aureus* bacterial counts initially decreased during the first 3 days of treatment in both groups. At day 5, bacterial counts continued to decrease in the steroid-treated group, but bacterial counts increased in the vehicle-treated group. There were no reported clinical signs of bacterial superinfection in either the steroid or vehicle groups. The study concluded that WWD were useful in treatment of exacerbated AD, with applications of topical corticosteroids showing better efficacy than steroid-free emollients. (Schnopp et al. 2002)

Devillers et al. (2002) evaluated the use of WWD in refractory AD in 12 adults and 14 children. WWD were applied daily and re-wettted every 2-3 hours for 1 week in an inpatient setting. Patients used 5% dilution of FP cream under WWD on affected areas of the face. As for the body, a side-to-side comparison study was performed, in which adults applied 10% and 25% dilutions of FP cream and children applied 5% and 10% dilutions of FP cream. Disease severity improved dramatically during the one week of inpatient therapy. There was no difference in improvement between dilutions applied to each side of the body. Following inpatient therapy, 8 adults and 13 children continued treatment at home with less potent dilutions of FP cream. Exacerbation of AD occurred in 3 adults and 2 children. Infectious complications included localized folliculitis (4 reported cases), secondary impetigo (2 reported cases), localized *Pseudomonas aeruginosa* infection, cellulitis of the left cheek in a patient without a facial mask, and purulent conjunctivitis in a patient with a facial mask. These complications may be attributed to variations in standard protocal for WWD application, such as prolonged (>8 hours) occlusion and the frequent rewetting procedure. (Devillers et al. 2002)

McGowan et al. (2003) examined the effects of WWD therapy using topical corticosteroids on short-term growth and bone turnover in 8 prepubertal children, ranging from 3-8 years of age. Tubular bandages were applied over 10% or 25% dilutions of beclomethasone dipropionate for 24 hours each day for 2 weeks. After 2 weeks, frequency of tubular bandages was reduced to overnight use for one week and then as required for the remainder of the treatment period. Occlusive dressings were applied for a median duration of 12 weeks (range 2 - 18 weeks). Short-term growth was assessed by measuring lower leg length velocity by knemometry, while bone turnover was assessed by urinary deoxypyridinoline excretion. (McGowan et al. 2003) (See Section 3.4 Cutaneous and Systemic Side Effects for further discussion of this study)

In randomized control trial, Beattie and Lewis-Jones (2004) compared the use of 1% hydrocortisone under WWD to conventional open therapy in 19 children with moderate, widespread AD. The control group applied 1% hydrocortisone twice daily for 2 weeks, without WWD. In the study group, patients applied 1% hydrocortisone once in the morning for 2 weeks, with WWD twice daily for the first week and then only at night for the second week. Both groups were allowed to apply non-steroidal emollients as often as necessary. Beattie and Lewis Jones (2004) found no difference in clinical improvement between the control group and the study group. The authors, therefore, concluded that conventional open therapy using 1% hydrocortisone and emollients alone appeared to be as effective as using 1% hydrocortisone under WWD for moderate AD. Despite these findings, it is important to note that the use of 1% hydrocortisone is a less potent choice than what is generally used in clinical practice when treating moderate AD. If the authors had evaluated the use of a mid-potency topical corticosteroid under WWD, the degree of improvement between the study and control groups might have been markedly different. In terms of health related quality of life, Beattie and Lewis-Jones (2004) found greater improvements in the non-WWD control group than the WWD group for both the child and the family. Children in the non-WWD control group also reported more sleep than the WWD group, but there was no significant difference for itch between treatment groups. In regards to infections, 2 of the 10 (20%) children in the WWD group experienced folliculitis, one of which had to be withdrawal from the study. There were no reported clinical infections in the non-WWD control group. (Beattie and Lewis-Jones 2004)

Foelster-Holst et al. (2006) conducted a randomized, controlled study of 24 adults and children with acute episodes of AD. This was left-right comparison study, in which patients had skin lesions symmetrically affecting both arms or legs. One arm or leg was randomly treated with the topical prednicarbat (a medium potency corticosteroid), with WWD using a tubular bandage. The other extremity received topical prednicarbat alone. After 48-72 hours of therapy, both groups showed improvement of the local SCORAD, but the improvement in the WWD group was significantly better. No adverse effects were observed in either treatment group. (Foelster-Holst et al. 2006)

Hindley et al. (2006) carried a randomized, control trial to investigate the efficacy of WWD as compared to conventional topically applied corticosteroids. This 4-week study consisted of a total of 50 children with moderate-to-severe eczema. In the conventional treatment group, patients had emollients applied as needed and 1% hydrocortisone ointment (or more potent topical steroids, if necessary) applied twice daily. In the WWD treatment group, patients had wet wraps applied daily for a 24-hour period over 1% hydrocortisone ointment (or more potent topical steroids, if necessary) during the first week, followed by wet wraps applied for a 12- or 24-hour period depending on disease progress for the remaining three weeks. When wet wraps were applied for only a 12-hour period, 1% hydrocortisone and emollients were used during the non-wet wrap period. Both treatment groups demonstrated improvement in overall SCORAD scores; however, there was no significant difference between the conventional and WWD treatment groups. Five out of 23 (22%) children in the WWD treatment group required antibiotics for skin infections, as compared to none of the children in the conventional treatment group. The authors conclude that 4-weeks of maintenance WWD treatment may be associated with more skin infections than conventional treatment. (Hindley et al. 2006) However, it is important to realize that in clinical practice, physicians usually do not use WWD for maintenance therapy of AD over a 4-week duration. Instead, physicians are more likely to use WWD in settings of acute generalized eczematous flares for 3-7 days to induce disease remission. (Williams 2006) Lee et al. (2007) examined the therapeutic efficacy of WWD and the mechanism behind its therapeutic efficacy in treatment of AD. Ten patients with severe AD received WWD (without steroid treatment) for 7–14 days. SCORAD was used to assess AD severity, immediately following the end of treatment and 7 days after termination of treatment. Transepidermal water loss, water content in the corneum, and lipid amount of skin surface were also measured. The SCORAD was significantly reduced after WWD therapy. Additionally, epidermal water content was increased and transepidermal water loss was decreased following WWD therapy; these results were maintained 1 week after terminating therapy. In atopic lesions, increased release of lamellar bodies and restoration of intercellular lipid lamellar structure was observed. The authors speculated that increased secretion of lamellar bodies induced with WWD occlusion may lead to recovery of the abnormal epidermal barrier and clinical improvement in AD. (Lee et al. 2007)

In a clinical study of six children with moderate to severe AD, Hon et al. (2007) tested the efficiacy of WWD occlusion using Tubifast® garments with mometasone furoate 0.1% cream. Short-term use of WWD occlusion over 3 days demonstrated improvement in disease severity based on SCORAD. In addition, a wrist motion monitor was used to measure nocturnal itch, which showed that average scratching activity was significantly reduced by 20–60% on day 3 of treatment. Furthermore, WWD was effective in improving quality of life in these children. (Hon et al. 2007)

Since its introduction by Goodyear et al. (1991) nearly two decades ago, WWD occlusion has been extensively used as a relatively safe and effective treatment modality for children with acute erythrodermic AD and those with severe and/or refractory AD. The most effective topical corticosteroid to be used is still uncertain, but 10% dilutions of potent topical corcorticosteroid are most commonly used. Protocols on adminstration and duration of WWD occlusion can vary between studies. (Oranje et al. 2006) (See Table 3)

Advantages of WWD occlusion include a rapid therapeutic response, reduction in itch and sleep disturbances, and a possible decreased topical corticosteroid use. Disadvantages include high cost, the need for specialized training, increased potential for topical corticosteroid absorption, and increased incidences of folliculitis and other cutaneous infections. (Oranje et al. 2006)

However, the application of WWD has become less time-consuming and more feasible for home use with development of Tubifast® garments manufactured by Medlock Medical®

(available since 2003). With the introduction of these garments, wet wrapping can be done in 20–25 minutes. Tubifast garments® are available as tights for babies aged 6–24 months, vests for children 6 months through 14 years, and socks and leggings in all sizes. These washable garments are absorbent, holding enough water to remain moist for hours, and are elastic and able to conform to the contours of the body. (Page 2005)

1. Choose the appropriate width of the tubular bandages and cut these to size to fit the affected body areas (i.e. arms, legs, trunk). Alternatively, Tubifast® garments can be used.
2. Apply the appropriate dilution of topical corticosteroids (e.g. fluticasone propionate 0.05% cream, mometasone furoate 0.1% cream) on the involved skin. In general, diluted steroids in emollients of 1:9 are applied to the face of all patients and body of infants, while diluted steroids in emollients of 1:9 or 1:3 are applied on the body of adults.
3. Wet the pieces of tubular bandage in lukewarm water. Alternatively, if Tubifast® garments are used, then the inner garment is moistened using a plant sprayer.
4. Apply the first layer of wet tubular bandages. Connect the arm and leg pieces to the trunk. Apply the facial mask, if necessary. Alternatively, if Tubifast® garments are used, the inner garment is moistened using a plant spray.
5. Apply the second layer of dry tubular bandage. Again, connect the arm and leg pieces to the trunk. Apply the facial mask, if necessary. Alternatively, if Tubifast® garments are used, a second dry Tubifast® garment is placed over the wet one.
6. Re-wet the tubular bandages every 2-3 hours. Alternatively, if Tubifast® garments are used, re-wet the inner Tubifast® garment every 2-3 hours.
7. Repeat procedures #1-6 (described above) daily.
8. After 7 days of occlusive therapy, the dilution of topical corticosteroids (e.g. fluticasone propionate 0.05% cream, mometasone furoate 0.1% cream) is applied on the involved skin for 4-7 consecutive days.

Table 3. Protocol for Wet Wrap Dressing occlusion

Finally, in a review article, Devillers and Oranje (2006) made the following conclusions regarding WWD occlusion with a grade C of recommendation. 1) WWD using cream or ointment and a double layer of cotton bandages, with a moist first layer and a dry second layer, is an efficacious short-term treatment for children with severe and/or refractory AD.2) The use of WWD with diluted topical corticosteroids is a more efficacious treatment than wet-wrap dressings with emollients only for children with severe and/or refractory AD. 3) The use of WWD with diluted topical corticosteroids is a safe intervention treatment for children with severe and/or refractory AD for up to 14 days, with temporary systemic bioactivity of the corticosteroids as the only reported serious adverse effect. 4) Lowering the absolute amount of applied topical corticosteroid to once daily application and further dilution can reduce potential risks. (Devillers and Oranje 2006)

3.2 Dry wrap dressings

DWD occlusion in AD has been less well studied (Table 4). Specifically, Rajka et al. (1981) examined the effect of dry occlusion on skin microbial flora. Occlusion using plastic film was applied to 10 patients with AD. A significant increase in the density of *S. aureus* was observed after 24 hours of dry occlusion. Notably, 2 of the 10 patients had tiny pustules or crusts following dry occlusion. But, there were no reports of AD exacerbation. (Rajka et al. 1981)

Study Design	Results		Adverse Events		
	Response to therapy	Additional Information	Infection	Skin Atrophy	Systemic
Rajka et al., 1981 (Prospective)	N/A	No reports of AD exacerbation	Increased *S. aureus* density, 2/10 (20%) with pustules or crusts	N/A	N/A
Geraldez et al. 1989 (RCT)	Significantly greater improvement in pruritus and lichenifiction in non-occlusive control group		Control group: none reported, versus Treatment group: 2/30 (7%) with pustular lesions and 1/30 (3%) with erythema	N/A	N/A
Volden et al., 1992 (Prospective)	44/48 (92%) complete resolution, 4/48 (8%) partial remission (>50% clearance)	Instant relief from scratching	Mild folliculitus reported in 2/48 (4%) of adults.	None	N/A
Gauger et al., 2003 (Prospective)	Improved SCORAD, versus constant in control group		Decreased *S. aureus* density in silver-coated textile group, versus constant or increased in control group	N/A	N/A

Table 4. Outcomes of Studies on Dry Wrap Dressing Occlusion

Geraldez et al. (1989), in a randomized controlled study of 60 patients with lichen simplex chronicus, observed more infections and other adverse events in patients treated with diflucortolone valerate 0.3% ointment under occlusion as compared those treated without occlusion. Among the patients using dry occlusion, 2 patients (7%) developed pustular lesions surrounding the affected sites, one (3%) had erythema, and one (3%) had hyperpigmentation. None in the control group experienced any side effects. The control group also reported greater improvements in both pruritus and lichenication. The authors noted that the difference in the observed efficacy may be due to poorer absorption of the ointment that tended to adhere to the plastic occlusive material. Furthermore, the adverse events seen in the treatment group may have resulted from the combination of both the ointment vehicle and the nature of the plastic occlusive material that created an over-occlusive environment, thereby favoring microbial proliferation and/or contact sensitization. (Geraldez et al. 1989)

Volden et al. (1992) treated 48 patients with chronic, therapy-resistant AD, with once-weekly application of clobetasol propionate lotion under hydrocolloid (Duoderm®) occlusive dressings. Of the 48 patients, 44 (92%) had complete resolution of lesions, and 4 (8%) had partial response (defined as >50% clearance). There were also 2 (4%) patients with mild folliculitis. The authors conclude that adverse events were both mild and infrequent. (Volden 1992)

Gauger et al. (2003) further addressed the concern of skin colonization with *S. aureus* using occlusion therapy for AD. A side-to-side comparative study of 15 patients with generalized or localized AD was performed, in which the flexures of the elbows were covered with silver-coated textiles on one arm and cotton on the other arm for one week. The study found a significant decrease in *S. aureus* colonization on the lesions covered with silver-coated textile just 2 days after initiation of therapy and lasting until the end of the treatment. Additional, a significantly less amount of *S. aureus* was observed on the silver-coated textile sites than the cotton sites at the end of the treatment. Clinical improvement further correlated with the reduction of bacterial colonization. Thus, the silver-coated textile appeared to not only improve active lesions of AD, but also mitigate the potential pro-microbial effects of dry occlusion alone. (Gauger et al. 2003)

Ultimately, DWD occlusion appears to improve disease severity and is perhaps most beneficial in chronic treatment-resistant eczematous lesions. However, there is too little data to determine whether occlusion, in particular DWD occlusion, predisposes skin bacterial growth. But, it seems reasonable to conclude that the addition of antimicrobial topical agents (e.g. antiseptic or silver preparations) to occlusive therapy might be helpful in countering the potential risk of infection. (Abeck et al. 1999; Gauger 2006)

3.3 Hydrogel patch

In a pilot study of 15 patients, Park et al. (2011) evaluated the efficacy and safety of a hydrogel patch for AD treatment. The hydrogel patch used in this study was composed of an adhesive, thin, flexible, hydrogel layer on an impermeable urethane surface. Unlike hydrocolloid dressings (e.g. Duoderm®) with low water content, the hydrogel patch consisted of approximately 50% water. In this 6-week study, patients applied the hydrogel patch over one lesion for 6-8 hours daily and triamcinolone (TAC) 0.1% cream twice daily to another lesion. Erythema, induration, lichenification, excoriation, and total EASI scores significantly improved compared to baseline in both the hydrogel patch and TAC groups.

Improvement in pruritis was observed in both treatment groups, but was only statistically significant in the TAC group. At week 4, there was no significant difference in all sub-scores between the patch and TAC groups (except pruritus, as stated above). Improvement was maintained after discontinuing treatment for 2 weeks. No adverse events from steroid use occurred. This study appears to demonstrate that instant correction of the dysfunctional skin barrier with the hydrogel patch can improve signs and symptoms of AD comparable to TAC 0.1% cream. Thus, the hydrogel patch may provide a new approach to occlusive therapy without the potential risks of topical corticosteroid use (Park et al. 2011)

3.4 Cutaneous and systemic side effects

Topical corticosteroid use can cause both cutaneous and systemic side effects, most significantly laboratory adrenal insufficiency. Risk factors include the use of high potency corticosteroids, occlusive or prolonged therapy, and application to thin- or barrier-compromised skin lesions. (Levin and Maibach 2002) Occlusive therapy with topical corticosteroids does not appear to be associated with an increased incidence of local non-infectious side effects, such as skin atrophy and striae. This is most likely because nearly all studies have examined limited treatment durations and diluted topical corticosteroids. However, several studies demonstrated either lowering of morning cortisol levels (Hartmann and Lahmann 1977; Goodyear et al. 1991), loss of diurnal cortisol rhythm (Hartmann and Lahmann 1977), or overt laboratory HPA suppression with WWD (Wolkerstorfer et al. 2000; Devillers et al. 2002). Importantly, nearly all cases of decreased cortisol levels proved to be transient, returning to normal ranges within weeks of discontinuing therapy.

Specifically, Goodyear et al. (1991) found that 0900 hour cortisol levels were suppressed immediately after treatment with WWD, but returned to normal 2 weeks following therapy. Following this observation by Goodyear et al. (1991) of a transient lowering of morning cortisol levels (Goodyear et al. 1991), Wolkerstorfer et al. (2000) decided to examine the effects of different corticosteroid dilutions under WWD occlusion on HPA axis supression in children with severe refractory AD. Only 3 out of the 18 children in the first treatment group (i.e. 50% dilution of FP cream) and none of the 5 children in the second treatment group (i.e. 10%, 25% and 50% dilutions of FP cream) demonstrated HPA axis suppression based on 0900 hour serum cortisol measurements following 2 weeks of WWD occlusion. In the third treatment group (i.e. 0%, 5%, 10%, or 25% dilutions of FP cream applied to the whole body), children demonstrated HPA axis suppression based on 0600 hour serum cortisol measurements, which was associated with the absolute amount of applied corticosteroid. To be more specific, a dose-response relationship was observed with an absolute amount of topical corticosteroid applied. Patients using 800 μg m^{-2} daily (equivalent to 1.6 g FP 0.05% cream) had an approximately 80% improvement, while patients using absolute amounts >957 μg m^{-2} daily had no greater improvement. Patients using absolute amounts ≤800 μg m^{-2} daily had no suppression of the HPA axis. This suggests that weaker dilutions of topical corticosteroid may have a lower risk of HPA axis suppression, while still maintaining comparable efficacy to more potent dilutions of topical corticosteroid. (Wolkerstorfer et al. 2000)

Similarly, Devillers et al. (2002) found a significant decrease in early-morning serum cortisol levels following 1-week of inpatient WWD therapy. Transient cortisol levels below the normal range were observed after 4 days in 3 children and after one week in 2 adults. One adult, who also taking inhaled steroids, developed prolonged suppression of the HPA axis, in combination with several abdominal striae. (Devillers et al. 2002)

As for the effect of occlusive therapy using topical corticosteroids on bone development, McGowan et al. (2003) examined short-term growth and bone turnover in prepubertal children undergoing WWD occlusion for AD. Knemometry, a technique estimating the distance between the heel and knee of the sitting child, was used as a non-invasive measurement of lower leg length, in combination with 24-hour urinary deoxypyridinoline excretion to evaluate bone turnover. Lower leg length and urinary deoxypyridinoline levels for all children remained similar in pre-treatment measurements and during therapy. This suggests that WWD occlusion for a limited duration does not impact growth parameters. (McGowan et al. 2003)

4. Occlusion in clinical practice

Occlusive therapy, in particular WWD occlusion, can be useful as a 'stepped-up' therapy in controlling acute erythrodermic AD or as a second-line therapy for severe and/or refractory disease. There is limited convincing data that WWD occlusion is superior to conventional open application of topical corticosteroids. However, occlusive therapy represents an important alternative to currently available, but often undesirable standard treatment modalities for AD. A few drawbacks of standard therapies include dependency on super-potent topical corticosteroids, frequent and inconvenient sessions of phototherapy, and serious systemic side effects with oral medications (e.g. nephrotoxicity with cyclosporine use).

Based on the studies on occlusive therapy, it appears that the greatest benefits of topical corticosteroids under occlusion is achieved during the first week of therapy. This suggests that if used as 'rescue' therapy for acute flares or intermittently for maintenance, durations of up to 1 week might be adequate (Wolkerstorfer et al. 2000; Pei et al. 2001). Anecdotally, long-term effects are thought to be sustained when WWD occlusion are continued with emollients for 2-4 more weeks to improve skin hydration (Nicol 1987). Variations in protocol regarding duration of WWD occlusion and rewetting procedures possibly contributed to differences observed in efficacy and incidence of infection. It may, therefore, be advisable to limit occlusion to less than 8 hours duration, apply WWD no more than twice daily, and avoid rewetting procedures.

It is difficult to ascertain the extent to which occlusion may promote bacterial colonization. However, the use of anti-bacterial agents, when applied alone or under occlusion, appears to not only inhibit bacterial colonization, but also reduce disease severity. (Abeck et al. 1999; Brockow et al. 1999; Gauger 2006) Thus, it seems logical that antibacterials, whether topical or systemic, might be a beneficial adjunct to occlusive therapy helping to decrease the potential risk of clinical infection. As such, topical antibacterials in combination with topical corticosteroids under occlusion may be useful when treating small areas of skin for a limited period of time, while systemic antibacterials in combination with topical corticosteroid under occlusion may more be appropriate when treating larger areas of involvement. Yet, the use of antibacterials must be weighed against the potential risk of antimicrobial resistance and contact sensitization. (Williams 2000; Zhai and Maibach 2001)

More specifically, according to Williams (2000), there are three categories of patients with AD: 1) those with obvious clinical infection, in whom anti-staphylococcal therapy is essential, 2) those with mild disease and a lower density of S. aureus colonization, in whom no evidence supports additional benefit of anti-staphylococcal therapy, and 3) those with fissured or cracked eczema without overt signs of infection such as crusting or folliculitis. (Williams 2000) While the latter group of patients carry an intermediate to high levels of *S. aureus*, studies are contradictory regarding the clinical benefits of anti-staphylococcal therapy in these patients. Clinicians may choose to institute antimicrobial therapy, in combination with topical corticosteroids under occlusion. If poorly responsive to WWD occlusion, addition of corticosteroid with topical or oral antibiotics has been helpful anecdotally, suggesting that subclinical infection or heavy colonization may impede response to topical corticosteroids. (Nicol 1987) Despite half a century of topical corticosteroid use in eczematous skin, the clinical criteria for the addition of a topical antimicrobial agents remains to be determined.

In terms of the concern for adrenal suppression with topical corticosteroids under occlusion, the minimal available data suggests that a decrease in cortisol levels can occur, but these effects are generally transient. The use of mid- or high-potency corticosteroid, an ointment vehicle, occlusion, and a disrupted skin barrier are all contributing factors that can increase the risk of systemic side effects including this possibilty of adrenal suppression. Of note, there has been only one suggested fatal case of adrenal insuffiency from topical corticosteroid use. However, the details of this case are limited. It is known that the patient was an 11-year old girl with generalized psoriasis being treated with betamethasone cream under occlusion for a prolonged durations. However, the concentration and the exact quantity of betamethasone cream applied, as well as the duration of therapy are unknown. (Levin and Maibach 2002)

Several strategies may be used to limit the potential for such complications. Possible options include using occlusive therapy only intermittently, reducing topical corticosteroid potency gradually as inflamed skin improves, and applying occlusion only once-daily. Studies have demonstrated that twice-daily application of topical corticosteroids to be no more effective than once-daily regimens and more prone to systemic side effects. (Lagos and Maibach 1998; Green et al. 2005) In addition, diluting topical corticosteroids may be helpful in reducing the risk of serious side effects. However, such preparations may alter the physiochemical properties of the agent and may not serve to reduce disease activity. (Haigh and Smith 1991; Gao and Li Wan Po 1994; Ohtani et al. 2002; Kizu et al. 2004) Furthermore, the application of a hydrogel patch, which appeared to have similar efficacy as topical corticosteroid use, may potentially serve as an ideal method of treating AD while avoiding topical corticosteroids. (Park et al. 2011) But, additional studies on the efficacy of the hydrogel patch in the treatment of AD are needed. Ultimately, if prolonged topical corticosteroid use is required in certain patients with refractory disease, adrenal function may be monitored using morning plasma cortisol and urinary steroid levels, in combination with rapid ACTH stimulation testing, while evaluating the patient for cutaneous atrophy or Cushingoid features (Levin and Maibach 2002). But, the rare occurence of topical corticosteroid-induced Addison's disease makes this suggestion impractical for most patients.

Topical immunosuppressive agents such as pimecrolimus or tacrolimus under occlusion have not yet been studied extensively. These agents might represent a valuable non-steroidal alternative, though systemic absorption should be measured to confirm that immunosuppressive levels have not been reached. An open-label study evaluating topical pimecrolimus cream 1% in the treatment of chronic hand dermatitis showed that twice-daily application under occlusion was safe and effective, resulting in low pimecrolimus blood levels. (Thaci et al. 2003) Beyeler et al. (2006) reported a case of a female patient treated with tacrolimus 0.1% ointment under occlusion with Unna's paste boots (zinc bandages), whose serum levels had reached 12.9 μg/l after 5 days of treatment, corresponding to high-dose immunosuppression. Beyeler et al. (2006) attributed the increased systemic absorption to the combination of severely damaged skin barrier function, application of tacrolimus to a large surface area, and occlusion under zinc bandages. (Beyerler et al. 2006)

The wide variation in occlusive techniques and predominance of uncontrolled trials with small sample sizes make direct comparison of studies evaluating the safety and efficacy of occlusive therapy difficult. Limited numbers of studies using control groups restricts the conclusions that can be drawn regarding the benefit of occlusive therapy versus conventional therapies. However, it can be concluded that occlusive therapy has been shown, both formally and anecdotally, to be very effective in severe or exacerbated AD. It, therefore, offers an important alternative or adjunct therapy to more commonly used approaches. The randomized controlled trials described in this chapter resulted in divergent outcomes regarding infectious complications and efficacy. Differences could be related to the study populations (i.e. exacerbated versus moderate AD) or different topical corticosteroid application regimens.

While the exact mechanism of action of occlusive therapy is still unknown, a recent pilot study demonstrated significant down-regulation of 7 serum chemokines following WWD occlusion for 1 week in 6 children with severe AD. Of these, 4 chemokines are considered to be potential serum markers for the disease activity of AD. (Ong et al. 2008) In another study evaluating WWD occlusion using diluted tacrolimus and fluticasone propionate cream in APOC1 mice with AD, WWD occlusion improved transepidermal water loss, reinforcing that this may be one of the therapeutic aspects of occlusive therapy. (Oranje et al. 2009)

Future studies should evaluate the efficacy of occlusive therapy versus open topical corticosteroid application with measurements on the differences in systemic absorption. Studies should also investigate the impact of varying the durations of occlusive therapy. Given the number of protocols utilizing inpatient or specialized nurse-assisted visits, it would be useful to understand the contribution of professional supervised application. To our knowledge, no studies to date have evaluated occlusion as preventive therapy (i.e., to prevent disease flares and maintain cutaneous hydration).

5. Conclusion

WWD occlusion may be a reasonable first-line therapy for acute exacerbations of AD and second-line therapy for refractory disease. DWD occlusion appears to be efficacious having relatively low risk of infectious complications and may be particularly useful in treatment of chronic AD lesions. However, it remains unclear if occlusive therapy offers significant advantageous over conventional open therapy. The risk of infection associated with occlusive therapy, while greater than open therapies, seems to be manageable and may be mitigated by limiting the duration of occlusion, avoiding rewetting and perhaps adding antibacterial agents. Transient changes in morning cortisol levels and rare clinical HPA suppression seen with the use of topical corticosteroids under occlusion are concerning side effects, but are likely related to corticosteroid potency and the absolute amount applied. The hydrogel patch offers an innovative approach to the treatment of AD instantly correcting the barrier defect, and it may have similar efficacy as topical corticosteroids without the systemic risks. Further controlled studies are needed to better evaluate the risks and benefits of these occlusive modalities in the treatment of AD.

6. References

Abeck, D., K. Brockow, et al. (1999). Treatment of acute exacerbated atopic eczema with emollient-antiseptic preparations using the "wet wrap" ("wet pajama") technique. *Hautarzt*, 50(6): 418-421.

Aly, R., C. Shirley, et al. (1978). Effect of prolonged occlusion on the microbial flora, pH, carbon dioxide and transepidermal water loss on human skin. *J Invest Dermatol*, 71(6): 378-381.

Arikawa, J., M. Ishibashi, et al. (2002). Decreased levels of sphingosine, a natural antimicrobial agent, may be associated with vulnerability of the stratum corneum from patients with atopic dermatitis to colonization by Staphylococcus aureus. *J Invest Dermatol*, 119(2): 433-439.

Beattie, P. E. and M. S. Lewis-Jones (2004). A pilot study on the use of wet wraps in infants with moderate atopic eczema. *Clin Exp Dermatol*, 29(4): 348-353.

Beyerler, M., P. Schmid-Grendelmeier, et al. (2006). Significantly elevated systemic levels after occlusive application of topical tacrolimus in atopic dermatitis. *Dermatology*, 212(3): 260-261.

Bridgman, A. (1995). The use of wet wrap dressings for eczema. *Paediatr Nurs*, 7(2): 24-27.

Brockow, K., P. Grabenhorst, et al. (1999). Effect of gentian violet, corticosteroid and tar preparations in Staphylococcus-aureus-colonized atopic eczema. *Dermatology*, 199(3): 231-236.

Devillers, A. C., F. B. de Waard-van der Spek, et al. (2002). Treatment of refractory atopic dermatitis using 'wet-wrap' dressings and diluted corticosteroids: results of standardized treatment in both children and adults. *Dermatology*, 204(1): 50-55.

Devillers, A. C. and A. P. Oranje (2006). Efficacy and safety of 'wet-wrap' dressings as an intervention treatment in children with severe and/or refractory atopic dermatitis: a critical review of the literature. *Br J Dermatol*, 154(4): 579-585.

Foelster-Holst, R., F. Nagel, et al. (2006). Efficacy of crisis intervention treatment with topical corticosteroid prednicarbat with and without partial wet-wrap dressing in atopic dermatitis. *Dermatology*, 212(1): 66-69.

Gao, H. Y. and A. Li Wan Po (1994). Topical formulations of fluocinolone acetonide. Are creams, gels and ointments bioequivalent and does dilution affect activity? *Eur J Clin Pharmacol*, 46(1): 71-75.

Gauger, A. (2006). Silver-coated textiles in the therapy of atopic eczema. *Curr Probl Dermatol*, 33: 152-164.

Gauger, A., M. Mempel, et al. (2003). Silver-coated textiles reduce Staphylococcus aureus colonization in patients with atopic eczema. *Dermatology*, 207(1): 15-21.

Geraldez, M. C., M. Carreon-Gavino, et al. (1989). Diflucortolone valerate ointment with and without occlusion in lichen simplex chronicus. *Int J Dermatol*, 28(9): 603-604.

Goodyear, H. M., K. Spowart, et al. (1991). Wet-wrap' dressings for the treatment of atopic eczema in children. *Br J Dermatol*, 125(6): 604.

Green, C., J. L. Colquitt, et al. (2005). Topical corticosteroids for atopic eczema: clinical and cost effectiveness of once-daily vs. more frequent use. *Br J Dermatol*, 152(1): 130-141.

Haigh, J. M. and E. W. Smith (1991). Topical corticosteroid-induced skin blanching measurement: eye or instrument? *Arch Dermatol*, 127(7): 1065.

Hartmann, F. and J. J. Lahmann (1977). Effect of the external use of triamcinolone acetonide under foil occlussive dressings on the plasma cortisol level and on the diurnal rhythm of plasma cortisol. *Hautarzt*, 28(4): 198-202.

Hindley, D., G. Galloway, et al. (2006). A randomised study of "wet wraps" versus conventional treatment for atopic eczema. *Arch Dis Child*, 91(2): 164-168.

Hon, K. L., K. Y. Wong, et al. (2007). Efficacy and problems associated with using a wet-wrap garment for children with severe atopic dermatitis. *J Dermatolog Treat*, 18(5): 301-305.

Kizu, J., W. Ichihara, et al. (2004). Survey of mixing commercially available corticosteroid ointments with other ointments and the anti-inflammatory activity of the admixtures. *Yakugaku Zasshi*, 124(2): 93-97.

Krakowski, A. C., L. F. Eichenfield, et al. (2008). Management of atopic dermatitis in the pediatric population. *Pediatrics*, 122(4): 812-824.

Lagos, B. R. and H. I. Maibach (1998). Frequency of application of topical corticosteroids: an overview. *Br J Dermatol*, 139(5): 763-766.

Lee, J. H., S. J. Lee, et al. (2007). The effect of wet-wrap dressing on epidermal barrier in patients with atopic dermatitis. *J Eur Acad Dermatol Venereol*, 21(10): 1360-1368.

Levin, C. and H. I. Maibach (2002). Topical corticosteroid-induced adrenocortical insufficiency: clinical implications. *Am J Clin Dermatol*, 3(3): 141-147.

Mallon, E., S. Powell, et al. (1994). Wet wrap' dressings for the treatment of atopic ezcema in the community. *J Dermatolog Treat*, (5): 97-87.

McGowan, R., P. Tucker, et al. (2003). Short-term growth and bone turnover in children undergoing occlusive steroid ('Wet-Wrap') dressings for treatment of atopic eczema. *J Dermatolog Treat*, 14(3): 149-152.

Nicol, N. H. (1987). Atopic dermatitis: the (wet) wrap-up. *Am J Nurs*, 87(12): 1560-1563.

Ohtani, M., N. Yamada, et al. (2002). Effect of admixture of commercially available corticosteroid ointments and/or creams on vasoconstrictor activity. *Yakugaku Zasshi*, 122(1): 107-112.

Ong, P. Y., R. M. Ferdman, et al. (2008). Down-regulation of atopic dermatitis-associated serum chemokines by wet-wrap treatment: a pilot study. *Ann Allergy Asthma Immunol*, 100(3): 286-287.

Ong, P. Y., T. Ohtake, et al. (2002). Endogenous antimicrobial peptides and skin infections in atopic dermatitis. *N Engl J Med*, 347(15): 1151-1160.

Oranje, A. P., A. C. Devillers, et al. (2006). Treatment of patients with atopic dermatitis using wet-wrap dressings with diluted steroids and/or emollients. An expert panel's opinion and review of the literature. *J Eur Acad Dermatol Venereol*, 20(10): 1277-1286.

Oranje, A. P., R. Verbeek, et al. (2009). Wet-wrap treatment using dilutions of tacrolimus ointment and fluticasone propionate cream in human APOC1 (+/+) mice with atopic dermatitis. *Br J Dermatol*, 160(1): 54-61.

Page, B. (2005). The benefits of Tubifast Garments in the management of atopic eczema. *Br J Nurs*, 14(5): 289-290, 292.

Park, K., F. Kamangar, et al. (2011). Instant Barrier Repair: A Pilot Study Investigating Occlusion with a New Hydrogel Patch for the Treatment of Atopic Dermatitis. *J Dermatolog Treat*, Accepted for publication.

Pei, A. Y., H. H. Chan, et al. (2001). The effectiveness of wet wrap dressings using 0.1% mometasone furoate and 0.005% fluticasone proprionate ointments in the treatment of moderate to severe atopic dermatitis in children. *Pediatr Dermatol,* 18(4): 343-348.

Rajka, G., R. Aly, et al. (1981). The effect of short-term occlusion on the cutaneous flora in atopic dermatitis and psoriasis. *Acta Derm Venereol,* 61(2): 150-153.

Schnopp, C., C. Holtmann, et al. (2002). Topical steroids under wet-wrap dressings in atopic dermatitis--a vehicle-controlled trial. *Dermatology,* 204(1): 56-59.

Tang, W. Y. (2000). Diluted steroid facial wet wraps for childhood atopic eczema. *Dermatology,* 200(4): 338-339.

Thaci, D., K. Steinmeyer, et al. (2003). Occlusive treatment of chronic hand dermatitis with pimecrolimus cream 1% results in low systemic exposure, is well tolerated, safe, and effective. An open study. *Dermatology,* 207(1): 37-42.

Volden, G. (1992). Successful treatment of therapy-resistant atopic dermatitis with clobetasol propionate and a hydrocolloid occlusive dressing. *Acta Derm Venereol Suppl (Stockh),* 176: 126-128.

Williams, H. (2006). Wet wrap bandages for 4 weeks did not differ from topical ointments but increased skin infections in paediatric atopic eczema. *Evid Based Med,* 11(4): 108.

Williams, R. E. (2000). The antibacterial-corticosteroid combination. What is its role in atopic dermatitis? *Am J Clin Dermatol,* 1(4): 211-215.

Wolkerstorfer, A., R. L. Visser, et al. (2000). Efficacy and safety of wet-wrap dressings in children with severe atopic dermatitis: influence of corticosteroid dilution. *Br J Dermatol,* 143(5): 999-1004.

Zhai, H. and H. I. Maibach (2001). Effects of skin occlusion on percutaneous absorption: an overview. *Skin Pharmacol Appl Skin Physiol,* 14(1): 1-10.

19

Improvement of Atopic Dermatitis by Human Sebaceous Fatty Acids and Related Lipids

Hiroyuki Araki, Yoshiya Sugai and Hirofumi Takigawa
Tochigi Research Laboratories, Kao Corporation
Japan

1. Introduction

Our bodies are protected against a variety of external factors such as transient pathogens and can preserve homeostasis. This defense mechanism consists of many components, including antimicrobial lipids such as *cis*-6-hexadecenoic acid (C16:1Δ6) (Wille & Kydonieus, 2003) and sphingosine (Arikawa et al., 2002), as well as antimicrobial peptides such as β-defensins and cathelicidin (Harder et al., 2010; Hsu et al., 2009; Tay et al., 2011). The levels of these antimicrobial components in the skin of atopic dermatitis (AD) patients are lower than those of healthy subjects (Arikawa et al., 2002; Harder et al., 2010; Takigawa et al., 2005). It has been reported that the uncommon lipid C16:1Δ6 is present as a major component of sebaceous lipids in human skin and hair but that it is not generally included in plant or animal oils. We have focused on this very unique unsaturated fatty acid, and have been investigating the relationship between this fatty acid and the resident flora of human skin as well as transient pathogens. In the course of that research, we found a correlation between C16:1Δ6 and AD, and have developed a method for the production of C16:1Δ6 on an industrial-scale (Araki et al., 2007; Koike et al., 2000a, 2000b; Takeuchi et al., 1990). In addition, we have made further progress in antimicrobial research involving C16:1Δ6 (Araki et al., 2005) and have selected fatty acid derivatives (oxa-fatty acids) with higher activity by means of analyses of structure-activity relationships (Sugai et al., in preparation).
In this chapter, we introduce our research into fatty acids, and we also review approaches to normalizing AD from a microbiological point of view.

2. Function of human sebaceous fatty acid "C16:1Δ6"

Human skin lipids, including sphingosine and C16:1Δ6, provide a defense against external factors and function to maintain homeostasis. It is well established that human skin lipids contribute to the defense mechanism termed "self-sterilization" (Wille & Kydonieus, 2003) and the antimicrobial activities of each lipid component have been evaluated (Arikawa et al., 2002; Harder et al., 2010). A significant difference was found in the fatty acid composition of sebum lipids between AD patients and healthy controls (Takigawa et al., 2005). We describe the results of our investigation in the section below.

2.1 *Cis*-6-hexadecenoic acid (C16:1Δ6)

Cis-6-hexadecenoic acid, termed sapienic acid, is unique in the animal kingdom, being a 16-carbon mono-unsaturated fatty acid with a *cis*-double bond located at the sixth carbon from the carboxyl terminal (Fig. 1).

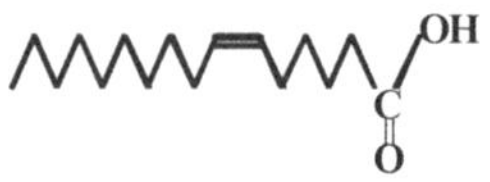

Fig. 1. Structure of *cis*-6-hexadecenoic acid (C16:1Δ6)

This fatty acid is an isomer of palmitoleic acid (*cis*-9-hexadecenoic acid (C16:1Δ9)), which is a common constituent of the glyceride of human adipose tissue. In addition, C16:1Δ6 is a major component of sebaceous wax esters, triacyl glycerols, and of free fatty acids found in skin and hair (Downing & Strauss, 1974; Morello & Downing 1976; Yamamoto et al., 1987). Sapienic acid represents 85% of the lipid in *Thunbergia alata* seed oil, and is obtained either by extraction of this plant or by chemical synthesis (Spencer et al., 1971).

2.2 Relationship between human sebaceous fatty acid C16:1Δ6 and AD

The composition of free fatty acids in the sebum at the recovery level is shown in Figure 2 (Takigawa et al., 2005). The level of C16:1Δ6 in healthy control skin ranged from 0.43 to 5.38 μg/cm² with a mean of 2.0 μg/cm² (4.9 to 16.8% with a mean of 12.9% in percent of total)

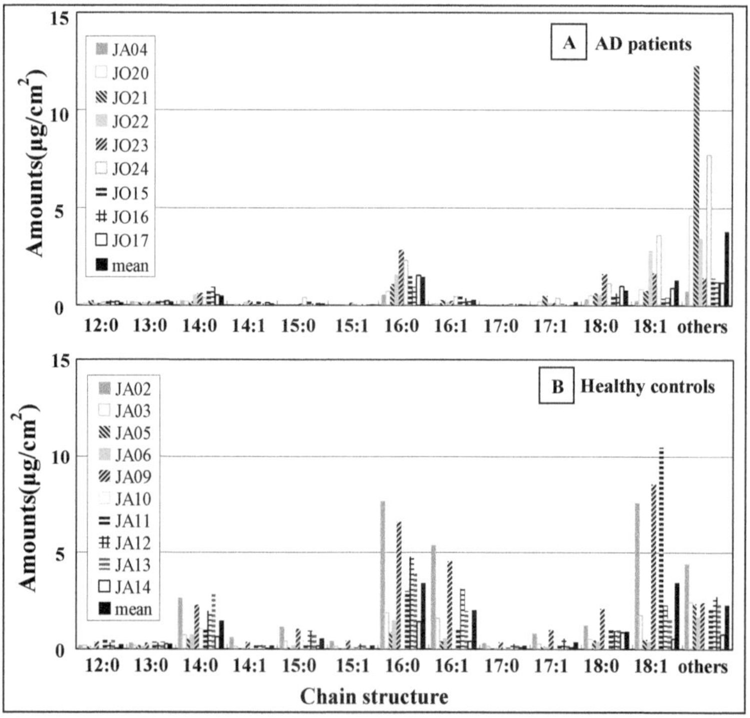

Fig. 2. Amount of free fatty acid in sebum from AD patients (upper panel) and from healthy controls (lower panel). Sebum was analyzed at the recovery level.

and the total level of C16:0 ranged from 0.88 to 7.64 μg/cm² with a mean of 3.43 μg/cm² (14.9 to 28.2% with a mean of 22.1% in percent of total). In contrast, the level of C16:1Δ6 (0.08 to 0.53 μg/cm² with a mean of 0.26 μg/cm²) and the percent of total (1.1 to 8.7% with a mean of 3.0% in percent of total) in the skin of AD patients were lower than in the healthy controls, although the amounts of C16:0 (0.53 to 2.84 μg/cm² with a mean of 1.44 μg/cm²) and the percent of total (6.8 to 30.7% with a mean of 16.5% in percent of total) were similar to those of the healthy controls. A significant decrease in free C16:1Δ6 content in nonlesional skin from AD patients compared with healthy controls was found.

2.3 Antibacterial activity of C16:1Δ6: Selective antibacterial activity

Colonization of *S. aureus* has been reported in AD patients and is regarded as an exacerbation factor (Akiyama et al., 1996). Antimicrobial agents, including C16:1Δ6, inhibited the growth of *S. aureus* at a final concentration of 100 mg/l in the following order; Benzalkonium chloride = Triclosan > C16:1Δ6 > Trichlorocarbanilide, while they inhibited the growth of *S. epidermidis* in the following order; Benzalkonium chloride = Triclosan> C16:1Δ6 = Trichlorocarbanilide (Fig. 3). Whereas C16:1Δ6 could inhibit the growth of *S. aureus* over a concentration range from 100 to 1000 ppm, it did not greatly inhibit *S. epidermidis*.

In addition, the antibacterial mechanism of C16:1Δ6 against *S. aureus* and *S. epidermidis* was investigated using protoplasts treated with lysostaphin. The results of this experiment indicated that there was no difference in the effectiveness of C16:1Δ6 against *S. aureus* and *S. epidermidis*, and suggested that the antibacterial action of C16:1Δ6 against Staphylococcal bacteria was caused by disruption of the cell membrane, not disruption of the cell wall, and that this disruption resulted in leakage of bacterial components (Data not shown).

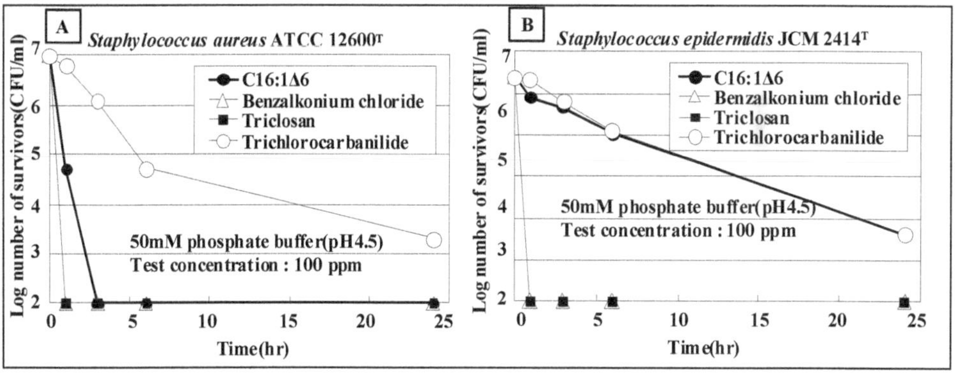

Fig. 3. Comparison of the antimicrobial effects of C16:1Δ6 against *Staphylococcus aureus* ATCC 12600T (left panel) and *Staphylococcus epidermidis* JCM 2414T (right panel).

2.4 Topical application of C16:1Δ6 to AD patients

An inverse correlation between *S. aureus* colonization and the level of C16:1Δ6 in AD patients was found (Fig. 4). In addition, the colonization of *S. aureus* was reduced by topical application of C16:1Δ6 to the skin of six to eight AD patients in a small-scale clinical study. Based on these investigations, it was considered that the decreased level of

C16:1Δ6 in AD patients may be one of the factors that contribute to the colonization of *S. aureus* (Takigawa et al., 2005).
We have confirmed that C16:1Δ6 functions as a natural antibacterial component and has very unique properties including "selective antibacterial activity", in which it shows effective antibacterial activity against transient *S. aureus* but not against residential *S. epidermidis*. By topical application of this fatty acid to AD patients, the colonization of *S. aureus*, which is believed to be an exacerbation factor for this disease, was repressed, thereby indicating the effectiveness of this fatty acid. From the results of these investigations, a new approach for improvement of skin disorders, based on normalization of the microflora on human skin, was proposed using the selective antibacterial activity of C16:1Δ6.

3. Proposed industrial production of C16:1Δ6 using a bioreactor

Microbial production of various materials has a number of advantages over chemical synthesis such as cost effectiveness, ease of production and regiospecific production. Considering the unique function of C16:1Δ6, and its potential therapeutic usefulness, we investigated the possibility of microbiologically producing C16:1Δ6.
There are many reports regarding microbial production of polyunsaturated fatty acids under simple and mild conditions. The production of γ-linoleic acid and arachidonic acid by species of the fungus *Mortierella* is a valuable product for many applications, and the triglyceride esters of poly unsaturated fatty acids that are produced in a fermentation process are used in skin care products (Certik & Shimizu, 1999a; Suzuki, 1987, 1988; Yamada et al., 1987) and baby formula (Certik & Shimizu, 1999b; Shinmen et al., 1989; Yamada, 1988). We isolated an alkane-assimilating *Rhodococcus* sp. strain from a soil sample and found that a mutant was capable of introducing a *cis*-double bond into various aliphatic substrates. We used this mutant for production of C16:1Δ6, investigated the production process, and further constructed a bioreactor system for its industrial production.

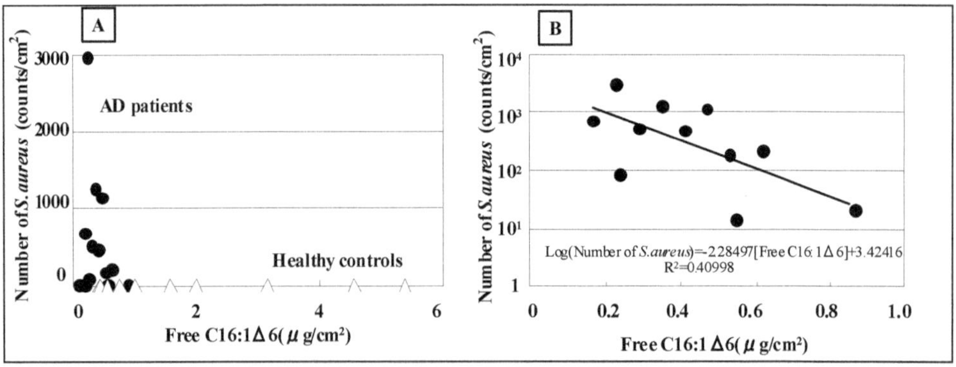

Fig. 4. Relationship between free C16:1Δ6 and *S. aureus* in the skin. A: in the skin of AD patients and Healthy Controls; B: in the skin of AD patients who exhibited more than 10 counts/cm² of *S. aureus*. AD patients; (•), Healthy Controls; (Δ)

3.1 Desaturation reaction of aliphatic substrates by a mutant strain of alkane-assimilating *Rhodococcus* sp.

We found that the double mutant designated *Rhodococcus* sp. KSM-MT66 had the ability to desaturate various aliphatic compounds such as alkanes, chloro alkanes and fatty acid esters, and that this mutant strain produced unsaturated compounds extracellularly. When hexadecanoic acid esters such as methyl, propyl, isopropyl, and isobutylester were supplied as substrates to the resting cells, their corresponding *cis*-desaturated compounds were produced at a concentration of 0.5, 20, 53 and 7 g/l in 3 days. The enzyme(s) responsible for the desaturation reaction appears to recognize mainly the sixth carbon from the carbonyl carbons (Fig. 5). The bioproduction of C16:1Δ6 esters has not been previously reported (Koike et al., 1999). When alkanes were supplied to this mutant strain, the main products had a double bond at the ninth carbon from the terminal methyl group. These experiments indicated that the unsaturated position differed according to differences in the supplied substrates (Koike et al., 2000a).

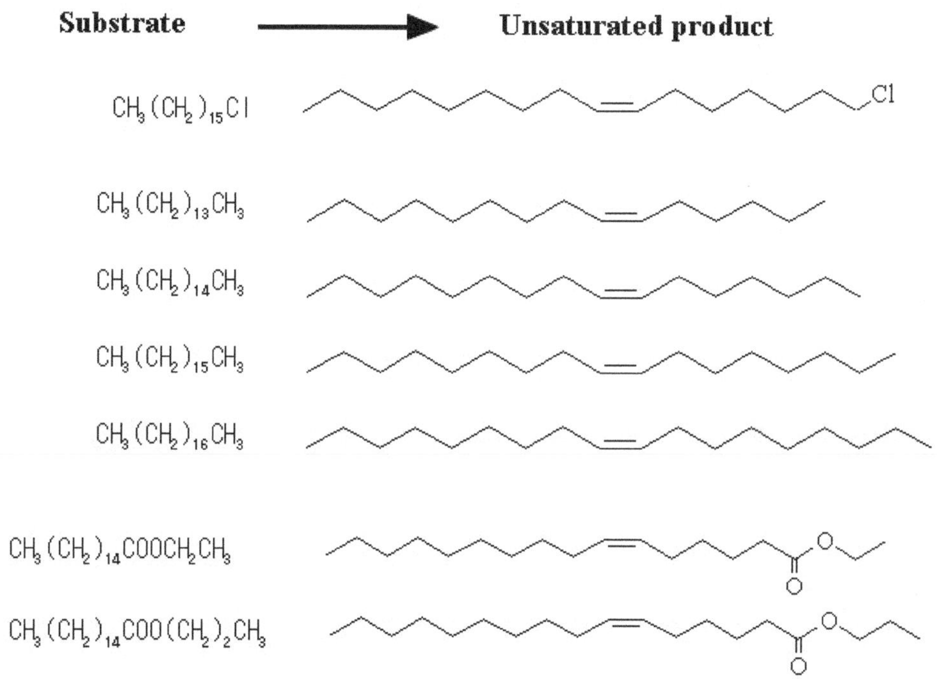

Fig. 5. The patterns of regiospecific desaturation of aliphatic substrates by *Rhodococcus* sp. strain KSM-MT66 cells.

3.2 Production of a C16:1Δ6 ester by resting cells of *Rhodococcus* sp. KSM-MT66

We determined the condition with resting cells of the *Rhodococcus* sp. KSM-MT66 strain to produce C16:1Δ6. The reaction mixture contained 20% (w/v) hexadecanoic acid isopropyl ester (IP-C16:0), 0.25 M phosphate buffer (pH 7.0), 1.0% (w/v) monosodium glutamate, 2 mM thiamine, 2 mM $MgSO_4$, and 5% (wet w/v) resting cells. Bioconversion was performed using a 1.0 l working volume in a 2.6 l bioreactor at 26 °C with aeration and agitation. Glutamate, thiamine, and $MgSO_4$ prevented cell damage of this strain during repeat-batch bioconversion, and optimum concentrations of these factors were maintained in the reaction mixture. Under optimum conditions, about 50 g/l of C16:1Δ6 isopropyl ester (IP-C16:1Δ6) was produced extracellularly in 3 days.

Since this reaction mixture consisted of water, oil and cells, we considered that this may make it difficult to separate the products. We therefore designed a new process to recover the products. Thus, the oil in water (O/W-type) emulsified reaction mixture was kept without agitation for 20 hours, the water layer was drained out, an appropriate volume of substrate, IP-C16:0, was added to the reaction mixture to invert the emulsion phase to a W/O-type, and the product, IP-C16:1Δ6, in the continuous oil phase was recovered through a hydrophobic hollow-fiber module (Fig. 6). The hydrophobic cells were concentrated in the oil phase. It was then possible to start the next batch by adding fresh medium to these cells (Koike et al., 2000b; Takeuchi et al., 1990). This system allows repeat-batch reactions without having to use an organic solvent to recover the products.

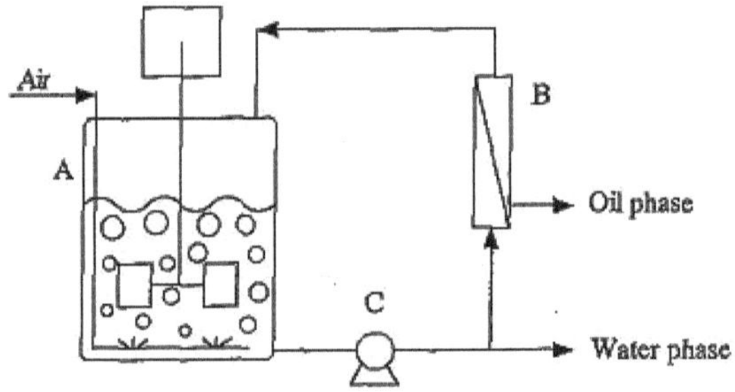

Fig. 6. Schematic diagram of the membrane bioreactor system for Rhodococcal bioconversion. (A) Reactor vessel; (B) Hydrophobic hollow-fiber module; (C) Circulation pump.

3.3 Repeat-batch production of the C16:1Δ6 ester

The reason for the decline in late production during repeat batch production may be due to various factors such as accumulation of some inhibitory products, cell damage and/or exhaustion of some nutrients. Since monosodium glutamate was found to reduce cell damage, we investigated the effect of monitoring and adjusting the concentration of monosodium glutamate on productivity during repeat batch production (see sec. 3-2). The results of this experiment showed that a productivity of 0.8 g/l was attained over the course of 13 cycles (300 hours) by maintaining the concentration of monosodium glutamate between 0.5 and 1.5% (Fig. 7). It was possible to recover the produced IP-C16:1Δ6 using the hollow-fiber system, and IP-C16:1Δ6 was then purified by urea adduct treatment, evaporated and applied to a silica gel column. The total yield of IP-C16:1Δ6 using this procedure was 79% and the purity was over 97%. Long term operation of C16:1Δ6 ester production was achieved using a 2.6 l fermentor (Koike et al., 2000b).

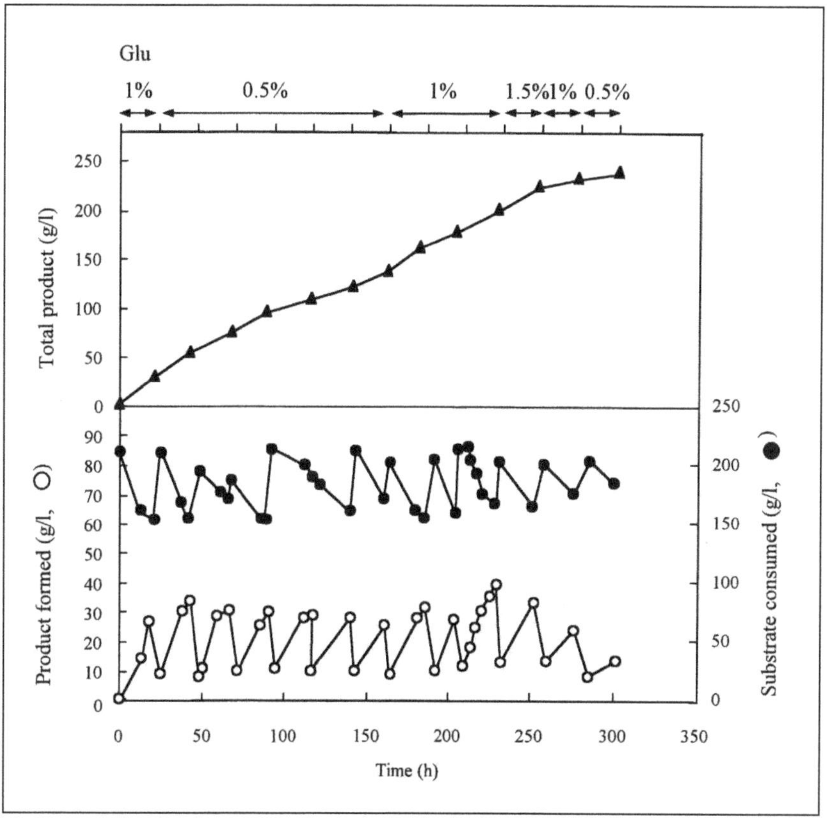

Fig. 7. Repeat-batch reaction using a membrane bioreactor system with a phase inversion for the production of IP-C16:1Δ6 by the resting cells of *Rhodococcus* sp. KSM-MT66.

3.4 Fermentative production of IP-C16:1Δ6 using growing cells of the mutant *Rhodococcus* sp. KSM-MT66

The resting cell production of IP-C16:1Δ6 described above includes four complicated steps; (i) cell growth, (ii) cell harvesting, (iii) incubation of cells with substrate and (iv) phase-inversed separation of the product using a hydrophobic fiber membrane system.

In order to develop a more convenient production process we therefore investigated production of IP-C16:1Δ6 using a fermentation process. We first established a basal medium for *Rhodococcus* sp. KSM-MT66. When production was performed under resting cell conditions, 18 g/l of IP-C16:1Δ6 was produced over 3 days of cultivation. Optimization of the concentrations of metal ions greatly improved production of IP-C16:1Δ6, resulting in production of 52 g/l over 4 days of cultivation (see sec. 3.5).

3.5 Fermentative production of IP-C16:1Δ6 using the mutant *Rhodococcus* sp. KSM-T64

Since there was a possibility that the IP-C16:1Δ6 product might be degraded by esterases present in the *Rhodococcus* sp. KSM-MT66, we attempted to create *Rhodococcus* mutants with reduced esterase activity by UV irradiation. Of the colonies which showed lower growth than KSM-MT66 on the minimum agar containing IP-C16:0, one mutant, designated KSM-T64, displayed 40% of the esterase activity of KSM-MT66.

Using this mutant strain T64, and optimizing culture conditions, more than 60 g/l of IP-C16:1Δ6 could be produced in a flask (Table 1). Optimization of culture conditions in a 30 l jar fermentor, resulted in production of 50 g/l over 4 days of cultivation (Fig. 8). Furthermore, C16:1Δ6 can be easily obtained by simple hydrolysis of IP-C16:1Δ6 (Araki et al., 2007).

Reaction condition			KSM- MT66	KSM-T64
Reaction process			Resting	Growing
Reaction ingredient	Monosodium glutamate		1.0%	2.0%
	Metal	$MgSO_4 \cdot 7H_2O$	2 mM	2 mM
		$MnSO_4 \cdot 6H_2O$	-[a]	2 μM
		$FeSO_4 \cdot 7H_2O$	-	60 μM
		$CuSO_4 \cdot 5H_2O$	-	5 μM
		$ZnSO_4 \cdot 7H_2O$	-	-
	Thiamine		2 mM	-
	Yeast extract (P-21)		-	0.8%
	Phosphate buffer		250 mM	350 mM
			pH 7	pH 7.3
	IP-C16:0		20%	22%
IP-C16:1 productivity			50 g l^{-1}	61 g l^{-1}

a Not added.

Table 1. Production of IP-C16:1Δ6 by *Rhodococcus* sp. KSM-MT66 and KSM-T64.

4. The production of C16:1Δ6 by genetically modified bacteria: Cloning and expression of two novel desaturases from *Rhodococcus* sp.

4.1 Review of desaturase studies

An enzyme that removes hydrogen atoms from a fatty acid derivative, thereby creating a double bond, is called a desaturase, and desaturases are key enzymes for the maintenance of cell life cycles. Desaturases are divided into three types based on substrate specificity; acyl-CoA, acyl-ACP, and acyl-lipid types (Fox et al., 2004). Desaturases are further sub-divided into membrane-bound and soluble types. Membrane-bound enzymes are very unstable and are known to be very difficult to purify. However, recently a very interesting report has been published regarding the purification of human stearoyl-CoA desaturase (Gorden & Fox, 2008). In contrast, there have been some reports regarding the purification and clarification of the crystal structure of the soluble types of enzymes (Lindqvist et al., 1996).

Delta 6-desaturases have been reported to be obtained from animals, plants, fungi and cyanobacteria (Aki et al., 1999; Cahoon et al., 1994; Inagaki et al., 2003; Okayasu et al., 1981; Reddy & Thomas, 1996; Zhan et al., 2004). Human and rat fatty acid desaturase 2 (FADS2) -encoding delta 6-desaturases recognize a saturated fatty acid as a substrate under some conditions (Ge et al., 2003; Guillou et al., 2003), and a human delta 6-desaturase gene has been reported to be expressed only in the sebaceous gland. Regarding microbial delta 6-desaturases, industrial producers of unsaturated fatty acids have focused mainly on fungi of the *Mortierella* spp., especially *Mortierella alpina* and *Mortierella cincinelloides*. Two types of delta 6-desaturases have been reported to be expressed by *Mortierella alpina*. The corresponding genes were isolated and the sequences and functions of these genes have been analyzed (Huang et al., 1999; Sakuradani et al., 1999; Sakuradani & Shimizu, 2003). However, even though many delta 6-desaturase genes have been obtained, no delta 6-desaturase genes have been purified from *Rhodococcus* sp.
We aimed to obtain delta 6-desaturase genes from the *Rhodococcus* sp. KSM-T64 strain, which shows 40% of the esterase activity of the parent strain, KSM-MT66.

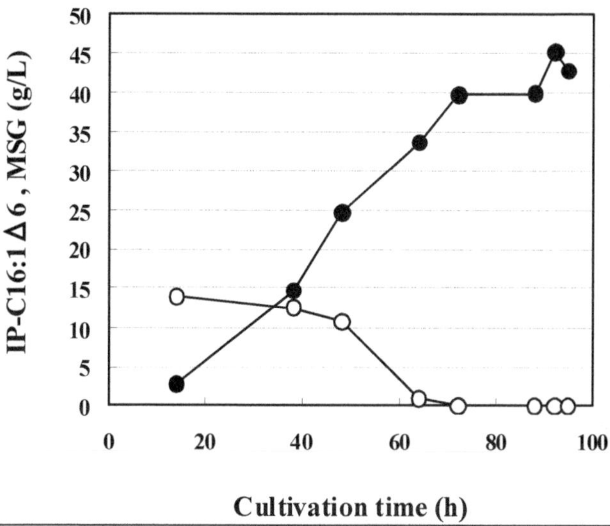

Fig. 8. Production of IP-C16:1Δ6 in a 30 l-jar fermentor under optimized conditions.

IP-C16:1Δ6 (•), monosodium glutamate (MSG) (○). Cultivation was performed at 26 °C, with agitation at 350 rpm, aeration at 0.3 vvm and pressure at 0.2 kg/cm^2. The *Rhodococcus* sp. KSM-T64 was used.

4.2 Cloning of delta 6-desaturase genes from the *Rhodococcus* sp. KSM-T64 strain

The production of IP-C16:1Δ6 by *Rhodococcus* sp. was improved by the addition of metal ions as mentioned above. We therefore targeted the membrane-bound delta 6-desaturase and attempted to clone a gene whose encoded protein could introduce a *cis*-double bond. We cloned the delta 6-desaturase gene on the basis of previously reported conserved sequences. Histidine motifs (Shanklin & Fox, 1994; Shanklin, 2009) that bind to ferric ions and whose sequences are known to be conserved in membrane-bound desaturases in a number of species including worms, borages, *Mucor* sp. and *Mortierella* sp., were targeted for primer design for PCR amplification (Fig. 9). These primers were used for degenerated PCR and nested PCR. In addition, inverse PCR was performed using the obtained PCR products. Approximately 5.5 kbp of sequence was obtained using these methods. Within this sequence, there were sequences that corresponded to two tandem desaturase-like proteins; the first ORF (Rdes1) was comprised of 420 amino acids and the second ORF (Rdes2) was comprised of 413 amino acids from inffered start codons individually. The estimated molecular mass of the Rdes1 protein was 47985 Da and that of Rdes2 was 46951 Da. Three histidine motifs that are established consensus sequences in desaturase proteins were found in these ORF sequences (Fig. 10).

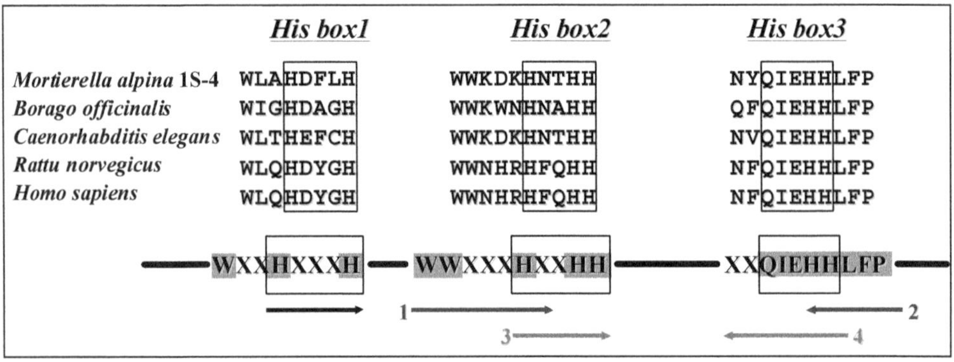

Fig. 9. Construction of PCR primers based on the histidine motifs that are conserved among delta 6-desaturases obtained from various organisms.
The sequence of primers 1, 2, 3, and 4 was; 5′-YTGGTGGAAGGRYAABCAYAA-3′, 5′-RGGGAAVARRTGGTG-3′, 5′-CAYAAYNMDCAYCA-3′, and 5′-RGGGAAVARRTGGTG-3′ respectively. Y, R, B, N, M, D, V, and W were mixed primers of C/T, AA/G, C/T/G, A/C/G/T, A/C, A/G, A/C/G and A/T respectively.

Among the membrane-bound delta 6-desaturases which were clarified the function except for putative and probable delta 6-desaturases, Rdes1 and Rdes2 had about 30% to *Homo sapiens* as an amino acid sequence. An unknown ORF whose function has not yet been clarified is present upstream of these two delta 6-desaturase genes. A domain search revealed that this ORF had an oxidoreductase NAD-binding domain, an oxidoreductase FAD-binding domain, a 2Fe-2S iron-sulfur cluster domain and a ferric reductase domain (data not shown).

4.3 Expression of delta 6-desaturase genes in *Escherichia coli*

Plasmids incorporating the delta 6-desaturase genes Rdes1 and Rdes2 were individually introduced into competent *E. coli* BL21 (DE3) cells, and the corresponding proteins were produced by IPTG induction. Production of very high amounts of these proteins was confirmed using SDS-PAGE. The molecular mass of each of these expressed proteins was 45 kDa. These proteins were identified by comparison with a control cell lysate which was prepared from cells transformed with vector alone.

Fatty acids extracted from *E.coli* transformants that expressed Rdes1 and Rdes2 were analyzed using GC and GC/MS. The level of C16:1Δ6 was increased 2.5-fold in the Rdes1-expressing transformant and 4.8-fold in the Rdes2-expressing transformant, over that of control.

Although the level of C16:1Δ6 fatty acids in the transformants was higher than that of control, it was unclear if these delta 6-desaturase genes of the *Rhodococcus* sp. produced extracellular IP-C16:1Δ6 or not (Araki et al., 2005).

```
ORF1(mature)   1:VAITDIKEFSHLTEADVEALGRELDQIRLDIEDSRGIRDARYIRRVIRVQRALELGGRIA 60
ORF2(mature)   1:MAIADVKEYAHLTDADIEALGRELDAIRRDIEESRGEKDARYVRNVIRLQRSLEIGGRAV 60
                  ** * **  *** ** ******** ** *** ***  **** * *** ** ** ***

ORF1(mature)  61:LFGSRYRPAWLVGTTLLSLSKIIENMELGHNVMHGQWDWMNDPEIHSVSWEWDQTGPSEH 120
ORF2(mature)  61:LFASRRRPAWLAGVGLLTLSKIIENMELGHNVMHGQWDWMNDPEIHSTSWEWDVTGPSAH 120
                 ** ** ***** *  ** ***************************** ***** **** *
                                             His box1
ORF1(mature) 121:WKRAHNYQHHTYTNVVGMDEDLGFGILRMTRDEPWKPINLFQPIANVILAATFEWGIALH 180
ORF2(mature) 121:WKQTHNYLHHKYTNVLGMDDDVGYGLLRVTRDQRWKPFNAGNLVYNTLLALFFEYGIAAQ 180
                 **  *** ** **** *** * * * ** ***  *** *      *  **  ** ***
                    His box2
ORF1(mature) 181:DLTAAAELEGAE-KGQLNSQANKDFARKIFRQVGKDFILFPALTGPAWKSTMSANATANL 239
ORF2(mature) 181:HLELGKVAKGRADKEETQRKLRE-VGEKIGKQVLRDYVIYPAITGPAWKSTLSANFTANT 239
                  *       *   *             **  **  *    ** ******** *** ***

ORF1(mature) 240:VRNLWAYVVIFCGHFPDGAEKFTVAEFEQETRHEWYLRQMLGSANFNSGKLMGLMSGNLS 299
ORF2(mature) 240:LRNVWTNAVIFCGHFPDGAEKFTKEDIDKETQAQWYLRQMLGSANIEGSALMDFMTGNLS 299
                  ** *   ***************      **   ***********     **  * ****

ORF1(mature) 300:YQIEHHVFPDLPSNRYPEIAVKMRALCEKFDLPYTTGSLFKQYLLALRTIHKLALPDKWL 359
ORF2(mature) 300:YQIEHHLFPDLPSNRYKDIAVTVRQLADKYDLPYTTGPLAVQYAKSWRTIAKLSLPNKYL 359
                 ****** *********  ***  * *  * ******* *  **    *** ** ** * *
                 His box3
ORF1(mature) 360:TATSDNAPETSSELRFRDSGFRDAAMAMVEDLRTDPITGKRLGLLTALKSQARS---R-- 414
ORF2(mature) 360:KDTVDNAPETASERMFD------GELTS--TV--DPVTGRRSGLKSAIARKRKSGKLRSL 409
                   * ****** **  *                  ** ** * **  *      *   *

ORF1(mature) 415:MPKRRK                                                       420
ORF2(mature) 410:LGLR--                                                       413
                    *
```

Fig. 10. Sequence homology of the proteins encoded by Rdes1 (ORF1) and Rdes2 (ORF2).

The homology search was performed using Genetyx Win ver.6.1. The gap penalty score was set at -10 as an insert and -3 as an extend. The three histidine rich regions (Histidine motifs) that are conserved in membrane binding desaturases are boxed.

5. Further investigation of human sebaceous fatty acids combined with chemical synthesis: Structure-activity relationship of oxa-fatty acids

C16:1Δ6 has a double bond and, consequently, its stability is a concern, which raises doubts regarding adequate stability of C16:1Δ6 in products. The stability of C16:1Δ6 can be improved by replacing the unsaturated fatty acids with the corresponding oxa-fatty acids (Alkoxy fatty acids). Such a change would also be expected to lead to an improvement in antimicrobial properties of the fatty acid. We describe the results of our investigations regarding such a replacement in the section below.

5.1 Review of the antimicrobial activities of oxa-fatty acids

Although oxa-fatty acids are widely used as intermediate chemicals in fine chemical fields such as medicine, agriculture and fragrance, there have only been a few reports of the antimicrobial activity of oxa-fatty acids. N-alkoxyacetic acid and its methyl ester showed good antifungal activity against *Aspergillus niger, Myrothecium verrucaria,* and *Trichoderma viride* (Gershon et al., 1979). In addition, 4-oxatetradecanoic acid, which is an inducer of myristic acid β-oxidation, displayed antifungal activity against *Cryptococcus neoformans* and also antiviral activity against human immunodeficiency virus I (Langner et al., 1992). These studies indicate that oxa-fatty acids of C16:1Δ6, in which the double bond has been replaced with an ether bond (7-oxaheptadecanoic acid or 6-decyloxy hexanoic acid), will maintain their antibacterial activity and will also have a novel function, that is antifungal activity.

5.2 Synthesis and evaluation of a C16 oxa-fatty acid

An oxygen-containing analog of C16:1Δ6 (oxa-fatty acid:7-oxaheptadecanoic acid) was synthesized by condensation of *n*-decanol with 6-bromo-hexanoic acid under alkaline conditions. The antimicrobial activities of purified 7-oxaheptadecanoic acid were then compared with those of C16:1Δ6. The oxa-fatty acid analog of C16:1Δ6, 7-oxaheptadecanoic acid, retained the selective antimicrobial activity of C16:1Δ6, being effective against *S. aureus* but not against *S. epidermidis* (Fig. 11), and, displayed similar activity to C16:1Δ6 against *Propinibacterium acnes*, which is associated with AD (Ishibashi et al., 2009). In addition, 7-oxaheptadecanoic acid had gained an additional anti-yeast activity against *Malassezia*, which is associated with skin disorders such as seborrhea dermatitis and AD (Tajima et al., 2008). Moreover, the best molecule for treatment of skin disorders such as seborrhea dermatitis and AD could be selected by means of structure-activity relationships (Sugai et al., in preparation).

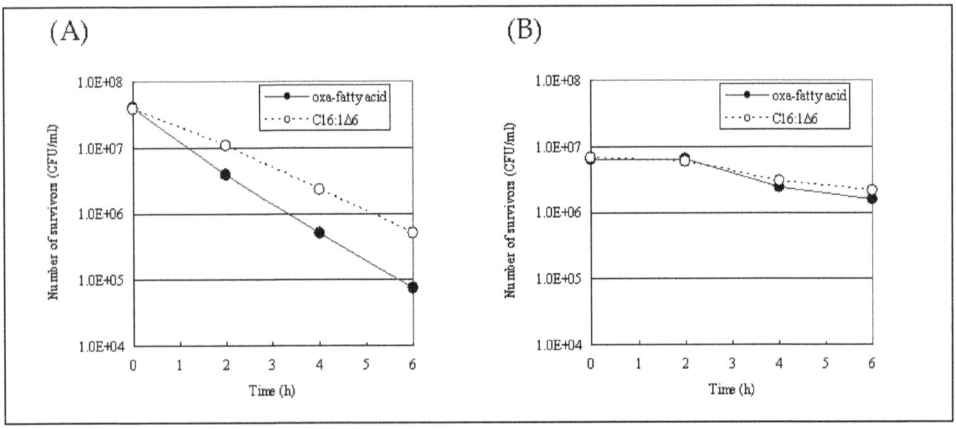

Fig. 11. Antibacterial activity of 7-oxaheptadecanoic acid. A: *S. aureus*; B: *S. epidermidis*

6. Conclusion

We found that *cis*-6-hexadecenoic acid (C16:1Δ6) displayed a selective antimicrobial activity that was unique among human sebaceous lipids. It was suggested that topical application of C16:1Δ6 to the skin of AD patients, who have lower levels of C16:1Δ6 in skin lipids than healthy controls, was effective for treatment of this skin condition. We proposed an industrial process for the production of C16:1Δ6 using *Rhodococcus* sp. An oxygen-containing analog of C16:1Δ6 (7-oxaheptadecanoic acid) was found to be more effective against microorganisms such as *S.aureus* and *Malassezia* sp. that are associated with skin disorders. It was proposed that the best oxa-fatty acid derivative of C16:1Δ6 could be selected by analysis of structure-activity relationships.

7. References

Aki, T., Inagai, K., Higashimoto, H., Kawamoto, S., Shigeta, S., Ono, K., & Suzuki, O. (1999). Molecular cloning and functional characterization of rat delta-6 fatty acid desaturase, Biochem. Biophys. Res. Commun., 255, pp. 575-579

Akiyama, H., Ueda, M., Toi, Y., Kanzeki, H., Tada, J., & Arata, J. (1996). Comparison of the severity of atopic dermatitis lesions and the density of *Staphylocossus aureus* on the lesions after antistaphylococcus treatment, J. Infect. Chemother., 2, pp. 70

Araki, H. (2005). Gene cloning novel two delta 6-fatty acid desaturases from *Rhodococcus* strain, Annual meeting of Japan Society for Bioscience, Biotechnology, and Agrochemistry, Sapporo, Japan

Araki H., Hagihara H., Takigawa H., Kotan i N., Tujino Y., Koike K., Kawai S., Ozaki K., & Ito S. (2007). Hyperproduction of sebaceous *cis*-6-hexadecenoic acid by esterase-reduced mutant of *Rhodococcus* sp. strain, J. Biosci. Bioeng., 104, 4, pp. 300-303

Arikawa, J., Ishibashi, M., Kawashima, M., Takagi, Y., Ichikawa, Y., & Imokawa, G. (2002). Decrease levels of sphingosine, a natural antimicrobial agent, may be associated with vulnerability of the stratum corneum from patients with atopic dermatitis to colonization by *Staphylococcus aureus*, J. Invest. Dermatol., 119, pp. 433-39

Cahoon, E. B., Cranmer, A. M., Shanklin, J., & Ohlrogge, J. B. (1994). Delta 6 hexadecenoic acid is synthesized by the activity of a soluble delta 6 palmitoyl-acyl carrier protein desaturase in *Thunbergia alata* endosperm, J. Biol. Chem., 269, pp. 27519-27526

Certik, M. & Shimizu, S. (1999a). Biosynthesis and regulation of microbial polyunsaturated fatty acid production, J. Biosci. Bioeng., 87, pp. 1-14

Certik, M. & Shimizu, S. (1999b). Production and application of single cell oils, Agro. Food Ind. Hi-Technol., 10, pp. 26-32

Fox, B. G., Lyle, K. S., & Rogge, C. E. (2004). Reactions of the diiron enzyme stearoyl-acyl carrier protein desaturase, Acc. Chem. Res., 37, pp. 421-429

Ge, L., Gordon, J. S., Hsuan, C., Stenn, K., & Prouty, S. M. (2003). Identification of the delta-6 desaturase of human sebaceous glands: expression and enzyme activity, J. Invest. dermatol., 120, pp. 707-714

Gershon, H., Shanks, L., & DeAngelis, A. (1979). Antifungal properties of n-alkoxyacetic acids and their methyl esters, J. Pharm. Sci., 68, pp. 82-84

Gorden, M. A., & Fox, B. G. (2008). Wheat germ cell-free translation, purification, and assembly of a functional human stearoyl-CoA desaturase complex, Protein Expression Purif., 62, pp. 171-178

Guillou, H., Rioux, V., Catheline, D., Thibault, J. N., Bouriel, M., Jan, S., D'Andrea, S., & Legrand, P. (2003). Conversion of hexadecanoic acid to hexadecenoic acid by rat Delta 6-desaturase, J. Lipid Res., 44, pp. 450-454

Harder, J., Dressel, S., Wittersheim, M., Cordes, J., Meyer-Hoffert, U., Mrowietz, U., Főlster-Holst, U., Proksch, E., Schröder, J. M., Schwarz, T., & Gläser, R. (2010). Enhanced expression and secretion of antimicrobial peptides in atopic dermatitis and after superficial skin injury, J. Invest. Dermatol., 130, pp. 1355-1364

Hsu, K. H., Pei, C., Yeh, J. Y., Shih, C. H., Chung, Y. C., Hung, L. T., & Ou, B. R. (2009). Production of bioactive human alpha-defensin 5 in *Pichia pastoris*, J. Gen. Appl. Microbiol., 55, pp. 395-401

Huang, Y. S., Chaudhary, S., Thurmond, J. M., Bobik, E. G. Jr., Yuan, L., Chan, G. M., Kichner, S. J., Mukerji, P., & Knutzon, D. S. (1999). Cloning of delta12- and delta6-desaturases from *Mortierella alpina* and recombinant production of gamma-linolenic acid in *Saccharomyces cerevisiae*, Lipids, 34, pp. 649-659

Inagaki, K., Aki, T., Shiota, T., Kawamoto, S., Shigeta, S., Suzuki, O., & Ono, K. (2003). Evidence of isozymes for delta6 fatty acid desaturase in rat hepatocytes, Biosci. Biotechnol. Biochem., 67, pp. 451-454

Ishibashi, Y., Katoh, H, Asahi Y., Sugita, T., Nishikawa, A. (2009). Identification of the major allergen of *Malassezia globosa* relevant for atopic dermatitis, J. Dermatol. Sci., 55, pp. 185-192

Koike, K., Ara, K., Adachi, S., Takigawa, H., Mori, H., Inoue, S., Kimura, Y., & Ito, S. (1999). Regiospecific internal desaturation of aliphatic compounds by a mutant *Rhodococcus* strain, Appl. Environ. Microbiol., 65, pp. 5636-5638

Koike, K., Takaiwa, M., Ara, K., Inoue, S., Kimura, Y., & Ito, S. (2000a). Production of isopropyl *cis*-6-hexadecenoate by regiospecific desaturation of isopropyl palmitate by a double mutant of a *Rhodococcus* strain, Biosci. Biotechnol. Biochem., 64, 399-404

Koike, K., Takeuchi, K., Mino, H., Takaiwa, M., Tohoh, T., Tadokoro, T., Tsutoh, K., & Ito, S. (2000b). A repeat-batch membrane bioreactor with a phase inversion for desaturation of isopropyl palmitate by a mutant *Rhodococcus* strain, J. Biotechnol., 80, pp. 101-107

Langner, C. A., Lodge, J. K., Travis, S. J., Caldwell, J. E., Lu, T., Li, Q., Bryant, M. L., Devadas, B., Gokel, G. W., Kobayashi, G. S., & Gordon, J. I. (1992). 4-oxatetradecanoic acid is fungicidal for *Cryptococcus neoformans* and inhibits replication of human immunodeficiency virus I, J. Biol. Chem., 267(24), pp. 17159-17169

Lindqvist, Y., Huang, W., Schneider, G., & Shanklin, J. (1996). Crystal structure of delta9 stearoyl-acyl carrier protein desaturase from castor seed and its relationship to other di-iron proteins, EMBO J., 15, pp. 4081-4092

Okayasu, T., Nagao, M., Ishibashi, T., & Imai, Y. (1981). Purification and partial characterization of linoleoyl-CoA deaturase from rat liver microsomes, Arch. Biochem. Biophys., 206, pp. 21-28

Reddy, A. S., & Thomas, T. L. (1996). Expression of a cyanobacterial delta 6-desaturase gene results in gamma-linolenic acid production in transgenic plants, Nat. Biotechnol., 14, pp. 639-642

Sakuradani, E., Kobayashi, M., & Shimizu, S. (1999). Delta6-fatty acid desaturase from an arachidonic acid-producing *Mortierella* fungus, Gene, 238, pp. 445-453

Sakuradani, E., & Shimizu, S. (2003). Gene cloning and functional analysis of a second delta 6-fatty acid desaturase from an arachidonic acid-producing *Mortierella* fungus, Biosci. Biotechnol. Biochem., 67, pp. 704-711

Shanklin, J., Whittle, E., & Fox, B. G. (1994). Eight histidine residues are catalitically essential in a membrane-associated iron enzyme, stearoyl-CoA desaturase, and are conserved in alkane hydroxylase and xylene monooxygenase, Biochemistry, 33, pp. 12787-12794

Shanklin, J., Guy, J. E., Mishra, G., & Lindqvist, Y. (2009). Desaturase: Emerging models for understanding functional diversification of diiron-containing enzymes, J. Biol. Chem., 284, pp. 18559-18563

Shinmen, Y., Shimizu, S., Akimoto, K., Kawashima, H., & Yamada, H. (1989). Production of arachidonic acid by *Mortierella* fungi, Appl. Microbiol. Biotechnol., 31, 11-16

Spencer, G. F., Kleiman, R., Miller R. W., & Earle, F. R. (1971). Occurrence of *cis*-6-hexadecenoic acid as the major component of *Thunbergia alata* seed oil, Lipids, 6, pp. 712-714

Sugai, Y., et al., In preparation.

Suzuki, O. (1987). Production of gamma-linoleic acid by fungi and its industrialization. Proceeding of world conference on biotechnology for the fats and oils industry, AOCS., pp. 110-116

Suzuki, O. (1988). Production of γ-linoleic acid by fungi and its industrialization, p. 110-116. In Applewhite, T. H. (ed.), Proceedings of World Conference on Biotechnology for the Fats and Oils Industry, Hamburg, Germany, 1987. American Oil Chemists' Society, Champaign

Tajima, M., Sugita, T., Nishikawa, A., Tsuboi, R. (2008). Molecular analysis of *Malassezia* microflora in seborrheic dermatitis patients: Comparison with other diseases and healthy subjects, J. Invest. Dermatol., 128, pp. 345-351

Takeuchi, K., Koike, K., & Ito, S. (1990). Production of *cis*-unsaturated hydrocarbons by a strain of *Rhodococcus* in repeated batch culture with a phase-inversion, hollow-fiber, J. Biotechnol., 14, pp. 179-186

Takigawa, H., Nakagawa, H., Kuzukawa, M., Mori, H., & Imokawa, G. (2005). Deficient production of hexadecenoic acid in the skin is associated in part with the vulnerability of atopic dermatitis patients to colonization by *Staphylococcus aureus*, Dermatology, 211, pp. 240-248

Tay, D. K., Rajagopalan, G., Li, X., Chen, Y., Lua, L. H., Leong, S. S. (2011). A new bioproduction route for a novel antimicrobial peptide, Biotechnol. Bioeng., 108, pp. 572–581

Wille, J. J., & Kydonieus, A., (2003). Palmitoleic acid isomer (C16: 1 delta6) in human skin sebum is effective against gram-positive bacteria, Skin Pharmacol. Appl. Skin Physiol., 16, pp. 176-187

Yamada, H., Shimizu, S., & Shinmen, Y. (1987). Production of arachidonic acid by *Mortierella elongata* 1S-5, Agric. Biol. Chem., 51, pp. 785-790

Yamada, H. (1988). Production of arachidonic acid and eicosapentaenoic acid by microorganisms, p. 173-177. In Applewhite, T. H. (ed.), Proceedings of World Conference on Biotechnology for the Fats and Oils Industry, Hamburg, Germany, 1987. American Oil Chemists' Society, Champaign

Zhan, Q., Li, M., Ma, H., Sun, Y., & Xing, L. (2004). Idenitification and characterization of a novel Delta6-fatty acid desaturase gene from *Rhizopus arrhizus*, FEBS Lett., 556, pp. 81-85

20

Probiotics and Atopic Dermatitis

Feriel Hacini-Rachinel, Ivana Jankovic,
Anurag Singh and Annick Mercenier
Nestlé Research Center, Lausanne
Switzerland

1. Introduction

The term "probiotic" was only coined starting from 1953 and means "for life" ("pro = for" and "bios = life") as opposed to "antibiotics". Yet, the related concept dates back to the early 1900s when Tissier and Metchnikoff pioneered the notion that not all bacteria are detrimental and that some may even be ingested for benefit of health and longevity (Tissier, 1906; Metchnikoff, 1908). Since then, over 9000 articles and 700 clinical trials have been devoted to document and unravel the beneficial effects attributed to probiotic strains and the mechanisms of action that may be involved. The health benefits attributed to probiotics are numerous (Nomoto, 2005; Nova et al., 2007; O'Hara and Shanahan, 2007; Parvez et al., 2006; Salminen et al., 2005; Sanders, 2008; Santosa et al., 2006) but the level of proof supporting them is highly variable depending on the benefit and more importantly on the studied strain. In view of the large diversity and the high number of probiotic candidate strains it is important to stress that most observations are strictly strain specific which means that data obtained on a given strain may not be extrapolated to all strains belonging to the corresponding bacterial species and genus. This renders a global analysis of the field quite difficult and general conclusions often lack accuracy.

2. Human gut microbiota

The adult human gastro-intestinal tract (GIT) houses about 10^{14} microbial cells, that outnumber by a factor of 10 the number of cells that compose the human body. This complex microbiota contains over 1000 bacterial types whose number and composition vary along the GIT as a consequence of the different biochemical conditions in the intestine, nutrient availability, age and health status of the host. Of note, the corresponding pool of genes (microbiome) is 150 times larger than the human genome (Eckburg et al., 2005). For this reason, the gut microbiota is sometimes referred to as an organ by itself. It is well established today that this complex microbial community plays an essential role in health and well being. Research conducted with germ-free or gnotobiotic (*i.e.* germ-free animals that were colonized by known bacteria) rodents has unambiguously demonstrated that even if germ free animals are viable when housed in specific conditions and fed with a very nutritious diet, the gut microbiota plays a critical role for normal growth and development (Kelly et al., 2007; Sjogren et al., 2009).

The GIT of mammals is sterile at birth but it becomes rapidly colonized by maternal and environmental bacteria during the delivery. The successive installation of bacterial species has been well studied (Fanaro et al., 2003; Salminen and Gueimonde, 2005) and was shown to be influenced by several factors such as the mode of delivery and the neonate's diet (Laubereau et al., 2004; Martindale et al., 2005; Negele et al., 2004; Sicherer and Burks, 2008; Zutavern et al., 2006). The next critical phase of bacterial colonization occurs around weaning, when new foods are progressively introduced in the infant's diet. A more complex microbiota is then established that evolves towards the typical adult one over the following years. The progressive bacterial population of the infant intestines has been shown to be of prime importance in the development of a mature gut ecosystem and a functional mucosal immune system. The GIT corresponds to a huge mucosal surface (close to 200 m^2 in the adult) that is constantly challenged by external factors such as food components, microbes, toxic compounds, chemicals *etc.* and as such is one of the principal point of entry of pathogens. The GIT thus developed into a sophisticated organ that is able to discriminate between harmful and harmless agents, with an immune system that rapidly mounts defensive responses against infectious microbes while being able to tolerate food or self antigens. This exquisite level of regulation is progressively established as a result of bacterial stimulus including gut microbial colonization in early stages of life. The "hygiene hypothesis" postulates that the lack of adequate microbial challenge linked to modern living conditions in westernized countries is at the origin of the increasing prevalence of chronic immune dysfunctions such as inflammatory bowel disease and allergy (Ege et al., 2008; Schaub et al., 2006; Waser et al., 2007). This postulate is the rationale behind the use of probiotic microorganisms to promote, restore or maintain a healthy status in humans and animals.

3. Probiotics and health related benefits

Probiotics have been defined by a FAO/WHO expert group as « live microorganisms which when administered in adequate amounts confer a health benefit on the host » (2001). This is the most widely accepted definition even if others - that are relatively similar- can be found in literature. This definition implies that the microorganisms are not restricted to bacteria, and yeasts such as *Saccharomyces boulardii/cerevisiae* for example have been studied for their health promoting properties. Typically *S. boulardii* probiotic preparations are commercialized as over the counter (OTC) products to fight diarrhea. Yet, most of the probiotic research has been conducted with lactobacilli and bifidobacteria, even though one strain of *Escherichia coli, E. coli Nissle* 1917, and a few strains of *Enterococcus* and *Bacillus* have also been well studied during the last decades. Today, the search for new health promoting microorganisms is extending beyond bacteria isolated from humans to strains originating from fermented food and feed products such as *Pediococcus, Propionobacterium* and *Lactococcus spp*. The bacterial genera *Lactobacillus, Enterococcus, Pedicoccus, Propionibacterium, Streptococcus* and *Lactococcus* belong to the family of lactic acid bacteria (LAB) which - as indicated by their name - are able to rapidly transform fermentable carbohydrates in substantial amounts of lactic acid, eventually accompanied by acetic and propionic acid, and butyrate. The capacity of lowering the environmental pH and thus creating an unfavorable milieu for specific pathogens is at the origin of the use of LAB for the preparation and preservation of fermented food and feed products since time immemorial. As a consequence, several LAB species have a "generally-recognised-as-safe" (GRAS) status in the food industry due to their long history of safe human consumption. Several species are also part on the endogenous mammal microbiota and can naturally be found in the oral, intestinal and urogenital tracts of healthy individuals. The number of specific genera of LAB varies along the gastro-intestinal ecosystem and lactobacilli are typically dominant members of the human vaginal microbiota where they play a key protective role against infections (Falagas et al., 2007).

The health benefits addressed by probiotic research are ranging from their anti-microbial properties to the impact probiotics may have on the host immune system and gut barrier, and on the metabolism and composition of the endogenous microbiota, and as a consequence on the host physiology. The applications are nowadays extending to extra-intestinal sites such as the skin, the oral cavity, the urogenital tract and importantly the gut-brain axis. Targeted diseases include bacterial and viral infections, chronic immune disorders such as allergy, inflammatory bowel disease and autoimmune diseases, irritable bowel syndrome, energy and weight management, mood disorders, stress and even psychological disorders such as autism (Asahara et al., 2001; Bin-Nun et al., 2005; Brenner et al., 2009; Carroll et al., 2007; Chapat et al., 2004; Cryan and O'Mahony, 2011; Dani et al., 2002; Iovieno et al., 2008; Madsen et al., 2001; Zareie et al., 2006). From an experimental point of view, the major challenge is to select the most appropriate candidate probiotic strain(s) to reach the selected aim. Therefore, a series of *in vitro* and *ex vivo* assays are used before testing a limited number of strains in animal models mimicking the human disease. Even if time consuming this preclinical research is aiming at facilitating the clinical studies that are mandatory to support the health claim that may be attributed to a probiotic strain. In the past several selection criteria have been applied such as origin of the strain, acid and bile resistance, adhesion to epithelial cells *etc.*, which today rather serve for characterization of candidate probiotic strains (Mercenier et al., 2008). Nowadays, safety and stability of the strains are considered as the main criteria that may lead to exclusion of strains for further applications (Delgado et al., 2008; Grimoud et al., 2010; Gueimonde and Salminen, 2006; Kalliomaki et al., 2010; Niers et al., 2007).

4. Probiotics and immune modulation

Probiotics are able to interact at different levels with the host intestinal ecosystem. They may exert effects in the gut lumen via the release of soluble active compounds (metabolites, enzymes), by co-aggregation with pathogens and by intensive cross-talk with the endogenous microbiota (Ait-Belgnaoui et al., 2006; Boirivant and Strober, 2007; Ewaschuk et al., 2008; Haller et al., 2001). They are also known to interact with the intestinal epithelial barrier and its associated mucus, and to initiate immune signaling (Vesterlund et al., 2006; Ohland and MacNaughton, 2010). Specific probiotics are able to exert an effect beyond the gut, influencing the systemic immune system as well as other cell and organ systems, such as liver and brain. For example, certain strains were shown to interact with the enteric nervous system and as such to trigger the gut-brain axis (Cryan and O'Mahony, 2011; Duncker et al., 2008).

Even though we are far from having identified all active compounds that may mediate these interactions, it has been undoubtedly established that bacterial cell surface associated molecules are recognized by the gut immune system. The cell wall of gram-positive bacteria - to which most probiotic bacteria belong - differs from that of gram-negative bacteria by a higher content in peptidoglycan, by the absence of lipopolysaccharides (LPS) and presence of a variety of lipoteichoic acids (LTA) or wall teichoic acids (WTA) instead. In both gram-positive and gram-negative bacteria the cell surface may also be decorated by exopolysaccharides (EPS) and/or glycosylated proteins. Altogether these cell surface components correspond to Microbial Associated Molecular Patterns or MAMPs (also named PAMPS for pathogenic microbes) that may differ substantially from one strain to another. MAMPS are known to bind to specific receptors, the pattern recognition receptors or PRRs, which are expressed by many immune cells and tissues such as the gut epithelium. The binding of MAMPs to PRRs explains how probiotic, commensal or pathogenic bacteria can elicit innate and adaptive immune responses in the host by triggering signaling cascades that in turn lead to the production of cytokines, chemokines and other innate effectors (Abreu, 2010; Kawai and Akira, 2010; Wells et al., 2010). The PRRs belong to three major families: the Toll-like receptors (TLRs), retinoic acid inducible gene I (RIG-I)-like receptors and nucleotide oligomerization domain-like (NOD) receptors (Kawai and Akira, 2010). The TLR and NOD receptors have been shown to play a role in immune activation by probiotics and commensals and so to influence skewing of naïve T cells, regulation of regulatory T cells (Tregs) and activation of antigen presenting cells (APCs) such as dendritic cells (DCs) and macrophages. Activated DCs produce different cytokines in response to different bacterial stimuli and this has consequences for the induction of different T cell subtypes (Baba et al., 2008; Mohamadzadeh et al., 2005). In this sense it is not surprising that different candidate probiotic strains exhibit different immune modulation specificities as they may carry varying MAMPs (Wells, 2011).

Several studies have demonstrated that *in vitro* cytokine profiles elicited from PBMCs, DCs or macrophages vary substantially depending on the species but importantly also on the strain (Wells et al., 2011). Typically, Meijerink *et al.* recently compared the DC response to stimulation by 42 *Lactobacillus plantarum* strains and amounts of IL-10 and IL-12 levels showed up to 39 and 600 fold differences, respectively (Meijerink et al., 2010). This indicates that multiple factors play a role in determining the immune phenotype of a strain. Using genome comparison of *L. plantarum* strains and gene deletion techniques, bacterial genetic loci involved in these specific immune properties could be identified (Marco et al., 2009; Meijerink et al., 2010).

The impact of the LTA has also been highlighted by genetic studies dealing with different *Lactobacillus* species, for example the composition of LTA in *L. plantarum* NCIMB8826 and *Lactobacillus rhamnosus* GG (Grangette et al., 2005; Perea et al., 2007), and presence/absence of LTA in *Lactobacillus acidophilus* NCK56 (Mohamadzadeh et al., 2011) was shown to influence the pro- or anti-inflammatory properties of the wild type and mutant strains. These are examples of studies that combined bacterial physiology and genetics with *in vitro* immune assays in order to generate a hypothesis that could be tested in animal models. They illustrate a nowadays quite active and rapidly evolving field of research. Recent reviews have captured the information that has been gathered on how probiotics can signal through TLR2, TLR2/6, TLR4, TLR9, NOD 1 & 2, and other signaling pathways (Lebeer et al., 2010; Wells et al., 2011).

Different lactobacilli and bifidobacteria have been reported to enhance or restore the barrier function (Resta-Lenert and Barrett, 2003; Ulluwishewa et al., 2011). *In vivo* data support these observations, which were recently reinforced in a human study showing that tight junction proteins of the gut epithelium (biopsies) were regulated upon perfusion of *L. plantarum* WCFS1 in the duodenum of healthy volunteers (Karczewski et al., 2010).

Even though a lot of research has been dedicated to identify which cell surface molecules are operational in the probiotic-host interaction, other molecules such as DNA (Rachmilewitz et al., 2002; Rachmilewitz et al., 2004), metabolites or secreted soluble factors have also been established to play a key role. For example, soluble factors of *Bifidobacterium breve* C50 were demonstrated to participate to the anti-inflammatory properties of the strain and to impact on intestinal ion channels (Heuvelin et al., 2010).

While providing an exhaustive review of this area is beyond the scope of the chapter, it might be concluded that the use of a variety of *in vitro* and *in vivo* immune models linked to a good knowledge of bacterial physiology and genetics allowed progress in understanding the mechanisms of action of specific probiotic strains and identification of certain effector molecules. Nevertheless, efforts should be continued in this area while it will also be necessary to fill the major gap that remains between preclinical and clinical research.

5. Atopic dermatitis (AD): Physiopathology of AD

Atopic dermatitis or atopic eczema (AD/AE) is a chronic inflammatory disease of the skin, which usually occurs in the early years of life. The skin in AD is extremely dry and itchy and is inflamed - this leads to the characteristic redness, swelling, and scaling pattern often seen in the face and at flexural surfaces of the extremities of patients suffering from AD. AD has been divided in at least 2 different forms: (i) IgE associated or extrinsic dermatitis; (ii) non-IgE associated or intrinsic dermatitis.

Based on epidemiological and immunological studies, the natural history of AD seems to follow three phases: an initial non-atopic (non-IgE associated) form of eczema occurring in the early infancy followed in 60 to 80% of the cases by a sensitization to food and /or environmental allergens with the development of associated IgE (true AD). Finally, an IgE sensitization to self-proteins is observed in a high proportion of children and adults with AD due to molecular mimicry (Bieber, 2008).

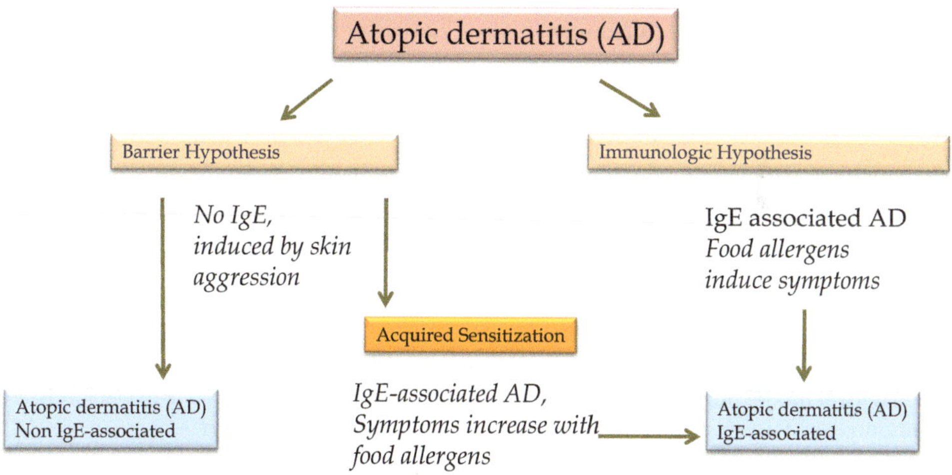

Fig. 1. AD classification (Bieber, 2008)

AD is often the first disorder to manifest in the relay of allergies, usually referred to as the Atopic March (Hahn and Bacharier, 2005; Illi et al., 2004; Spergel and Paller, 2003; Zheng et al., 2011). The prevalence of the disorder has increased dramatically in the last two decades similar to other allergies such as allergic rhinitis and asthma. AD affects mostly infants and young children and according to recent epidemiological studies, 5-20% of children are affected in developed countries (Asher et al., 2006; Williams et al., 1999). The treatment of AD is mainly symptomatic and includes emollients to moisturize the skin, and topical corticosteroids along with a switch to an elimination diet (BuBmann et al., 2009; Peserico et al., 2008).

AD has a complex etiology. Recent investigations into mechanisms that drive the inflammatory response in AD have highlighted the crucial role of genetic predisposition. Many mutations have been associated to the development of AD. These mutations are located in two subsets of genes, in structural protein genes involved in the epidermal-barrier function or in genes involved in IgE production (Bieber, 2008; Demehri et al., 2009; Hsu et al., 2008; Suzuki et al., 2011). Also, environmental factors can contribute to the development of AD. As such, AD can be classified into IgE-mediated and non IgE-mediated subtypes (Fig. 1.).

As mentioned above, it has been postulated ("hygiene hypothesis") that the pattern of bacterial colonization of the gut during the early months after birth can contribute to the development of AD (Vael and Desager, 2009). During the first year of life the newborn immune system is still under development while exposure to novel dietary foods is increasing, especially around the weaning period. These multifactorial events in concert contribute to the establishment of oral tolerance, *i.e.* prevention or development of atopic sensitization to common foods such as cow's milk, eggs, wheat and nuts that predispose to the development of AD (Garcia et al., 2007; Gonzalez, I et al., 1971; Han et al., 2004; Heratizadeh et al., 2011).

6. Animal models of allergy and preclinical studies with probiotics

Even though animal models do not completely recapitulate all clinical, histological and immunological features of human AD, they can offer valuable tools (i) to evaluate candidate probiotic strains and their ability to prevent/alleviate AD and (ii) to elucidate their cellular and molecular mechanisms of action. Indeed, assessing the effect of probiotic candidate strains directly in human trials is expensive and time-consuming. Moreover, the number of candidate strains, the importance of their preparation/formulation, the dose, routes and possible administration regimens/schedules increase the number of parameters to be evaluated before to launch a clinical trial. Also, food and safety agencies recommend to better characterize the mechanism of action of potential probiotics. Since access to biological materials other than blood is limited and functional studies are difficult to perform in human trials, research on probiotics may benefit from preclinical animal models (Kalliomaki et al., 2010).

In the context of AD, several animal models are used nowadays (Jin et al., 2009) (table 1). The historical model of Nc/Nga mice that spontaneously develop AD-like features has been commonly used to evaluate the capacity of candidate strains to prevent/manage AD (Matsuda et al., 1997). In this model, Nc/Nga mice housed under specific pathogen free conditions are protected from AD. Once these mice are transferred to air-unregulated conventional environment, they exhibit AD-like lesions by 7-8 weeks. Feeding (heat-treated) *Lactobacillus rhamnosus* GG or live *Lactobacillus johnsonii* NCC533 around weaning period prevented or delayed the onset of AD (Sawada et al., 2007; Tanaka et al., 2008). Offsprings exhibited lower clinical scores with shorter scratching duration/frequency, a reduced total IgE serum titer and a decreased number of mast cells infiltrating skin lesions. One of the caveats of the model of Nc/Nga mice is that the allergen is unknown. To circumvent this

Animals	Models	Examples	Common features with human AD/rationale	Ref.
Rodents	Spontaneous dermatitis	Nc/Nga mice	Mice develop AD-like lesions when housed in non-sterile (conventional) environment. Closely mimics human AD features: scratching behavior, skin thickening,dermal infiltration of eosinophils and mononuclear cells, elevation of total IgE	Matsuda et al., 1997
		DS-Nh mice	AD develops in conventional conditions with elevation of total IgE. The skin is colonized with *Staphylococcus aureus*	Hikita et al., 2002
	Epicutaneous sensitization	Skin injury and epicutaneous sensitization with ovalbumin	Skin barrier disruption, mimics skin injury inflicted by scratching in patients with AD: epidermal and dermal thickening, infiltration of $CD4^+$ T cells and eosinophils, upregulation of Th2 cytokines, production of specific IgE	Spergel et al., 1998
		Epicutaneous sensitization with aero-allergens (house dust mite, *Aspergillus fumigatus*)	Majority of patients with allergic rhinitis have pre-existing atopic disease. Mimics skin hyperplasia, infiltration of $CD4^+$ T cells and eosinophils, upregulation of Th2 cytokines, elevation of total IgE	Huang et al., 2003b; Akei et al., 2005
		Epicutaneous sensitization with Th2-inducing hapten (oxazolone, trinitrochlorobenzene)	Mimics exposure to allergen via a breach in the skin barrier: epidermal hyperplasia, elevation of transepidermal water loss, infiltration of $CD4^+$ T cells, mast cells and eosinophils, upregulation of Th2 cytokines	Matsumoto et al., 2004; Man et al., 2008
		Food hypersensitivity-induced AD (allergen + cholera toxin)	Supports the role of food allergy in a subset of patients with AD: scratching is one of the possible clinical symptoms	Li et al., 2001
		Superantigen-induced AD	Mimics the exacerbation of AD by *S. aureus*	Laouini et al., 2003
		Mice overexpressing IL-4	IL-4 Tg mice develop dermatitis with infiltration of mononuclear cells, mast cells, and eosinophils	Chan et al., 2001
		Mice overexpressing TSLP, Retinoid X Receptor $RXR\alpha\beta^{ep-/-}$ mice	Mice overexpress the cytokine thymic stromal lymphopoietin (TSLP), known to be produced in epidermal keratinocytes of AD patients, and develop AD-like skin and systemic abnormalities	Yoo et al., 2005; Li et al., 2005

Animals	Models	Examples	Common features with human AD/rationale	Ref.
	Genetically modified mice	IL-31 transgenic mice	IL-31 overexpression reproduces skin histological lesions with no IgE increase or systemic Th2 cytokines	Dillon et al., 2004
		Stratum corneum (SC) chymotripic enzyme overexpresssing transgenic mice	The SC chymotrypic enzyme, a serine protease has been shown to be overexpressed in chronic lesion of AD. The SC chymotrypic enzyme transgenic mice develop AD-like skin lesions	Hansson et al., 2002
		Cathepsin E-deficient mice	The cathepsin E (Cat E) proteinase is preferentially expressed in the antigen-presenting cells. The Cat E°/° mice develop pruritic and skin lesions, infiltration of $CD4^+$ T cells and eosinophils, upregulation of Th2 cytokines, elevation of total IgE	Tsukuba et al., 2003
		Caspase-1 or IL-18 transgenic mice	IL-18 precursor becomes active after cleavage with capase-1 (CASP1). Its expression is increased in human AD skin lesions and IL-18 and CASP1 transgenic mice develop AD-like skin inflammation with scratching behavior. They have a spontaneous Th2-bias, elevated seric IgG1and IgE and histamine levels, and an increased number of skin mast cells	Konishi et al., 2002
		APOC1 transgenic mice	APOC1 (Apolipoprotein C1) is expressed in the skin and involved in lipoprotein metabolism. In the APOC1 the transgenic mice there is an impairment of the skin barrier function that leads to increased total IgE and dermatitis. Both can be suppressed by topical corticoid treatment	Nagelkerken et al., 2008
Dogs	Spontaneous dermatitis	Beagles	This model reproduces human AD clinically, histologically with an epidermal barrier dysfunction. Immunologically, AD dogs' PBMC exhibit a Th2 cytokine profile	Marsella and Girolomoni, 2009

Table 1. Common preclinical models of AD (adapted from (Jin et al., 2009))

drawback, modified models have been set up. Repeated application of house dust mite *Dermatophagoides farina* extract induces human-like atopic skin lesions (Huang et al., 2003a). In this model, oral administration of live *Lactobacillus plantarum* from Kimchi, a traditional Korean fermented food (Won et al., 2011), or of live *L. johnsonii* NCC533 alleviated AD symptoms (Inoue et al., 2007). In another Nc/Nga-derived model, mice were sensitized by epicutaneous application of the hapten picryl chloride, and oral administration of heat-treated *Lactobacillus breve* SBC8803 delayed the development of AD (Segawa et al., 2008). It is noteworthy that most of these experiments have been performed in young mice with administration of probiotics around weaning. However recent papers started to investigate the impact of different intervention periods. In this respect, a protective effect of live *L. rhamnosus* LPR was observed when the strain was fed to pregnant dams and their pups for 12 weeks. Protection was equally seen when probiotic treatment started at weaning but not when it was initiated one week after the onset of the disease (Tanaka et al., 2009).

The general hypothesis evoked to explain the beneficial effect of specific probiotic strains in allergy mouse models is their capacity to establish or restore the Th1/Th2 balance. Indeed, allergic disorders such as AD are characterized by an immune response that is Th2-biased with increased production of cytokines IL-4, IL-5 and IL-13. Investigators working in the probiotic field thus started to screen strains according to their ability to polarize T cells responses into Th1 responses (with IL-12 and INFγ production) (Mohamadzadeh et al., 2005) and to induce regulatory T cells (Hacini-Rachinel et al., 2009).

Alternative models such as the canine model of AD might be of interest as the latter, for ex., displays features similar to human AD. Of note, Marsella et al. evaluated the efficacy of *L. rhamnosus* GG in the prevention of canine AD but no significant decrease in clinical symptoms was observed (Marsella, 2009).

7. Probiotics and allergy: Clinical studies

Studies have been conducted comparing the gut microbiota of infants with AD or food allergy to non-allergic infants and in these studies it was observed that allergic infants had reduced numbers of lactobacilli and bifidobacteria species in their gut (Adlerberth et al., 2007; Kirjavainen et al., 2002; Penders et al., 2007). A little more than a decade ago the first studies were published testing the hypothesis that probiotic intervention either in the pre- or post- natal period (pregnant women, offsprings or both) could influence the incidence of AD in the early years of life. Over 25 published studies have investigated similar hypotheses since then. However, these studies have largely differed in the choice of probiotic strain investigated, duration of administration of the strain, the population treated (mothers vs. newborns vs. both mothers and newborns) and in selecting the primary outcome addressing the efficacy of the trial. We have grouped the studies into 2 types- those in which the probiotic is given as a prevention strategy *i.e.* in at risk population (history of atopy in the family) and the others in which probiotics are administered as a therapeutic entity in subjects diagnosed with AD to better manage their symptoms.

7.1 Prevention of AD

Around 15 clinical trials have investigated the efficacy of probiotic in prevention of AD (summarized in Table 2). We highlight some of the more relevant well designed trials that raised key questions in the field of probiotics. Kalliomaki *et al.* conducted the first long-term preventive study on probiotics in AD and found that supplementation with the *L. rhamnosus*

Ref.	Study design	Probiotic daily dose	Intervention	Population	Biological effect
Kim et al., 2010	R, DB, PC	1) *B. bifidum* BGN4, *B. lactis* AD011, *L. acidophilus* AD030 each at 1.6e9 cfu/day in powder 2) Placebo powder (maltodextrin and alpha-corn)	Given to mothers from 8 weeks before delivery until 3 months post-delivery, then to infants from 4 until 6 months	68 Infants at high risk of eczema; Korea	The cumulative incidence of eczema during the first 12 months was reduced significantly in probiotic group
Morisset et al., 2011	R, DB, PC	1) Infant formula fermented with *B. breve* C50 (4.2e9 cfu/100g)+ *S. thermophilus* 065 (3.8e7 cfu/100g) 2) Placebo: infant formula	1 year from birth	129 Infants and children at high risk of atopy (0-24 months), France	No effect between the groups
Niers et al., 2009	R, DB, PC	1) *B. bifidum* W23, *B lactis* W52, *L lactis* W58 (Ecologic® Panda) 3e9 cfu/day (1e9 of each); freeze dried powder; in sachet 2) Placebo: rice starch + maltodextran in sachet	During last 6 weeks of pregnancy and postnatally for 12 months to infant	98 Pregnant women with history of allergy, Netherland	Severity of atopic dermatitis decreased in probiotic treated-group during first 3 months
Taylor et al., 2007	R, DB, PC	1) *L. acidophilus*, LAVRI-A1 3e9 cfu/day lyophilised 2) Placebo: maltodextrin	6 months	178 Infants (< 6 months) with allergic disease history, Australia	No effect on incidence of atopic dermatitis
Ortiz-Andrellucchi et al., 2008	R, DB, PC	1) *L. casei* DN-114001 in milk (fermentation, dose not given) 2) Placebo (the same fermented milk b-irradiated)	45 days post delivery to mother	104 Prenatal, mother (18-40 y), Spain	No difference in the incidence of infant atopic dermatitis at 6 months
West et al., 2009	R; DB, PC	1) *L. paracasei* F19 lyophilised in cereals (rice and wheat based + milk proteins) 1e8 cfu/day 2) Placebo: cereals	9 months	171 Infants (subpopulation of at risk), Sweden	The cumulative incidence of atopic dermatitis was lower in probiotic treated-group
Abrahamsson et al., 2007	R, DB, PC	1) *L. reuteri* ATCC55730 1e8 cfu/day in coconut and peanut oil 2) Placebo: Same oil	4 weeks before delivery, 1 year mother and infant, 1 year follow up	188 Prenatal with allergic disease history, Sweden	Less IgE associated eczema at 2 years. Less skin prick test reactivity
Kopp et al., 2008	R, DB, PC	1) *L. rhamnosus* GG 1e10 cfu/day lyophilised in capsules 2) Placebo: microcrystalline cellulose in capsules	4-6 weeks before delivery + 6 months postnatally (first 3 months through the mothers/breastfeeding)	94 Pregnant women/ babies with familial atopic disease, Germany	No effect on the severity of atopic dermatitis

Ref.	Study design	Probiotic daily dose	Intervention	Population	Biological effect
Kalliomaki et al., 2001; Kalliomaki et al., 2003; Kalliomaki et al., 2007	R, DB, PC	1) *L. rhamnosus* GG 1e10 cfu/day lyophilised in capsules 2) Placebo: microcrystalline cellulose in capsules	2-4 weeks before delivery 6 months post natal	132 Prenatal with history of atopic disease, Finland	Incidence of eczema decreased during first 2, 4 and 7 years of life, respectively
Rautava et al., 2002	R, DB, PC	1) *L. rhamnosus* GG (Valio) 2e10 cfu/day lyophilised 2) Placebo: microcrystalline cellulose	4 weeks before giving birth and during breastfeeding	62 Mother/ Infant with history of atopic disease, Finland	Significant reduction in development of atopic eczema during first 2 years in probiotic treated-group
Huurre et al., 2008	R, DB, PC	1) *L. rhamnosus* GG, *B lactis* Bb12 1e10 cfu/day lyophilised (to the mother) 2) Placebo: crystalline cellulose	Middle pregnancy to end, breastfeeding	171 Prenatal with allergic history, Finland	Reduction of sensitization at 12 months in probiotic treated-group
Soh et al., 2009	R, DB, PC	1) *B. longum* BL999 1e8, *L. rhamnosus* LPR 2e8 cfu/day in formula 2) Placebo: formula	6 months	253 Infants (<6m) with history of allergic disease, Singapore	No effect on atopic senistisation and eczema at 1 year
Wickens et al., 2008	R, DB, PC	1) *L. rhamnosus* HN001, 6e9 cfu/day freeze-dried in capsules 2) *B. lactis* HN019 (Fonterra), 9e9 cfu/day freeze-dried in capsules 3) Placebo: capsules (dextran, salt, yeast extract)	Mothers: from 35 weeks gestation to 6 months postpartum. Infants: from birth to 2 years	446 Pregnant women with familial atopic disease, New Zealand	Reduction of eczema and of developing SCORAD by 2 years for *L. rhamnosus*, no effect on atopy; no effect of *B. lactis* HN019
Kuitunen et al., 2009	R, DB, PC	1) *L. rhamnosus* GG and LC705, .*B breve* Bb99, *P. freudenreichii* JS 1e10, 4e8, 4e9 cfu/day resp lyophilised (Valio mix 1) + GOS 2) Placebo: Microcrystalline cellulose	4 weeks before delivery 6 months to infant	891 Pregnant women/ babies with familial atopic disease, Finland	Reduction of IgE-associated allergic disease in cesarean-delivered infants only as secondary outcome
Kukkonen et al., 2007; Kukkonen et al., 2008; Kukkonen et al., 2010	R, DB, PC	1) *L. rhamnosus* GG 1e10, *L. rhamnosus* LC705 1e10, *B. breve* Bb99 4e8, *P. freudenreichii* 4e9 cfu/day + GOS lyophilised in capsules (Valio mix 1) 2) placebo: microcrystalline cellulose in capsules	2-4 wks before delivery 6 months to the infant	1223 Pregnant women with familial atopic disease, Finland	Probiotic treatment showed no effect on the incidence of all allergic diseases by age 2 years but prevented atopic eczema

Table 2. Prevention Studies in AD with Probiotics (R= randomized; DB= double blinded; PC= placebo controlled)

GG strain both to mothers (history of atopic diseases) prenatally in the last 2-4 weeks of pregnancy and subsequently to infants from birth to 6 months significantly reduced the incidence of AD at 2 years of age, *i.e.* 15/64 subjects were confirmed AD patients in the probiotic group compared to 31/68 in the placebo control group. Interestingly enough, IgE levels and skin prick test (SPT) reactivity to common food- and aero-allergens were not different between the groups at 2 years (Kalliomaki et al., 2001). The same authors conducted a follow-up of the subjects till 4 and 7 years of age and documented the incidence of other allergic disorders (allergic rhinitis, asthma) in addition to the long term effect of probiotic treatment on AD incidence. At both the follow up time-points, *i.e.* 4 and 7 years, the incidence of AD was lower in the probiotic treated group compared to the placebo group (Kalliomaki et al., 2003; Kalliomaki et al., 2007). Yet, the incidence of respiratory allergies at the follow-up time periods seemed to be higher in the probiotic treated group. The link between probiotic administration early on in life and the development of later onset of allergies deserves to be further investigated. A subsequent study evaluating the *L. rhamnosus* GG strain in similar clinical trial settings reported no preventive effect on the development of AD at 2 years of age (Kopp et al., 2008). Possibly the beneficial effects of probiotic strains are influenced by variants such as diet and genetic heterogeneity in the target population or the strain preparation/formulation.

With the increasing interest in the field of probiotics, various strains were reported to display established or potential benefit for allergy management. In this scope, it may become important to compare the efficacy of different strains in the same clinical trial. Wickens *et al.* did exactly that and compared the efficacy of *L. rhamnosus* HN001 and *B. lactis* HN109 to a placebo; reduction in the incidence of AD at 2 years of age was observed with *L. rhamnosus* HN001 but not with *B. lactis* HN109 in comparison to the placebo, which constitutes a quite convincing result (Wickens et al., 2008). Combinations of multiple strains have also been attempted in AD clinical trials; Soh *et al.* combined two strains *B. longum* BL999 and *L. rhamnosus* GG (LPR), and found that in comparison to the placebo there was no significant effect in the reduction of AD incidence at 1 year of age (Soh et al., 2009). It should be emphasized that combination of different probiotic candidates or increasing the probiotic dose does not necessarily lead to an increased beneficial effect.

7.2 Therapy: Management of AD symptoms

Compared to prevention studies, probiotic trials in management of AD are relatively of shorter duration (typically 4-12 weeks) and aim at reducing the severity of AD. The primary outcome selected is often a change in SCORAD index which is a validated clinical scoring system that evaluates the intensity, severity of disease and quality of life parameters associated with AD symptoms. AD usually manifests at around 3-4 months of age and resolves in about 50% of the AD subjects by 2-3 years of age. As such it is often a challenge to demonstrate superiority of treatment compared to the placebo in these trials, as the baseline parameters improve spontaneously in part of the enrolled subjects since they are already on eviction diet and standardized treatments. Current data with probiotics in the management of AD is limited even though the first studies were reported almost 15 years ago (Majamaa and Isolauri, 1997).

Most studies supplement infant formulas that are extensively hydrolyzed with their choice of probiotic strains to demonstrate efficacy of probiotics over placebo (non supplemented formula). Extensively hydrolyzed formulas are a common dietary recommendation for

Ref.	Study design	Probiotic daily dose	Intervention	Population	Biological effect
Miniello et al., 2010	R, DB, PC	1) *L. reuteri* ATCC 55730 1e8 cfu/day in a chewable tablet 2) Placebo: identical table without probiotics	8 weeks	51 Children with atopic or non atopic eczema (4-10y), Italy	No improvement in SCORAD index by the probiotic treatment
van der Aa et al., 2010	R, DB, PC	1) *B. breve* M-16V 1.3e9 cfu/100ml + GOS/FOS mixture (Immunofortis) in an extensively hydrolyzed formula 2) Placebo: extensively hydrolyzed formula	12 weeks	90 Infants with atopic dermatitis, Netherlands	Synbiotic-treatment lowered the SCORAD index only in the IgE-positive subgroup
Isolauri et al., 2000	R, DB, PC	1) *L. rhamnosus* GG 3e8 2) *B lactis* Bb12 1e9 cfu/g in hydrolyzed formula 3) Placebo: hydrolyzed formula	2 months	27 Infants (mean 4.6m) exclusively breast fed with atopic eczema, Finland	Severity of atopic eczema, decreased in both probiotic treated-groups
Hol et al., 2008	R, DB, PC	1) *L. casei* CRL431, *B lactis* Bb12 1e9-1e10 cfu/day in formula 2) Placebo: formula	12 months	119 Infants with cow's milk allergy, Netherlands	No difference in cumulative percent of tolerance to cow's milk
Weston et al., 2005	R, DB, PC	1) *L. fermentum* VRI-033 PCC 2e9 cfu/day lyophilised 2) Placebo: maltodextrin	8 weeks treatment 8 weeks follow up	56 Infant (6-18m) with atopic dermatitis, Australia	Reduction in SCORAD index by the probiotic treatment
Rosenfeldt et al., 2003	R, DB, PC CO	1) *L. rhamnosus* 19070, *L reuteri* DSM12246, 1e10 cfu/day lyophilised in bags 2) Placebo: skim mlik protein and dextrose anhydrate in bags	6 weeks treatment with 6 weeks wash out between	41 Children (1-13y) with moderate to severe atopic dermatitis, Denmark	No change in SCORAD index but improvement in patients's subjective evaluation of eczema in probiotic treated-group
Kirjavainen et al., 2003	R, DB, PC	1) *L. rhamnosus* GG 3e10 cfu/day/kg body weight in an extensively hydrolysed milk formula, 2) Heat-killed LGG in the same formula 3) Placebo: same formula	Mean duration 7.5 weeks	35 Infants (mean age 5.5 mths) with atopic eczema and cow's milk allergy, Finland	All treatments including placebo caused a reduction in SCORAD index. Heat-inactivated GG caused adverse GIT symptoms. Study stopped because of adverse effects

Ref.	Study design	Probiotic daily dose	Intervention	Population	Biological effect
Brouwer et al., 2006	R, DB, PC	1) *L. rhamnosus* GG 5e8 cfu in an extensively hydrolysed milk formula 2) *L. rhamnosus* Lrh 5e8 cfu in an extensively hydrolysed milk formula 3) Placebo: extensively hydrolysed milk formula	3 months	50 formula-fed Infants (<5months) with atopic dermatitis, suspected with cow's milk allergy, Netherlands	No effect on SCORAD index
Folster-Holst et al., 2006	R, DB, PC	1) *L. rhamnosus* GG 1e10 cfu/day lyophilised in capsules 2) Placebo: cristalline cellulose	8 weeks	54 Infants (1-55 months) with moderate to severe atopic dermatitis, Germany	No difference for the clinical symptoms of atopic dermatitis (SCORAD, pruritus, sleep loss)
Gruber et al., 2007	R, DB, PC	1) *L. rhamnosus* GG 1e10 cfu/day lyophilised in capsuless 2) Placebo: cellulose + saccharose + magnesium	12 weeks	102 Infants (3-12m) with atopic dermatitis , Germany	No effect on atopic dermatitis symptoms, consumption of rescue medication, seric IgE and the quality of life
Majamaa and Isolauri, 1997	R, DB, PC	1) *L. rhamnosus* GG, 5e8 cfu/g of hydrolysed formula 2) Placebo: hydrolysed formula 3) *L. rhamnosus* GG 2e10 cfu/day given to nursing mother	1 month	37 Infants (2-16 months) with atopic dermatitis, CMA suspected, Finland	Severity of atopic dermatitis, decreased in probiotic treated-infants
Sistek et al., 2006	R, DB, PC	1) *L. rhamnosus* and *B. lactis* HN019 (Fonterra) 2e10 cfu/day lyophilised in capsules 2) Placebo: microcrystalline cellulose in capsules	12 weeks	59 Children (1-10 years) with atopic dermatitis, UK	Severity of atopic dermatitis decreased only among children sensitized to foods in probiotic treated-group
Passeron et al., 2006	R, DB, PC	1) *L. rhamnosus* Lcr 35/ 3e9 cfu/day + prebiotic + fermentation broth lyophilised 2) Placebo: prebiotic	3 months	39 Children (2-12 years) with atopic dermatitis, France	No difference in SCORAD scores
Woo et al., 2010	R, DB, PC	1) *L. sakei* KCTC 10755BP/ 1e10 cfu/day freeze-dried in a sachet 2) Placebo: microcrystalline cellulose in a sachet	12 weeks	88 Children with atopic dermatitis(2-10 years), Korea	Severity of atopic dermatitis decreased in probiotic treated-group

Ref.	Study design	Probiotic daily dose	Intervention	Population	Biological effect
Viljanen et al., 2005	R, DB, PC	1) *L. rhamnosus* GG 1e10 2) MIX: GG + *L. rhamnosus* LC705 1e10, *B. breve* BBi99 4e8, *P. freudenreichii* 4e9 cfu/day lyophilised 3) Placebo: microcrystalline cellulose	4 weeks	230 Infants (<12 months) with suspected cow's milk allergy, Finland	Severity of atopic dermatitis decreased in IgE-sensitized infants with LGG treatment
Roessler et al., 2008	R, DB, PC CO	1) .*L paracasei* Lpc-37 8e10, *L. acidophilus* 74-2 6e6, *B. lactis* DGCC420 1e7 cfu/day in yoghurt drink 2) Placebo: yoghurt drink (fermented with *S. thermophilus*)	8 weeks treatment with 2weeks wash out between	15 Adults with atopic dermatitis, Germany	No difference in SCORAD scores
Torii et al., 2011	R, DB, PC	1) Heat-killed *L. acidophilus* L92 1.5e11 Eq cfu/day+dextrin 2) Placebo: dextrin	8 weeks	60 Children (1-12 yrs) with atopic dermatitis, Japan	Improvement of symptom-medication-score in probiotic treated-group
Moroi et al., 2011	Prospective, R, DB, PC	1) Heat-killed *L. paracasei* K71 2e11 Eq cfu/day+dextrin 2) Placebo: dextrin	12 weeks	33 Adult atopic dermatitis patients managed with topical corticosteroid and tacrolimus treatment; Japan	Probiotic but not the placebo significantly decreases the skin severity score from baseline. However there was no intergroup (probiotic vs placebo) difference
Nermes et al., 2011	R, DB, PC	1) LGG 3.4e9 cfu/day + extensively hydrolysed milk formula 2) Placebo: extensively hydrolysed milk formula	3 months	39 Children with atopic dermatitis, Finland	No effect on SCORAD severity

Table 3. Management studies in AD with probiotics (R= randomized; DB= double blinded; PC= placebo controlled)

infants with AD manifestations linked to cow's milk allergy and are largely effective in reducing the severity of AD. To demonstrate an improvement with probiotic supplementation is by itself a challenging primary outcome. Different strains have been evaluated in pilot clinical trials (Table 3) with mixed results. Isolauri *et al.* showed that both *L. rhamnosus* LGG and *B. lactis* Bb12 were effective in reducing the severity of AD (Isolauri et al., 2000). Interestingly, in a recent publication LGG was however shown to have no effect on AD severity (Nermes et al., 2011).

The selection of the target population also plays a major role in the success of these trials. Weston *et al.* demonstrated the efficacy of *L. fermentum* PCC in a cohort of subjects with moderate to severe AD while other studies have typically selected mild to moderate AD subjects and have not succeeded in showing the efficacy of the probiotic strains (Weston et al., 2005). Combinations, with other strains or with prebiotics have been attempted with a variable success. For example, van der Aa *et al.* evaluated a combination of *B. breve* M-16V with a prebiotic mixture. After 12 weeks, the severity of atopic dermatitis (AD) did not differ between the two groups, indicating no superiority of the synbiotic combination of (pro- and pre-biotic) over placebo (van der Aa et al., 2010).

8. Conclusion

Probiotics in general are widely available and advertised for numerous health benefits ranging from infectious and inflammatory disorders - including allergy -, gut health to cognitive performance and skin health. However, the level of available or supporting scientific evidence varies widely depending on the studied probiotic strain and its proposed health benefit. Since numerous pre-clinical studies and clinical trials have examined the efficacy of candidate strains in different models and target populations, it is not possible to make the general conclusion that "probiotics" work at large for this or that purpose. As discussed in the chapter, health benefits or immune effects are strikingly strain specific, which means that observations made on one strain cannot be extrapolated, unless proven, to any other strain. As reviewed recently by Kalliomäki *et al.* (Kalliomaki et al., 2010), particularly for AD, taking into account the pre-clinical studies and clinical trials done, it is too early for the scientific community to recommend a general use of probiotics in routine clinical practice, even though specific strains have been developed with success. The meta-analyses that have been performed on probiotics and health benefits often include results of clinical trials conducted with different strains in different formats (probiotic powders or strains included in a fermented food), in different settings (prevention or treatment) targeting different populations (at risk or diseased people, varying age populations) and relying on different administration regimes (dose, timing, length of the treatment). Yet, a beneficial effect has been reported typically in the case of necrotizing enterocolitis or antibiotic-associated diarrheas. For allergy, the situation is complicated by the fact that this disease corresponds to a syndrome covering multiple manifestations that are influenced by several factors -including environmental ones- that may impact on the onset or the perpetuation of the disease (Prescott and Bjorksten, 2007). The meta-analyses conducted so far diverge somewhat in their conclusions even if they agree on the fact that the evidence is better for allergy prevention than for treatment (Doege et al., 2011; Kalliomaki et al., 2010). In 2008, ILSI Europe organized an expert meeting to establish guidance for assessing the probiotic beneficial effects and to propose how to fill the gap in the areas of digestive system metabolism, chronic intestinal disorders, infections and allergic diseases and the conclusions of this work have been published (The journal of Nutrition, 140, Number 3S-I, supplement). Potential avenues for optimizing clinical trials in the field of probiotics and allergy, and caveats that may lead to misinterpretation of overall results were outlined (Kalliomaki et al., 2010).

A few studies point to the fact that probiotics may work only on IgE-mediated AD. These results although are based on (often retrospective) sub-grouping of the target population into IgE vs. non-IgE groups. Clinical trials are needed in the future specifically in large enough cohorts of IgE-mediated AD to substantiate this hypothesis.

Even though several probiotic candidate strains have been tested *in vitro* and in preclinical models of AD, it remains difficult to discuss the predictive value of these preclinical studies. Indeed there has not been sufficient alignment between the strains used for clinical trials and the ones used for preclinical studies. However, the preclinical models can certainly serve the purpose of (i) further understanding the mechanisms of action of specific strains that have been found to be beneficial in AD clinical trials, (ii) evaluating the best intervention window(s) (prenatal, perinatal, weaning, later in life), (iii) performing dose-response curves and (iv) analyzing the impact of probiotic preparation/formulation or inclusion in a final product, to assess combinations of anti-allergy ingredients, and (v) supporting the dossier to submit for approval by ethical committees for human trials.

In conclusion, when analyzing the results of past and ongoing clinical trials performed with probiotics and allergy, it should be kept in mind that AD is a complex multifactorial disease whose onset or outcome may strongly depend on the complex interplay between the host, in particular its genetic background, the status of the immune system and intestinal microbiota, and environmental factors. Nevertheless, additional efforts in the area deserve to be pursued as nutritional interventions remain by themselves an interesting approach to manage allergic manifestations.

9. Acknowledgements

We warmly thank Dr Carine Blanchard for critical review of the chapter and her suggestions.

10. References

Joint FAO/WHO Expert Consultation on Evaluation of Health and Nutritional Properties of Probiotics in Food Including Powder Milk with Live Lactic Acid Bacteria. Health and Nutritional Properties of Probiotics in Food including Powder Milk with Live Lactic Acid Bacteria. 2001. Ref Type: Report

Abrahamsson,T.R., Jakobsson,T., Bottcher,M.F., Fredrikson,M., Jenmalm,M.C., Bjorksten,B., and Oldaeus,G. (2007). Probiotics in prevention of IgE-associated eczema: a double-blind, randomized, placebo-controlled trial. J. Allergy Clin. Immunol. *119,* 1174-1180.

Abreu,M.T. (2010). Toll-like receptor signalling in the intestinal epithelium: how bacterial recognition shapes intestinal function. Nat. Rev. Immunol. *10,* 131-144.

Adlerberth,I., Strachan,D.P., Matricardi,P.M., Ahrne,S., Orfei,L., Aberg,N., Perkin,M.R., Tripodi,S., Hesselmar,B., Saalman,R., Coates,A.R., Bonanno,C.L., Panetta,V., and Wold,A.E. (2007). Gut microbiota and development of atopic eczema in 3 European birth cohorts. J. Allergy Clin. Immunol. *120,* 343-350.

Ait-Belgnaoui,A., Han,W., Lamine,F., Eutamene,H., Fioramonti,J., Bueno,L., and Theodorou,V. (2006). Lactobacillus farciminis treatment suppresses stress induced visceral hypersensitivity: a possible action through interaction with epithelial cell cytoskeleton contraction. Gut *55*, 1090-1094.

Akei,H.S., Mishra,A., Blanchard,C., and Rothenberg,M.E. (2005). Epicutaneous antigen exposure primes for experimental eosinophilic esophagitis in mice. Gastroenterology *129*, 985-994.

Asahara,T., Nomoto,K., Watanuki,M., and Yokokura,T. (2001). Antimicrobial activity of intraurethrally administered probiotic Lactobacillus casei in a murine model of Escherichia coli urinary tract infection. Antimicrob. Agents Chemother. *45*, 1751-1760.

Asher,M.I., Montefort,S., Bjorksten,B., Lai,C.K., Strachan,D.P., Weiland,S.K., and Williams,H. (2006). Worldwide time trends in the prevalence of symptoms of asthma, allergic rhinoconjunctivitis, and eczema in childhood: ISAAC Phases One and Three repeat multicountry cross-sectional surveys. Lancet *368*, 733-743.

Baba,N., Samson,S., Bourdet-Sicard,R., Rubio,M., and Sarfati,M. (2008). Commensal bacteria trigger a full dendritic cell maturation program that promotes the expansion of non-Tr1 suppressor T cells. J. Leukoc. Biol. *84*, 468-476.

Bieber,T. (2008). Atopic dermatitis. N. Engl. J. Med. *358*, 1483-1494.

Bin-Nun,A., Bromiker,R., Wilschanski,M., Kaplan,M., Rudensky,B., Caplan,M., and Hammerman,C. (2005). Oral probiotics prevent necrotizing enterocolitis in very low birth weight neonates. J. Pediatr. *147*, 192-196.

Boirivant,M. and Strober,W. (2007). The mechanism of action of probiotics. Curr. Opin. Gastroenterol. *23*, 679-692.

Brenner,D.M., Moeller,M.J., Chey,W.D., and Schoenfeld,P.S. (2009). The utility of probiotics in the treatment of irritable bowel syndrome: a systematic review. Am. J. Gastroenterol. *104*, 1033-1049.

Brouwer,M.L., Wolt-Plompen,S.A., Dubois,A.E., van der Heide,S., Jansen,D.F., Hoijer,M.A., Kauffman,H.F., and Duiverman,E.J. (2006). No effects of probiotics on atopic dermatitis in infancy: a randomized placebo-controlled trial. Clin. Exp. Allergy *36*, 899-906.

BuBmann,C., Bieber,T., and Novak,N. (2009). Systemic therapeutic options for severe atopic dermatitis. J. Dtsch. Dermatol. Ges. *7*, 205-219.

Carroll,I.M., Andrus,J.M., Bruno-Barcena,J.M., Klaenhammer,T.R., Hassan,H.M., and Threadgill,D.S. (2007). Anti-inflammatory properties of Lactobacillus gasseri expressing manganese superoxide dismutase using the interleukin 10-deficient mouse model of colitis. Am. J. Physiol Gastrointest. Liver Physiol *293*, G729-G738.

Chan,L.S., Robinson,N., and Xu,L. (2001). Expression of interleukin-4 in the epidermis of transgenic mice results in a pruritic inflammatory skin disease: an experimental animal model to study atopic dermatitis. J. Invest Dermatol. *117*, 977-983.

Chapat,L., Chemin,K., Dubois,B., Bourdet-Sicard,R., and Kaiserlian,D. (2004). Lactobacillus casei reduces CD8+ T cell-mediated skin inflammation. Eur. J. Immunol. *34*, 2520-2528.

Cryan,J.F. and O'Mahony,S.M. (2011). The microbiome-gut-brain axis: from bowel to behavior. Neurogastroenterol. Motil. *23*, 187-192.

Dani,C., Biadaioli,R., Bertini,G., Martelli,E., and Rubaltelli,F.F. (2002). Probiotics feeding in prevention of urinary tract infection, bacterial sepsis and necrotizing enterocolitis in preterm infants. A prospective double-blind study. Biol. Neonate *82*, 103-108.

Delgado,S., O'Sullivan,E., Fitzgerald,G., and Mayo,B. (2008). In vitro evaluation of the probiotic properties of human intestinal Bifidobacterium species and selection of new probiotic candidates. J. Appl. Microbiol. *104*, 1119-1127.

Demehri,S., Morimoto,M., Holtzman,M.J., and Kopan,R. (2009). Skin-derived TSLP triggers progression from epidermal-barrier defects to asthma. PLoS. Biol. *7*, e1000067.

Dillon,S.R., Sprecher,C., Hammond,A., Bilsborough,J., Rosenfeld-Franklin,M., Presnell,S.R., Haugen,H.S., Maurer,M., Harder,B., Johnston,J., Bort,S., Mudri,S., Kuijper,J.L., Bukowski,T., Shea,P., Dong,D.L., Dasovich,M., Grant,F.J., Lockwood,L., Levin,S.D., LeCiel,C., Waggie,K., Day,H., Topouzis,S., Kramer,J., Kuestner,R., Chen,Z., Foster,D., Parrish-Novak,J., and Gross,J.A. (2004). Interleukin 31, a cytokine produced by activated T cells, induces dermatitis in mice. Nat. Immunol. *5*, 752-760.

Doege,K., Grajecki,D., Zyriax,B.C., Detinkina,E., Zu,E.C., and Buhling,K.J. (2011). Impact of maternal supplementation with probiotics during pregnancy on atopic eczema in childhood - a meta-analysis. Br. J. Nutr. 1-6.

Duncker,S.C., Wang,L., Hols,P., and Bienenstock,J. (2008). The d-alanine content of lipoteichoic acid is crucial for Lactobacillus plantarum-mediated protection from visceral pain perception in a rat colorectal distension model. Neurogastroenterol. Motil.

Eckburg,P.B., Bik,E.M., Bernstein,C.N., Purdom,E., Dethlefsen,L., Sargent,M., Gill,S.R., Nelson,K.E., and Relman,D.A. (2005). Diversity of the human intestinal microbial flora. Science *308*, 1635-1638.

Ege,M.J., Herzum,I., Buchele,G., Krauss-Etschmann,S., Lauener,R.P., Roponen,M., Hyvarinen,A., Vuitton,D.A., Riedler,J., Brunekreef,B., Dalphin,J.C., Braun-Fahrlander,C., Pekkanen,J., Renz,H., and von Mutius,E. (2008). Prenatal exposure to a farm environment modifies atopic sensitization at birth. J. Allergy Clin. Immunol. *122*, 407-12, 412.

Ewaschuk,J.B., Diaz,H., Meddings,L., Diederichs,B., Dmytrash,A., Backer,J., Looijer-van,L.M., and Madsen,K.L. (2008). Secreted bioactive factors from Bifidobacterium infantis enhance epithelial cell barrier function. Am. J. Physiol Gastrointest. Liver Physiol *295*, G1025-G1034.

Falagas,M.E., Betsi,G.I., and Athanasiou,S. (2007). Probiotics for the treatment of women with bacterial vaginosis. Clin. Microbiol. Infect. *13*, 657-664.

Fanaro,S., Chierici,R., Guerrini,P., and Vigi,V. (2003). Intestinal microflora in early infancy: composition and development. Acta Paediatr. Suppl *91*, 48-55.

Folster-Holst,R., Muller,F., Schnopp,N., Abeck,D., Kreiselmaier,I., Lenz,T., von,R.U., Schrezenmeir,J., Christophers,E., and Weichenthal,M. (2006). Prospective, randomized controlled trial on Lactobacillus rhamnosus in infants with moderate to severe atopic dermatitis. Br. J Dermatol. *155*, 1256-1261.

Garcia,C., El-Qutob,D., Martorell,A., Febrer,I., Rodriguez,M., Cerda,J.C., and Felix,R. (2007). Sensitization in early age to food allergens in children with atopic dermatitis. Allergol. Immunopathol. (Madr.) *35*, 15-20.

Gonzalez,d.l.R., I, Inigo,J.F., and Oehling,A. (1971). The importance of food sensitization in atopic dermatitis. Dermatologica *143*, 288-291.

Grangette,C., Nutten,S., Palumbo,E., Morath,S., Hermann,C., Dewulf,J., Pot,B., Hartung,T., Hols,P., and Mercenier,A. (2005). Enhanced antiinflammatory capacity of a Lactobacillus plantarum mutant synthesizing modified teichoic acids. Proc. Natl. Acad. Sci. U. S. A *102*, 10321-10326.

Grimoud,J., Durand,H., de,S.S., Monsan,P., Ouarne,F., Theodorou,V., and Roques,C. (2010). In vitro screening of probiotics and synbiotics according to anti-inflammatory and anti-proliferative effects. Int. J. Food Microbiol. *144*, 42-50.

Gruber,C., Wendt,M., Sulser,C., Lau,S., Kulig,M., Wahn,U., Werfel,T., and Niggemann,B. (2007). Randomized, placebo-controlled trial of Lactobacillus rhamnosus GG as treatment of atopic dermatitis in infancy. Allergy *62*, 1270-1276.

Gueimonde,M. and Salminen,S. (2006). New methods for selecting and evaluating probiotics. Dig. Liver Dis. *38 Suppl 2*, S242-S247.

Hacini-Rachinel,F., Gheit,H., Le Luduec,J.B., Dif,F., Nancey,S., and Kaiserlian,D. (2009). Oral probiotic control skin inflammation by acting on both effector and regulatory T cells. PLoS. ONE. *4*, e4903.

Hahn,E.L. and Bacharier,L.B. (2005). The atopic march: the pattern of allergic disease development in childhood. Immunol. Allergy Clin. North Am. *25*, 231-46, v.

Haller,D., Colbus,H., Ganzle,M.G., Scherenbacher,P., Bode,C., and Hammes,W.P. (2001). Metabolic and functional properties of lactic acid bacteria in the gastro-intestinal ecosystem: a comparative in vitro study between bacteria of intestinal and fermented food origin. Syst. Appl. Microbiol. *24*, 218-226.

Han,D.K., Kim,M.K., Yoo,J.E., Choi,S.Y., Kwon,B.C., Sohn,M.H., Kim,K.E., and Lee,S.Y. (2004). Food sensitization in infants and young children with atopic dermatitis. Yonsei Med. J. *45*, 803-809.

Hansson,L., Backman,A., Ny,A., Edlund,M., Ekholm,E., Ekstrand,H.B., Tornell,J., Wallbrandt,P., Wennbo,H., and Egelrud,T. (2002). Epidermal overexpression of stratum corneum chymotryptic enzyme in mice: a model for chronic itchy dermatitis. J. Invest Dermatol. *118*, 444-449.

Heratizadeh,A., Wichmann,K., and Werfel,T. (2011). Food allergy and atopic dermatitis: how are they connected? Curr. Allergy Asthma Rep. *11*, 284-291.

Heuvelin,E., Lebreton,C., Bichara,M., Cerf-Bensussan,N., and Heyman,M. (2010). A Bifidobacterium probiotic strain and its soluble factors alleviate chloride secretion by human intestinal epithelial cells. J. Nutr. *140*, 7-11.

Hikita,I., Yoshioka,T., Mizoguchi,T., Tsukahara,K., Tsuru,K., Nagai,H., Hirasawa,T., Tsuruta,Y., Suzuki,R., Ichihashi,M., and Horikawa,T. (2002). Characterization of dermatitis arising spontaneously in DS-Nh mice maintained under conventional conditions: another possible model for atopic dermatitis. J. Dermatol. Sci. *30*, 142-153.

Hol,J., van Leer,E.H., Elink Schuurman,B.E., de Ruiter,L.F., Samsom,J.N., Hop,W., Neijens,H.J., de Jongste,J.C., and Nieuwenhuis,E.E. (2008). The acquisition of tolerance toward cow's milk through probiotic supplementation: a randomized, controlled trial. J. Allergy Clin. Immunol. *121*, 1448-1454.

Hsu,C.K., Akiyama,M., and Shimizu,H. (2008). Filaggrin: an emerging star in atopic march. J. Formos. Med. Assoc. *107*, 429-431.

Huang,C.H., Kuo,I.C., Xu,H., Lee,Y.S., and Chua,K.Y. (2003a). Mite allergen induces allergic dermatitis with concomitant neurogenic inflammation in mouse. J. Invest Dermatol. *121*, 289-293.

Huang,C.H., Kuo,I.C., Xu,H., Lee,Y.S., and Chua,K.Y. (2003b). Mite allergen induces allergic dermatitis with concomitant neurogenic inflammation in mouse. J. Invest Dermatol. *121*, 289-293.

Huurre,A., Laitinen,K., Rautava,S., Korkeamaki,M., and Isolauri,E. (2008). Impact of maternal atopy and probiotic supplementation during pregnancy on infant sensitization: a double-blind placebo-controlled study. Clin. Exp. Allergy *38*, 1342-1348.

Illi,S., von,M.E., Lau,S., Nickel,R., Gruber,C., Niggemann,B., and Wahn,U. (2004). The natural course of atopic dermatitis from birth to age 7 years and the association with asthma. J. Allergy Clin. Immunol. *113*, 925-931.

Inoue,R., Otsuka,M., Nishio,A., and Ushida,K. (2007). Primary administration of Lactobacillus johnsonii NCC533 in weaning period suppresses the elevation of proinflammatory cytokines and CD86 gene expressions in skin lesions in NC/Nga mice. FEMS Immunol Med. Microbiol. *50*, 67-76.

Iovieno,A., Lambiase,A., Sacchetti,M., Stampachiacchiere,B., Micera,A., and Bonini,S. (2008). Preliminary evidence of the efficacy of probiotic eye-drop treatment in patients with vernal keratoconjunctivitis. Graefes Arch. Clin. Exp. Ophthalmol. *246*, 435-441.

Isolauri,E., Arvola,T., Sutas,Y., Moilanen,E., and Salminen,S. (2000). Probiotics in the management of atopic eczema. Clin. Exp. Allergy *30*, 1604-1610.

Jin,H., He,R., Oyoshi,M., and Geha,R.S. (2009). Animal models of atopic dermatitis. J. Invest Dermatol. *129*, 31-40.

Kalliomaki,M., Antoine,J.M., Herz,U., Rijkers,G.T., Wells,J.M., and Mercenier,A. (2010). Guidance for substantiating the evidence for beneficial effects of probiotics: prevention and management of allergic diseases by probiotics. J. Nutr. *140*, 713S-721S.

Kalliomaki,M., Salminen,S., Arvilommi,H., Kero,P., Koskinen,P., and Isolauri,E. (2001). Probiotics in primary prevention of atopic disease: a randomised placebo-controlled trial. Lancet *357*, 1076-1079.

Kalliomaki,M., Salminen,S., Poussa,T., Arvilommi,H., and Isolauri,E. (2003). Probiotics and prevention of atopic disease: 4-year follow-up of a randomised placebo-controlled trial. Lancet *361*, 1869-1871.

Kalliomaki,M., Salminen,S., Poussa,T., and Isolauri,E. (2007). Probiotics during the first 7 years of life: a cumulative risk reduction of eczema in a randomized, placebo-controlled trial. J. Allergy Clin. Immunol. *119*, 1019-1021.

Karczewski,J., Troost,F.J., Konings,I., Dekker,J., Kleerebezem,M., Brummer,R.J., and Wells,J.M. (2010). Regulation of human epithelial tight junction proteins by Lactobacillus plantarum in vivo and protective effects on the epithelial barrier. Am. J. Physiol Gastrointest. Liver Physiol *298*, G851-G859.

Kawai,T. and Akira,S. (2010). The role of pattern-recognition receptors in innate immunity: update on Toll-like receptors. Nat. Immunol. *11*, 373-384.

Kelly,D., King,T., and Aminov,R. (2007). Importance of microbial colonization of the gut in early life to the development of immunity. Mutat. Res. *622*, 58-69.

Kim,J.Y., Kwon,J.H., Ahn,S.H., Lee,S.I., Han,Y.S., Choi,Y.O., Lee,S.Y., Ahn,K.M., and Ji,G.E. (2010). Effect of probiotic mix (Bifidobacterium bifidum, Bifidobacterium lactis, Lactobacillus acidophilus) in the primary prevention of eczema: a double-blind, randomized, placebo-controlled trial. Pediatr. Allergy Immunol. *21*, e386-e393.

Kirjavainen,P.V., Arvola,T., Salminen,S.J., and Isolauri,E. (2002). Aberrant composition of gut microbiota of allergic infants: a target of bifidobacterial therapy at weaning? Gut *51*, 51-55.

Kirjavainen,P.V., Salminen,S.J., and Isolauri,E. (2003). Probiotic bacteria in the management of atopic disease: underscoring the importance of viability. J. Pediatr. Gastroenterol. Nutr. *36*, 223-227.

Konishi,H., Tsutsui,H., Murakami,T., Yumikura-Futatsugi,S., Yamanaka,K., Tanaka,M., Iwakura,Y., Suzuki,N., Takeda,K., Akira,S., Nakanishi,K., and Mizutani,H. (2002). IL-18 contributes to the spontaneous development of atopic dermatitis-like inflammatory skin lesion independently of IgE/stat6 under specific pathogen-free conditions. Proc. Natl. Acad. Sci. U. S. A *99*, 11340-11345.

Kopp,M.V., Hennemuth,I., Heinzmann,A., and Urbanek,R. (2008). Randomized, double-blind, placebo-controlled trial of probiotics for primary prevention: no clinical effects of Lactobacillus GG supplementation. Pediatrics *121*, e850-e856.

Kuitunen,M., Kukkonen,K., Juntunen-Backman,K., Korpela,R., Poussa,T., Tuure,T., Haahtela,T., and Savilahti,E. (2009). Probiotics prevent IgE-associated allergy until age 5 years in cesarean-delivered children but not in the total cohort. J. Allergy Clin. Immunol. *123*, 335-341.

Kukkonen,K., Kuitunen,M., Haahtela,T., Korpela,R., Poussa,T., and Savilahti,E. (2010). High intestinal IgA associates with reduced risk of IgE-associated allergic diseases. Pediatr. Allergy Immunol. *21*, 67-73.

Kukkonen,K., Savilahti,E., Haahtela,T., Juntunen-Backman,K., Korpela,R., Poussa,T., Tuure,T., and Kuitunen,M. (2007). Probiotics and prebiotic galacto-oligosaccharides in the prevention of allergic diseases: a randomized, double-blind, placebo-controlled trial. J Allergy Clin. Immunol *119*, 192-198.

Kukkonen,K., Savilahti,E., Haahtela,T., Juntunen-Backman,K., Korpela,R., Poussa,T., Tuure,T., and Kuitunen,M. (2008). Long-term safety and impact on infection rates of postnatal probiotic and prebiotic (synbiotic) treatment: randomized, double-blind, placebo-controlled trial. Pediatrics *122*, 8-12.

Laouini,D., Kawamoto,S., Yalcindag,A., Bryce,P., Mizoguchi,E., Oettgen,H., and Geha,R.S. (2003). Epicutaneous sensitization with superantigen induces allergic skin inflammation. J. Allergy Clin. Immunol. *112*, 981-987.

Laubereau,B., Filipiak-Pittroff,B., von Berg,A., Grubl,A., Reinhardt,D., Wichmann,H.E., and Koletzko,S. (2004). Caesarean section and gastrointestinal symptoms, atopic dermatitis, and sensitisation during the first year of life. Arch. Dis. Child *89*, 993-997.

Lebeer,S., Vanderleyden,J., and De Keersmaecker,S.C. (2010). Host interactions of probiotic bacterial surface molecules: comparison with commensals and pathogens. Nat. Rev. Microbiol. *8*, 171-184.

Li,M., Messaddeq,N., Teletin,M., Pasquali,J.L., Metzger,D., and Chambon,P. (2005). Retinoid X receptor ablation in adult mouse keratinocytes generates an atopic dermatitis triggered by thymic stromal lymphopoietin. Proc. Natl. Acad. Sci. U. S. A *102*, 14795-14800.

Li,X.M., Kleiner,G., Huang,C.K., Lee,S.Y., Schofield,B., Soter,N.A., and Sampson,H.A. (2001). Murine model of atopic dermatitis associated with food hypersensitivity. J. Allergy Clin. Immunol. *107,* 693-702.

Madsen,K., Cornish,A., Soper,P., McKaigney,C., Jijon,H., Yachimec,C., Doyle,J., Jewell,L., and De Simone,C. (2001). Probiotic bacteria enhance murine and human intestinal epithelial barrier function. Gastroenterology *121,* 580-591.

Majamaa,H. and Isolauri,E. (1997). Probiotics: a novel approach in the management of food allergy. J. Allergy Clin. Immunol. *99,* 179-185.

Man,M.Q., Hatano,Y., Lee,S.H., Man,M., Chang,S., Feingold,K.R., Leung,D.Y., Holleran,W., Uchida,Y., and Elias,P.M. (2008). Characterization of a hapten-induced, murine model with multiple features of atopic dermatitis: structural, immunologic, and biochemical changes following single versus multiple oxazolone challenges. J. Invest Dermatol. *128,* 79-86.

Marco,M.L., Peters,T.H., Bongers,R.S., Molenaar,D., van,H.S., Sonnenburg,J.L., Gordon,J.I., and Kleerebezem,M. (2009). Lifestyle of Lactobacillus plantarum in the mouse caecum. Environ. Microbiol. *11,* 2747-2757.

Marsella,R. (2009). Evaluation of Lactobacillus rhamnosus strain GG for the prevention of atopic dermatitis in dogs. Am. J. Vet. Res. *70,* 735-740.

Marsella,R. and Girolomoni,G. (2009). Canine models of atopic dermatitis: a useful tool with untapped potential. J. Invest Dermatol. *129,* 2351-2357.

Martindale,S., McNeill,G., Devereux,G., Campbell,D., Russell,G., and Seaton,A. (2005). Antioxidant intake in pregnancy in relation to wheeze and eczema in the first two years of life. Am. J. Respir. Crit Care Med. *171,* 121-128.

Matsuda,H., Watanabe,N., Geba,G.P., Sperl,J., Tsudzuki,M., Hiroi,J., Matsumoto,M., Ushio,H., Saito,S., Askenase,P.W., and Ra,C. (1997). Development of atopic dermatitis-like skin lesion with IgE hyperproduction in NC/Nga mice. Int Immunol *9,* 461-466.

Matsumoto,K., Mizukoshi,K., Oyobikawa,M., Ohshima,H., and Tagami,H. (2004). Establishment of an atopic dermatitis-like skin model in a hairless mouse by repeated elicitation of contact hypersensitivity that enables to conduct functional analyses of the stratum corneum with various non-invasive biophysical instruments. Skin Res. Technol. *10,* 122-129.

Meijerink,M., van,H.S., Taverne,N., Wels,M., de,V.P., Bron,P.A., Savelkoul,H.F., van,B.J., Kleerebezem,M., and Wells,J.M. (2010). Identification of genetic loci in Lactobacillus plantarum that modulate the immune response of dendritic cells using comparative genome hybridization. PLoS. ONE. *5,* e10632.

Mercenier,A., Lenoir-Wijnkoop,I., and Sanders,M.E. (2008). Physiological and Functional Properties of Probiotics. Bulletin of International Dairy Federation.

Metchnikoff,E. (1908). Optimistic studies. Putman's Sons 161-183.

Miniello,V.L., Brunetti,L., Tesse,R., Natile,M., Armenio,L., and Francavilla,R. (2010). Lactobacillus reuteri modulates cytokines production in exhaled breath condensate of children with atopic dermatitis. J. Pediatr. Gastroenterol. Nutr. *50,* 573-576.

Mohamadzadeh,M., Olson,S., Kalina,W.V., Ruthel,G., Demmin,G.L., Warfield,K.L., Bavari,S., and Klaenhammer,T.R. (2005). Lactobacilli activate human dendritic cells that skew T cells toward T helper 1 polarization. Proc. Natl. Acad. Sci. U. S. A *102,* 2880-2885.

Mohamadzadeh,M., Pfeiler,E.A., Brown,J.B., Zadeh,M., Gramarossa,M., Managlia,E., Bere,P., Sarraj,B., Khan,M.W., Pakanati,K.C., Ansari,M.J., O'Flaherty,S., Barrett,T., and Klaenhammer,T.R. (2011). Regulation of induced colonic inflammation by Lactobacillus acidophilus deficient in lipoteichoic acid. Proc. Natl. Acad. Sci. U. S. A *108 Suppl 1*, 4623-4630.

Morisset,M., Aubert-Jacquin,C., Soulaines,P., Moneret-Vautrin,D.A., and Dupont,C. (2011). A non-hydrolyzed, fermented milk formula reduces digestive and respiratory events in infants at high risk of allergy. Eur. J. Clin. Nutr. *65*, 175-183.

Moroi,M., Uchi,S., Nakamura,K., Sato,S., Shimizu,N., Fujii,M., Kumagai,T., Saito,M., Uchiyama,K., Watanabe,T., Yamaguchi,H., Yamamoto,T., Takeuchi,S., and Furue,M. (2011). Beneficial effect of a diet containing heat-killed Lactobacillus paracasei K71 on adult type atopic dermatitis. J. Dermatol. *38*, 131-139.

Nagelkerken,L., Verzaal,P., Lagerweij,T., Persoon-Deen,C., Berbee,J.F., Prens,E.P., Havekes,L.M., and Oranje,A.P. (2008). Development of atopic dermatitis in mice transgenic for human apolipoprotein C1. J. Invest Dermatol. *128*, 1165-1172.

Negele,K., Heinrich,J., Borte,M., von Berg,A., Schaaf,B., Lehmann,I., Wichmann,H.E., and Bolte,G. (2004). Mode of delivery and development of atopic disease during the first 2 years of life. Pediatr. Allergy Immunol. *15*, 48-54.

Nermes,M., Kantele,J.M., Atosuo,T.J., Salminen,S., and Isolauri,E. (2011). Interaction of orally administered Lactobacillus rhamnosus GG with skin and gut microbiota and humoral immunity in infants with atopic dermatitis. Clin. Exp. Allergy *41*, 370-377.

Niers,L., Martin,R., Rijkers,G., Sengers,F., Timmerman,H., van,U.N., Smidt,H., Kimpen,J., and Hoekstra,M. (2009). The effects of selected probiotic strains on the development of eczema (the PandA study). Allergy *64*, 1349-1358.

Niers,L.E., Hoekstra,M.O., Timmerman,H.M., van Uden,N.O., de Graaf,P.M., Smits,H.H., Kimpen,J.L., and Rijkers,G.T. (2007). Selection of probiotic bacteria for prevention of allergic diseases: immunomodulation of neonatal dendritic cells. Clin. Exp. Immunol. *149*, 344-352.

Nomoto,K. (2005). Prevention of infections by probiotics. J. Biosci. Bioeng. *100*, 583-592.

Nova,E., Warnberg,J., Gomez-Martinez,S., Diaz,L.E., Romeo,J., and Marcos,A. (2007). Immunomodulatory effects of probiotics in different stages of life. Br. J. Nutr. *98 Suppl 1*, S90-S95.

O'Hara,A.M. and Shanahan,F. (2007). Mechanisms of action of probiotics in intestinal diseases. ScientificWorldJournal. *7*, 31-46.

Ohland,C.L. and MacNaughton,W.K. (2010). Probiotic bacteria and intestinal epithelial barrier function. Am. J. Physiol Gastrointest. Liver Physiol *298*, G807-G819.

Ortiz-Andrellucchi,A., Sanchez-Villegas,A., Rodriguez-Gallego,C., Lemes,A., Molero,T., Soria,A., Pena-Quintana,L., Santana,M., Ramirez,O., Garcia,J., Cabrera,F., Cobo,J., and Serra-Majem,L. (2008). Immunomodulatory effects of the intake of fermented milk with Lactobacillus casei DN114001 in lactating mothers and their children. Br. J. Nutr. 1-12.

Parvez,S., Malik,K.A., Ah,K.S., and Kim,H.Y. (2006). Probiotics and their fermented food products are beneficial for health. J. Appl. Microbiol. *100*, 1171-1185.

Passeron,T., Lacour,J.P., Fontas,E., and Ortonne,J.P. (2006). Prebiotics and synbiotics: two promising approaches for the treatment of atopic dermatitis in children above 2 years. Allergy *61,* 431-437.

Penders,J., Stobberingh,E.E., van den Brandt,P.A., and Thijs,C. (2007). The role of the intestinal microbiota in the development of atopic disorders. Allergy *62,* 1223-1236.

Perea,V.M., Verhoeven,T.L., Draing,C., Von,A.S., Pfitzenmaier,M., Geyer,A., Lambrichts,I., Grangette,C., Pot,B., Vanderleyden,J., and De Keersmaecker,S.C. (2007). Functional analysis of D-alanylation of lipoteichoic acid in the probiotic strain Lactobacillus rhamnosus GG. Appl. Environ. Microbiol. *73,* 3595-3604.

Peserico,A., Stadtler,G., Sebastian,M., Fernandez,R.S., Vick,K., and Bieber,T. (2008). Reduction of relapses of atopic dermatitis with methylprednisolone aceponate cream twice weekly in addition to maintenance treatment with emollient: a multicentre, randomized, double-blind, controlled study. Br. J. Dermatol. *158,* 801-807.

Prescott,S.L. and Bjorksten,B. (2007). Probiotics for the prevention or treatment of allergic diseases. J. Allergy Clin. Immunol. *120,* 255-262.

Rachmilewitz,D., Karmeli,F., Takabayashi,K., Hayashi,T., Leider-Trejo,L., Lee,J., Leoni,L.M., and Raz,E. (2002). Immunostimulatory DNA ameliorates experimental and spontaneous murine colitis. Gastroenterology *122,* 1428-1441.

Rachmilewitz,D., Katakura,K., Karmeli,F., Hayashi,T., Reinus,C., Rudensky,B., Akira,S., Takeda,K., Lee,J., Takabayashi,K., and Raz,E. (2004). Toll-like receptor 9 signaling mediates the anti-inflammatory effects of probiotics in murine experimental colitis. Gastroenterology *126,* 520-528.

Rautava,S., Kalliomaki,M., and Isolauri,E. (2002). Probiotics during pregnancy and breast-feeding might confer immunomodulatory protection against atopic disease in the infant. J. Allergy Clin. Immunol. *109,* 119-121.

Resta-Lenert,S. and Barrett,K.E. (2003). Live probiotics protect intestinal epithelial cells from the effects of infection with enteroinvasive Escherichia coli (EIEC). Gut *52,* 988-997.

Roessler,A., Friedrich,U., Vogelsang,H., Bauer,A., Kaatz,M., Hipler,U.C., Schmidt,I., and Jahreis,G. (2008). The immune system in healthy adults and patients with atopic dermatitis seems to be affected differently by a probiotic intervention. Clin. Exp. Allergy *38,* 93-102.

Rosenfeldt,V., Benfeldt,E., Nielsen,S.D., Michaelsen,K.F., Jeppesen,D.L., Valerius,N.H., and Paerregaard,A. (2003). Effect of probiotic Lactobacillus strains in children with atopic dermatitis. J. Allergy Clin. Immunol. *111,* 389-395.

Salminen,S. and Gueimonde,M. (2005). Gut microbiota in infants between 6 and 24 months of age. Nestle. Nutr. Workshop Ser. Pediatr. Program. *56,* 43-51.

Salminen,S.J., Gueimonde,M., and Isolauri,E. (2005). Probiotics that modify disease risk. J. Nutr. *135,* 1294-1298.

Sanders,M.E. (2008). Use of probiotics and yogurts in maintenance of health. J. Clin. Gastroenterol. *42 Suppl 2,* S71-S74.

Santosa,S., Farnworth,E., and Jones,P.J. (2006). Probiotics and their potential health claims. Nutr. Rev. *64,* 265-274.

Sawada,J., Morita,H., Tanaka,A., Salminen,S., He,F., and Matsuda,H. (2007). Ingestion of heat-treated Lactobacillus rhamnosus GG prevents development of atopic dermatitis in NC/Nga mice. Clin. Exp. Allergy *37,* 296-303.

Schaub,B., Lauener,R., and von Mutius,E. (2006). The many faces of the hygiene hypothesis. J. Allergy Clin. Immunol. *117*, 969-977.

Segawa,S., Hayashi,A., Nakakita,Y., Kaneda,H., Watari,J., and Yasui,H. (2008). Oral administration of heat-killed Lactobacillus brevis SBC8803 ameliorates the development of dermatitis and inhibits immunoglobulin E production in atopic dermatitis model NC/Nga mice. Biol. Pharm. Bull. *31*, 884-889.

Sicherer,S.H. and Burks,A.W. (2008). Maternal and infant diets for prevention of allergic diseases: understanding menu changes in 2008. J. Allergy Clin. Immunol. *122*, 29-33.

Sistek,D., Kelly,R., Wickens,K., Stanley,T., Fitzharris,P., and Crane,J. (2006). Is the effect of probiotics on atopic dermatitis confined to food sensitized children? Clin. Exp. Allergy *36*, 629-633.

Sjogren,Y.M., Tomicic,S., Lundberg,A., Bottcher,M.F., Bjorksten,B., Sverremark-Ekstrom,E., and Jenmalm,M.C. (2009). Influence of early gut microbiota on the maturation of childhood mucosal and systemic immune responses. Clin. Exp. Allergy *39*, 1842-1851.

Soh,S.E., Aw,M., Gerez,I., Chong,Y.S., Rauff,M., Ng,Y.P., Wong,H.B., Pai,N., Lee,B.W., and Shek,L.P. (2009). Probiotic supplementation in the first 6 months of life in at risk Asian infants--effects on eczema and atopic sensitization at the age of 1 year. Clin. Exp. Allergy *39*, 571-578.

Spergel,J.M., Mizoguchi,E., Brewer,J.P., Martin,T.R., Bhan,A.K., and Geha,R.S. (1998). Epicutaneous sensitization with protein antigen induces localized allergic dermatitis and hyperresponsiveness to methacholine after single exposure to aerosolized antigen in mice. J. Clin. Invest *101*, 1614-1622.

Spergel,J.M. and Paller,A.S. (2003). Atopic dermatitis and the atopic march. J. Allergy Clin. Immunol. *112*, S118-S127.

Suzuki,Y., Kodama,M., and Asano,K. (2011). Skin barrier-related molecules and pathophysiology of asthma. Allergol. Int. *60*, 11-15.

Tanaka,A., Fukushima,Y., Benyacoub,J., Blum,S., and Matsuda,H. (2008). Prophylactic effect of oral administration of Lactobacillus johnsonii NCC533 (La1) during the weaning period on atopic dermatitis in NC/NgaTnd mice. Eur. J. Dermatol. *18*, 136-140.

Tanaka,A., Jung,K., Benyacoub,J., Prioult,G., Okamoto,N., Ohmori,K., Blum,S., Mercenier,A., and Matsuda,H. (2009). Oral supplementation with Lactobacillus rhamnosus CGMCC 1.3724 prevents development of atopic dermatitis in NC/NgaTnd mice possibly by modulating local production of IFN-gamma. Exp. Dermatol. *18*, 1022-1027.

Taylor,A.L., Dunstan,J.A., and Prescott,S.L. (2007). Probiotic supplementation for the first 6 months of life fails to reduce the risk of atopic dermatitis and increases the risk of allergen sensitization in high-risk children: a randomized controlled trial. J. Allergy Clin. Immunol. *119*, 184-191.

Tissier,H. (1906). CR. Soc Biol *60*, 359.

Torii,S., Torii,A., Itoh,K., Urisu,A., Terada,A., Fujisawa,T., Yamada,K., Suzuki,H., Ishida,Y., Nakamura,F., Kanzato,H., Sawada,D., Nonaka,A., Hatanaka,M., and Fujiwara,S. (2011). Effects of oral administration of Lactobacillus acidophilus L-92 on the symptoms and serum markers of atopic dermatitis in children. Int. Arch. Allergy Immunol. *154*, 236-245.

Tsukuba,T., Okamoto,K., Okamoto,Y., Yanagawa,M., Kohmura,K., Yasuda,Y., Uchi,H., Nakahara,T., Furue,M., Nakayama,K., Kadowaki,T., Yamamoto,K., and Nakayama,K.I. (2003). Association of cathepsin E deficiency with development of atopic dermatitis. J. Biochem. *134*, 893-902.

Ulluwishewa,D., Anderson,R.C., McNabb,W.C., Moughan,P.J., Wells,J.M., and Roy,N.C. (2011). Regulation of tight junction permeability by intestinal bacteria and dietary components. J. Nutr. *141*, 769-776.

Vael,C. and Desager,K. (2009). The importance of the development of the intestinal microbiota in infancy. Curr. Opin. Pediatr. *21*, 794-800.

van der Aa,L.B., Heymans,H.S., van Aalderen,W.M., Sillevis Smitt,J.H., Knol,J., Ben,A.K., Goossens,D.A., and Sprikkelman,A.B. (2010). Effect of a new synbiotic mixture on atopic dermatitis in infants: a randomized-controlled trial. Clin. Exp. Allergy *40*, 795-804.

Vesterlund,S., Karp,M., Salminen,S., and Ouwehand,A.C. (2006). Staphylococcus aureus adheres to human intestinal mucus but can be displaced by certain lactic acid bacteria. Microbiology *152*, 1819-1826.

Viljanen,M., Savilahti,E., Haahtela,T., Juntunen-Backman,K., Korpela,R., Poussa,T., Tuure,T., and Kuitunen,M. (2005). Probiotics in the treatment of atopic eczema/dermatitis syndrome in infants: a double-blind placebo-controlled trial. Allergy *60*, 494-500.

Waser,M., Michels,K.B., Bieli,C., Floistrup,H., Pershagen,G., von Mutius,E., Ege,M., Riedler,J., Schram-Bijkerk,D., Brunekreef,B., van Hage,M., Lauener,R., and Braun-Fahrlander,C. (2007). Inverse association of farm milk consumption with asthma and allergy in rural and suburban populations across Europe. Clin. Exp. Allergy *37*, 661-670.

Wells, J. M. Immunomodulatory mechanisms of lactobacilli. Microbial Cell Factories . 2011. 10(S1):S17.

Wells,J.M., Loonen,L.M., and Karczewski,J.M. (2010). The role of innate signaling in the homeostasis of tolerance and immunity in the intestine. Int. J. Med. Microbiol. *300*, 41-48.

Wells,J.M., Rossi,O., Meijerink,M., and Van Baarlen,P. (2011). Epithelial crosstalk at the microbiota-mucosal interface. Proc. Natl. Acad. Sci. U. S. A *108 Suppl 1*, 4607-4614.

West,C.E., Hammarstrom,M.L., and Hernell,O. (2009). Probiotics during weaning reduce the incidence of eczema. Pediatr. Allergy Immunol. *20*, 430-437.

Weston,S., Halbert,A., Richmond,P., and Prescott,S.L. (2005). Effects of probiotics on atopic dermatitis: a randomised controlled trial. Arch. Dis. Child *90*, 892-897.

Wickens,K., Black,P.N., Stanley,T.V., Mitchell,E., Fitzharris,P., Tannock,G.W., Purdie,G., and Crane,J. (2008). A differential effect of 2 probiotics in the prevention of eczema and atopy: A double-blind, randomized, placebo-controlled trial. J. Allergy Clin. Immunol.

Williams,H., Robertson,C., Stewart,A., Ait-Khaled,N., Anabwani,G., Anderson,R., Asher,I., Beasley,R., Bjorksten,B., Burr,M., Clayton,T., Crane,J., Ellwood,P., Keil,U., Lai,C., Mallol,J., Martinez,F., Mitchell,E., Montefort,S., Pearce,N., Shah,J., Sibbald,B., Strachan,D., von,M.E., and Weiland,S.K. (1999). Worldwide variations in the prevalence of symptoms of atopic eczema in the International Study of Asthma and Allergies in Childhood. J. Allergy Clin. Immunol. *103*, 125-138.

Won,T.J., Kim,B., Lim,Y.T., Song,D.S., Park,S.Y., Park,E.S., Lee,D.I., and Hwang,K.W. (2011). Oral administration of Lactobacillus strains from Kimchi inhibits atopic dermatitis in NC / Nga mice. J. Appl. Microbiol. *110,* 1195-1202.

Woo,S.I., Kim,J.Y., Lee,Y.J., Kim,N.S., and Hahn,Y.S. (2010). Effect of Lactobacillus sakei supplementation in children with atopic eczema-dermatitis syndrome. Ann. Allergy Asthma Immunol. *104,* 343-348.

Yoo,J., Omori,M., Gyarmati,D., Zhou,B., Aye,T., Brewer,A., Comeau,M.R., Campbell,D.J., and Ziegler,S.F. (2005). Spontaneous atopic dermatitis in mice expressing an inducible thymic stromal lymphopoietin transgene specifically in the skin. J. Exp. Med. *202,* 541-549.

Zareie,M., Johnson-Henry,K.C., Jury,J., Yang,P.C., Ngan,B.Y., McKay,D.M., Soderholm,J.D., Perdue,M.H., and Sherman,P.M. (2006). Probiotics prevent bacterial translocation and improve intestinal barrier function in rats following chronic psychological stress. Gut.

Zheng,T., Yu,J., Oh,M.H., and Zhu,Z. (2011). The atopic march: progression from atopic dermatitis to allergic rhinitis and asthma. Allergy Asthma Immunol. Res. *3,* 67-73.

Zutavern,A., Brockow,I., Schaaf,B., Bolte,G., von Berg,A., Diez,U., Borte,M., Herbarth,O., Wichmann,H.E., and Heinrich,J. (2006). Timing of solid food introduction in relation to atopic dermatitis and atopic sensitization: results from a prospective birth cohort study. Pediatrics *117,* 401-411.

21

The Role of Probiotics in Atopic Dermatitis Prevention and Therapy

Öner Özdemir
Republic of Turkey, Ministry of Health, İstanbul Medeniyet University
Göztepe Research / Training Hospital
Turkey

1. Introduction

Development of the child's immune system tends to be directed toward a T-helper 2 (Th2) phenotype in infants, whereas postnatal maturation is associated with gradual inhibition of Th2 and increasing Th1 affinity [1]. Thus, immature Th2-dominant neonatal responses must undergo environment-driven maturation via microbial contact in the early postnatal period to prevent development of childhood allergic diseases. Nevertheless, nowadays the increased use of antimicrobial medication, the consumption of sterile food, and reduced family size that result in lower rates of infection during childhood also reduce early contact to microbes. Consequentially, at an early age the infant`s immune system results in subsequent polarization toward a Th2 phenotype during postnatal maturation. Among several other phenomena, the present increase in allergic diseases seen in the industrialized countries has been attributed, to a relative lack of microbial stimulation of the infantile gut immune system and the exaggerated hygiene of the typical western lifestyle during early childhood. And this is known as the hygiene hypothesis [2].

The newborn is first colonized by microbes at birth. The colonization of the gut that begins promptly after birth is affected by mode of delivery, early feeding strategies and the hygienic conditions around the child (the early environment). The colonizing bacteria originate mainly from the mother's gut and vaginal tract [3]. For instance, children born by cesarean section are colonized with Bifidobacteria and Lactobacilli later than vaginally delivered children, and are shown to have more frequent respiratory allergies [4]. After delivery, breastfeeding continues to enhance the original inoculum by the introduction of specific lactic acid bacteria, Bifidobacteria and bacteria from the mother's skin, all of which enable the infant gut microbiota that is dominated by Bifidobacteria. Breast milk also contains plentiful indigestible oligosaccharides, which pass through the whole intestine and promote the growth and activity of commensal bacteria; composed mainly of Bifidobacteria [5]. These bacteria set the basis for gut microbiota development and modulation, along with environmental exposures such as antibiotic administration.

The greatest differences between breast-fed and formula-fed infants appear to be in lactic acid bacteria and Bifidobacteria colonization. Usually, Bifidobacteria appear after birth and, within a week, are reported as the dominant bacterial group, with Bifidobacterium (Bfdbm) infantis / longum / breve being the most common species in breast-fed infants [6]. In addition, Lactobacillus (Lctbs) acidophilus is the most common Lctbs in the feces of breast-

fed infants. Formula-fed infants, on the other hand, tend to have a flora that is more complex, consisting mostly of Coliforms and Bacteroides, with significantly lower the prevalence of Bifidobacteria [7]. After weaning, the microflora of children begins to resemble that of adults, with increased Bacteroides, Veillonella, and Fusobacterium [8].
Epidemiologic data showed that atopic children have a different intestinal flora from that of healthy ones, with higher levels of Clostridia and lower levels of Bifidobacteria. Furthermore, other studies have also shown that early colonization with potentially more pathogenic bacteria such as Clostridium difficile and Staph. aureus is more likely to occur in children who go on to develop allergy. In contrast, lactic acid bacteria and Bifidobacteria are found more commonly in the composition of the intestinal flora of non-allergic children. The enhanced presence of these probiotic bacteria in the intestinal microbiota seems to correlate with protection against atopy [9,10]. Based on these data, "harmless" microbial agents that are probiotics have been presently tested for their efficacy in the prevention and therapy of allergy in infants [11-14].
The interest in probiotic therapeutic potential in allergic disorders stemmed from the fact that they have been shown to improve intestinal permeability and reduce inflammatory cytokines. Such effects would be desirable in treating allergic disorders including atopic dermatitis (AD). Therefore, several studies have been designed to examine the efficacy of probiotics in many allergic conditions, such as eczema and food allergies [13,14]. Including the first publication in 1997, over 30 randomized, double-blind, placebo-controlled clinical trials have been conducted to study the effects of various probiotics on treatment and prevention of allergic diseases. In total, almost 3000 individuals (including those in placebo groups) have participated in these studies so far. In the first-time study done by Majamaa and Isolauri in 1997, the administration of LGG to highly selected patients (age <2 years, challenge-proven cow's milk allergy, and mild-to- moderate eczema) significantly improved the total SCORAD score [15]. Later the Finnish study of Kalliomaki was the first report to describe that the frequency of AD in neonates treated with Lctbs rhamnosus GG (LGG) was half that of the placebo [16]. However, these results recently have been questioned by other trials, which reported no difference in the development and therapy of AD in neonates supplemented with LGG or other probiotics. Therefore, an allergen-preventive or therapeutic effect of probiotics in AD could not be consistently established. The aims of this chapter are to comprehensively define probiotic properties and to characterize current knowledge of probiotics, including the key mechanisms of probiotic effects as well as their preventative/ therapeutic role in AD at last.

1.1 What are probiotics?

The year 2011 marks the 104nd year since Eli Metchnikoff suggested that the consumption of lactic acid bacteria may benefit the human host's immune system [11]. However, not until the mid-1960 did the term probiotic become the trend. Probiotics means "for life" and is defined by the World Health Organization and the Food and Agriculture Organization of the United Nations as "live microorganisms which, when administered in adequate amounts as part of food, confer a beneficial health effect by producing gut microflora on the host." These probiotics are mainly represented by lactic acid bacteria [12]. Simply; probiotics are ingested live microbes that can modify intestinal microbial populations in a way that benefits the host.

Characteristics of probiotics

There are several generally accepted characteristics that define probiotic bacteria. Probiotics:

- are microbial organisms;

- remain viable and stable after culture, manipulation, and storage before utilization;
- survive gastric, biliary, and pancreatic digestion;
- are able to induce a host response once they enter the intestinal microbial ecosystem; and
- yield a functional or clinical benefit to the host when consumed [10-16].

1.2 Atopic dermatitis (eczema)

Atopic dermatitis (AD) is the most common chronic skin condition in infants and children, with a prevalence of 10- 20% in population. Geographic location affects the prevalence of this disease, with the highest prevalence in the United States and Europe [17]. Important factors in the susceptibility to develop AD include a genetic basis and environmental factors. Eczema refers to a chronic or relapsing itchy skin inflammation with typical lesions and locations. AD has been linked to food hypersensitivity, especially milk and egg proteins. However, 40-60% of children with AD may not develop IgE sensitization [18]. The term eczema has been recently proposed, but for practical purposes, both AD and eczema will be used in this chapter.

There have been several proposed methods for classifying the severity of AD in various research studies mentioned in this chapter, but only the Scoring of AD Severity Index (SCORAD), established by the European Task Force on AD, has been validated for reproducibility and accuracy in assessing therapeutic response [17,18]. The SCORAD combines objective measures, such as extent and severity of skin lesions, and subjective criteria, such as pruritus and sleep loss. Children with AD can be further classified as having mild: (≤25), moderate: (25-50), or severe: (≥50) disease based on their SCORAD score.

2. Experimental and clinical essentials of preventative and therapeutic probiotic use in AD

As briefly mentioned above, there is a good experimental and clinical theoretical basis for using probiotics in the prevention and therapy of AD. Germ-free animal models demonstrate that bacterial gut colonization is essential for maturation of immune function and induction of oral tolerance. It has been proposed that a similar but more subtle process may be occurring in human beings with progressively cleaner environments. Probiotic intestinal flora is arguably the most abundant source of early immune stimulation and contributes significantly to microbial burden in early life. A number of studies have suggested differences in the early colonization patterns of infants who go on to develop allergic disease. These studies strongly suggest that the pattern of colonization in the first weeks of life may influence the patterns of immune development [19,20]. These notions have been supported by observations that gut flora can influence local and systemic immune responses. There has been speculation that intestinal flora may influence the maturing precursor cells that circulate through the gut before they home to other tissues. This may explain how probiotic species can influence systemic immune responses and IgA production in distal sites, such as the respiratory tract. Together with reported clinical effects in early allergic disease, this has logically led to a growing interest in the role of probiotics in allergy prevention [13,14].

The gastrointestinal tract of the newborn baby is sterile. Soon after birth, however, it is colonized by many different microorganisms. Colonization is complete after around one week, but the numbers and species of intestinal bacteria fluctuate markedly during the first several months of life. The composition of the gut microbiota differs between healthy and allergic infants and even in countries with a high and low prevalence of allergies [21]. Mode of delivery, either vaginal or through caesarean section, also has a major impact on early colonization patterns of the infant gut [4]. In the case of allergy, the rationale for modulating the intestinal microbiota is supported by observations that allergic children have a different microbiota composition than healthy infants. The main changes associated with allergic trait are less frequent colonization with Lactobacilli and lower counts of Bifidobacteria [9,22]. In addition to these quantitative differences in the Bfdbm microbiota, qualitative differences have also been observed. Infants with AD have been found to have a more adult type Bfdbm microbiota with high prevalence of Bfdbm adolescentis. Healthy infants, on the other hand, were found to be colonized mainly by Bfdbm bifidum, typical for breast-fed infants [7,8]. The Bifidobacteria from infants with AD were found to induce a higher secretion of proinflammatory cytokines in vitro, whereas the Bifidobacteria from healthy infants induced the secretion of more antiinflammatory cytokines. Also, Bifidobacteria of dairy origin stimulated more antiinflammatory and less inflammatory cytokines than Bifidobacteria from allergic infants. In addition to differing in their induction of cytokines, Bifidobacteria from allergic and healthy infants also exhibited different in vitro adhesion to Caco-2 tissue culture cells and intestinal mucus. This difference in adhesion to the intestinal mucosa may result in a different or reduced stimulation of the immune system through the gut-associated lymphoid tissue [23]. Lower counts of Bifidobacteria have been reported in atopic vs nonatopic children preceding allergen sensitization. Bifidobacteria are hypothesized to more effectively promote tolerance to nonbacterial antigens, primarily by inhibiting the development of a Th2-type (proallergic) response. In a recent study, a positive change in stool colonization in atopic infants supplemented with Bfdbm lactis has been shown with a decrease of Bacteroides and E coli in the stool. Most interestingly, serum IgE correlated with E coli counts, and in highly sensitized infants, IgE correlated with Bacteroides counts [24]. Thus, certain probiotics seem to influence the gut's allergen-stimulated inflammatory response and provide a barrier effect against antigens that might otherwise ultimately lead to systemic allergic symptoms (such as eczema).

A recent prospective study from 3 European birth cohorts found, however, no differences in gut microbiota by culture-dependent analysis of fecal samples among infants developing or not developing atopic eczema and food allergy. On the contrary, a subgroup analysis of the cohort by cultivation independent techniques indicated a significantly lower diversity in the gut microbiota of 1-week-old neonates who later manifested atopic eczema than in neonates remaining healthy during the first 18 months of life, highlighting once more that classical microbiological plating techniques are inappropriate for extensive characterization of the gut microbiota [25]. Similarly, less diverse microbial communities were found among 5-year-old allergic children than among nonallergic children by using another culture-independent technique. The same study demonstrated that Bfdbm catenulatum /pseudocatenulatum prevail in nonallergic children [26]. On the contrary, this particular Bifidobacterial species was associated with atopic eczema in a nested case-control study conducted in a different age group, country, and disease population, highlighting the complexity of the situation. As the immune modulation properties of bacteria seem to be distinctly strain specific, it cannot be ruled out that the nature of the immune response induced by a specific strain plays a more important role than its classification.

Probiotic intestinal flora contributes to microbial antigen exposure in early life and is one of the most abundant sources of early immune stimulation. Because allergic immune responses manifest early in life, there has been obvious interest in the potential benefits of modifying the gastrointestinal flora by using probiotic supplementation. However, the value of probiotics for primary prevention is controversial [13,14]. So far, there have been only several studies to address the role of probiotics in primary prevention, with a reported suspicious reduction in the incidence of eczema. The role of probiotics in allergy prevention has remained controversial, and there has been an urgent call for similar studies to address this further. This chapter will try to highlight the issues with probiotics in the therapy / prevention of AD and future of this therapy. Here, firstly newly described mechanisms of probiotic effects will be defined. Later, under the light of recent literature probiotic use in AD therapy and prevention is being discussed in detail.

2.1 Experimental (animal) and clinical (human) studies showing mechanisms of probiotics` effects in atopic diseases including eczema

Although the beneficial effects of probiotics on wide variety of atopic diseases have been suggested, little is known about how probiotics modulate the immune system and atopic disease development. Currently, only limited publications are available defining the effects of probiotics in murine or human models of AD. Therefore, it is important to explore the effect of probiotics in various experimental and clinical atopic disease models.

2.1.1 Maturing gut barrier: Probiotic regulation in intestinal epithelium and upregulation of host immune responses

Recent data indicate that commensal intestinal microbiota represents a major modulator of intestinal homeostasis. Dysregulation of the symbiotic interaction between intestinal microbiota and the mucosa may result in a pathological condition with potential clinical repercussions. For instance, it is shown that mice reared in germ-free conditions have an underdeveloped immune system and have no oral tolerance. In contrast, pathogen-free mice are capable of reconstituting the bacterial flora with Bifidobacteria and tolerance development [27].

In addition to providing maturational signals for the gut-associated lymphoid tissue, probiotics balance the generation of pro- and anti-inflammatory cytokines in the gut. After probiotic consumption, decrease in fecal α-1 antitrypsin, serum TNF-α, and changes in TGF-β and other cytokines point to down-regulation of inflammatory mediators [28]. For instance, after a challenge study in infants allergic to cow's milk, fecal IgA levels were detected to be higher and TNF-α levels were lower in the Lctbs rhamnosus GG (LGG) applied group compared to the placebo [29]. Similarly, another study by Kirjavainen et al suggested that Bfdbm lactis Bb12 might modify gut microflora to alleviate early onset atopic eczema. And this modification was found to be compatible with reductions of serum TNF-α and fecal α-1-antitrypsin levels as well as an increase in fecal IgA level [23].

Moreover, probiotic bacteria may counteract the inflammatory process by stabilizing the gut microbial environment and the permeability barrier of the intestine, and by enhancing the degradation of enteral antigens and altering their immunogenicity [30]. This gut-stabilizing effect of probiotics could be explained by the improvement by probiotics of the immunological barrier of the intestine through intestinal IgA responses, specifically [31,32]. Consistent with these explanations, in children with food allergies, probiotics are shown to reverse increased intestinal permeability and to enhance frequently defective IgA responses [33].

2.1.2 Immunomodulation: Th1/Th2 balance, IgE production and cytokines

In addition to maturing gut barrier, certain strains of Lactobacilli and Bifidobacteria modulate the production of cytokines by monocytes and lymphocytes, and may divert the immune system in a regulatory or tolerant mode [27,34]. Nonetheless, there are still some studies showing no significant effects of probiotics on either Th1 or Th2 cell responses to allergens. Although the cytokine stimulation profiles of different probiotic strains vary, the strains isolated from healthy infants mainly stimulate non-inflammatory cytokines [35]. Therefore, it seems that changes in cytokine profile induced by probiotics may be probiotic strain- or site-specific and dependent on the experimental system used. For instance, Lctbs reuteri induced proinflammatory and Th1 cytokines; and Bfdbm bifidum/infantis and Lctbs lactis reduced Th2 cytokines [36].

Several studies have shown the immunomodulatory effects of probiotic bacteria. In one study, Bfdbm bifidum / infantis and Lctbs lactis reduced Th2 cytokines and acted as potent inducers of IL-10 production in different peripheral blood mononuclear cell cultures [37]. In another study, eight common Lctbs strains were studied with respect to induction of cytokines by the murine gut mucosa in response to a parenterally administered antigen. Lctbs reuteri induced proinflammatory and Th1 cytokines; however, Lctbs casei tended to induce IL-10 / IL-4 [38]. Yet on the contrary, in some children receiving probiotics, reduced IL-10 responsiveness to house dust mites allergens was observed [39]. In a study, the effects of feeding Lctbs F19 were evaluated during weaning on the incidence of eczema and Th1/Th2 balance. In a double-blind, placebo-controlled randomized intervention trial, infants were fed cereals with (n:89) or without Lctbs F19 (n:90) from 4 to 13 months of age. At 13 months of age, the IFN-γ/ IL-4 mRNA ratio was significantly higher in the probiotic compared with the placebo group. The higher Th1/Th2 ratio in the probiotic compared with the placebo group suggests enhancing effects of Lctbs F19 on the T cell-mediated immune response. And probiotics also increased Th1 cytokines and inhibited allergen-induced IgE and Th2 cytokines in some atopic children [40,41].

In a mouse model, effect of oral probiotics administration, including Bfdbm lactis/bifidum and Lctbs acidophilus, on mice with ovalbumin (OVA)-induced food allergy was studied. The mice treated with probiotics suppressed production of the OVA-specific IgE, IgG1, and IgA. Additionally, the level of IL-4 was significantly lower, and the levels of INF-γ and IL-10 were significantly higher in the mice treated with probiotics than that in the nontreated mice [42]. Another murine model showed that oral administration of an immunostimulatory DNA sequence from Bfdbm longum suppressed Th2 immune responses in mice and inhibited IgE production in vitro [43]. A final study showed that the administration of either Bfdbm lactis Bb-12 or LGG suppressed antigen-specific IgE production too [44].

A decrease in the secretion of pro-inflammatory cytokines, IFN-γ, TNF-α and IL-12 has been demonstrated. Consistently, in an experimental study, probiotic supplementation decreased the severity of allergic skin responses in allergen-sensitized pigs with a corresponding increase in IFN-γ expression [45]. However, the study by Rosenfeldt et al. demonstrated no significant changes in serum cytokines (IL-2, IL-4, IL-10 and IFN-γ) during 6 weeks of probiotic treatment [46]. Another study by Brouwer et al. showed no statistically significant effects of probiotic supplementation on cytokine production (IL-4, IL-5 and IFN-γ) as well [47]. These results differ from those of Pohjavuori et al, who were able to demonstrate an increase of IFN-γ production in peripheral blood mononuclear cell in infants with AD treated with LGG instead of placebo [48]. Additionally, the improvement in AD severity of very young children with probiotic treatment was detected to be associated with significant

increases in the capacity for Th1 IFN-γ responses and altered responses to skin and enteric flora. This effect was still evident 2 months after the supplementation was ceased [49].
Reduction in serum soluble CD4 as a marker of T-cell activation described by Isolauri et al. They also found significant changes in indirect markers of allergic inflammation, such as sCD4 in the serum of infants with AD supplemented with Bfdbm lactis and LGG [50].
In a randomized controlled trial by Boyle et al showed that LGG treatment during pregnancy (prenatal) for the prevention of eczema was not associated with any change in cord blood immune markers such as TGF-β, IL-10, IL-12, IL-13, IFN-γ and TNF-α as well as Dendritic and Treg cell numbers [51].
Twelve human studies were included in a review and 67% showed a positive association with TGF-β1 or TGF-β2 demonstrating protection against allergy-related outcomes in infancy and early childhood. High variability in concentrations of TGF-β was noted between and within studies, some of it explained by maternal history of atopy or by consumption of probiotics. Human milk TGF-β appears to be essential in developing and maintaining appropriate immune responses in infants and may provide protection against adverse immunological outcomes, corroborating findings from experimental animal studies. In a study, aim was to evaluate the effect of probiotic supplementation on the immunological composition of breast milk and colostrum in relation to sensitization and eczema in the babies. Total IgA, secretory IgA, TGF-β1, TGF-β2, IL-10, TNF-α, and soluble CD14 were analyzed in colostrum and mature milk obtained from women treated with probiotics from gestational week 36 until delivery. The total IgA, secretory IgA, TGF-β1, TNF-α, and sCD14 in breast milk were not affected by the intake of probiotics. Supplementation of probiotics during pregnancy was associated with low levels of TGF-β2 and slightly increased levels of IL-10 in colostrum. Infants receiving breast milk with low levels of TGF-β2 were less likely to become sensitized and possibly less IgE-associated eczema in breast-fed infants during their first 2 yr of life [52]. However, another trial by Boyle et al showed that LGG treatment during pregnancy (prenatal) for the prevention of eczema was associated with decreased breast milk soluble CD14 and IgA levels, not TGF-β [51]. The difference between these studies looks probiotic species, which may affect the immunological composition of breast milk.

2.1.3 Anti-inflammatory effects: Their effects on serum inflammatory parameters

The anti-inflammatory effect of probiotics has been attributed to increased production of IL-10 by immune cells in the lamina propria, Peyer's patches and the spleen of treated animals [35-38]. Oral administration of LGG resulted in elevated IL-10 concentrations in atopic children, indicating that specific probiotics may have anti-inflammatory effects in vivo and possible enhancing regulatory or tolerance-inducing mechanisms as well. A review of the evidence from randomized controlled trials by Betsi et al about probiotics for the treatment or prevention of AD: the results of 13 relevant randomized (placebo)-controlled trials (RCTs) were reviewed: 10 of which evaluated probiotics as treatment and 3 for prevention of AD. In four of these six RCTs, clinical improvement was associated with a change in some inflammatory markers [53]. Another randomized, double-blind, placebo-controlled study conducted by Brouwer et al showed no statistically significant effects of probiotic supplementation on inflammatory parameters [47].
Some probiotics have been reported to reduce proinflammatory cytokines through Th17 cells. Suppression of this newly discovered subset of T cells by probiotics might explain effects observed in different experimental models that all involve inflammatory responses. For instance, Lctb casei suppressed inflammation reducing proinflammatory cytokines released from Th17 cells [54]. Also, in a study administration of the probiotics mixture

(Lctbs acidophilus, Lctbs casei, Lctbs reuteri, Bfdbm bifidum, and Streptococcus thermophilus) induced both T-cell and B-cell hyporesponsiveness and down-regulated Th1, Th2, and Th17 cytokines [55].
A study by Woo et al evaluated the effect of Lctbs sakei supplementation in children with atopic eczema-dermatitis syndrome. In this study, compared with placebo, probiotic administration was associated with lower pretreatment-adjusted serum levels of chemokines such as CCL17 and CCL27, which were significantly correlated with SCORAD total score [56].
Probiotic-induced chronic low-grade inflammation characterized by elevation of CRP, IgE, IgA, and IL-10 was shown in some studies, the changes typically observed in helminth infection-associated induction of regulatory mechanisms. The association of increased CRP with a decreased risk of eczema at 2 years of age in allergy-prone children supports the view that chronic, low-grade inflammation protects from eczema. The findings emphasize the role of chronic microbial exposure as an immune modulator protecting from allergy [57].
A study by Rosenfeldt et al, 2 probiotic Lctbs strains (lyophilized Lctbs rhamnosus 19070-2 and Lctbs reuteri DSM 122460) were given in combination for 6 weeks to 1- to 13-year-old children with AD. During active treatment, serum eosinophil cationic protein (ECP) levels significantly decreased. A combination of Lctbs rhamnosus and Lctbs reuteri was beneficial in the management of AD and the effect was more pronounced in atopic eczema patients [46]. Another study was conducted by Brouwer et al showed, during Lctbs species supplementation, a moderate but significant reduction in soluble ECP levels was found. ECP, a cytotoxic protein released from activated eosinophils, has been used to monitor disease activity in AD. Thus sECP might be a more sensitive marker in acute exacerbations of the eczema than a marker of disease activity per se [47]. Although this study by Brouwer et al revealed no statistically significant effects of probiotic supplementation on eosinophil protein X (EPX) in urine, Isolauri et al found significant changes in EPX in the urine of infants supplemented with Bfdbm lactis and LGG [15].

2.1.4 Development of tolerogenic Dendritic cells

Selected species of the Bfdbm genus were demonstrated to prime in vitro cultured neonatal Dendritic cell (DC)s to polarize T cell responses and may therefore be used as candidates in primary prevention of allergic diseases. Bfdbm bifidum was found to be most potent polarizer in vitro-cultured DCs to drive Th1-cell responses involving increased IFN-γ producing T cells concomitant with reduction of IL-4-producing T-cells [58]. In addition, T-cells stimulated by Bfdbm bifidum matured DCs as producers of more IL-10 [59]. Moreover, Lctbs rhamnosus, member of another genus of probiotic bacteria, modulates DC function to induce a novel form of T-cell hyporesponsiveness [60]. Lctbs reuteri/casei have been also shown to prime monocyte-derived DCs through the C-type lectin DC-specific intercellular adhesion molecule 3-grabbing non-integrin (DC-SIGN) to drive the development of Treg cells [61]. These Treg cells produce increased levels of IL-10 and are capable of inhibiting the proliferation of bystander T cells. This study suggests that the targeting of DC-SIGN by certain probiotic bacteria might explain their beneficial effect in the treatment of a number of inflammatory diseases, including AD.

2.1.5 Immunoregulation by T regulatory (Treg) cells

As mentioned earlier, Lctbs reuteri / casei have been also shown to prime monocyte-derived DCs through the DC-SIGN to drive the development of Treg cells [61]. And the probiotic combinations are alleged to cause a paradoxic Th2 stimulation and to induce chronic low-grade inflammation, practically the same as in chronic and balanced helminth infection, which is associated with activation of Treg cells suppressing allergic inflammation. Since the colonization is yet transient, the induction of Treg cells is not permanent. Thus when these immunologic effects no longer operate, the clinical effect is simultaneously lost. For instance, when helminth infections are treated, the prevalence of allergic sensitization increases rapidly. This is a plausible explanation for the fading probiotic effect as well [57].

Recent studies also provided evidence that one effect of probiotics may involve induction of differentiation of IL-10-dependent, TGF-β-bearing Tregs. In a food allergy mouse model, oral administration of Bfdbm bifidum and Lctbs acidophilus suppressed OVA-specific IgE production, which was caused by inducing Treg -associated TGF-β production [62]. Another study demonstrated that neonatal application of probiotic bacteria inhibits subsequent allergic sensitization and airway disease in a murine model of asthma by induction of Treg cells and TGF-β production [63].

Generation of CD4+/Foxp3+ Treg cells by probiotics administration suppresses immune and allergic disorders. Recently, two studies reported that oral administration of a certain probiotic strain could increase Foxp3+ Tregs [55]. It is known that the lower percentage of epidermal or dermal Foxp3+ cells in eczematous dermatitis might contribute to their pathogenesis [64]. In a recent study, a mixture of probiotics (Lctbs acidophilus, Lctbs casei, Lctbs reuteri, Bfdbm bifidium, and Streptococcus thermophilus) was identified that up-regulates CD4+/Foxp3+ Treg cells. Administration of the probiotics mixture induced both T-cell and B-cell hyporesponsiveness and down-regulated Th1, Th2, and Th17 cytokines [55,65]. It also induced generation of CD4+/Foxp3+ Tregs from the CD4+/25- population and increased the suppressor activity of naturally occurring CD4+/25+ Tregs. Conversion of T cells into Foxp3+ Tregs is directly mediated by regulatory DCs that express high levels of IL-10 and TGF-β. In a murine AD model, treatment with this probiotic mixture significantly inhibited the clinical symptoms of AD progression by reducing IgE levels [total and specific IgE levels], infiltrated lymphocytes and granulocytes, and levels of AD-associated cytokines [55]. Lctbs casei treatment enhanced the frequency of FoxP3(+) Treg in the skin and increased the production of IL-10 by CD4+/25+ Treg cells in skin draining lymph nodes of hapten-sensitized mice. These data demonstrate that orally administered Lctbs casei (DN-114 001) efficiently alleviate T cell-mediated skin inflammation without causing immune suppression, via mechanisms that include control of CD8+ effector T cells and involve regulatory CD4+ T cells. Lctbs casei may thus represent a probiotic of potential interest for immunomodulation of T cell-mediated allergic skin diseases in human [66]. However, another study showed that Foxp3 mRNA expression at 6 months of age is higher in infants having AD, but it is not affected by giving probiotics from birth [67].

2.1.6 Lymphocyte subpopulations

Several studies reveal that the probiotics differently modulate peripheral blood immune parameters in healthy subjects and patients with AD.

Gerasimov et al conducted a study to assess the clinical efficacy and impact of Lctbs acidophilus DDS-1, Bfdbm lactis UABLA-12 with fructo-oligosaccharide on peripheral blood lymphocyte subsets in preschool children with moderate-to-severe AD. The percentage of CD4, and the percentage and absolute count of CD25 decreased, and the percentage and absolute count of CD8 increased in the probiotic group at week 8, compared with placebo (p:< 0.007). They found a significant correlation between CD4 percentage, CD25 percentage,

CD25 absolute count, and SCORAD values in the probiotic group at week 8. The administration of a probiotic mixture and fructo-oligosaccharide was correlated with significant clinical improvement in children with AD, with corresponding lymphocyte subpopulation changes in peripheral blood [68].

However, in another study major lymphocyte subsets were not affected by the probiotic intervention. The expression of CD4+/25+ T cells was similar in healthy subjects and AD patients, whereas CD4+/54+ decreased significantly in patients with AD and remained uninfluenced in healthy subjects. The purpose of a study by Roessler et al was to elucidate the influence of a probiotic drink containing a combination of the probiotics Lctbs paracasei Lpc-37, Lctbs acidophilus 74-2 and Bfdbm animalis subsp. lactis DGCC 420 (Bfdbm lactis 420) in healthy volunteers and in patients with AD on clinical and immunological parameters and their detection in feces. In a double-blind, randomized cross-over study was conducted in 15 healthy adults and 15 patients with AD. The probiotic product or placebo was given over 2 months. In AD patients, the SCORAD tended to decrease by 15.5% (P:0.08). However, CD57+ increased significantly in healthy subjects after probiotic intake and was not changed in patients [69].

2.1.7 Toll-like receptor (TLR) stimulation

A number of experiments indicate that infectious agents can promote protection from ADs through mechanisms independent of their constitutive antigens, leading to stimulation of non-antigen specific receptors such as TLRs. A family of pattern recognition receptors such as TLRs on gut lymphoid and epithelial cells mediates innate immune responses to bacterial molecular patterns and, thereby, orchestrates acquired immunity. The transient protection offered by probiotics against IgE-associated allergic diseases is based on stimulation of TLRs, which produce mediators such as IL-6; these further induce IgA differentiation from naive B cells. Both these events were shown to to occur after probiotic administration to infants with eczema, as well as in infants who showed increased levels of serum CRP, IL-10, and IgE at age 6 months.

Similarly, TLR stimulation was also thought to happen after probiotic administration in infants with eczema who showed increased levels of serum CRP, IL-10, and IgE [57]. This probiotic-induced low-grade inflammation was characterized by elevation of CRP, IgE, IgA, and IL-10, the changes typically observed in helminth infection-associated induction of regulatory mechanisms. Moreover, the association of increased CRP with a decreased risk of eczema at 2 years of age in allergy-prone children supports the view that chronic, low-grade inflammation protects from eczema. The findings emphasize the role of chronic microbial exposure as an immune modulator protecting from allergy thru activation of Treg cells. Consistently, lactic acid bacteria species such as Bfdbm bifidum / infantis and Lctbs salivarius were shown to be capable of activating TLR-2 [70]. Oral administration of Lctbs reuteri attenuated major characteristics of an asthmatic response, including airway eosinophilia, local cytokine responses, and hyperresponsiveness to methacholine. This effect of Lctbs reuteri on the allergic airway response was found to be dependent on TLR-9 [71].

In summary, local influences of probiotics potentially include reduction of gut permeability and systemic penetration of antigens, increased local IgA production, and alteration of local inflammation or tolerance induction. Some possible systemic effects consist of anti-inflammatory effects mediated by TLRs, Th1 skewing of responses to allergens, and activation of tolerogenic DCs, in addition to Treg cell production. [The various effects of different probiotic strains in atopic diseases as well as in AD are summarized in table 1].

References	Probiotic Strain	Effect of probiotic	Outcome
		Maturing Gut Barrier	
Sudo et al 27	Bfdbm	Oral tolerance	↑
Isolauri et al 15,29,50,76	LGG	Fecal IgA levels	↑
Isolauri et al 15,29,50,76	Lctbs rhamnosus GG (LGG)	Gut-stabilizing effect	↑
Malin et al 31	LGG	Gut defense	↑
Kaila et al 33	Lctbs	Intestinal permeability	↓
		Immunomodulation	
Niers et al 37,58,82	Bfdbm bifidum / infantis; Lctbs lactis	Th2 Cytokines	↓
Niers et al 37,58,82	Bfdbm bifidum / infantis; Lctbs lactis	IL-10 Production	↑
Maassen et al 38,105	Lctbs casei	IL-10 Production	↑
Maassen et al 38,105	Lctbs reuteri	Th1 Cytokines	↑
Maassen et al 38,105	Lctbs casei	IL-4 Production	↑
Kim et al 42,62,83	Bfdbm lactis/ bifidum; Lctbs acidophilus	IL-10 Production	↑
Kim et al 42,62,83	Bfdbm lactis/ bifidum; Lctbs acidophilus	IL-4 Production	↓
Kim et al 42,62,83	Bfdbm lactis/ bifidum; Lctbs acidophilus	IFN-γ Production	↑
Kim et al 42,62,83	Bfdbm lactis/ bifidum; Lctbs acidophilus	IgE Production	↓
Takahashi 43	Bfdbm longum	Th2 Cytokines	↓
Takahashi 43	Bfdbm longum	IgE Production	↓
Sistek et al 41	Lctbs rhamnosus GG (LGG)	IL-10 Production	↑
Kruisselbrink et al 39	Lctbs plantarum	IL-10 Production	↓
Hart et al 59	Bfdbm bifidum	IL-10 Production	↑
		Th1/Th2 balance	
Niers et al 58	Bfdbm bifidum	Most potent Dendritic cell polarizer in vitro	↑
Hart et al 59	Bfdbm bifidum	Human Dendritic cell phenotype modulator	↑
Braat et al 60	Lctbs rhamnosus	Dendritic cell function modulator	↑
Smits et al 61	Lctbs reuteri / casei	Prime monocyte-derived Dendritic cell	↑
		Serum Inflammatory Parameters	

References	Probiotic Strain	Effect of probiotic	Outcome
Maassen et al 38,105	Lctbs reuteri	Immunomodulation	↑
Sistek et al 41	Lctbs rhamnosus GG (LGG)	Immunomodulation	↓
		Development of Tolerogenic Dendritic Cells	
Niers et al 37,58,82	Bfdbm	Prime neonatal Dendritic cell	↑
Braat et al 60	Lctbs rhamnosus	Modulates Dendritic cell function	↑
Smits et al 61	Lctbs reuteri / casei	Prime monocyte-derived Dendritic cell	↑
		Toll-like Receptor Stimulation	
Hoarau et al 70	Bfdbm bifidum / infantis; Lctbs salivarius	Activate TLR-2	↑
Forsythe et al 71	Lctbs reuteri	Activate TLR-9	↑
		T-regulatory Cell Production	
Smits et al 61	Lctbs reuteri / casei	Prime monocyte-derived Dendritic cell	↑
Kim et al 42,62,83	Bfdbm bifidum; Lctbs acidophilus	TGF-β production	↑
Feleszko 63	LGG, Bfdbm lactis (Bb-12)	TGF-β production	↑
		T-cell Hyporesponsiveness	
Kruisselbrink et al 39	Lctbs plantarum	Inhibits specific T-cell responses	↑
Braat et al 60	Lctbs rhamnosus	Modulates Dendritic cell function	↑

Abbreviations: Lctbs = Lactobacillus; Bfdbm = Bifidobacterium; LGG= Lactobacillus rhamnosus GG; ↑= increase in symptoms or negative effect; ↓= decrease in symptoms or positive effect; ↔ = No change in symptoms or no effect

Table 1. Various mechanisms for effects of probiotic strains in atopic disorders including eczema are shown from experimental (animal) and clinical (human) studies referred in the chapter text.

3. The role of probiotics in the prevention and treatment of AD

The increased prevalence of atopic diseases is nowadays defined as an epidemic. AD is known as the earliest of these conditions, might act as an indicator for the development of IgE-mediated atopic manifestations. Thus, being aware of possible measures, such as probiotic use, to prevent and/or heal atopic disease is essential for the practicing allergist. Here, their role in the prevention and therapy of AD under the recent literature gathered from Medline and Pubmed are discussed. The various effects of different probiotic strains in AD are summarized in table 2.

References	Probiotic Species	Type of Atopic Dermattis	Outcome
		Atopic (IgE-associated) Eczema	
Isolauri et al 15,29,50,76	Bfdbm or Lctbs	Food (cow's milk) Allergy	↓
Wickens et al 81	Lctbs rhamnosus	IgE-associated eczema	↓
Viljanen et al 28,72	LGG	Atopic eczema/dermatitis syndrome	↓
Sistek et al 41	Lctbs rhamnosus + Bfdbm lactis	Eczema , food-sensitized atopy	↓
Kuitunen et al 74	Lctbs+ Bfdbm+ Propionibacteria	IgE-associated allergy	↓
Majamaa et al 15	LGG	Food-sensitized eczema	↓
Rosenfeldt et al 49	Lctbs rhamnosus + Lctbs reuteri	Atopic eczema	↓
Kukkonen et al 73, 108	Mix (LGG, Lctbs rhamnosus LC705, Bfdbm breve, Propionibacterium)	Atopic eczema	↓
Abrahamsson et al 75	Lctbs reuteri ATCC 55730	Atopic eczema	↓
		Non-atopic Eczema	
Kalliomäki et al 16	LGG	Atopic dermatitis	↓
Woo et al 56	Lctbs sakei	Atopic dermatitis	↓
Weston et al 78	Lctbs fermentum	Atopic dermatitis	↓
Hoang et al 79	Lctbs rhamnosus	Atopic dermatitis	↓
Hattori et al 80	Bfdbm breve	Atopic dermatitis	↓
Wickens et al 81	Lctbs rhamnosus, Bfdbm animalis (Bb–12)	Atopic dermatitis	↓
Marschan et al 57	Mix (LGG, Lctbs rhamnosus LC705, Bfdbm breve, Propionibacterium)	Atopic dermatitis	↓
Niers et al 37,58,82	Bfdbm bifidum, Bfdbm lactis, Lactococcus lactis	Atopic dermatitis	↓
Kim et al 42,62,83	Bfdbm bifidum, Bfdbm lactis, Lctbs acidophilus	Atopic dermatitis	↓
Dotterud et al 84	LGG, Lctbs acidophilus, Bfdbm animalis (Bb–12)	Atopic dermatitis	↓
Böttcher et al 52	Lctbs reuteri	Atopic dermatitis (sensitization)	↓
West et al 40	Lctbs casei F19	Atopic dermatitis	↓
Lodinova-Zadnikova et al 85	Escherichia coli	Atopic dermatitis (IgE allergies)	↓
Gerasimov et al 68	Lctbs acidophilus, Bfdbm lactis	Atopic dermatitis	↓

References	Probiotic Species	Type of Atopic Dermattis	Outcome
		Eczema (atopic dermatitis)	
Kopp et al 88	LGG	Atopic dermatitis (wheezing)	↔, (↑)
Taylor et al 87	LGG or Lctbs acidophilus	Atopic dermatitis (cow's milk allergy)	↔, (↑)
Boyle RJ et al 51	LGG	Atopic dermatitis	↔
Gruber et al 89	LGG	Atopic dermatitis	↔
Soh et al 91	Bfdbm longum + Lctbcs rhamnosus	Eczema and atopic sensitization	↔
Lee et al 95	Various	Atopic dermatitis	↔
Brouwer et al 47	Lctbs rhamnosus	Atopic dermatitis	↔
Kuitunen et al 74	Lctbs+ Bfdbm+ Propionibacteria	Atopic dermatitis	↔
Fölster-Holst et al 90	LGG	Atopic dermatitis	↔

Abbreviations: Lctbs = Lactobacillus; Bfdbm = Bifidobacterium; LGG= Lactobacillus rhamnosus GG; ↑= increase in symptoms or negative effect; ↓= decrease in symptoms or positive effect; ↔ = No change in symptoms or no effect

Table 2. The various effects of different probiotic strains, referred in the chapter text, in atopic and non-atopic eczema are shown.

Any difference for IgE-sensitized (atopic) vs. non-IgE-sensitized (non-atopic) eczema groups?
A number of studies could only relate probiotic benefits to a certain subset of AD patients. In support of the efficacy of probiotics in IgE-sensitized children, some other studies also demonstrated comparable results as well. In brief: treatment with Lctbs rhamnosus for the first 2 years of life was associated with a significant reduction in the prevalence of any IgE-associated eczema by about a half [16]. Another study demonstrated that LGG alleviated atopic eczema/dermatitis syndrome symptoms in IgE-sensitized infants [28]. In food-sensitized atopic children, the efficacy of the probiotics such as Lctbs rhamnosus and Bfdbm lactis was demonstrated too [40].This effect was more pronounced in patients with a positive skin prick test and increased IgE levels.

Yet, some other studies failed to demonstrate that the severity and frequency of AD were decreased with the supplementation of probiotics, regardless of their IgE sensitization status. For instance; Boyle et al and others could not show any effect even for LGG in infants with AD [51]. A few meta-analyses also could not confirm that IgE sensitization was indeed a factor in determining the efficacy of probiotics in atopic children. However, the heterogeneity between studies may be attributable to probiotic strain-specific effects and other factors as well, meaning that some probiotic strains may still have a therapeutic role in eczema [13,14].

3.1 IgE-sensitized (atopic) eczema therapy and prevention

Recently published one of the largest studies by Viljanen et al to date compared LGG or a probiotic mix (LGG, Lctbs rhamnosus LC705, Bfdbm breve Bb99, and Propionibacterium freudenreichii ssp. shermanii JS) with placebo. In this study, 230 Finnish children with AD were treated for 4 weeks with LGG, a mixture of four probiotic strains or placebo. With supplementation with probiotics (LGG), Viljanen et al found significant improvement on the SCORAD index only in "IgE-sensitized -cow's milk -allergic- infants of the atopic eczema/dermatitis syndrome (AEDS). Only in the subgroup of IgE-sensitized children, did the LGG group show a greater reduction in SCORAD than the placebo group but this effect could have been due to a higher baseline score in this subgroup. There was no difference between the groups at the end of 4-week therapy and 4 weeks after therapy was discontinued. Contrary to what would be expected, improvement was seen 4 weeks after discontinuation of therapy rather than during treatment [28,72]. Rosenfeldt et al from Denmark in a study, 2 lyophilized probiotic Lctbs strains (lyophilized Lctbs rhamnosus 19070-2 and Lctbs reuteri DSM 122460) were given in combination for 6 weeks to 1- to 13-year-old (mean age, 5.2 years) children with AD. This study used 2 different Lctbs species in older children. A combination of these was beneficial in the management of AD. Statistically significant improvement in SCORAD score was seen only in a subset of children with positive skin prick test results and elevated IgE levels [46]. Another study by Sistek et al showed the efficacy of the probiotics Lctbs rhamnosus and Bfdbm lactis in food-sensitized children [41].

A study by Finnish group used the same probiotic mixture with prebiotic. Kukkonen et al in a trial using probiotic mix (Lctbs rhamnosus GG, Lctbs rhamnosus LC705, Bfdbm breve Bb99; and Propionibacterium freudenreichii ssp. shermanii JS) and prebiotic galacto-oligosaccharides demonstrated that the prevention of atopic eczema in high-risk Finnish infants is possible by modulating the infant's gut microbiota with probiotics and prebiotics. Probiotic treatment compared with placebo reduced IgE-associated (atopic) diseases. Probiotic treatment also reduced eczema and atopic eczema [73].

In 2009, in a study by Kuitunen et al 1223 Finnish mothers were randomized with infants at high risk for allergy to receive the same probiotic mixture (2 Lactobacilli, Bifidobacteria, and propionibacteria) or placebo during the last month of pregnancy and their infants to receive it from birth until age 6 months. Infants also received a prebiotic galacto-oligosaccharide or placebo. At 5 years, the cumulative incidence of allergic diseases (eczema, food allergy, allergic rhinitis, and asthma) and IgE sensitization were evaluated. Frequencies of allergic and IgE-associated allergic disease and sensitization in the probiotic and placebo groups were similar. However, less IgE-associated allergic disease occurred in cesarean-delivered children receiving probiotics. No allergy-preventive effect that extended to age 5 years was achieved with perinatal supplementation of probiotic bacteria to high-risk mothers and children. It conferred protection only to cesarean-delivered children [74].

Similarly; Abrahamsson et al could not confirm a preventive effect of probiotics (Lctbs reuteri ATCC 55730) on infant eczema in a recently published study. However, he observed that the treated infants had less IgE-associated eczema at 2 years. Moreover, skin prick test reactivity was also less common in the treated group than in the placebo group, but this difference reached significance only for infants with allergic Swedish mothers [75].

In conclusion; all of these studies taken together demonstrate that probiotics are might not be effective and /or therapeutic for all children with AD, but offer benefit in a subset of IgE-sensitized children.

3.2 Non-IgE-sensitized (non-atopic) eczema therapy and prevention

Until now, several clinical studies have been published that have focused on the use of probiotics for therapy and primary prevention of atopic diseases. To date, the results of at least 15 prospective preventive studies with different Lctbs or Bfdbm strains (or mixture) in children at high risk for allergic diseases have been published.

The first study in the literature by Isolauri et al analyzed a benefit of LGG in mild AD disease in 1997. They observed 27 exclusively breastfed infants (median age 4-6 months) with mild AD (median SCORAD score of 16), receiving extensively hydrolysed whey formula with (LGG or Bfdbm strain) or without probiotics (placebo) for 8 weeks. They showed a reduction in the SCORAD by 15 points (from 16 to 1) for the LGG and by 16 points (from 16 to 0) for the Bfdbm arm, as compared with a reduction of 2-6 points (from 16 to 13-4) in the placebo arm. However, one month after therapy, SCORAD scores were comparable with those of placebo. Therefore, the probiotic effect was limited to acceleration of improvement in infants with mild disease [15]. The same investigators subsequently published 2 additional studies. One of these studies compared LGG with Bfdbm lactis Bb-12, both of which showed a significant improvement in SCORAD score over placebo. However, after 6 months, the median SCORAD score was zero in all groups, again suggesting that the effect is limited to rapid initiation of improvement [76]. The other study underlined the importance of viability for probiotic species. The use of heat inactivated LGG resulted in adverse gastrointestinal symptoms with diarrhea, and study recruitment was halted. They concluded that supplementation of infant formulas with viable but not heat-inactivated LGG was found to be a potential approach for the management of atopic eczema and cow's milk allergy [77].

In an earlier study by Viljanen et al probiotics have been suggested to be useful in children with AEDS. In 2010, a study by Woo et al was performed to assess the clinical effect of Lctbs sakei supplementation in children with AEDS. In this study, children aged 2 to 10 years with AEDS with a minimum SCORAD score of 25 were randomized to receive either daily Lctbs sakei KCTC 10755BP or daily placebo supplementation for 12 weeks. At week 12, SCORAD total scores adjusted by pretreatment values were lower after probiotic treatment than after placebo treatment. There was a 31% improvement in mean disease activity with probiotic use compared with a 13% improvement with placebo use. Therefore significant differences in favor of probiotic treatment were also observed in proportions of patients achieving improvement of at least 30% and 50%. Interestingly, clinical improvement in this study was not just observed in the subgroup of IgE-sensitized children, contrary to Viljanen et al study, and it was regardless of IgE sensitization [56]. Weston et al from Australia published their experience with using Lctbs fermentum VRI-003 PCC for 8 weeks in 53 infants with AD. After 16 weeks the probiotic group had significant reduction of SCORAD scores while the placebo group did not. Lctbs fermentum caused a significant reduction in SCORAD scores. Although the change in SCORAD score from baseline in the probiotic group was significant, the difference between the probiotic and placebo groups did not reach significance by week 16 [78]. In a study by Hoang et al, they followed 14 cases of pediatric patients (ages of 8 months to 64 months) with a history of resistant eczema for a period of at least 6 months. All of these children received Lctbs rhamnosus cell lysate daily as an immunobiotic supplement. The results of this open label non-randomized clinical observation showed a substantial improvement in quality of life, skin symptoms and day- and nighttime irritation scores in children with the supplementation of Lctbs rhamnosus lysate. There were no intolerance or adverse reactions observed in these children. Lctbs rhamnosus cell lysate may thus be used as a safe and effective immunobiotic for the treatment and prevention of childhood eczema [79]. Bfdbm breve has been reported by Hattori et al to improve cutaneous symptoms of AD patients. Fifteen children with AD who had Bfdbm-deficient microflora were selected for this study. Eight subjects in the Bifidobacteria -administered group were given oral administration of lyophilized Bfdbm breve M-16V strain. In the Bifidobacteria -administered group, the proportion of Bfdbm in the fecal microflora was increased and the proportion of aerobic bacteria was decreased after 1 month of administration. Furthermore, significant improvement of allergic symptoms (in cutaneous symptom and total allergic scores) was also observed in the Bifidobacteria -administered group. The tendency of allergic symptom improvement was remarkable compared with the control group; however there was no correlation between changes in fecal microflora and allergic symptoms [80].

The Finnish study of Kalliomäki et al was the first report to describe that the frequency of AD in the probiotic group was half that of the placebo. This hallmark study demonstrated that administration of LGG for 1 month before and 6 months after birth to their infants was associated with a significant reduction in the cumulative incidence of eczema during the first 7 year of life. The effect of probiotics on preventing AD has been demonstrated in infants of Finnish pregnant mothers with a strong family history of eczema, allergic rhinitis or asthma. The frequency of developing AD in the offspring was significantly reduced by 2, 4, and 7 years, by 50%, 44%, and 36%; respectively. But there were no preventive effects on atopic sensitization and onset of respiratory allergic diseases [16].

Wickens et al studied a differential effect of 2 probiotics in the prevention of eczema and atopy. Infants receiving Lctbs rhamnosus had a significantly reduced risk of eczema, compared with placebo, but this was not the case for B animalis subsp lactis. In a double-blind, randomized placebo-controlled trial of infants at risk of allergic disease, pregnant women were randomized to take Lctbs rhamnosus HN001, Bfdbm animalis subsp lactis strain HN019 or placebo daily from 35 weeks gestation until 6 months if breastfeeding, and their infants were randomized to receive the same treatment from birth to 2 years (n:474). Infants receiving Lctbs rhamnosus had a significantly reduced risk of eczema compared with placebo, but this was not the case for Bfdbm animalis subsp lactis. There was no significant effect of Lctbs rhamnosus or Bfdbm animalis subsp lactis on atopy. Lctbs rhamnosus (71.5%) was more likely than Bfdbm animalis subsp lactis (22.6%) to be present in the feces at 3 months, although detection rates were similar by 24 months. The authors found out that supplementation with Lctbs rhamnosus, but not Bfdbm animalis subsp lactis, substantially reduced the cumulative prevalence of eczema, but not atopy, by 2 years [81].

In a randomized double-blind study by Marschan et al, probiotic bacteria (Lctbs rhamnosus GG (ATCC 53103), Lctbs rhamnosus LC705, Bfdbm breve Bb99, and Propionibacterium freudenreichii ssp. Shermanii JS) or placebo were given for 1 month before delivery to mothers and for 6 months to infants with a family history of allergy. Infants receiving probiotic bacteria had higher plasma levels of CRP, total IgA, total IgE, and IL-10 than infants in the placebo group. Increased plasma CRP level at age 6 months was associated with a decreased risk of eczema and with a decreased risk of allergic disease at age 2 years, when adjusted with probiotic use. The association of CRP with a decreased risk of eczema at 2 years of age in allergy-prone children supports the view that chronic, low-grade inflammation protects from eczema. Probiotic-induced low-grade inflammation was characterized by elevation of IgE, IgA, and IL-10, the changes typically observed in helminth infection-associated induction of regulatory mechanisms [57] (please see the section: mechanisms of probiotics` effects).

In the PandA study of Niers et al administered a mixture of probiotic bacteria (Bfdbm bifidum W23, Bfdbm lactis W52, and Lactococcus lactis W58; Ecologic Panda) for 6 week prenatally to mothers of high-risk children and to their offspring for the first 12 months of life. Although cumulative incidence of atopic eczema and IgE levels were similar in both treated and placebo groups, the parental reported eczema was significantly lower during the first 3 months of life in infants receiving probiotics. This particular combination of probiotic bacteria showed a preventive effect on the incidence of eczema in high-risk children, which seems to be sustained during the first 2 years of life. In addition to previous studies, the preventive effect appeared to be established within the first 3 months of life in this study [82].

In a trial by Kim et al, 112 pregnant women with a family history of allergic diseases received a mixture of Bfdbm bifidum BGN4, Bfdbm lactis AD011, and Lctbs acidophilus AD031, starting at 4-8 wks before delivery and continuing until 6 months after delivery. The cumulative incidence of eczema during the first 12 months was reduced significantly in probiotic group; however, there was no difference in serum total IgE level or the sensitization against food allergens between the two groups. Prenatal and postnatal supplementation with a mixture of probiotics is an effective approach in preventing the development of eczema in infants at high risk of allergy during the first year of life [83].

In a randomized, double-blind trial by Dotterud et al, probiotics was given in pregnant women to prevent allergic disease. In this study children from a nonselected maternal population, women received probiotic milk or placebo from 36 weeks of gestation to 3 months postnatally during breastfeeding. The probiotic milk contained Lctbs rhamnosus GG, Lctbs acidophilus La-5 and Bfdbm animalis subsp. lactis Bb-12. At 2 years of age, all children were assessed for atopic sensitization, AD, asthma and allergic rhinoconjunctivitis. Probiotics given to nonselected mothers reduced the cumulative incidence of AD, but had no effect on asthma or atopic sensitization [84].

Böttcher et al's study demonstrated that Lctbs reuteri supplementation during pregnancy associated with reduced risk of sensitization during infancy. Swedish pregnant women were treated with Lctbs reuteri (n:54) or placebo (n:55) from gestational week 36 until delivery. The infants were followed prospectively for 2 years regarding development of eczema and sensitization as defined by a positive skin prick test and/or circulating allergen-specific IgE antibodies at 6, 12, and 24 months of age [52].

Of note, another recently published Swedish study demonstrated that administration of Lctbs casei F19 during weaning significantly reduced the incidence of eczema, indicating that proper timing of the probiotic intervention is a critical factor. This study also supports the notion that there is more than a single window of opportunity to manage allergic diseases. This study evaluated the effects of feeding with Lctbs F19 during weaning period on the incidence of eczema and Th1/Th2 balance. In this intervention trial by West et al, infants were fed cereals with (n:89) or without Lctbs F19 (n:90) from 4-13 months of age. The cumulative incidence of eczema at 13 months was 11% and 22% in the probiotic and placebo groups, respectively ($p:<0.05$). At 13 months of age, the IFN-γ / IL-4 mRNA ratio was significantly higher in the probiotic compared with the placebo group. The higher Th1/Th2 ratio in the probiotic compared with the placebo group suggests enhancing effects of Lctbs F19 on the T cell-mediated immune response. In contrast, there were no differences between groups in serum IgE concentrations. As a result, feeding Lctbs F19 during weaning could be an effective tool in the prevention of early manifestation of allergy such as eczema [40].

Oral administration of probiotic Escherichia coli after birth in the early postnatal period by Lodinova-Zadnikova et al reduced frequency of serum specific IgE allergies later in life (after 10 and 20 years) [85].
Gerasimov et al conducted a study to assess the clinical efficacy and impact of Lctbs acidophilus DDS-1, Bfdbm lactis UABLA-12 with fructo-oligosaccharide on peripheral blood lymphocyte subsets in preschool children with moderate-to-severe AD. In a randomized, double-blind, placebo-controlled, prospective trial of 90 children aged 1-3 years with moderate-to-severe AD who were treated with a mixture of probiotics with fructo-oligosaccharide for 8 weeks versus placebo. At the final visit, the percentage significant decrease in SCORAD was 33.7% in the probiotic group compared with 19.4% in the placebo group. Children receiving probiotic showed a greater decrease in the mean SCORAD score than did children from the placebo group at week 8. The administration of a probiotic mixture and fructo-oligosaccharide was associated with significant clinical improvement in children with AD, with corresponding lymphocyte subset changes in peripheral blood [68].
In conclusion; here probiotics were more likely to be effective in treating moderately severe AD as well as mild atopic disease. Although not every study result above was significant, the effect of probiotics did not seem to be greater just in the IgE-sensitized group than in the non–IgE-sensitized group. Nevertheless, there have been several reports in the literature showing no effect of probiotics, which are being discussed the section below.

3.3 No therapeutic or preventive effect of probiotics in AD regardless of IgE sensitization

It is striking that the proportion of children with AD and allergic sensitization such as in the study of Taylor and Huurre et al was significantly higher in the probiotic group [86]. In Taylor et al's trial probiotic supplementation postnatally failed to reduce the risk of AD and increased the risk of allergen sensitization in high-risk children. Newborns of women with allergy (n:231) received either Lctbs acidophilus (LAVRI-A1) or placebo daily for the first 6 months of life. Children were assessed for AD and other symptoms at 6 and 12 months and had allergen skin prick tests at 12 months of age. At 6 and 12 months, AD rates were similar in the probiotic and placebo groups. At 12 months, the rate of sensitization was significantly higher in the probiotic group. The presence of culturable Lactobacilli or Bfdbm in stools in the first month of life was not associated with the risk of subsequent sensitization or disease; however, the presence of Lctbs at 6 months of age was associated with increased risk of subsequent cow's milk sensitization. Early probiotic supplementation with Lctbs acidophilus did not reduce the risk of AD in high-risk infants and was associated with increased allergen sensitization in infants receiving supplements. There were 3 major differences between Taylor's study and the others. The type of probiotic product (Lctbs acidophilus), the supplementation period (1 year) as well as the timing of the introduction of the probiotic were different. Taylor et al administered the probiotic supplement postnatally, while other studies administered probiotics before and after birth. Prenatal supplementation may prove to be crucial for the preventive benefit of probiotics in this disorder. The data from the Taylor et al's study point in the same direction regarding allergic sensitization, also suggesting that the use of probiotics for primary prevention must be exercised with caution [87].
Similarly, a randomized, double-blind, placebo-controlled prospective trial by Kopp et al of probiotics for primary prevention did show no clinical effects of LGG supplementation. 105 pregnant women from families with ≥1 member (mother, father, or child) with an atopic

disease were randomly assigned to receive either the probiotic LGG or pacebo. The supplementation period started 4 to 6 weeks before expected delivery, followed by a postnatal period of 6 months. The primary end point was the occurrence of AD at the age of 2 years. Secondary outcomes were severity of AD, recurrent episodes of wheezing bronchitis, and allergic sensitization at the age of 2 years. Notably, children with recurrent (≥5) episodes of wheezing bronchitis were more frequent in the LGG group (26%), as compared with the placebo group (9%). As a result, supplementation with LGG during pregnancy and early infancy neither reduced the incidence of AD nor altered the severity of AD in affected children but was associated with an increased rate of recurrent episodes of wheezing bronchitis. No difference was observed between both groups in total Ig E concentrations or numbers of specific sensitization to inhalant allergens [88].

Furthermore; prenatal probiotic LGG treatment during pregnancy was not associated with reduced risk of eczema or IgE-associated eczema in a randomized controlled trial by Boyle RJ [51]. In a recent study, 250 pregnant women were recruited carrying infants at high risk of allergic disease to a randomized controlled trial of probiotic supplementation (LGG) from 36 weeks gestation until delivery. Gruber et al's study also did not show any effect for LGG in infants with AD regardless of their IgE sensitization status [89].

However, a study from the Netherlands by Brouwer et al and another study from Germany by Folster-Holst et al showed no effect of LGG in infants with AD regardless of their IgE sensitization status. In a study conducted by Brouwer et al, after 4–6 weeks of baseline and double-blind, placebo-controlled challenges for diagnosis of cow's milk allergy, infants less than 5 months old with AD received a hydrolysed whey-based formula as placebo (n:17), or supplemented with either Lctbs rhamnosus (n:17) or LGG (n:16) for 3 months. No statistically significant effects of probiotic supplementation on SCORAD, sensitization, inflammatory parameters or cytokine production between groups were found. No clinical or immunological effect of the probiotic bacteria used in infants with AD [47]. A similar prospective study by Fölster-Holst et al was performed to reassess the efficacy of orally administered LGG in infants with AD. In a randomized, double-blind, placebo-controlled study, 54 infants aged 1–55 months with moderate to severe AD were randomized to receive LGG or to placebo during an 8-week intervention phase. At the end of treatment there were no significant differences between the groups with respect to clinical symptoms (SCORAD, pruritus, and sleep loss), immunological parameters, or health-related quality of life of the parents [90]. Additionally; Soh et al in a clinical trial involving 253 infants with a family history of allergic disease utilized probiotic supplementation (Bfdbm longum + Lctbs rhamnosus) in the first 6 months of life in Asian infants at risk and evaluated the effects on eczema and atopic sensitization at the age of 1 year. Early life administration of a cow's milk formula supplemented with probiotics showed no effect on prevention of eczema or allergen sensitization in the first year of life in Asian infants at risk of allergic disease [91].

In conclusion; LGG was mostly used probiotic species in these studies. Firstly used by Kalliomaki et al [16] with a success however, other groups including Brouwer, Boyle, Kopp, Gruber, and Fölster -Holst et al [47,51,87,88,90] could not demonstrate any benefit in AD. For instance: Kopp et al have shown that the probiotic LGG has no preventive effect on the development or the severity of AD at the age of 2 years in a German population of infants at high risk. Instead, there was a significantly higher risk of ≥5 episodes with wheezing bronchitis during the first 2 years in the LGG group, as compared with placebo. There were several methodological differences between these studies: Kopp et al adapted the protocol of Kalliomäki et al and continued to supplement LGG for 3 months after birth to the breastfeeding mothers and the following 3 months only to the neonates. This modification was made to achieve a more consistent probiotic delivery. Second, Finnish mothers received supplementation during the last 4 weeks of pregnancy, whereas pregnant women in this population commenced with LGG or placebo for 4 to 6 weeks. They extended the prenatal supplementation period, because a 4-week period is thought to possibly be too short for suspected in utero effects of LGG supplementation. Also, population in this study by Kopp et al was being of higher risk compared with the Finnish population, which might account for the differing results. And more infants with older siblings were recruited compared with the Finnish study. Lastly, the Finnish and German populations are of different genetic background.

4. Recent metaanalyses and reviews from literature

A metaanalysis of the evidence from randomized controlled trials by Betsi et al on probiotics for the treatment or prevention of AD: the results of 13 relevant randomized (placebo)-controlled trials were reviewed: 10 of which evaluated probiotics as treatment and 3 for prevention of AD. Four RCTs suggested that there was a statistically significant decrease in SCORAD after probiotic administration to infants or children with AD for 1 or 2 months compared with that after placebo. While in two RCTs SCORAD was significantly reduced after treatment with Lactobacilli only in children with IgE-associated AD. In three RCTs, the change in SCORAD was not statistically significant between probiotic- and placebo-treated children, although in one of these trials SCORAD was significantly lower after probiotic than with placebo treatment in food-sensitized children. As a result; probiotics, especially Lctbs rhamnosus GG, seem to be effective for the prevention of AD and they were also found to reduce the severity of AD in approximately half of the RCTs evaluated [53]. Likewise, Zhu et al did a metaanalysis of lactic acid bacteria as probiotics for the primary prevention of infantile eczema. The data from this metaanalysis suggested that lactic acid probiotics combined with other probiotics play a role in the prevention of infantile eczema. Conversely, another recent meta-analysis did not show a therapeutic difference among children receiving probiotics. This analysis excluded six of the ten studies published, making the validity of the report questionable [92].

In a review article; atopic disease and / or food hypersensitivity outcomes were assessed by Osborn et al in 6 studies enrolling 2080 infants, but outcomes for only 1549 infants were reported. Meta-analysis of five studies reporting the outcomes of 1477 infants found a significant reduction in infantile eczema. When the analysis was restricted to studies reporting atopic eczema (confirmed by skin prick test or specific IgE), the findings were no longer significant. All studies reporting significant benefits used probiotic supplements containing Lctbs rhamnosus and enrolled infants at high risk of allergy [93]. Another recent meta-analysis suggested that probiotics may benefit children and infants with the disorder. The metaanalysis identified 10 randomized, controlled trials. A significant overall benefit was demonstrated after the use of probiotics, resulting in a reduction of the SCORAD scores compared to placebo. LGG appeared to be more effective than other probiotic preparations and children with more severe disease were more likely to benefit from the use of probiotics [94]. This remarkable meta-analysis was done to determine whether probiotics are efficacious in treating AD and to explore whether type of probiotic used, duration of therapy, patient age, severity of disease, and IgE sensitization are factors in determining efficacy. For this meta-analysis of randomized controlled trials describing the efficacy of probiotics in AD, a comprehensive search was performed of databases through January 2008. Eleven studies were identified, and data from 10 studies (n: ≥678) were available to analyze. There was an overall statistically significant difference favoring probiotics compared with placebo in reducing the SCORAD index. Children with moderately severe disease were more likely to benefit. Duration of probiotic administration, age, and type of probiotic used did not affect outcome. Data from this meta-analysis suggest a modest role for probiotics in pediatric AD and the effect is seen in moderately severe rather than mild disease [94]. Lee et al meta-analyzed 10 double-blind randomized controlled clinical trials. And they found out that current evidence was more convincing for probiotics' efficacy in prevention than treatment of pediatric AD [95].

However, in a Cochrane Review by Boyle et al concluded that the evidence suggests that probiotics are not an effective treatment for eczema, and probiotic treatment carries a small risk of adverse events [96]. Another review of 13 studies of probiotics for treating established eczema by Williams at al did not show convincing evidence of a clinically worthwhile benefit [97].

Taken together, most of these metaanalytic studies show a mild-moderate benefit over placebo for the treatment and/or preventionof AD. However, several of the studies still show no benefit. Some probiotics appeared to be more effective than other probiotic preparations and in children with more severe disease. It seems that duration of probiotic administration, age, and type of probiotic used did not affect outcome. Although there was a reduction in clinical eczema score in infants, this effect was not consistent between studies and caution is advised in view of methodological concerns regarding included studies.

5. Affecting factors coexisting in various studies and why inconsistent results in some studies?

Most of the studies have been conducted in small numbers of patients and results have varied considerably, even with the same strain of probiotics. When compared to the hallmark Finnish Kalliomaki study, there were also a number of other key differences between these studies that could contribute to the disparity in clinical findings. **Firstly** (biological difference of probiotic strains), different probiotic species were used in various studies. Lctbs rhamnosus GG is the strain that has been most studied. Probiotic doses have also varied considerably between the studies. Although there are noted biological differences between strains, various strains have been observed to have different immunologic effects both in vivo and in vitro [35]. Thus, the effects of preparations differ markedly, and the concept itself might be misleading in these studies and could be changed: continuous change in the supplemented strain could lead to continued immunologic stimulus and sustained and stronger effects. As a result, on the basis of these studies, immunologic effects expressed as chronic low-grade inflammation were more pronounced with LGG alone rather than with the mixture of 4 strains used in some prevention studies [57]. This might explain the more sustained preventive effect observed earlier. The results of various studies also demonstrate that findings from any probiotic bacteria cannot be extrapolated to other probiotic bacteria [20]. **Secondly** (use of probiotics in prenatal/intrauterine or postnatal or weaning period), Finnish mothers commenced supplementation during pregnancy, whereas some supplementation began in the first days of life. Prenatal/intrauterine use of probiotics would imply a direct immune effect in utero rather than any effect on postnatal colonization. However, it seems unlikely that supplementation for only a few weeks in the antenatal period alone would account for such significant differences in study outcomes, although this remains a possibility. **Thirdly** (intervention methods), in most studies all babies received the supplement directly, regardless of feeding method, whereas in the Finnish and other studies, the mother took the probiotics if babies were breast-fed. Therefore, the Finnish probiotic group and others included breast-fed infants who did not receive probiotics directly in addition to the bottle-fed infants who received probiotics for 6 months. **Fourthly** (postnatal assessment time), some researchers assessed clinical outcomes at 12 months of age, whereas the effects on AD in the Finnish or other studies were reported at 2, 4 and subsequently at 7 years of age. AD typically begins in the first year of life, and it is possible that more children could become affected in their second year of life. And in young infants, the immune system is still developing. There is still a possibility to direct it toward tolerance. In older children, the allergic phenotype is already established, and here one may only be able to relieve the symptoms. **Fifthly** (atopy risk and host factors of targeted group), some studies were performed in high-risk population all had maternal allergic disease confirmed by SPT, whereas the Finnish and other population included children with maternal, paternal, or sibling allergy. This may lead to some population being of slightly higher risk, compared with the Finnish and other population at the same age. Explanations for varied study results include host factors such as genetic susceptibility, environmental factors such as geographic region and diet [98]. Genotyping of study patients in relation to different genes predisposing to allergic diseases may help to find patients that might especially benefit from probiotic intervention. For example, 2 independent mutations in the gene encoding the epidermal protein filaggrin have been shown to be strong predisposing factors for childhood eczema [99]. Of note, these same mutations have recently been demonstrated to be associated not only with eczema-associated asthma susceptibility but also with asthma severity independent of eczema status. More generally, any means to better stratify or select defined subpopulations of subjects (e.g. patients with food allergy as a separate group) would help in clarifying the potency and limits of probiotic interventions against atopic diseases. **Sixthly** (other methodological set-up), there may be still due to differences in the clinical and methodological set-up (additional treatments such as topical treatment or feeding hydrolyzed infant formulae and importantly, different probiotic preparations or formulations or combinations). Other differences include age (6–18 months) of the studied children and an intervention period (16 weeks) of time. **Seventhly** (nomenclature of the disease), to date, randomized clinical trials of probiotics in allergic diseases have mostly focused on children with eczema and atopic eczema. The definitions of the disease have recently been revised by an international expert group [17-19]. In many of the studies published before the revision of the nomenclature, different definitions have been used, making direct comparisons between the studies difficult. The severity of AD at the start of an intervention may influence the outcome as well, as you imagine.

6. Safety

Probiotics available as food ingredients or dietary supplements that contain microorganisms have been used extensively in food processing for years, with a long history of safety and no adverse effects on metabolism. However, when considering the safety of probiotics, potential adverse effects include systemic infections, altered metabolism, and gene transfer [100]. A recent report has identified Lctbs septicemia in 2 children with short bowel syndrome who were receiving LGG supplementation for control of bacterial overgrowth

[101]. Land et al recently reported LGG probiotic sepsis occurring in immunocompromised infants and children [102]. A medically fragile infant 6 weeks of age became septic with a strain of LGG that was being provided as a supplement. Molecular DNA fingerprinting confirmed that the LGG probiotic supplement was the bacterial isolate from the infant. Neonatal sepsis and meningitis that were apparently associated with the administration of a probiotic supplement were also reported [103,104]. Children with abnormal immune function, premature infants, and those with indwelling central lines should use these products with caution, because many species such as Lactobacilli, streptococci, and enterococci are potential opportunistic pathogens. Owing to the theoretical risk of immunomodulation, especially in immunocompromised hosts or those with autoimmune disorders, few reports of probiotic-related disease have been reported [105].

Bifidobacteria have also been consumed in infant formulas for ≥15 years worldwide and have not been associated with any pathologic or adverse event. In particular, studies have documented safety and adequate growth with Bfdbm lactis in infants from birth and in vulnerable populations, including preterm infants, malnourished infants, and infants born to mothers with HIV disease. From the safety point of view, according to current available information, Bifidobacteria, particularly Bfdbm lactis, has a uniquely strong safety profile, making it a good probiotic candidate for newborns and young infants [106]. Lactobacilli, particularly Lctbs rhamnosus (LGG), also seem generally safe and may be a probiotic appropriate for older infants and children [107]. Until adequate data are available for each specific probiotic bacterium, use of probiotics in general cannot be recommended in immunocompromised populations. However, as safety is better documented for specific bacteria, we may be able to use them in certain populations (such as premature infants) that may stand to benefit the most from probiotic use.

Another consideration is that cow's milk protein allergy is one of the common food allergies in infants. Culture conditions used in growing several probiotic products may contain cow's milk protein. There have been reports of severe adverse reactions when pediatric patients with cow's milk protein allergy ingested probiotics. Therefore, caution should be used in prescribing such probiotic products in sensitized children to avoid significant reactions. There is also a study worth mentioning by Taylor et al using Lctbs acidophilus daily for the first 6 months of life in newborns of women with allergy. The presence of Lctbs in the body at 6 months of age was associated with increased risk of subsequent cow's milk sensitization as well [87]. Nevertheless other studies have examined the effect of probiotic consumption on sensitization to several allergens (e.g. peanut, hen's egg, soy, wheat, milk, cat, dog), as determined by specific IgE production or skin prick test. The authors could not find a difference before and after the treatment. Interesting another trial by Kopp et al demonstrated that supplementation with LGG during pregnancy and early infancy in affected children it might be associated with an increased rate of recurrent episodes of wheezing bronchitis [88]. However, a recent study was done by Kukkonen et al evaluating airway inflammation in probiotic-treated children at 5 years in 1018 children. Early intervention with probiotics and prebiotics did not affect airway inflammation later in childhood [108].

Furthermore, similarly certain probiotics are known to stimulate Th1 immunity, which has been suggested as one of the mechanisms by which they can suppress Th2-mediated allergic diseases. However, this presumed excessive immunostimulation might aggravate or induce Th1-mediated immune responses and diseases such as type 1 diabetes, multiple sclerosis; and it might cause an additional safety issue [105]. Consequence of over-activation of the immune system by probiotics in hosts with immune dysfunctions, such as individuals genetically predisposed to autoimmunity, has raised some concerns too. With respect to the association between bacterial antigens and autoimmune responses and the adjuvant activity of lactic acid bacteria strains, the involvement of lactic acid bacteria in the pathogenesis of some models of autoimmunity in experimental animals and possibly in humans has been suggested [109]. Thus, from a safety point of view, the potential of probiotic bacteria (especially the immunostimulatory strains), to induce destructive inflammation or autoimmunity needs to be investigated. For instance, it has been experimentally demonstrated that Lctbs casei cell wall components (given intraperitoneally) are able to induce cardioangitis (an autoimmunity-associated heart disease) in mice [110].

7. Conclusion

As mentioned above, there is a large amount of conflicting data on the preventive/therapeutic effects of probiotics in AD. Results from metaanalyses and systematic reviews that combine results of studies from different types of probiotics to examine the effects in any disease should be interpreted with caution. One may quickly recognize the degree of heterogeneity among the different probiotic studies. As mentioned, very few studies were similar in design. Several different probiotic strains with different dosing regimens were used, and many studies showed similarity in efficacy to placebo shortly after probiotic therapy was discontinued. Some probiotic studies suggest short-term statistically significant improvement in SCORAD scores and no sustained benefit from continued ingestion. Therefore, subgroup analysis became critical in understanding the outcomes of the studies. Not all children receiving the probiotic agent benefited, but subsets of these patients, mainly those with moderate disease activity and IgE-associated disease (atopic eczema), seemed to have benefited the most. There are also difficulties of recognizing etiology and pathogenesis of AD in which have many mechanisms involved. Similarly, with various strains, especially e.g. in Kopp and Taylor et al's study, development and/or stimulation of Th2-mediated immune responses have been described [87,88]. Additionally, if probiotics are used in patients with ADs for any reason -therapy or prevention- cautionary approach ought to be taken. Thus, probiotics cannot be recommended generally for primary prevention of ADs. Any probiotics should not be used especially in immune-compromised children; even they have at risk for ADs. Finally, there is insufficient but fairly promising evidence to recommend the addition of probiotics to foods for prevention and treatment of AD [111].

8. Five-year view and future expectations

Involvement of commensal enteric microflora and its components with strong immunoactivating properties in etiopathogenetic mechanism of multifactorial diseases, including atopic diseases has been recently suggested. Regulation of intestinal microflora composition (e.g. by probiotics) offers the possibility to influence the development of mucosal and systemic immunity as well as it can play a role also in prevention and treatment of AD. Progress has been made by the identification of receptors and pathways through which gut microbes influence development of the immune system. Such mechanistic data have moved a field that was once regarded as being on the scientific fringe to the mainstream, and support increased funding to advance this promising area of research in the hope that it might deliver the long awaited answer of how to safely prevent AD.

Better understanding of the effects of different probiotic strains and a deeper insight into the mechanisms of the heterogeneous manifestations of AD are needed for the validation of specific strains carrying anti-allergic potential. Therefore, research activities are currently focusing on identification of specific probiotic strains with immunomodulatory potential and on how dietary content interacts with the most efficacious probiotic strains. Moreover, the selection of the most beneficial probiotic strain, the dose, and the timing of supplementation still need to be determined. Further studies should also clarify if any susceptible groups of AD exist and how these groups benefit from supplementation with certain probiotic strains.

Some studies in the management of AD suggest that therapeutic benefit requires a combination of probiotic species (as with VSL#3 or Lacto-mix) or that the component(s) responsible for the anti-inflammatory effect in combination preparations have specific properties that monotherapy probiotics do not [112]. This concept also supports the use of prebiotics that increase concentrations of several commensal immunoregulatory bacteria. Prebiotic use was shown to be associated with a reduction in the faecal concentration of Bacteroides fragilis, but had no effect on Lactobacilli or Bifidobacteria. Genetically modified probiotics will be tested for their ability to attenuate AD thru secreting regulatory cytokines in experimental models as well [113]. In near future, the researchers will look for more appropriate combinations of probiotic species or modified probiotics with/without prebiotic and test them in human/experimental AD models.

Additionally, side effects are very low and they might not be nonexistent, as shown in a set of patients with different diseases. However, probiotics should not be considered as totally harmless, particularly in the immunodeficient host, and more safety studies are needed. As imagined, probiotics may have unpredictable behaviour like all microorganisms, such as unanticipated gene expression in nonnative host environment, or acquired mutations occurring spontaneously via bacterial DNA-transfer mechanisms [114]. And certain probiotics are known to stimulate Th1 immunity, which has been suggested as one of the mechanisms by which they can suppress Th2-mediated allergic diseases [110].

9. Key issues

- Since conclusions on probiotics are limited to specific strains and models, they should not be generalized [20,35].
- Probiotics should not be considered as completely harmless, particularly in the immunodeficient host, and more safety studies are needed [100-110, 115,116].
- Physiological use (normal route, normal dose, normal growth phase, specific strain or substrain/species) is studied in all cases, so as not to overwhelm (high dose) or circumvent natural immune processing [100-110].
- Do probiotics really induce/exacerbate Th1 and / or Th2- mediated diseases? Such as being reported an increased rate of recurrent wheezing episodes, an augmented rate of atopic disorders, increased sensitization to allergens as well as autoimmune disorders. Lactobacilli and Bifidobacteria have specific dose- and duration- dependent immunomodulatory effects on the proliferation of B-/T-lymphocytes [108-110].
- The researchers ought to look for more appropriate and safe combinations of probiotic species (as with VSL#3 or Lacto-mix) or modified probiotics with/without prebiotic and test them in human/experimental AD models [112].
- Research activities are currently focusing on identification of specific probiotic strains with immunomodulatory potential and on how dietary content interacts with the most

efficacious probiotic strains. Further studies should be made for the identification of receptors and pathways through which gut microbes influence development of the immune system [117,118].

10. References

[1] Prescott SL, Macaubas C, Holt BJ, Smallacombe TB, Loh R, Sly PD, Holt PG. Transplacental priming of the human immune system to environmental allergens: universal skewing of initial T cell responses toward the Th2 cytokine profile. J Immunol 1998; 160: 4730-7.

[2] Cabana MD, McKean M, Wong AR, Chao C, Caughey AB. Examining the hygiene hypothesis: the Trial of infant probiotic supplementation. Paediatr Perinat Epidemiol 2007; 21 Suppl 3: 23-8.

[3] Björkstén B, Sepp E, Julge K, Voor T, Mikelsaar M. Allergy development and the intestinal microflora during the first year of life. J Allergy Clin Immunol 2001; 108: 516-20.

[4] Renz-Polster H, David MR, Buist AS, Vollmer WM, O'Connor EA, Frazier EA, Wall MA. Caesarean section delivery and the risk of allergic disorders in childhood. Clin Exp Allergy 2005; 35: 1466-72.

[5] Newburg DS. Oligosaccharides in human milk and bacterial colonization. J Pediatr Gastroenterol Nutr 2000; 30(suppl 2): S8-17.

[6] Matsuki T, Watanabe K, Tanaka R, Fukuda M, Oyaizu H. Distribution of bifidobacterial species in human intestinal microflora examined with 16S rRNA-gene-targeted species-specific primers. Appl Environ Microbiol 1999; 65: 4506-12.

[7] Harmsen HJ, Wildeboer-Veloo AC, Raangs GC, Wagendorp AA, Klijn N, Bindels JG, Welling GW. Analysis of intestinal flora development in breast-fed and formula-fed infants by using molecular identification and detection methods. J Pediatr Gastroenterol Nutr 2000; 30: 61-7.

[8] Yoshioka H, Iseki K, Fujita K. Development and differences of intestinal flora in the neonatal period in breast-fed and bottle-fed infants. Pediatrics 1983; 72: 317-21.

[9] Kalliomaki M, Kirjavainen P, Eerola E, Kero P, Salminen S, Isolauri E. Distinct patterns of neonatal gut microflora in infants in whom atopy was and was not developing. J Allergy Clin Immunol 2001; 107: 129-34.

[10] Gareau MG, Sherman PM, Walker WA. Probiotics and the gut microbiota in intestinal health and disease.Nat Rev Gastroenterol Hepatol. 2010; 7(9): 503-14.

[11] Metchnikoff E. The Prolongation of Life: Optimistic Studies. London: G. P. Putnam & Sons; 1907.

[12] Food and Agriculture Organization, World Health Organization. Report of Joint FAO/WHO expert consultation on evaluation of health and nutritional properties of probiotics in food including powder milk with live lactic acid bacteria. FAO/WHO Report No. 10-1-2001.

[13] Özdemir Ö. Various effects of different probiotic strains in allergic disorders: an update from laboratory and clinical data. Clin Exp Immunol. 2010; 160(3), 295-304.

[14] Özdemir Ö. Any Benefits of Probiotics in Allergic Disorders? Allergy Asthma Proc 2010; 31, 103-11.

[15] Majamaa H, Isolauri E. Probiotics. A novel approach in the management of food allergy. J Allergy Clin Immunol 1997; 99: 179-85.

[16] Kalliomäki M, Salminen S, Poussa T, Isolauri E. Probiotics during the first 7 years of life: a cumulative risk reduction of eczema in a randomized, placebo- controlled trial. J Allergy Clin Immunol 2007, 119(4):1019-21.

[17] Darsow U, Wollenberg A, Simon D, Taïeb A, Werfel T, Oranje A, et al. ETFAD/EADV eczema task force 2009 position paper on diagnosis and treatment of atopic dermatitis. J Eur Acad Dermatol Venereol. 2010; 24(3): 317-28. doi: 10.1111/j.1468-3083.2009.03415.x

[18] Colin R Simpson, John Newton, Julia Hippisley-Cox, Aziz Sheikh. Trends in the epidemiology and prescribing of medication for eczema in England. J R Soc Med 2009: 102: 108–117. doi: 10.1258/jrsm.2009.080211.

[19] Bongaerts GP, Severijnen RS. Preventive and curative effects of probiotics in atopic patients. Med Hypotheses. 2005;64(6):1089-92.

[20] Walker WA. Mechanisms of action of probiotics. Clin Infect Dis 2008; 46 Suppl 2:S87-91; discussion S144-51.

[21] Björkstén B, Naaber P, Sepp E, Mikelsaar M. The intestinal microflora in allergic Estonian and Swedish 2-year-old children. Clin Exp Allergy. 1999; 29(3): 342–6.

[22] Watanabe S, Narisawa Y, Arase S, Okamatsu H, Ikenaga T, Tajiri Y, Kumemura M. Differences in fecal microflora between patients with atopic dermatitis and healthy control subjects. J Allergy Clin Immunol 2005, 111(3): 587-91.

[23] Kirjavainen PV, Arvola T, Salminen SJ, Isolauri E. Aberrant composition of gut microbiota of allergic infants: a target of bifidobacterial therapy at weaning? Gut 2002; 51–55.

[24] Sepp E, Julge K, Mikelsaar M, Björkstén B. Intestinal microbiota and immunoglobulin E responses in 5-year-old Estonian children. Clin Exp Allergy 2005, 35(9): 1141-6.

[25] Adlerberth I, Strachan DP, Matricardi PM, Ahrné S, Orfei L, Aberg N, et al. Gut microbiota and development of atopic eczema in 3 European birth cohorts. J Allergy Clin Immunol 2007, 120(2): 343-50.

[26] Penders J, Stobberingh EE, Thijs C, Adams H, Vink C, van Ree R, van den Brandt PA et al. Molecular finger printing of the intestinal microbiota of infants in whom atopic eczema was or was not developing. Clin Exp Allergy 2006, 36(12): 1602-8.

[27] Sudo N, Sawamura S, Tanaka K, Aiba Y, Kubo C, Koga Y. The requirement of intestinal bacterial flora for the development of an IgE production system fully susceptible to oral tolerance induction. J Immunol 1997; 159: 1739–45.

[28] Viljanen M, Kuitunen M, Haahtela T, Juntunen-Backman K, Korpela R, Savilahti E. Probiotic effects on faecal inflammatory markers and on faecal IgA in food allergic atopic eczema/dermatitis syndrome infants. Pediatr Allergy Immunol 2005; 16: 65-71.

[29] Isolauri E. Studies on Lactobacillus GG in food hypersensitivity disorders. Nutr Today Suppl 1996; 31: 285–315.

[30] Cebra JJ. Influences of microbiota on intestinal immune system development. Am J Clin Nutr 1999; 69: 1046S–1051S.

[31] Malin MV, Korhonen H, Syvaoja EL, et al. Dietary therapy with lactobacillus GG, bovine colostrum or bovine immune colostrum in patients with juvenile chronic arthritis: evaluation of effect on gut defense mechanisms. Inflammopharmacology 1997; 5: 219-36.

[32] Pessi T, Isolauri E, Sutas Y, Kankaanranta H, Moilanen E, Hurme M. Suppression of T cell activation by Lactobacillus rhamnosus GG-degraded bovine casein. Immunopharmacology 2001; 1: 211–8.
[33] Kaila M, Isolauri E, Soppi E, Virtanen E, Laine S, Arvilommi H. Enhancement of the circulating antibody secreting cell response in human diarrhea by a human Lactobacillus strain. Pediatr Res 1992; 32: 141–4.
[34] Ruemmele FM, Bier D, Marteau P, Rechkemmer G, Bourdet-Sicard R, Walker WA, Goulet O. Clinical evidence for immunomodulatory effects of probiotic bacteria. J Pediatr Gastroenterol Nutr 2009; 48: 126-41.
[35] Christensen HR, Frokiaer H, Pestka JJ. Lactobacilli differentially modulate expression of cytokines and maturation surface markers in murine dendritic cells. J Immunol 2002; 168: 171–8.
[36] Salminen SJ, Gueimonde M, Isolauri E. Probiotics that modify disease risk. J Nutr 2005; 135: 1294-8.
[37] Niers LE, Timmerman HM, Rijkers GT et al. Identification of strong interleukin-10 inducing lactic acid bacteria which downregulate T helper type 2 cytokines. Clin Exp Allergy 2005; 35: 1481–9.
[38] Maassen CB, van Holten-Neelen C, Balk F, den Bak-Glashouwer MJ, Leer RJ, Laman JD, Boersma WJ, Claassen E. Strain-dependent induction of cytokine profiles in the gut by orally administered Lactobacillus strains. Vaccine 2000; 18: 2613–23.
[39] Kruisselbrink A, Heijne Den Bak-Glashouwer MJ, Havenith CE, Thole JE, Janssen R. Recombinant Lactobacillus plantarum inhibits house dust mite-specific T-cell responses. Clin Exp Immunol 2001; 126: 2–8.
[40] West CE, Hammarström ML, Hernell O. Probiotics during weaning reduce the incidence of eczema. Pediatr Allergy Immunol. 2009;20(5):430-7.
[41] Sistek D, Kelly R, Wickens K, Stanley T, Fitzharris P, Crane J. Is the effect of probiotics on atopic dermatitis confined to food sensitized children? Clin Exp Allergy 2006; 36: 629-33.
[42] Kim JY, Choi YO, Ji GE. Effect of oral probiotics (Bifidobacterium lactis AD011 and Lactobacillus acidophilus AD031) administration on ovalbumin-induced food allergy mouse model. J Microbiol Biotechnol 2008; 18: 1393-1400.
[43] Takahashi N, Kitazawa H, Iwabuchi N, Xiao JZ, Miyaji K, Iwatsuki K, Saito T. Immunostimulatory oligodeoxynucleotide from Bifidobacterium longum suppresses Th2 immune responses in a murine model. Clin Exp Immunol 2006; 145:130-8.
[44] Shida K, Makino K, Morishita A. Lactobacillus casei inhibits antigen induced IgE secretion through regulation of cytokine production in murine splenocyte cultures. Int Arch Allergy Immunol 1998;115:278-87.
[45] Thomas DJ, Husmann RJ, Villamar M, Winship TR, Buck RH, Zuckermann FA. Lactobacillus rhamnosus HN001 attenuates allergy development in a pig model. PLoS One. 2011; 6(2): e16577.
[46] Rosenfeldt V, Benfeldt E, Nielsen SD, Michaelsen KF, Jeppesen DL, Valerius NH, Paerregaard A. Effect of probiotic Lactobacillus strains in children with atopic dermatitis. J Allergy Clin Immunol 2003; 111: 389-95.

[47] Brouwer ML, Wolt-Plompen SA, Dubois AE, van der Heide S, Jansen DF, Hoijer MA, Kauffman HF, Duiverman EJ. No effects of probiotics on atopic dermatitis in infancy: a randomized placebo-controlled trial. Clin Exp Allergy. 2006; 36(7): 899-906.
[48] Pohjavuori E, Viljanen M, Korpela R, Kuitunen M, Tiittanen M, Vaarala O, Savilahti E.Lactobacillus GG effect in increasing IFN-gamma production in infants with cow's milk allergy. J Allergy Clin Immunol. 2004; 114(1): 131-6.
[49] Prescott SL, Dunstan JA, Hale J, Breckler L, Lehmann H, Weston S, Richmond P. Clinical effects of probiotics are associated with increased interferon-gamma responses in very young children with atopic dermatitis. Clin Exp Allergy. 2005; 35(12): 1557-64.
[50] Isolauri E, Arvola T, Sütas Y, Moilanen E, Salminen S. Probiotics in the management of atopic eczema. Clin Exp Allergy. 2000; 30(11):1604-10.
[51] Boyle RJ, Ismail IH, Kivivuori S, Licciardi PV, Robins-Browne RM, Mah LJ, et al. Lactobacillus GG treatment during pregnancy for the prevention of eczema: a randomized controlled trial. Allergy. 2011;66(4):509-16. doi: 10.1111/j.1398-9995.2010.02507.x.
[52] Böttcher MF, Abrahamsson TR, Fredriksson M, Jakobsson T, Björkstén B.Low breast milk TGF-beta2 is induced by Lactobacillus reuteri supplementation and associates with reduced risk of sensitization during infancy. Pediatr Allergy Immunol. 2008;19(6):497-504.
[53] Betsi GI, Papadavid E, Falagas ME. Probiotics for the treatment or prevention of atopic dermatitis: a review of the evidence from randomized controlled trials. Am J Clin Dermatol 2008; 9: 93-103.
[54] Chiba Y, Shida K, Nagata S, Wada M, Bian L, Wang C, et al. Well-controlled proinflammatory cytokine responses of Peyer's patch cells to probiotic Lactobacillus casei. Immunology. 2010; 130(3):352-62.
[55] Lavasani S, Dzhambazov B, Nouri M, Fåk F, Buske S, Molin G, Thorlacius H, Alenfall J, Jeppsson B, Weström B. A novel probiotic mixture exerts a therapeutic effect on experimental autoimmune encephalomyelitis mediated by IL-10 producing regulatory T cells. PLoS One. 2010; 5(2): e9009.
[56] Woo SI, Kim JY, Lee YJ, Kim NS, Hahn YS. Effect of Lactobacillus sakei supplementation in children with atopic eczema-dermatitis syndrome.Ann Allergy Asthma Immunol. 2010; 104(4): 343-8.
[57] Marschan E, Kuitunen M, Kukkonen K, Poussa T, Sarnesto A, Haahtela T, Korpela R, Savilahti E, Vaarala O. Probiotics in infancy induce protective immune profiles that are characteristic for chronic low-grade inflammation. Clin Exp Allergy. 2008; 38(4): 611-8.
[58] Niers LE, Hoekstra MO, Timmerman HM, van Uden NO, de Graaf PM, Smits HH, Kimpen JL, Rijkers GT. Selection of probiotic bacteria for prevention of allergic diseases: immunomodulation of neonatal dendritic cells. Clin Exp Immunol 2007; 149: 344-52.
[59] Hart AL, Lammers K, Brigidi P et al. Modulation of human dendritic cell phenotype and function by probiotic bacteria. Gut 2004; 53: 1602–9.
[60] Braat H, van den Brande J, van Tol E, Hommes D, Peppelenbosch M, van Deventer S. Lactobacillus rhamnosus induces peripheral hyporesponsiveness in stimulated

CD4+ T cells via modulation of dendritic cell function. Am J Clin Nutr 2004; 80: 1618–25.

[61] Smits HH, Engering A, van der Kleij D et al. Selective probiotic bacteria induce IL-10-producing regulatory T cells in vitro by modulating dendritic cell function through dendritic cell-specific intercellular adhesion molecule 3-grabbing nonintegrin. J Allergy Clin Immunol 2005; 115: 1260–7.

[62] Kim JY, Choi YO, Ji GE. Effect of oral probiotics (Bifidobacterium lactis AD011 and Lactobacillus acidophilus AD031) administration on ovalbumin-induced food allergy mouse model.J Microbiol Biotechnol. 2008;18(8):1393-400.

[63] Feleszko W, Jaworska J, Rha RD et al. Probiotic-induced suppression of allergic sensitization and airway inflammation is associated with an increase of T regulatory-dependent mechanisms in a murine model of asthma. Clin Exp Allergy 2007; 37: 498-505.

[64] Fujimura T, Okuyama R, Ito Y, Aiba S. Profiles of Foxp3+ regulatory T cells in eczematous dermatitis, psoriasis vulgaris and mycosis fungoides. Br J Dermatol. 2008; 158(6): 1256-63.

[65] Kwon HK, Lee CG, So JS, Chae CS, Hwang JS, Sahoo A, et al. Generation of regulatory dendritic cells and CD4+Foxp3+ T cells by probiotics administration suppresses immune disorders. Proc Natl Acad Sci USA 2010; 107(5): 2159-64.

[66] Hacini-Rachinel F, Gheit H, Le Luduec JB, Dif F, Nancey S, Kaiserlian D. Oral probiotic control skin inflammation by acting on both effector and regulatory T cells. PLoS One. 2009; 4(3): e4903.

[67] Taylor AL, Hale J, Hales BJ, Dunstan JA, Thomas WR, Prescott SL. FOXP3 mRNA expression at 6 months of age is higher in infants who develop atopic dermatitis, but is not affected by giving probiotics from birth. Pediatr Allergy Immunol 2007, 18(1): 10-9.

[68] Gerasimov SV, Vasjuta VV, Myhovych OO, Bondarchuk LI. Probiotic supplement reduces atopic dermatitis in preschool children: a randomized, double-blind, placebo-controlled, clinical trial. Am J Clin Dermatol. 2010; 11(5): 351-61. doi: 10.2165/11531420-000000000-00000.

[69] Roessler A, Friedrich U, Vogelsang H, Bauer A, Kaatz M, Hipler UC, Schmidt I, Jahreis G. The immune system in healthy adults and patients with atopic dermatitis seems to be affected differently by a probiotic intervention. Clin Exp Allergy. 2008; 38(1): 93-102.

[70] Hoarau C, Lagaraine C, Martin L, Velge-Roussel F, Lebranchu Y. Supernatant of Bifidobacterium breve induces dendritic cell maturation, activation, and survival through a Toll-like receptor 2 pathway. J Allergy Clin Immunol 2006; 117: 696–702.

[71] Forsythe P, Inman MD, Bienenstock J. Oral treatment with live Lactobacillus reuteri inhibits the allergic airway response in mice. Am J Respir Crit Care Med. 2007;175(6):561-9.

[72] Viljanen M, Savilahti E, Haahtela T, Juntunen-Backman K, Korpela R, Poussa T, Tuure T, Kuitunen M. Probiotics in the treatment of atopic eczema/dermatitis syndrome in infants: a double-blind placebo-controlled trial. Allergy. 2005; 60(4): 494-500.

[73] Kukkonen K, Savilahti E, Haahtela T, et al. Probiotics and prebiotic galactooligosaccharides in the prevention of allergic diseases: a randomized, doubleblind, placebo-controlled trial. J Allergy Clin Immunol. 2007; 119(1): 192–8.

[74] Kuitunen M, Kukkonen K, Juntunen-Backman K, Korpela R, Poussa T, Tuure T, Haahtela T, Savilahti E. Probiotics prevent IgE-associated allergy until age 5 years in cesarean-delivered children but not in the total cohort. J Allergy Clin Immunol 2009; 123: 335-41.

[75] Abrahamsson TR, Jakobsson T, Bottcher MF, et al. Probiotics in prevention of IgE-associated eczema: a double-blind, randomized, placebo-controlled trial. J Allergy Clin Immunol. 2007; 119(5): 1174–1180.

[76] Isolauri E, Rautava S, Kalliomäki M, Kirjavainen P, Salminen S. Role of probiotics in food hypersensitivity. Curr Opin Allergy Clin Immunol 2002; 2: 263-71.

[77] Kirjavainen PV, Salminen SJ, Isolauri E. Probiotic bacteria in the management of atopic disease: underscoring the importance of viability. J Pediatr Gastroenterol Nutr. 2003; 36(2): 223-7.

[78] Weston S, Halbert A, Richmond P, Prescott SL. Effects of probiotics on atopic dermatitis. A randomised controlled trial. Arch Dis Child 2005, 90(9): 892-7.

[79] Hoang BX, Shaw G, Pham P, Levine SA. Lactobacillus rhamnosus cell lysate in the management of resistant childhood atopic eczema. Inflamm Allergy Drug Targets. 2010; 9(3): 192-6.

[80] Hattori K, Yamamoto A, Sasai M, Taniuchi S, Kojima T, KobayashiY, et al. Effects of administration of bifidobacteria on fecal microflora and clinical symptoms in infants with atopic dermatitis. Arerugi 2003; 52: 20–30.

[81] Wickens K, Black PN, Stanley TV, et al. A differential effect of 2 probiotics in the prevention of eczema and atopy: a double-blind, randomized, placebo-controlled trial. J Allergy Clin Immunol 2008; 122: 788-94.

[82] Niers L, Martín R, Rijkers G, Sengers F, Timmerman H, van Uden N, et al. The effects of selected probiotic strains on the development of eczema (the PandA study). Allergy. 2009; 64(9): 1349-58.

[83] Kim JY, Kwon JH, Ahn SH, Lee SI, Han YS, Choi YO, et al. Effect of probiotic mix (Bifidobacterium bifidum, Bifidobacterium lactis, Lactobacillus acidophilus) in the primary prevention of eczema: a double-blind, randomized, placebo-controlled trial. Pediatr Allergy Immunol. 2010; 21(2 Pt 2): e386-93.

[84] Dotterud CK, Storrø O, Johnsen R, Oien T. Probiotics in pregnant women to prevent allergic disease: a randomized, double-blind trial. Br J Dermatol. 2010; 163(3): 616-23. doi: 10.1111/j.1365-2133.2010.09889.x.

[85] Lodinova-Zadnikova R, Cukrowska B, Tlaskalova-Hogenova H. Oral administration of probiotic Escherichia coli after birth reduces frequency of allergies and repeated infections later in life (after 10 and 20 years). Int Arch Allergy Immunol 2003, 131(3): 209-11.

[86] Huurre A, Laitinen K, Rautava S, Korkeamäki M, Isolauri E. Impact of maternal atopy and probiotic supplementation during pregnancy on infant sensitization: a double-blind placebo-controlled study. Clin Exp Allergy. 2008; 38(8):1342-8.

[87] Taylor A, Dunstan J, Prescott S. Probiotic supplementation for the first 6 months of life fails to reduce the risk of atopic dermatitis and increases the risk of allergen sensitization in high-risk children: a randomized controlled trial. J Allergy Clin Immunol 2007; 119:184-91.

[88] Kopp MV, Isabell Hennemuth, Andrea Heinzmann, Radvan Urbanek. Randomized, double-blind, placebo-controlled trial of probiotics for primary prevention: No clinical effects of Lactobacillus GG supplementation. Pediatrics 2008; 121: e850-6.
[89] Grüber C, Wendt M, Sulser C, Lau S, Kulig M, Wahn U, Werfel T, Niggemann B. Randomized, placebo-controlled trial of Lactobacillus rhamnosus GG as treatment of atopic dermatitis in infancy. Allergy 2007; 62(11): 1270-6.
[90] Fölster-Holst R, Müller F, Schnopp N, Abeck D, Kreiselmaier I, Lenz T, von Rüden U, et al. Prospective, randomized controlled trial on Lactobacillus rhamnosus in infants with moderate to severe atopic dermatitis. Br J Dermatol 2006, 155(6): 1256-61.
[91] Soh SE, Aw M, Gerez I, et al. Probiotic supplementation in the first 6 months of life in at risk Asian infants--effects on eczema and atopic sensitization at the age of 1 year. Clin Exp Allergy 2009; 39: 571-8.
[92] Zhu DL, Yang WX, Yang HM. [Meta analysis of lactic acid bacteria as probiotics for the primary prevention of infantile eczema]. Zhongguo Dang Dai Er Ke Za Zhi. 2010; 12(9): 734-9.
[93] Osborn DA, Sinn JK. Probiotics in infants for prevention of allergic disease and food hypersensitivity. Cochrane Database Syst Rev 2007; 4:CD006475.
[94] Michail S, Onady G, Stolfi A, Johnson T. Efficacy of probiotics in treatment of pediatric atopic dermatitis a meta-analysis of randomized, controlled trials. 2008, 101(5): 508-16.
[95] Lee J, Seto D, Bielory L. Meta-analysis of clinical trials of probiotics for prevention and treatment of pediatric atopic dermatitis. J Allergy Clin Immunol 2008; 121:116-21.
[96] Boyle RJ, Bath-Hextall FJ, Leonardi-Bee J, Murrell DF, Tang ML. Probiotics for treating eczema. Cochrane Database Syst Rev. 2008; (4): CD006135.
[97] Williams HC, Grindlay DJ. What's new in atopic eczema? An analysis of systematic reviews published in 2007 and 2008. Part 2. Disease prevention and treatment. Clin Exp Dermatol. 2010; 35(3): 223-7.
[98] Ogden NS, Bielory L. Probiotics. A complementary approach in the treatment and prevention of pediatric atopic disease. Curr Opin Allergy Clin Immunol 2005, 5(2):179-84.
[99] Batchelor JM, Grindlay DJ, Williams HC. What's new in atopic eczema? An analysis of systematic reviews published in 2008 and 2009. Clin Exp Dermatol. 2010; 35(8): 823-7; quiz 827-8. doi: 10.1111/j.1365-2230.2010.03901.x.
[100] Ishibashi N, Yamazaki S. Probiotics and safety. Am J Clin Nutr. 2001; 73(Suppl): 465S- 470S.
[101] Kunz AN, Noel JM, Fairchok MP. Two cases of Lactobacillus bacteremia during probiotic treatment of short gut syndrome. J Pediatr Gastroenterol Nutr 2004; 38: 457-8.
[102] Land MH, Rouster-Stevens K, Woods CR, Cannon ML, Cnota J, Shetty AK. Lactobacillus sepsis associated with probiotic therapy. Pediatrics. 2005; 115(1): 178-81.
[103] Thompson C, McCarter YS, Krause PJ, Herson VC. Lactobacillus acidophilus sepsis in a neonate. J Perinatol. 2001; 21(4):258-60.
[104] Broughton RA, Gruber WC, Haffar AA, Baker CJ. Neonatal meningitis due to Lactobacillus. Pediatr Infect Dis. 1983; 2(5): 382–4.
[105] Maassen CB, Claassen E. Strain-dependent effects of probiotic lactobacilli on EAE autoimmunity.Vaccine. 2008; 26(17): 2056-7.

[106] Food and Agriculture Organization, World Health Organization. The Food and Agriculture Organization of the United Nations and the World Health Organization Joint FAO/WHO Working Group report on drafting guidelines for the evaluation of probiotics in food. FAO/WHO Report No. 4-30-2002.
[107] Salminen S, von Wright A, Morelli L et al. Demonstration of safety of probiotics: a review. Int J Food Microbiol 1998; 44:93–106.
[108] Kukkonen AK, Kuitunen M, Savilahti E, Pelkonen A, Malmberg P, Mäkelä M. Airway inflammation in probiotic-treated children at 5 years. Pediatr Allergy Immunol. 2011; 22(2): 249-51. doi: 10.1111/j.1399-3038.2010.01079.x
[109] Baken KA, Ezendam J, Gremmer ER, de Klerk A, Pennings JL, Matthee B, et al. Evaluation of immunomodulation by Lactobacillus casei Shirota: immune function, autoimmunity and gene expression. Int J Food Microbiol. 2006; 112(1): 8-18.
[110] Okitsu-Negishi S, Nakano I, Suzukim K, Hashira S, Abe T, Yoshino K. The induction of cardioangitis by Lactobacillus casei cell wall in mice: I. The cytokine production from murine macrophages by Lactobacillus casei cell wall extract. Clin. Immunol. Immunopathol. 1996; 78: 30-40.
[111] Prescott SL, Björkstén B. Probiotics for the prevention or treatment of allergic diseases. J Allergy Clin Immunol. 2007; 120(2): 255–262.
[112] Chapman CM, Gibson GR, Rowland I.Health benefits of probiotics: are mixtures more effective than single strains? Eur J Nutr. 2011; 50(1): 1-17.
[113] Van Huynegem K, Loos M, Steidler L. Immunomodulation by genetically engineered lactic acid bacteria. Front Biosci. 2009; 14: 4825-35.
[114] Egervärn M, Roos S, Lindmark H. Identification and characterization of antibiotic resistance genes in Lactobacillus reuteri and Lactobacillus plantarum. J Appl Microbiol. 2009; 107(5): 1658-68.
[115] Despande GC, Rao SC, Keil AD, Patole SK. Evidence based guidelines for use of probiotics in preterm neonates. BMC Med. 2011; 9(1): 92.
[116] Elias J, Bozzo P, Einarson A. Are probiotics safe for use during pregnancy and lactation? Can Fam Physician. 2011; 57(3): 299-301.
[117] Marko Kalliomäki, Jean-Michel Antoine, Udo Herz, Ger T. Rijkers, Jerry M. Wells, Annick Mercenier. Guidance for Substantiating the Evidence for Beneficial Effects of Probiotics: Prevention and Management of Allergic Diseases by Probiotics. J. Nutr. 2010; 140: 713S–721S.
[118] Shida K, Nanno M, Nagata S. Flexible cytokine production by macrophages and T cells in response to probiotic bacteria: a possible mechanism by which probiotics exert multifunctional immune regulatory activities. Gut Microbes. 2011; 2(2): 109-14.

22

Food Compounds Inhibit *Staphylococcus Aureus* Bacteria and the Toxicity of Staphylococcus Enterotoxin A (SEA) Associated with Atopic Dermatitis

Reuven Rasooly and Mendel Friedman
Western Regional Research Center, Agricultural Research Service, United States Department of Agriculture, Albany, California USA

1. Introduction

Enterotoxigenic *S. aureus* is a major bacterial pathogen that develops multi-drug resistance to antibiotics (Pereira et al., 2009; Pu et al., 2011; Rhee & Woo, 2010). The enterotoxigenic bacteria and secreted toxins have been reported to cause clinical infections, and it has also been reported that they contaminate a broad variety of foods, including breaded chicken products (Pepe et al., 2006), canned mushrooms (Anderson et al., 1996), cheeses (Ertas et al., 2010; Ostyn et al., 2010; Rosengren et al., 2010), raw milk (Fusco et al., 2011; Heidinger et al., 2009), pork meat (Wallin-Carlquist et al., 2010), and other foods (Balaban & Rasooly, 2000) as well contaminating handles of shopping carts (Mizumachi et al., 2011) causing many foodborne illnesses in the United States each year (Shinefield & Ruff, 2009). Staphylococcal food poisoning is due to the absorption from the digestive tract into the circulation of the enterotoxins preformed in food A toxin level of <1 μg may induce symptoms of food poisoning. This level is reached with a bacterial population of $>10^5$ CFU/g food (Stewart, 2005).

S. aureus produces the virulent staphylococcal enterotoxin A (SEA), a single chain protein that consists of 233 amino acid residues with a molecular weight of 27,078 Da. It has been estimated that staphylococcal enterotoxin A (SEA) secreted by the bacteria is associated with 78% of staphylococcal outbreaks (Vernozy-Rozand et al., 2004). Heat used to eliminate the pathogenic bacteria may not eliminate toxins already formed (Margosch et al., 2005; Pepe et al., 2006).

Staphylococcus enterotoxins (SEs) exhibit two separate biological activities: they cause gastroenteritis in the gastrointestinal tract and they act as a superantigen on the immune system. Previous research has shown that emetic activities and superantigenic activities of SEs are related (Shinefield & Ruff, 2009; Stewart, 2005).

Because SEA is present in contaminated foods and exerts adverse effects on the gastrointestinal tract, there is a need to find food-compatible safe conditions to inactivate it. Efforts to inhibit the toxin or its release from *S. aureus* include the use of electrolyzed water (Suzuki et al., 2002), high pressure and heat (Margosch et al., 2005), radiation and pulsed electric fields (Walkling-Ribeiro et al., 2008), condensed tannins (Choi et al., 2007) and other plant extracts (Carlos et al., 2010; Ifesan & Voravuthlkunchai, 2009), peptides (Wang et al.,

2008), phenolic compounds (Rúa et al., 2010), licochalcone A (Qiu et al., 2010), essential oils (de Souza et al., 2010; Friedman et al., 2004a; Nuñez et al., 2007; Parsaeimehr et al., 2010; Qiu et al., 2011), and toxin-specific antibodies (Larkin et al., 2010).
The objective of our research effort is to discover food-compatible ways to inhibit or inactivate both the pathogen and the toxin. In this chapter we will briefly summarize our finding in these two areas that are also relevant to atopic dermatitis.

2. Experimental procedures

The following experimental methods were used to create the data shown in the Tables and Figures.

2.1 Antibacterial activities of plant compounds against antibiotic-resistant *S. aureus*

The following procedure was adapted from Friedman et al. (2004b). Stock suspensions, 1 mg/mL, of cinnamon oil, oregano oil, thyme oil, carvacrol, and perillaldehyde were prepared by vigorous vortexing in phosphate-saline buffer at pH 7. Dilutions from stock solutions were revortexed, to ensure even mixing, before being further diluted or added to the cell suspension in the microtiter plate. The two solids (β-resorcylic acid and dopamine) formed clear solutions in the buffer. Each test substance was prepared fresh before use. Individual wells of a microtiter plate (Becton Dickinson, Oxford, UK) were filled with 100 ml of the test substance in phosphate-saline buffer and 50 ml of the culture. Triplicate wells were used for each concentration, with phosphate-saline used in the blank. The plates were shaken and then incubated at 37 °C for 1 h. The number of organisms remaining viable was then determined by a Nutrient Agar Spread Plate Technique on a 10-ml aliquot removed from each well. Plates were incubated overnight at 37 °C prior to counting.

2.2 Antibacterial activity of Phloxine B against *S. aureus*

The following procedure was adapted from Rasooly (2005). Bacteria (200 µL) grown in BHI broth were removed during the logarithmic growth phase (OD of 0.3 at 600 nm) and spread over the surface of a BHI agar plate with a bent glass rod. Various concentrations of Phloxine B (10, 5, 2.5, 1.25 and 0.62 µg) and 5 µg of chloramphenicol (10 units) and 1.5 µg of tetracycline (2.5 units) were added to the wells of these plates as antibiotic standards. Plates were then incubated for 16 h at 37 °C in the light and in the dark. The potency of Phloxine B was determined by measuring the diameter of the inhibition zone made compared to zone produced by the standard antibiotics.

2.3 Antibacterial activity of 4-hydroxytyrosol and Hidrox-12 against *S. aureus*

The procedure was adapted from Friedman et al. (2011). *S. aureus* bacteria were grown overnight at 37 °C under aerobic conditions maintained by shaking at 200 rpm in Lucia-Bertani agar (LB) medium. The effect of 4-hydroxytyrosol and Hidrox-12 on bacterial growth was studied by addition of a bacterial suspension (~10^4 diluted from ~10^8 bacteria/mL) to various concentrations of 4-hydroxytyrosol (range: 0.71-0.022 mg/mL) and Hidrox-12 suspension (range: 1.29-0.040 mg/mL) in phosphate buffer pH 7.0. After 60 minutes of incubation at 37 °C, 200 rpm, each dose/bacterial suspension was diluted 1/10 and then 20 µL of each dose/bacterial suspension were dropped at the top of a square LB plate with grids. The plates were tilted and the drops ran down the plate. The plates were dried (~10-15 min) and then incubated overnight 37 °C. Each dose was sampled in quadruplicate with control values ~100 colony forming units (CFUs).

2.4 Prophylactic vaccination of mice with *S. aureus*

The following procedure was adapted from Balaban et al. (1998). RAP (regulatory RNAIII activating protein, 10 µg) was injected with CFA (completer Freund's adjuvant) on first injection, followed with ICFA (incomplete Freund's adjuvant) on second and third injections subcutaneously into 4-week old immunocompetent hairless male mice on days 0, 7, and 21. Control mice were either injected with the adjuvant alone or not injected. Vaccinated and control mice were challenged on day 31 with 1.24 x 10^8 CFU of wild-type Smith diffuse strain (SD) of *S. aureus* subcutaneously together with 1 mg of Cytodex beads to induce local infection. The size of the lesion was measured daily. Fisher's exact probability test was used to compare proportions of mice developing lesions and mice developing RAP antibodies among the RAP vaccinated, CFA controls, and untreated control groups. Among animals that developed lesions after challenge with *S. aureus*, the size of the lesions was compared by single-factor analysis of variance. Post-hoc testing was done by Fisher's protected least significant difference.

2.5 Staphylococcus enterotoxin (SEA) activity assays

The procedure was adapted from Friedman et al. (2011). Spleen cells were placed in 96-well plates (1 X 10^6/mL, 0.2 mL) in Russ-10 medium and treated with various concentrations of SEA following incubation at 37 °C in a 5% CO_2 incubator. After incubation at various time points, cell proliferation was measured by adding bromodeoxyuridine (5-bromo-2-deoxyuridine, BrdU)-labeled DNA to each well 4 h before fixation as described by the instructions of the manufacturer. Spectroscopic measurements were made at 620 and 450 nm.
A second measure of inhibition activity of SEA activity was determined by an enzyme cleavage assay. Briefly, the glycyl-phenylalanyl-aminofluorocoumarin (GF-AFC) substrate (50 µL) was added to the wells. After mixing and incubation for 30 min at 37°C, this substrate enters intact cells. The live cell protease then cleaves GF-AFC, releasing AFC which generates a fluorescent signal. The resulting fluorescence was measured by a fluorescence plate reader (excitation at 355 nm and emission at 523 nm). We used 5 and 200 ng/mL of the toxin because at (a) < 5 ng/mL we did not detect cell proliferation induced by the toxin; and (b) at ~200 ng/mL proliferation of spleen cells reach a maximum. Results are expressed as representative data from triplicate wells from two different methods, BRDU and the enzyme cleavage GFA-AFC assays which work only with live cells.

3. Results and discussion

Here, we briefly describe our studies designed to demonstrate the potential of bioactive food ingredients to inhibit growth of *S. aureus* bacteria and to inactivate SEA produced by these bacteria. The results suggest that it may possible to reduce the toxic potential of these toxin-producing organisms with the aid of edible food ingredients.

3.1 Naturally occurring compounds inactivate antibiotic-resistant *Staphylococcus aureus*

Antibiotic resistant microorganisms often arise from the administration of sub-therapeutic levels of antibiotics in animal feeds. They are present in the animal waste, often contaminating groundwater, surface water, irrigation water, fruits, and vegetables. They can then disseminate through the food chain and enter the human intestinal tract after the produce or undercooked meat is eaten (Davis & Lederberg, 2001; Walsh, 2003).

We showed that the following natural substances have antibacterial activity against three resistant pathogens including Staphylococcus aureus (ATCC12715): cinnamon oil, oregano oil, thyme oil, carvacrol, (S)-perillaldehyde, 3,4-dihydroxybenzoic acid (β-resorcylic acid), and 3,4-dihydroxyphenethylamine (dopamine) (Friedman et al., 2004a). Exposure of pathogens to a dilution series of the test compounds revealed that oregano oil is the most active substance (Table 1). Activities of the test compounds were in the following approximate order: oregano oil > thyme oil ≈ carvacrol > cinnamon oil > perillaldehyde > dopamine > β-resorcylic acid. The order of susceptibilities of the pathogens to inactivation is: *B. cereus* (vegetative) >> *S. aureus* ≈ *E. coli* >> *B. cereus* (spores). Some of the test substances may be effective against antibiotic-resistant bacteria in foods and feeds and in hospital environments.

	Concentration in well (μg/ml)				
Compound	0 (control)	66.7	6.67	1.34	0.067
Oregano oil	4.6 ± 0.08[1]	<1.5	3.4 ± 0.12^{c}	4.6 ± 0.07^{ab}	4.6 ± 0.12^{b}
Thyme oil	4.6 ± 0.04	<1.5	4.5 ± 0.04^{b}	4.6 ± 0.09^{b}	4.6 ± 0.05^{b}
Cinnamon oil	4.6 ± 0.12	2.6 ± 0.58	4.6 ± 0.02^{b}	4.6 ± 0.07^{b}	4.7 ± 0.11^{ab}
Carvacrol	4.9 ± 0.12	0 ± 0	4.8 ± 0.21^{a}	4.8 ± 0.04^{a}	4.8 ± 0.12^{a}
Perillaldehyde	4.7 ± 0.05	4.1 ± 0.1	4.6 ± 0.11^{b}	4.6 ± 0.12^{b}	4.8 ± 0.02^{a}
	Concentration in well (μg/ml)				
	0 (control)	3330	670	330	67
Dopamine	4.6 ± 0.07	3.2 ± 0.33	4.5 ± 0.03	4.5 ± 0.11	4.6 ± 0.12
	Concentration in well (μg/ml)				
	Control	6000	5330	4670	3330
β-Resorcylic acid	4.8 ± 0.06	<1.5	<1.5	<1.5	4.6 ± 0.03

Table 1. Antibacterial activities of three plant essential oils (oregano, thyme, cinnamon), two essential oil compounds (carvacrol, perillaldehyde), dopamine, and the phenolic compound β-resorcylic acid) against antibiotic-resistant *S. aureus* (log CFU/ml; average ± SD, n=3). CFU = colony-forming-units or bacterial counts. Superscript letters not in common are not significantly different ($p<0.05$). Adapted from (Friedman et al. 2004a).

3.2 The food dye Phloxine B inactivates *S. aureus*

The dye Phloxine B has been approved by the Food and Drug Administration (FDA) for human consumption. It is used in food, drugs, and cosmetics. We found that Phloxine B exhibits strong antimicrobial activities against several pathogenic bacteria including *S. aureus* (Rasooly, 2005).

The diffusion assay we used to determine bactericidal effects shows that the activity of Phloxine B is similar to that of the medicinal antibiotics chloramphenicol and tetracycline (Figure 1). Figure 2 shows the dose-dependence of the inactivation in the range 25 to 100 μg/ml. A postulated mechanism of antimicrobial effects of the negatively charged dye is described in some detail in the legend of Figure 3. It is likely that related charged polyaromatic compounds, including naturally occurring polyphenolic compounds, may operate by similar mechanisms. The results suggest that Phloxine B has the potential to be used as an antimicrobial agent against *S. aureus* in pathogens and in veterinary and human medicine and against other pathogenic bacteria. Its possible use against atopic dermatitis in human patients merits study.

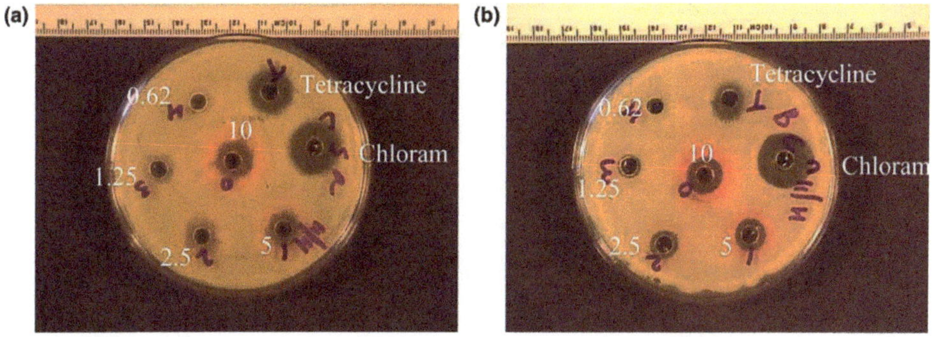

Fig. 1. Antibiotic potency of Phloxine B was determined by agar diffusion assay. Various concentrations of Phloxine B (10, 5, 2.5, 1.25, 0.62 µg) and 5 µg of chloramphenicol (10 units) and 1.5 µg tetracycline (2.5 units) were added to agar plates seeded with *S. aureus* (a), or *B. cereus* (b). Following incubation, the plates were examined for bacterial growth inhibition. Asdapted from (Rasooly, 2005).

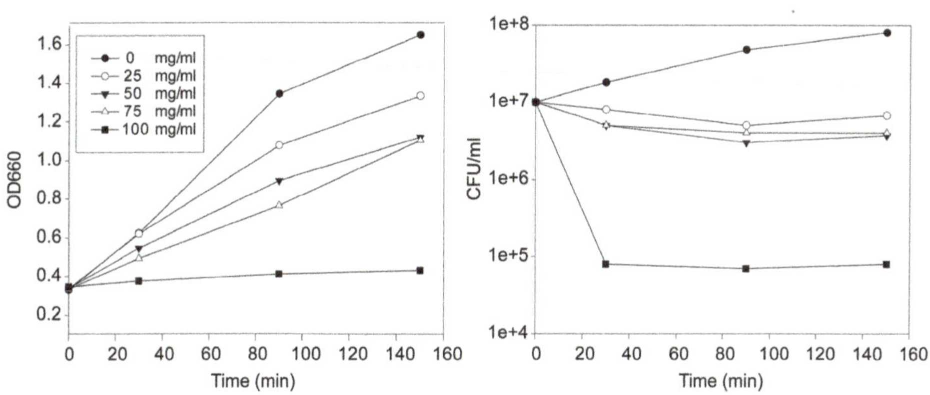

Fig. 2. Dose and time effect of Phloxine B (D&C Red#28) on *S. aureus*. Mid-log phase culture of *S. aureus* incubated with various concentrations of the dye. Turbidity of the media and bacteria viable cell count was measured at 20-minute intervals. Adapted from (Rasooly, 2005).

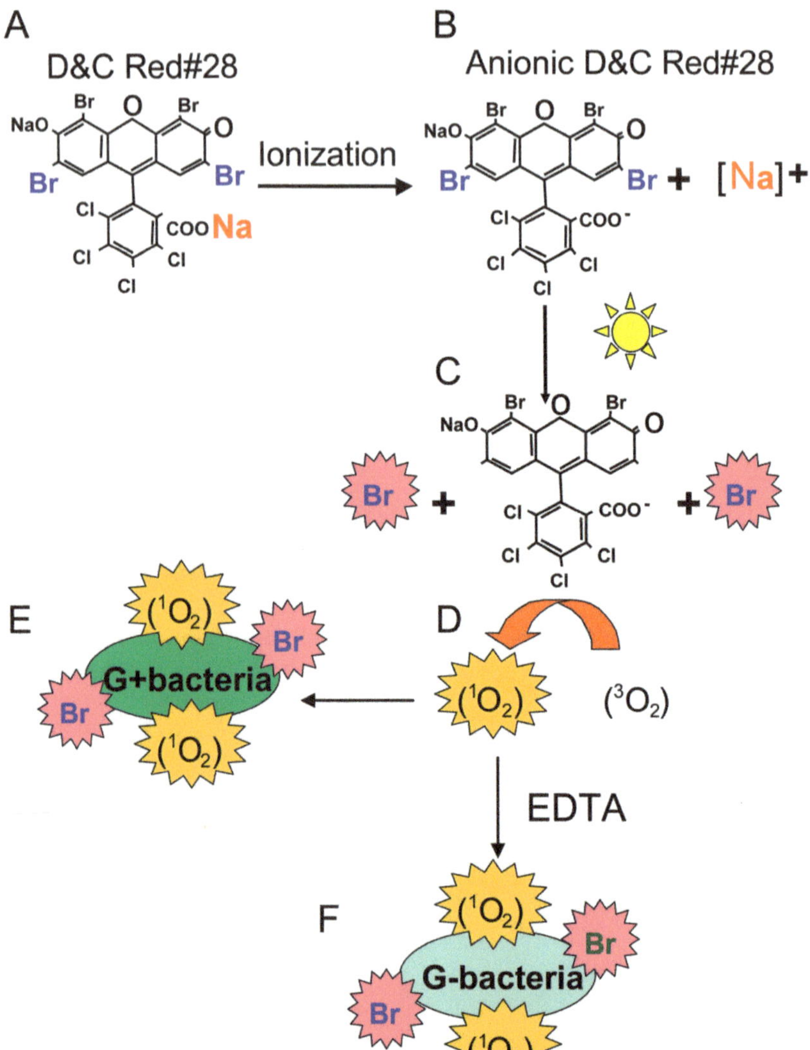

Fig. 3. The proposed mechanism of antimicrobial effects of the dye Phloxine B. Phloxine B (a) is ionized in water and (b) becomes negatively charged. The negatively charged anion (b) has a strong affinity for the positively charged cellular components such as proteins. Upon illumination (c), the photosensitized Phloxine B gains the energy associated with this light causing debromination and formation of free radicals and singlet oxygen ($^1O_2$) (d), which reacts with bacterial biomolecules (e), leading to cell death of the Gram-positive bacteria. The Gram-negative bacteria (f), which have highly negatively charged cell surfaces, repel the Phloxine B. Therefore, there is no binding and no antimicrobial effect between the dye and the Gram-negative bacteria. In the presence of EDTA, cell permeability increases, enabling dye penetration, leading to cell death. Adapted from (Rasooly, 2005).

3.3 Inhibition of SEA Release from *S. aureus* via autoinduction of virulence as a target for vaccine and therapy

With the increase in antibiotic resistance among staphylococci, there is an urgent need to develop vaccines to control bacterial infections. Although there are currently several vaccines at different stages of clinical development (Broughan et al., 2011), it seems that the development of a practical vaccine for which immunological responses can be monitored, thus enabling the prediction of its effectiveness in humans, is quite a challenging objective, not yet realized.

We believe that following novel approach we proposed merits further study (Balaban et al., 1998). The suggested approach is to interfere directly with bacterial virulence by interfering with transduction that leads to the production of toxins. This approach offers the possibility of transforming a toxin-producing pathogen to a non-pathogenic organism.

Antibiotic therapy against *S. aureus* is an important component of treatment for atopic dermatitis. However, the emergence of methicillin-resistant *S. aureus* (MRSA) presents new therapeutic challenges that suggest the need to develop new antimicrobial drugs and vaccines as an important objective. As mentioned earlier, the pathogenic effects of *S. aureus* are largely due to the production of bacterial toxins, especially SEA, which is regulated by the RNA molecule, RNAIII. The *S. aureus* protein called RAP activates RNAIII, and a peptide called RIP produced by non-pathogenic bacteria inhibits RNAIII. We discovered that mice vaccinated with RAP or treated with purified or synthetic RIP were protected against pathologic effects induced by *S. aureus*. (Table 2; Figure 4).

Treatment group	*No. of mice*	*No lesions*		*Lesions*		*Death*	
		n	*(%)*	*N*	*Mean size (mm2)*	*n*	*(%)*
Vaccination with RAP as an antigen							
RAP	24	17	(71)	6	96	1	(4)
RAP*	9	7	(78)	2	84	0	(0)
CFA	10	3	(30)	5	177	2	(20)
Untreated	12	0	(0)	9	370	3	(25)
RIP suppression of 8.5×10^7SD							
SD+RIP	4	3	(75)	1	33	0	(0)
SD+saline	4	1	(25)	3	39	0	(0)
RIP suppression of 1.4×10^8SD							
SD+RIP	8	4	(50)	4	45	0	(0)
SD+saline	6	0	(0)	6	100	0	(0)
RIP and Pep suppression of 1.4×10^9SD							
SD+RIP	10	3	(30)	3	39	4	(40)
SD+saline	10	2	(20)	6	160	2	(20)
SD+Pep	10	9	(90)	1	56	0	(0)
SD+DMSO	9	2	(20)	4	128	3	(22)

Table 2. Vaccination or suppression of *S. aureus* SD infections. Adapted from (Balaban et al., 1998).

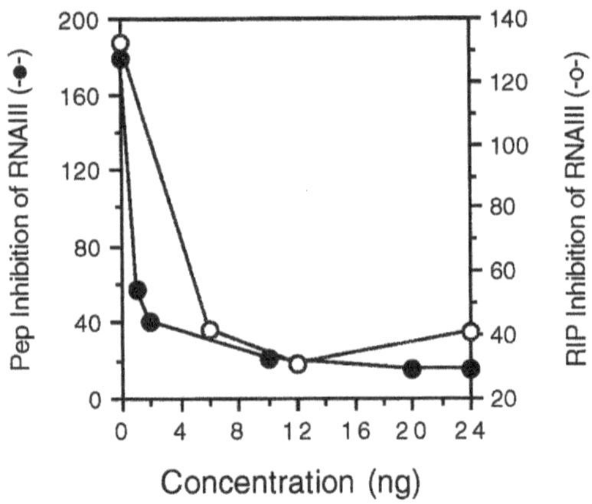

Fig. 4. Inhibition of RNAIII by native and synthetic RIP. Increasing amounts of RIP, which was purified on a C18 column or increasing amounts of synthetic peptide (Pep) were added to early exponential wild-type S. aureus and tested for the ability to inhibit RNAIII. Density of RNAIII is shown. $p<0.05$. Adapted from (Balaban et al., 1998).

Experimentally, we found that when we used increased inoculums of bacteria (1.4×10^8 cells per injection), four of eight animals were protected, and the remaining four developed a lesion that was 55% smaller than in control animals (Table 2). All the control animals (seven out of seven) challenged with SD and saline developed a lesion. When more bacteria were used (1.4×10), the synthetic RIP (0.5 mg of Pep) protected animals—90% (9 out of 10) of the animals showed no sign of disease (Table 2). These results suggest that the ratio between RIP and the bacteria is critical and helps determine the success of the host's immune response to eliminate the bacteria.

These observations suggest that targeting autoinducers of virulence or the signal transduction they activate may, therefore, be a unique and useful approach in preventing pathogenesis of toxin-producing *S. aureus* and possibly other toxin-producing pathogenic bacteria.

3.4 Apple polyphenols inhibit T-helper cell proliferation and cytokine production in spleen cells from C57BL/6 female mice

As mentioned earlier, *S. aureus* is a major bacterial pathogen that causes clinical infection and food-borne illnesses (Dinges et al., 2000). This bacterium produces a group of twenty-one known enterotoxins (SEs) that have two separate biological activities: they cause gastroenteritis in the gastrointestinal tract and act as a superantigen on the immune system. Functional enterotoxins bind to the alpha-helical regions of the major histocompatibility complex (MHC) class II molecules outside the peptide-binding groove of the antigen presenting cells (APC), and also to the variable region (Vß) on T-cell receptors. The toxin then forms a bridge between T cells and APCs. This event then initiates the proliferation of a large number (~20%) of T cells that induce the release of cytokines. At high concentrations, cytokines are involved in the etiology (causes) of several known human and animal diseases. These include atopic dermatitis and rheumatoid arthritis in humans (Lin et al., 2011; MacIas et al., 2011; Yeung et al., 2011).

Atopic dermatitis (eczema) is an inflammatory skin disease that affects 10-20% of children and 1-3% of adults (1-3). Antibiotics that suppress colonization of *S. aureus* are reported to mitigate the severity of atopic dermatitis disease. Most strains of *S. aureus* isolated from atopic skin lesions produce exotoxins with superantigen properties (Leung et al., 1993). It has been reported that staphylococcal superantigens can induce skin inflammation by several different mechanisms (Taskapan & Kumar, 2000). The reason we selected the superantigen for this study is that it is has been demonstrated to be an aggravating factor in atopic dermatitis, and because SEA is a representative antigen.

It has been previously reported that consumption of apple condensed tannins from unripe apples improve the symptoms associated with atopic dermatitis (Kojima et al., 2000). The mechanism of this improvement is largely unknown.

The main objective of our study was therefore to determine whether the beneficial effect of apple polyphenols is due to binding and inhibition of the superantigen and/or to inhibition of cell proliferation.

In the present study, we evaluated the ability of one commercial and two freshly prepared apple juices and of a commercial apple polyphenol preparation (Apple Poly®) to inhibit the biological activity of SEA. The results are depicted in Figures 5-9. Dilutions of freshly prepared apple juices and of Apple Poly® inhibited the biological activity of SEA without any significant cytotoxic effect on the spleen cells. Additional studies with antibody-coated immunomagnetic beads bearing specific antibodies against the toxin revealed that SEA added to apple juice appears to be largely irreversibly bound to the juice constituents (Fig. 8). The results suggest that food-compatible and safe anti-toxin phenolic compounds can be used to inactivate SEA in vitro and possibly also in vivo, even after the induction of T-cell proliferation by long-term exposure to SEA. The significance of the results for microbial food safety and human health is discussed.

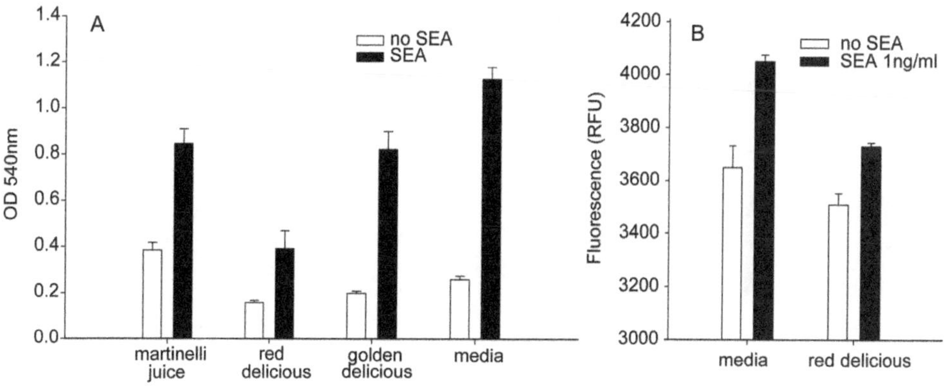

Fig. 5. Effect of apple juice on splenocyte proliferation. Apple juice and media used as a control with or without SEA (1 ng/mL) were incubated for 48 h with splenocyte cells followed by determining newly synthesized DNA (A) by cleavage of the peptide GF-AFC and (B) by use of live splenocytes. Error bars (n = 3) represent standard errors. Adapted from (Rasooly et al., 2010).

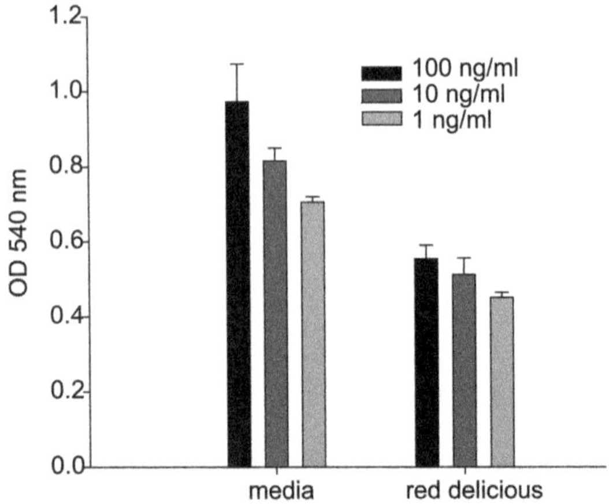

Fig. 6. Red Delicious apple juice inhibits high SEA concentrations. Three concentrations of SEA were incubated for 48 h with splenocyte cells followed by determining newly synthesized DNA. Error bars (n = 3) represent standard errors. Adapted from (Rasooly et al. 2010).

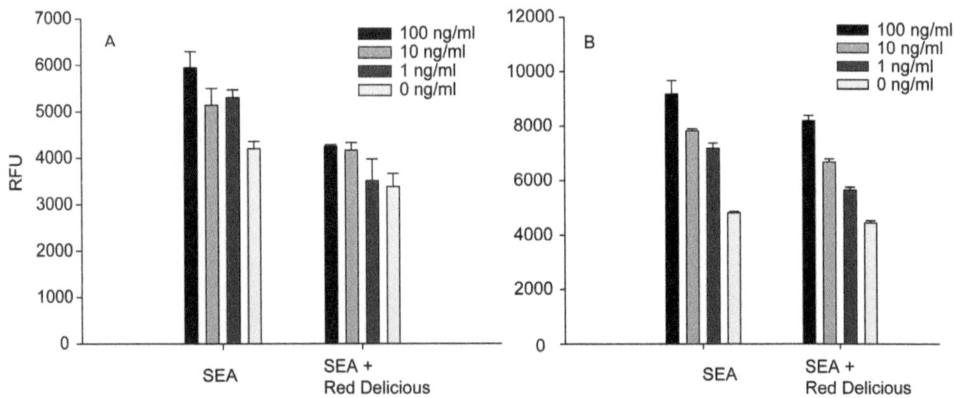

Fig. 7. Red Delicious apple juice reduces the activity of SEA after 24 or 48 h of incubation. Different amounts of SEA were added to the splenocytes, which were then incubated for 24 or 48 h. This was followed by the addition of Red Delicious apple juice and the determination of biological activity by cleavage of GF-AFC, produced by the live splenocyte cells after (A) 48 h or (B) 72 h. Error bars (n = 3) represent standard errors. Adapted from (Rasooly et al., 2010).

These observations suggest that Red Delicious juice has an inhibitory effect even after cell proliferation was initiated. We suggest that components of the juice disrupt the connection between antigen presenting cells (APCs) and T cells. Our results also imply that the mechanism by which consumed apple juice or apples may decrease the symptoms associated with atopic dermatitis is via inhibition of proliferation of T cells and the release of cytokines. The postulated mechanism that may govern the inhibition of the biological activity of SEA by apple compounds is visually illustrated in Figure 9.

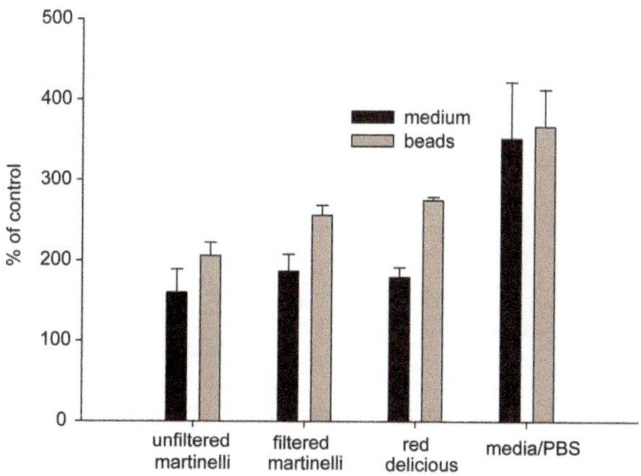

Fig. 8. Extraction and elution of SEA from apple juice treated with immunomagnetic beads. Apple juices were spiked with SEA (1 ng/mL) and incubated for 16 h with immunomagnetic beads. The toxin was dissociated from the beads and incubated with spleen cells. This was followed by the determination of newly synthesized DNA. Error bars (n = 3) represent standard errors. These results indicate that SEA added to apple juice appears to be largely irreversibly bound to the juice constituents. Adapted from (Rasooly et al. 2010).

The described findings suggest that apple juices and polyphenol-rich apple skin extracts have the potential to counteract adverse effects in animals and humans induced by SEA, and possibly also by the foodborne pathogen *S. aureus* that produces this virulent toxin. It would be of interest to find out whether or not the inhibited toxin in apple juice is reactivated in the digestive tracts of animals and humans and whether or not phenolic compounds present in other juices can concurrently inhibit the growth of *S. aureus* and other pathogens and the toxins produced by the pathogens.

In summary, our studies with apple juice and apples skin extracts demonstrated that apple polyphenols strongly inhibited superantigen-induced T-cell proliferation and cytokine production. The results also indicate that the low inhibitory action of freshly prepared Red Delicious apple juice is enhanced by added apple polyphenols. Further studies are needed to determine whether or not this combination may protect against animal and human diseases induced by high cytokine levels.

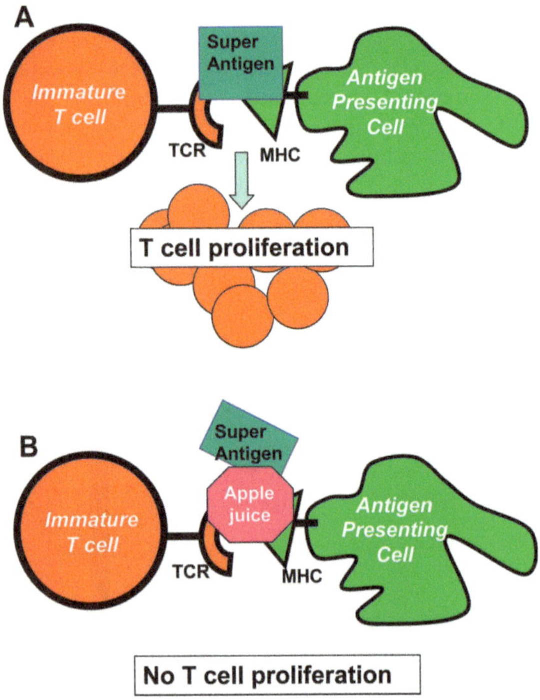

Fig. 9. A schematic representation of cellular events that lead to the inhibition of SEA-induced cell proliferation by apple juice. The individual steps in this scheme involve the (A) the formation of a bridge between APCs and T cells which results in induction of T-cell proliferation and (B) inhibition of T-cell proliferation by added pure apple juice that disrupts the connection between APCs and T cells. The net beneficial result of these events is the prevention of release and the consequent adverse effects induced by cytokines described in the Introduction. Abbreviations: MHC, major histocompatibility complex; TCR, T-cell receptor. Adapted from (Rasooly et al., 2010).

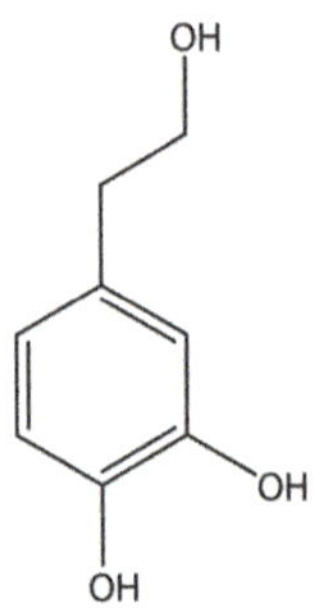

hydroxytyrosol
(4-(2-hydroxyethyl)benzene-1,2-diol)

Fig. 10. Structure of the olive compound, hydroxytyrosol that inhibits *S. aureus* and SEA.

3.5 The olive compound 4-hydroxytyrosol inactivates both *S. aureus* and inhibits the biological activity of SEA

Our observations that dilutions of freshly prepared apple juices and of a commercial apple skin preparation inhibited the biological activity of SEA in a spleen cell assay suggested that other natural plant-derived compounds and plant extracts have the potential to inhibit the growth of foodborne pathogens and the toxicological effects of toxins produced by some pathogens (Rasooly et al., 2010).

To further demonstrate this possibility, the objectives of another study were to determine whether the pure olive compound hydroxytyrosol (Figure 12) and a commercial olive powder named Hidrox-12 that contains hydroxytyrosol can inactivate *S. aureus* bacteria and inhibit the biological activity of SEA (Friedman et al., 2011). We found that olive ingredients also posses anti-*S. aureus* activity that reduced the counts of the bacteria in a dose-dependent manner. With hydroxytyrosol, the viable count of *S. aureus* bacteria after treatment at a concentration of 0.67 mg/ml for 60 min of contact, determined by plating on LB agar media, was decreased by 85%. We also found that dilutions of both test substances inactivated the pathogens.

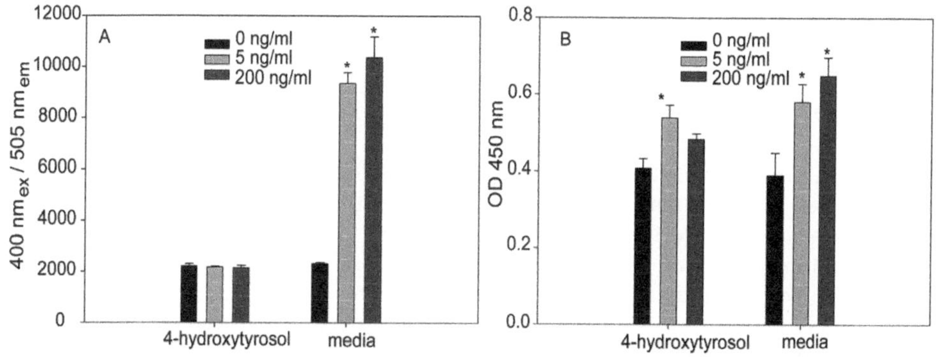

Fig. 11. Effect of hydroxytyrosol on splenocyte proliferation determined by two independent methods. Different concentrations of the toxin (0, 5, and 200 ng/mL) were exposed to hydroxytyrosol or the control (media) and were then incubated for 48 h with splenocyte cells followed by determining (A) GF-AFC cleavage by live cell protease (a measure of cellular activity) or (B) BrdU incorporation into newly synthesized DNA (a measure of cellular proliferation). Conditions: (A) GF-AFC substrate in intact cells is cleaved by live cell protease releasing the fluorescent AFC, quantified at an excitation wavelength of 355 nm and an emission wavelength of 523 nm. (B) BrdU (5-bromo-2-deoxyyridine)-labeled DNA was determined spectrophotometrically at absorbances of 620 nm and 450 nm. Error bars (n = 3) represent standard errors. Both assays show that hydroxytyrosol inhibited the biological activity of SEA. Error bars represent standard error (SEs), and an asterisk indicates significant differences ($P<0.05$) between treatments. Adapted from (Friedman et al., 2011).

Two independent cell assays (BrdU incorporation into newly synthesized DNA and glycyl-phenylalanyl-aminofluorocoumarin (GF-AFC) proteolysis) demonstrated that the olive compound also inhibits the biological activity of SEA. The described findings suggest that olive compounds have the potential to counteract adverse effects induced by SEA and by the foodborne pathogen *S. aureus* that produces this virulent toxin. To our knowledge, this is the first report that demonstrated with the aid of bactericidal and cell assays that the edible olive compound hydroxytyrosol can inactivate both *S. aureus* bacteria and SEA. The results suggest that food-compatible and safe anti-toxin olive compounds merit further study designed to demonstrate their potential to treat atopic dermatitis.

It would be of interest to extend these studies to the inactivation of other pathogens and toxins such as *E. coli* and Shiga toxin *in vitro* and in contaminated food such as meat, milk, and leafy greens.

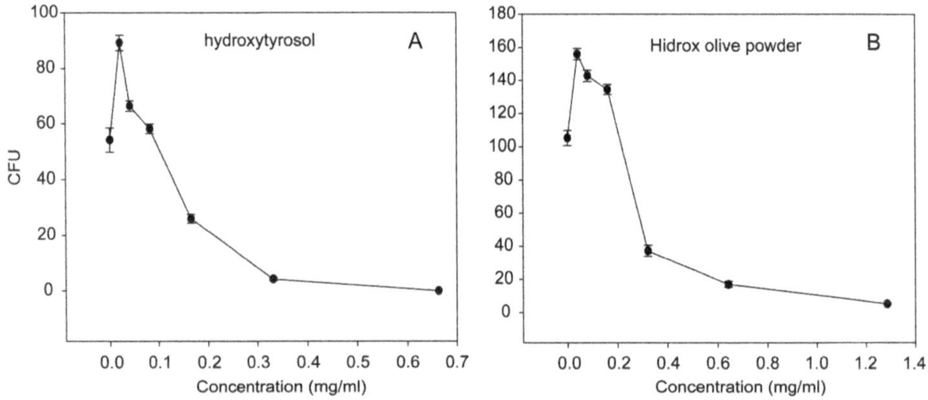

Fig. 12. (A) Antimicrobial activity of hydroxytyrosol against *S. aureus*. Conditions: bacteria were incubated with different concentrations of hydroxytyrosol. After incubation for 60 min, cells were plated and bacteria counted. (B) Antimicrobial activity of Hidrox-12 against *S. aureus*. Conditions: similar to those used for hydroxytyrosol. Error bars represent standard errors (n = 4). Both the pure olive compound and the olive extract inhibited the bacteria. The extent of inhibition by the extract was approximately equivalent to its content (12%) of hydroxytyrosol. Adapted from (Friedman et al. 2011).

4. Conclusion

S. aureus is a major bacterial pathogen that develops resistance to medical antibiotics. It has been reported to cause clinical infections and contamination of a broad variety of foods that may result in foodborne illness. These include canned mushroom, breaded chicken products, cheese, and raw milk as well on handles of shopping carts causing 185 000 cases of foodborne illnesses in the United States each year. *S. aureus* bacteria are present on the skin patients with atopic dermatitis. Many strains of *S. aureus* isolated from atopic skin lesions produce enterotoxins with superantigenic properties. *S. aureus* produces the virulent staphylococcal enterotoxin A, a single chain protein that consists of 233 amino acid residues. It has been estimated that the toxin that is secreted by the bacteria is associated with 78% of staphylococcal outbreaks. Our studies show that naturally occurring edible apple phenolic and olive compounds can both inactivate *S. aureus* bacteria and reduce the biological/toxicological properties of the toxin produced by these bacteria and that the food dye Phloxine B inhibits the release of SEA from the pathogens. Whether these novel approaches have therapeutic potential against atopic dermatitis and other diseases merits further study.

The described studies are part of a broader effort, the specific objective of which is to transform toxic proteins to nontoxic, digestible proteins in foods. For example, apple and other polyphenols present in numerous plant foods such as teas, sweet potatoes, and jujube fruits and seeds contain electron-rich aromatic structures and ionizable phenolic OH groups. These structures can in theory change the toxin via non-covalent binding to the toxin and/or by altering the distribution of ionic charges via H-bonding between OH groups and ionizable groups of the protein. We have no direct evidence for this theory, but note that in molecular simulation studies, we observed multiple hydrogen-bonding interactions between polyphenolic tea catechins and cell membranes that may result in anti-bactericidal effects due to disruption of the cell membranes followed by cell death (Sirk et al., 2009; Sirk et al., 2008; Sirk et al., 2011).

5. Acknowledgment

We thank our colleagues whose names appear on the cited publications and Carol E. Levin for facilitating the preparation of this chapter.

6. References

Anderson, J. E., Beelman, R. R., & Doores, S. (1996). Persistence of serological and biological activities of staphylococcal enterotoxin A in canned mushrooms. *Journal of Food Protection,* Vol.59, No. 12, pp. 1292-1299

Balaban, N., Goldkorn, T., Nhan, R. T., Dang, L. B., Scott, S., Ridgley, R. M., Rasooly, A., Wright, S. C., Larrick, J. W., Rasooly, R., & Carlson, J. R. (1998). Autoinducer of virulence as a target for vaccine and therapy against *Staphylococcus aureus*. *Science,* Vol.280, No. 5362, pp. 438-440

Balaban, N., & Rasooly, A. (2000). Staphylococcal enterotoxins. *International Journal of Food Microbiology,* Vol.61, No. 1, pp. 1-10

Broughan, J., Anderson, R., & Anderson, A. S. (2011). Strategies for and advances in the development of *Staphylococcus aureus* prophylactic vaccines. *Expert Review of Vaccines,* Vol.10, No. 5, pp. 695-708

Carlos, L. A., Amaral, K. A. S., Vieira, I. J. C., Mathias, L., Braz-Filho, R., Samarão, S. S., & Vieira-da-Motta, O. (2010). *Rauvolfia grandiflora* (apocynaceae) extract interferes with staphylococcal density, enterotoxin production and antimicrobial activity. *Brazilian Journal of Microbiology,* Vol.41, No. 3, pp. 612-620

Choi, O., Yahiro, K., Morinaga, N., Miyazaki, M., & Noda, M. (2007). Inhibitory effects of various plant polyphenols on the toxicity of Staphylococcal α-toxin. *Microbial Pathogenesis,* Vol.42, No. 5-6, pp. 215-224

Davis, J. R., & Lederberg, J. (Eds.). (2001). *Emerging infectious diseases from the global to local perspective: workshop summary,* National Academy of Sciences, ISBN 0-309-07184-4, Washington DC

de Souza, E. L., de Barros, J. C., de Oliveira, C. E. V., & da Conceição, M. L. (2010). Influence of *Origanum vulgare* L. essential oil on enterotoxin production, membrane permeability and surface characteristics of *Staphylococcus aureus*. *International Journal of Food Microbiology,* Vol.137, No. 2-3, pp. 308-311

Dinges, M. M., Orwin, P. M., & Schlievert, P. M. (2000). Exotoxins of *Staphylococcus aureus*. *Clinical Microbiology Reviews,* Vol.13, No. 1, pp. 16-34

Ertas, N., Gonulalan, Z., Yildirim, Y., & Kum, E. (2010). Detection of *Staphylococcus aureus* enterotoxins in sheep cheese and dairy desserts by multiplex PCR technique. *International Journal of Food Microbiology,* Vol.142, No. 1-2, pp. 74-77

Friedman, M., Buick, R., & Elliott, C. T. (2004a). Antibacterial activities of naturally occurring compounds against antibiotic-resistant *Bacillus cereus* vegetative cells and spores, *Escherichia coli,* and *Staphylococcus aureus. Journal of Food Protection,* Vol.67, No. 8, pp. 1774-1778

Friedman, M., Henika, P. R., Levin, C. E., & Mandrell, R. E. (2004b). Antibacterial activities of plant essential oils and their components against *Escherichia coli* O157:H7 and *Salmonella enterica* in apple juice. *Journal of Agricultural and Food Chemistry,* Vol.52, No. 19, pp. 6042-6048

Friedman, M., Rasooly, R., Do, P. M., & Henika, P. R. (2011). The olive compound hydroxytyrosol inactivates *Staphylococcus aureus* bacteria and Staphylococcal enterotoxin A (SEA). *Journal of Food Science (accepted)*

Fusco, V., Quero, G. M., Morea, M., Blaiotta, G., & Visconti, A. (2011). Rapid and reliable identification of *Staphylococcus aureus* harbouring the enterotoxin gene cluster (egc) and quantitative detection in raw milk by real time PCR. *International Journal of Food Microbiology,* Vol.144, No. 3, pp. 528-537

Heidinger, J. C., Winter, C. K., & Cullor, J. S. (2009). Quantitative microbial risk assessment for *Staphylococcus aureus* and *Staphylococcus* enterotoxin A in raw milk. *Journal of Food Protection,* Vol.72, No. 8, pp. 1641-1653

Ifesan, B. O. T., & Voravuthlkunchai, S. P. (2009). Effect of *Eleutherine americana* merr. Extract on enzymatic activity and enterotoxin production of *Staphylococcus aureus* in broth and cooked pork. *Foodborne Pathogens and Disease,* Vol.6, No. 6, pp. 699-704

Kojima, T., Akiyama, H., Sasai, M., Taniuchi, S., Goda, Y., Toyoda, M., & Kobayashi, Y. (2000). Anti-allergic effect of apple polyphenol on patients with atopic dermatitis: A pilot study. *Allergology International,* Vol.49, No. 1, pp. 69-73

Larkin, E. A., Stiles, B. G., & Ulrich, R. G. (2010). Inhibition of toxic shock by human monoclonal antibodies against staphylococcal enterotoxin B. *PLoS ONE,* Vol.5, No. 10, pp. e13253

Leung, D. Y. M., Harbeck, R., Bina, P., Reiser, R. F., Yang, E., Norris, D. A., Hanifin, J. M., & Sampson, H. A. (1993). Presence of IgE antibodies to staphylococcal exotoxins on the skin of patients with atopic dermatitis. Evidence for a new group of allergens. *Journal of Clinical Investigation,* Vol.92, No. 3, pp. 1374-1380

Lin, Y.-T., Wang, C.-T., Chao, P.-S., Lee, J.-H., Wang, L.-C., Yu, H.-H., Yang, Y.-H., & Chiang, B.-L. (2011). Skin-homing $CD4^+$ $Foxp3^+$ T cells exert Th2-like function after staphylococcal superantigen stimulation in atopic dermatitis patients. *Clinical and Experimental Allergy,* Vol.41, No. 4, pp. 516-525

Maclas, E. S., Pereira, F. A., Rietkerk, W., & Safai, B. (2011). Superantigens in dermatology. *Journal of the American Academy of Dermatology,* Vol.64, No. 3, pp. 455-472

Margosch, D., Moravek, M., Gaenzle, M. G., Maertlbauer, E., Vogel, R. F., & Ehrmann, M. A. (2005). Effect of high pressure and heat on bacterial toxins. *Food Technology and Biotechnology,* Vol.43, No. 3, pp. 211-217

Mizumachi, E., Kato, F., Hisatsune, J., Tsuruda, K., Uehara, Y., Seo, H., & Sugai, M. (2011). Clonal distribution of enterotoxigenic *Staphylococcus aureus* on handles of handheld shopping baskets in supermarkets. *Journal of Applied Microbiology,* Vol.110, No. 2, pp. 562-567

Nuñez, L., Moro, A., & D'Aquino, M. (2007). Staphylococcal enterotoxins and enzymes in presence of essential oils. *Ars Pharmaceutica,* Vol.48, No. 2, pp. 175-185

Ostyn, A., De Buyser, M. L., Guillier, F., Groult, J., Felix, B., Salah, S., Delmas, G., & Hennekinne, J. A. (2010). First evidence of a food poisoning outbreak due to staphylococcal enterotoxin type E, France, 2009. *Eurosurveillance,* Vol.15, No. 13, Article 3, pp. 1-4

Parsaeimehr, M., Basti, A. A., Radmehr, B., Misaghi, A., Abbasifar, A., Karim, G., Rokni, N., Motlagh, M. S., Gandomi, H., Noori, N., & Khanjari, A. (2010). Effect of *Zataria multiflora* boiss. Essential oil, nisin, and their combination on the production of enterotoxin C and α-hemolysin by *Staphylococcus aureus. Foodborne Pathogens and Disease,* Vol.7, No. 3, pp. 299-305

Pepe, O., Blaiotta, G., Bucci, F., Anastasio, M., Aponte, M., & Villani, F. (2006). *Staphylococcus aureus* and staphylococcal enterotoxin A in breaded chicken products: Detection and behavior during the cooking process. *Applied and Environmental Microbiology,* Vol.72, No. 11, pp. 7057-7062

Pereira, V., Lopes, C., Castro, A., Silva, J., Gibbs, P., & Teixeira, P. (2009). Characterization for enterotoxin production, virulence factors, and antibiotic susceptibility of *Staphylococcus aureus* isolates from various foods in Portugal. *Food Microbiology,* Vol.26, No. 3, pp. 278-282

Pu, S., Wang, F., & Ge, B. (2011). Characterization of toxin genes and antimicrobial susceptibility of *Staphylococcus aureus* isolates from Louisiana retail meats. *Foodborne Pathogens and Disease,* Vol.8, No. 2, pp. 299-306

Qiu, J., Feng, H., Xiang, H., Wang, D., Xia, L., Jiang, Y., Song, K., Lu, J., Yu, L., & Deng, X. (2010). Influence of subinhibitory concentrations of licochalcone A on the secretion of enterotoxins A and B by *Staphylococcus aureus. FEMS Microbiology Letters,* Vol.307, No. 2, pp. 135-141

Qiu, J., Wang, J., Luo, H., Du, X., Li, H., Luo, M., Dong, J., Chen, Z., & Deng, X. (2011). The effects of subinhibitory concentrations of costus oil on virulence factor production in *Staphylococcus aureus. Journal of Applied Microbiology,* Vol.110, No. 1, pp. 333-340

Rasooly, R. (2005). Expanding the bactericidal action of the food color additive phloxine B to gram-negative bacteria. *FEMS Immunology & Medical Microbiology,* Vol.45, No. 2, pp. 239-244

Rasooly, R., Do, P. M., & Friedman, M. (2010). Inhibition of biological activity of Staphylococcal Enterotoxin A (SEA) by apple juice and apple polyphenols. *Journal of Agricultural and Food Chemistry,* Vol.58, No. 9, pp. 5421–5426

Rhee, C. H., & Woo, G. J. (2010). Emergence and characterization of foodborne methicillin-resistant *Staphylococcus aureus* in Korea. *Journal of Food Protection,* Vol.73, No. 12, pp. 2285-2290

Rosengren, Å., Fabricius, A., Guss, B., Sylvén, S., & Lindqvist, R. (2010). Occurrence of foodborne pathogens and characterization of *Staphylococcus aureus* in cheese produced on farm-dairies. *International Journal of Food Microbiology,* Vol.144, No. 2, pp. 263-269

Rúa, J., Fernández-Álvarez, L., Gutiérrez-Larraínzar, M., Del Valle, P., De Arriaga, D., & García-Armesto, M. R. (2010). Screening of phenolic antioxidants for their inhibitory activity against foodborne *Staphylococcus aureus* strains. *Foodborne Pathogens and Disease,* Vol.7, No. 6, pp. 695-705

Shinefield, H. R., & Ruff, N. L. (2009). Staphylococcal infections: A historical perspective. *Infectious Disease Clinics of North America,* Vol.23, No. 1, pp. 1-15

Sirk, T. W., Brown, E. F., Friedman, M., & Sum, A. K. (2009). Molecular binding of catechins to biomembranes: Relationship to biological activity. *Journal of Agricultural and Food Chemistry,* Vol.57, No. 15, pp. 6720–6728

Sirk, T. W., Brown, E. F., Sum, A. K., & Friedman, M. (2008). Molecular dynamics study on the biophysical interactions of seven green tea catechins with lipid bilayers of cell membranes. *Journal of Agricultural and Food Chemistry,* Vol.56, No. 17, pp. 7750-7758

Sirk, T. W., Friedman, M., & Brown, E. F. (2011). Molecular binding of black tea theaflavins to biological membranes: Relationship to bioactivities. *Journal of Agricultural and Food Chemistry,* Vol.59, No. 8, pp. 3780-3787

Stewart, G. S. (2005). *Staphylococcus aureus,* In *Foodborne Pathogens - Microbiology and Molecular Biology,* P. M. Fratamico, A. K. Bhunia & J. L. Smith (Eds.), pp. 273-284, Caister Academic Press, ISBN 1-904455-00-X, Norfolk, UK

Suzuki, T., Itakura, J., Watanabe, M., Ohta, M., Sato, Y., & Yamaya, Y. (2002). Inactivation of staphylococcal enterotoxin-A with an electrolyzed anodic solution. *Journal of Agricultural and Food Chemistry,* Vol.50, No. 1, pp. 230-234

Taskapan, M. O., & Kumar, P. (2000). Role of staphylococcal superantigens in atopic dermatitis: From colonization to inflammation. *Annals of Allergy, Asthma and Immunology,* Vol.84, No. 1, pp. 3-12

Vernozy-Rozand, C., Mazuy-Cruchaudet, C., Bavai, C., & Richard, Y. (2004). Comparison of three immunological methods for detecting staphylococcal enterotoxins from food. *Letters in Applied Microbiology,* Vol.39, No. 6, pp. 490-494

Walkling-Ribeiro, M., Noci, F., Cronin, D. A., Riener, J., Lyng, J. G., & Morgan, D. J. (2008). Reduction of *Staphylococcus aureus* and quality changes in apple juice processed by ultraviolet irradiation, pre-heating, and pulsed electric fields. *Journal of Food Engineering,* Vol.89, pp. 267-273

Wallin-Carlquist, N., Marta, D., Borch, E., & Radstrom, P. (2010). Prolonged expression and production of *Staphylococcus aureus* enterotoxin A in processed pork meat. *International Journal of Food Microbiology,* Vol.141 Suppl 1, pp. S69-74

Walsh, C. (2003). *Antibiotics: Actions, Origins, Resistance,* ASM Press, ISBN 1-55581-254-6, Washington, D.C.

Wang, S., Li, Y., Xiong, H., & Cao, J. (2008). A broad-spectrum inhibitory peptide against staphylococcal enterotoxin superantigen SEA, SEB and SEC. *Immunology Letters,* Vol.121, No. 2, pp. 167-172

Yeung, M., Balma-Mena, A., Shear, N., Simor, A., Pope, E., Walsh, S., & McGavin, M. J. (2011). Identification of major clonal complexes and toxin producing strains among *Staphylococcus aureus* associated with atopic dermatitis. *Microbes and Infection,* Vol.13, No. 2, pp. 189-197

Permissions

The contributors of this book come from diverse backgrounds, making this book a truly international effort. This book will bring forth new frontiers with its revolutionizing research information and detailed analysis of the nascent developments around the world.

We would like to thank Itaru Dekio, MD, PhD, for lending his expertise to make the book truly unique. He has played a crucial role in the development of this book. Without his invaluable contribution this book wouldn't have been possible. He has made vital efforts to compile up to date information on the varied aspects of this subject to make this book a valuable addition to the collection of many professionals and students.

This book was conceptualized with the vision of imparting up-to-date information and advanced data in this field. To ensure the same, a matchless editorial board was set up. Every individual on the board went through rigorous rounds of assessment to prove their worth. After which they invested a large part of their time researching and compiling the most relevant data for our readers. Conferences and sessions were held from time to time between the editorial board and the contributing authors to present the data in the most comprehensible form. The editorial team has worked tirelessly to provide valuable and valid information to help people across the globe.

Every chapter published in this book has been scrutinized by our experts. Their significance has been extensively debated. The topics covered herein carry significant findings which will fuel the growth of the discipline. They may even be implemented as practical applications or may be referred to as a beginning point for another development. Chapters in this book were first published by InTech; hereby published with permission under the Creative Commons Attribution License or equivalent.

The editorial board has been involved in producing this book since its inception. They have spent rigorous hours researching and exploring the diverse topics which have resulted in the successful publishing of this book. They have passed on their knowledge of decades through this book. To expedite this challenging task, the publisher supported the team at every step. A small team of assistant editors was also appointed to further simplify the editing procedure and attain best results for the readers.

Our editorial team has been hand-picked from every corner of the world. Their multi-ethnicity adds dynamic inputs to the discussions which result in innovative outcomes. These outcomes are then further discussed with the researchers and contributors who give their valuable feedback and opinion regarding the same. The feedback is then collaborated with the researches and they are edited in a comprehensive manner to aid the understanding of the subject.

Apart from the editorial board, the designing team has also invested a significant amount of their time in understanding the subject and creating the most relevant covers. They scrutinized every image to scout for the most suitable representation of the subject and create an appropriate cover for the book.

The publishing team has been involved in this book since its early stages. They were actively engaged in every process, be it collecting the data, connecting with the contributors or procuring relevant information. The team has been an ardent support to the editorial, designing and production team. Their endless efforts to recruit the best for this project, has resulted in the accomplishment of this book. They are a veteran in the field of academics and their pool of knowledge is as vast as their experience in printing. Their expertise and guidance has proved useful at every step. Their uncompromising quality standards have made this book an exceptional effort. Their encouragement from time to time has been an inspiration for everyone.

The publisher and the editorial board hope that this book will prove to be a valuable piece of knowledge for researchers, students, practitioners and scholars across the globe.

List of Contributors

Hiromichi Yonekawa, Hiroshi Shitara and Choji Taya
Center for Basic Technology Research, Tokyo Metropolitan Institute of Medical Science, Tokyo, Japan

Toyoyuki Takada
Mammalian Genetics Laboratory, National Institute of Genetics, Mishima, Japan

Yoshibumi Matsushima
Research Institute for Clinical Oncology, Saitama Cancer Center, Saitama, Japan

Kunie Matsuoka and Yoshiaki Kikkawa
Mammalian Genetics Project, Tokyo Metropolitan Institute of Medical Science, Tokyo, Japan

Catharina Sagita Moniaga and Kenji Kabashima
Department of Dermatology, Kyoto University Graduate School of Medicine, Japan

Ulf Meyer-Hoffert
University Hospital Schleswig-Holstein, Campus Kiel, Department Dermatology, Germany

Kenji Izuhara, Hiroshi Shiraishi, Kazuhiko Arima and Shoichi Suzuki
Division of Medical Biochemistry, Department of Biomolecular Sciences, Japan

Shoichiro Ohta
Department of Laboratory Medicine, Saga Medical School, Japan

Tetsuya Honda
Department of Dermatology, Kyoto University Graduate School of Medicine, Kyoto, Japan

Susanne Stutte
Department of Microbiology and Immunobiology, Division of Immunology, Harvard Medical School, Boston, USA

Nancy Gerbitzki and Irmgard Förster
Molecular Immunology, IUF - Leibniz Research Institute for Environmental Medicine, Düsseldorf, Germany

Natalija Novak
Department of Dermatology and Allergy University of Bonn Medical Center, Bonn, Germany

Itaru Dekio
Department of Dermatology, Faculty of Medicine, Shimane University, Izumo, Japan

Takuji Nakashima and Yoshimi Niwano
Kitasato University, Tohoku University, Japan

Takashi Sugita and Takafumi Tanaka
Department of Microbiology, Meiji Pharmaceutical University, Kiyose, Tokyo, Japan

Yoshio Ishibashi and Akemi Nishikawa
Department of Immunobiology, Meiji Pharmaceutical University, Kiyose, Tokyo, Japan

Mami Tajima, Ryoji Tsuboi and Enshi Zhang
Department of Dermatology, Tokyo Medical University, Shinjuku, Tokyo, Japan

Nicola Fuiano
Paediatric Allergy Service, ASL Fg, Torremaggiore, Italy

Cristoforo Incorvaia
Allergy/Pulmonary rehabilitation, ICP Hospital, Milan, Italy

Zheng-Hong Di, Li Zhang, Ya-Ni Lv, Li-Ping Zhao, Hong-Duo Chen and Xing-Hua Gao
Department of Dermatology, No.1 hospital of China Medical University, China

Evmorfia Ladoyanni
Department of Dermatology, Dudley Group Hospitals, Corbett Hospital, Vicarage Road, Stourbridge, West Midlands, United Kingdom

Mitsuhiro Denda
Shiseido Research Center, Japan

Soheyla Mahdavian, Patty Ghazvini, Luis Pagan, Angela Singh and Todd Woodard
Florida A&M University College of Pharmacy and Pharmaceutical Sciences, USA

Jae Ho Lee
Department of Paediatrics, Chungnam National University, College of Medicine, Daejeon, Korea

Geunwoong Noh
Subdivision of Allergy and Clinical Immunology, Department of Paediatrics, Chungnam National University Hospital, Daejoen, Korea

S. Yoshihara, M. Ono, Y. Yamada, H. Fukuda, T. Abe and O. Arisaka
Department of Pediatrics, Dokkyo University School of Medicine, Tochigi, Japan

Massimo Milani
ALK Abellò Medical Department, Lainate, Milan, Italy

Misha M. Heller
University of Southern California, Keck School of Medicine, Los Angeles, California, USA

Eric S. Lee
University of Nebraska Medical Center, College of Medicine, Omaha, Nebraska, USA

Faranak Kamangar
University of California Davis, School of Medicine, Sacramento, California, USA

Wilson Liao and John Y. M. Koo
University of California San Francisco, Department of Dermatology, San Francisco, California, USA

Hiroyuki Araki, Yoshiya Sugai and Hirofumi Takigawa
Tochigi Research Laboratories, Kao Corporation, Japan

Feriel Hacini-Rachinel, Ivana Jankovic, Anurag Singh and Annick Mercenier
Nestlé Research Center, Lausanne, Switzerland

Öner Özdemir
Republic of Turkey, Ministry of Health, İstanbul Medeniyet University, Göztepe Research /Training Hospital, Turkey

Reuven Rasooly and Mendel Friedman
Western Regional Research Center, Agricultural Research Service, United States Department of Agriculture, Albany, California, USA